Office Care of Women

Office Care of Women

Edited by
Martin E. Olsen
East Tennessee State University, Johnson City, Tennessee
Botros Rizk
University of South Alabama, Mobile, Alabama

CAMBRIDGE
UNIVERSITY PRESS

CAMBRIDGE
UNIVERSITY PRESS

32 Avenue of the Americas, New York, NY 10013-2473, USA

Cambridge University Press is part of the University of Cambridge.

It furthers the University's mission by disseminating knowledge in the pursuit of education, learning, and research at the highest international levels of excellence.

www.cambridge.org
Information on this title: www.cambridge.org/9781107085701

First published 2016

Printed in the United States of America by Sheridan Books, Inc.

A catalog record for this publication is available from the British Library.

Library of Congress Cataloging in Publication Data
Olsen, Martin, editor. | Rizk, Botros, editor.
Office care of women / [edited by] Martin Olsen, Botros Rizk.
New York, NY : Cambridge University Press, 2016. | Includes bibliographical references.
LCCN 2015041401 | ISBN 9781107085701 (hardback)
| MESH: Women's Health. | Gynecology – methods. | Obstetrics – methods. | Patient-Centered Care – methods. | Physician's Practice Patterns. | Preventive Medicine – methods.
LCC RG101 | NLM WA 309 | DDC 618.1–dc23
LC record available at http://lccn.loc.gov/2015041401

ISBN 978-1-107-08570-1 Hardback

This book is dedicated to the physicians who serve patients in conflict areas. Your devotion to your patients is inspiring.

Contents

Section V–Reproductive endocrinology and infertility

Section VI–Nongynecologic conditions

Contributors

Khaled Afifi, MSc, MRCOG
Consultant Urogynaecologists and Obstetricians, Department of Obstetrics and Gynaecology, Royal Wolverhampton NHS Trust

Melanie Altizer
Assistant Professor Department of Obstetrics and Gynecology Virginia Tech

Sarah M. Appleton, MD
Assistant Professor, Department of Obstetrics and Gynecology University of Colorado School of Medicine

Norman A. Assad, MD
Associate Professor Department of Obstetrics and Gynecology East Tennessee State University

Anita Blanchard, MD
Professor Department Obstetrics and Gynecology, University of Chicago

Kari Braaten MD, MPH
Instructor, Department of Obstetrics, Gynecology, and Reproductive Biology Harvard Medical School

Brian Brocato, MD
Assistant Professor University of South Alabama

Randall Brown, MD, PhD, FASAM
Associate Professor, Department of Family Medicine UW School of Medicine and Public Health

Christinne Canela, MD
Assistant Professor Department of OB/GYN Carilion Clinic Virginia Tech Carilion School of Medicine

Megan Cheney, MD
Assistant Residency Program Director Banner Good Samaritan Hospital

Christine Conageski, MD
Assistant Professor, Department of Obstetrics and Gynecology University of Colorado School of Medicine

Charles Cox
Consultant Urogynaecologists and Obstetricians Department of Obstetrics and Gynaecology Royal Wolverhampton NHS Trust

Lee Dresang, MD
Professor, Department of Family Medicine UW School of Medicine and Public Health

Hal Elliott, MD
Associate Professor, Department of Psychiatry East Tennessee State University

Ibrahim El-Masri
Department of Obstetrics and Gynecology, University South Alabama College of Medicine and University of Balamand, Beirut, Lebanon

Ayman M. Elnaqa, MD, FRCOG
Consultant Urogynaecologists and Obstetricians Department of Obstetrics and Gynaecology Royal Wolverhampton NHS Trust#

John Ervin, MD
Department of Obstetrics and Gynecology Florida State University

Elizabeth A. Ferries-Rowe, MD, FACOG
Assistant Professor of Obstetrics and Gynecology Indiana University School of Medicine Chief of Service, Obstetrics and Gynecology Eskenazi Health Systems

Wing Kay Fok, MD
Instructor Department of Obstetrics and Gynecology Ohio State University

Beth Anne Fox, MD
Department of Family Medicine, East Tennessee State University

Jessica Francis, MD
Assistant Professor Department of Obstetrics and Gynecology Medical College of Wisconsin

Jennifer Frank, MD
ThedaCare Physicians

Nancy Gaba, MD
Department Obstetrics and Gynecology, George Washington University

Juan Garcia-Velasco, MD
Associate Professor, Department of Obstetrics Gynecolgy Rey Juan Carlos University

David Gregory
Associate Professor of Clinical Family Medicine, University of Virginia

Sarah Griffiths, BMedSci (Hons), BM BS, FRCA
Fellow in Obstetric Anaesthesia Queen Charlotte's and Chelsea Hospital Imperial College Healthcare NHS Trust

Ronald C. Hamdy, MD, FRCP, FACP
Professor Department of Internal Medicine, East Tennessee State University

Brigid Hayden MD, FRCOG
Consultant Obstetrician and Gynaecologist, Bolton, UK Committee Member of British Society for Paediatric and Adolescent Gynaecology

Sheri Holmes, MD
Department of Obstetrics & Gynecology East Tennessee State University

Joanna Hooper, MD
Assistant Professor, University of New Mexico

Jessica R. Jackson, MD
Maternal Fetal Medicine Fellow, Department of Obstetrics and Gynecology Florida State University

Julia V. Johnson, MD
Professor and Chair Department of Obstetrics and Gynecology, University of Massachusetts Medical School

Gail Joseph, MD
Resident Physician, Florida State University

Lisa M. Keder, MD, MPH
Associate Professor Department of Obstetrics and Gynecology Ohio State University

Elizabeth J. Kvach, MD, MA
Assistant Professor, Department of Family Medicine University of Colorado, Denver

Jeanette Lager, MD, MPH
Assistant Professor, University of California, San Francisco

Eduardo Lara-Torre MD, FACOG
Associate Professor of Obstetrics and Gynecology and Pediatrics Virginia Tech – Carilion School of Medicine

Lawrence Leeman, MD, MPH
Associate Professor, University of New Mexico

David Lewis, MD, MBA
Professor University of South Alabama

Jennifer Lesko MD, MPH
Assistant Professor, Department of Obstetrics and Gynecology George Washington University

Spiros A. Liatsikos, MD, PhD
Centre for Reproduction and Advanced Technology London, United Kingdom

Sharon Luent Seidel, MD
Clinical Assistant Professor, Department of Obstetrics and Gynecology Florida State University

Ondrea McKay, MD
Department of Medicine Rutgers, The State University of New Jersey, Rutgers New Jersey Medical School

Tristi W. Muir, MD
Professor, Department of Obstetrics and Gynecology Houston Methodist Hospital

Amanda B. Murchison MD, FACOG
Assistant Professor of Obstetrics and Gynecology Virginia Tech – Carilion School of Medicine

Geeta Nargund FRCOG
Centre for Reproduction and Advanced Technology London, United Kingdom

Lena Nguyen, DO
Education Chief Resident, Department of Obstetrics, Gynecology, and Women's Health Rutgers New Jersey Medical School

Martin E. Olsen, MD
Department of Obstetrics & Gynecology East Tennessee State University

Onyi Onuoha, MD, MPH
Assistant Professor Department of Anesthesiology and Critical Care University of Pennsylvania

Joseph E. Peterson, MD
Clinical Associate Professor, Department of Obstetrics and Gynecology Florida State University

BA Felicity Plaat, MBBS, FRCA
Consultant Anaesthetist Queen Charlotte's and Chelsea Hospital, Imperial College Healthcare NHS Trust

Jeffrey D. Quinlan, MD
Associate Professor Department of Family Medicine, Uniformed Services University of the Health Sciences

Botros Rizk
Department of Obstetrics and Gynecology, University South Alabama College of Medicine

Natalie E. Roche, MD
Assistant Professor, Department of Obstetrics, Gynecology, and Women's Health Rutgers New Jersey Medical School

Manjusha Sahni, MD
Assistant Professor, Department of Obstetrics/Gynecology, Virginia Tech Carilion School of Medicine

Catherine R. Salva, MD
Associate Professor of Clinical Obstetrics and Gynecology, Department of Obstetrics and Gynecology University of Pennsylvania

Karen E. Schetzina, MD, MPH, FAAP
Associate Professor and Director Division of Community Pediatrics Research Department of Pediatrics East Tennessee State University

Mark Schnee, MD
Department Obstetrics and Gynecology Indiana University

Karen M. Schneider, MD
Associate Professor, Department of Obstetrics and Gynecology Baylor College of Medicine

Jessica T. Servey, MD, Col, USAF, MC
Associate Professor of Family Medicine Uniformed Services University of the Health Sciences

Nancy Sokkary, MD
Assistant Professor Department of Obstetrics and Gynecology University of New Mexico School of Medicine

Elaine Stickrath, MD
Denver Health Medical Center Instructor, University of Colorado Denver

Meshell Stokes, MD
Resident Physician University of Tennessee, Chattanooga Unit

Laurie Swain, MD
Associate Professor, Baylor College of Medicine

Eric Swisher, MD
Assistant Professor Department of OB/GYN Virginia Tech Carilion School of Medicine Assistant Director of Minimally Invasive Gynecologic Surgery Carilion Roanoke Memorial Hospital

Theodore Tsaltas, MD
Assistant Professor University of Tennessee, Chattanooga Unit

Rola Turki
Department of Obstetrics and Gynecology, University South Alabama College of Medicine and King Abdulaziz University, Jeddah, Saudi Arabia

Julie Ware, MD, MPH, FAAP, FABM, IBCLC
Center for Breastfeeding Medicine Department of General and Community Pediatrics Cincinnati Children's Hospital Medical Center

Patrice M. Weiss, MD
Chair and Professor Department of OB/GYN Carilion Clinic Virginia Tech Carilion School of Medicine

Brett Worly, MD, FACOG
Assistant Professor, Department of Obstetrics/Gynecology Ohio State University Wexner Medical Center

Julie Zemaitis DeCesare, MD
Clinical Associate Professor, Florida State University College of Medicine

Preface

The care of women in the office setting is a key component of the global health care of female patients. Along with gynecology and obstetrics, office practice is one of the three key pillars of the practice by specialists in obstetrics/gynecology; office care of women is also a major component of the practices of family physicians, general practitioners, internal medicine doctors, and other health professionals.

By its nature, the health care of women requires complete attention to the entire patient. Comprehensive care involves assessment of multiple organ systems and specific issues; many issues are influenced by psychosocial and lifestyle contexts. This book brings together expertise from obstetrics and gynecology, family medicine, internal medicine, pediatrics, anesthesiology, and psychiatry to provide the clinician with knowledge to more accurately provide excellent care to women in the office or outpatient setting. The 50 chapters cover topics that are essential to clinicians who wish to competently provide excellence in the thorough diagnosis and management of the health issues facing their women patients in the outpatient office setting.

The wide range of topics covered in this book includes subjects that in many cases are extensive enough to warrant entire, distinct books. *Office Care of Women*, however, is written tightly and designed to be read from beginning to end so that the clinician can have a basic understanding that will be useful in the initial management of the vast majority of diagnoses seen in the outpatient clinical settings of women's health-care professionals. The basic knowledge gained from this book can then be used by the clinician to review the literature more knowledgeably when needed.

The provision of excellent health care to women is important not only to the patients served, but also to their families and to society at large. It is our hope that this book inspires readers to provide the finest health care possible to their patients.

Chapter 1

Preventive health care

Karen M. Schneider

Introduction

Preventive health-care centers on disease prevention and health maintenance. It encompasses routine health assessments of risk factors for the development of diseases, the early diagnosis of diseases, counseling regarding risk factors and disease identification, and other interventions or tests to prevent a health problem. Physical examination, screening tests, health education, and immunization programs are common examples of preventive health care. The common screening tests and recommendations for women are outlined and addressed in this chapter.

The annual examination

Every patient contact can be an opportunity to promote good health, but the annual exam should focus on disease prevention. A multitude of guidelines exist, and the American College of Obstetricians and Gynecologists (ACOG) recommends an annual well-woman visit that includes screening, evaluation, counseling, and immunizations based on age and risk factors (available at www.acog.org/wellwoman).[1] The latest screening guidelines are regularly updated and published on the US Preventive Services Task Force website: www.uspreventiveservicestaskforce.org. The Affordable Care Act (ACA) is intended to help Americans gain access to routine screening services and regular wellness visits. Health plans are required to cover certain preventive services with no cost sharing from the patient.[2] For women these include:

- well-woman exams on an annual basis
- gestational diabetes screening
- HPV DNA testing
- sexually transmitted infection counseling
- HIV screening and counseling
- contraception and contraceptive counseling
- breastfeeding counseling, support, and supplies
- domestic violence screening

Basic well-woman examination

At each well-woman visit, the patient's general health should be assessed along with investigation into risk factors for common and age-associated issues.

The patient's history should include:

- medical, surgical, mental, menstrual, and reproductive health
- family medical history
- use of medications
- use of tobacco, alcohol, or drugs
- sexual practices, including need for contraception
- abuse/neglect/violence
- diet and nutrition
- exercise and physical activity
- assessment of symptoms of age-related issues

The physical examination should include:

- height
- weight
- BMI calculation
- blood pressure
- neck: for adenopathy and thyroid assessment
- abdominal examination
- breasts: beginning at age 20, every one to three years; yearly after age 40
- pelvic: based on age or medical history
- other physical examination as clinically indicated

Laboratory, imaging, and other tests should be done based on age and risk factors (see www.acog.org/~/media/Departments/Annual%20Womens%20Health%20Care/PrimaryAndPreventiveCare.pdf).[3]

Office Care of Women, ed. Martin E. Olsen and Botros Rizk. Published by Cambridge University Press.

Pelvic examination

ACOG recommends a pelvic exam annually in women 21 years and older even though no evidence supports or refutes its use in asymptomatic, low-risk patients. The decision whether or not to perform a pelvic exam in an asymptomatic patient should be a shared decision between the patient and her physician. A pelvic exam should be done in women with symptoms of pelvic, genital tract, urological, or gastrointestinal problems.[1]

Cancer screening

Screening for certain cancers allows for early detection and improves cure and survival rates. Here we address screening for cancers that have shown a benefit toward improved outcomes with minimal harm from testing.

Breast cancer

Breast cancer is the most common cancer diagnosed in women in the United States, and screening has effectively reduced breast cancer mortality. General screening recommendations apply to women who are not at increased risk for breast cancer by virtue of a known genetic mutation or history of chest radiation. Genetic mutations account for a small percentage of women diagnosed with breast cancer annually; increasing age is the most important risk factor breast cancer.[4]

Mammography

In 2009 the US Preventive Serviced Task Force (USPSTF) recommended mammogram screening every two years for women aged 50 to 74 years, with individualization of biennial screening for younger women (aged 40 to 49 years) based on personal circumstances and values.[5] The American Cancer Society (ACS) and ACOG strongly recommend yearly screening with mammography beginning at age 40 years.

Life expectancy and medical comorbidities should be taken into account when screening women over the age of 75. The benefits of mammography decrease compared to the harms of overtreatment with advancing age. At age 75, women in consultation with their physician should decide whether to continue or stop screening.[4]

Clinical breast examination

A clinical breast exam should be done yearly for women 40 years and older and every one to three years for women aged 20 to 39 years.

Breast self-examination and breast self-awareness

Breast self-examination (BSE) is a method for women to examine their own breasts in a systematic way on a regular basis. BSE has not been proven to reduce morbidity or mortality related to breast cancer and may increase harm related to biopsies for false positive findings. ACOG and the ACS promote breast self-awareness. It focuses on women knowing what is normal for their own breasts so that any change, even a small one, can be recognized and reported to a health-care provider.

Enhanced screening for women at increased risk

Women with a known BRCA 1/2 mutation, 20% risk of breast cancer based on risk models, or personal history of breast cancer, as well as those who had thoracic radiation require enhanced surveillance for breast cancer. This includes twice yearly clinical breast exams, a yearly mammogram, a yearly breast MRI, and instruction on breast self-examination. For those women at risk due to thoracic radiation, screening should begin 8 to 10 years after they received treatment or at age 25, whichever occurs latest.[4]

Prevention of breast cancer in women at increased risk

Physicians should counsel and prescribe risk-reducing medications, such as tamoxifen or raloxifene, for women at increased risk for breast cancer and low risk for adverse medication effects.[6]

Cervical cancer

Routine screening with cervical cytology (Pap test) has reduced the incidence and mortality for cervical cancer in the United States by more than 50%.

Screening with cervical cytology should start at age 21, with Pap tests every three years through age 29. From age 30 to 65 years, women should have a Pap test simultaneously with a high-risk (oncogenic) human papillomavirus (HPV) test every five years or a Pap test alone every three years. Women aged 21 to 29 years should not be screened with HPV testing unless it is used to triage an abnormal result. Women younger than 21 years of age should not be screened regardless of the age of onset of sexual activity. Women who have undergone a hysterectomy and retain their cervix should continue routine age-based surveillance. Women with a previous history of CIN II or higher should continue to undergo routine age-based screening for 20 years beyond the initial post-treatment surveillance period even if that takes them beyond 65 years of age.

Woman with HIV infection should be screened twice a year in the first year after diagnosis, then annually thereafter. The Centers for Disease Control and Prevention (CDC) recommends initiating screening the year that diagnosis is made, even if the woman is younger than 21. There are no guidelines for screening in women who are immune-compromised due to other diseases or conditions, so beginning annual screenings at age 21 should be sufficient.

Colorectal cancer

Colorectal cancer (CRC) is the third leading cause of death among women in the United States. Although rectal bleeding is the most common symptom, most people diagnosed with colon cancer do not have symptoms. The American College of Gastroenterology (ACG) recommends both cancer prevention tests that can find cancer as well as polyps and cancer detection tests that have lower sensitivities for polyps and cancer (Table 1-1). Overall, the preferred screening method is colonoscopy every 10 years beginning at age 50, except for African Americans, who should begin screening at age 45. Detection tests may be used if a patient declines a prevention test or if prevention tests are not available to the patient. Women at higher risk for colon cancer due to strong family history, familial adenomatous polyposis (FAP) or hereditary non polyposis colorectal cancer (HNPCC) require more rigorous surveillance. Heavy cigarette smoking and obesity are linked to higher risk of CRC and occurrence at an earlier age. Therefore, consideration for earlier screening (possibly beginning at age 45) should be made on an individual basis for women who are heavy smokers or obese.[8]

Table 1-1 Colon cancer screening for the general population

Starting age	Tests	Frequency
50 years; 45 years for African Americans	**Prevention tests***	
	Colonoscopy**	Every 10 years
	Flexible Sigmoidoscopy	Every 5–10 years
	CT Colonography	Every 5 years
	Detection tests	
	Fecal Immunochemical Test for blood (FIT)***	Annually
	Fecal DNA	Every 3 years

* Prevention tests should be offered first.
** Colonoscopy is the preferred prevention test.
*** Preferred detection test. Hemoccult Sensa – 3 patient-collected samples.
Source: Compiled from Rex DK, Johnson DA, Anderson JC, et al. American College of Gastroenterology guidelines for colorectal cancer screening 2009. *Am J Gastroenterol* 2009 Mar;104(3):739–50.

Ovarian cancer

Routine screening for ovarian cancer in asymptomatic women is not recommended. Women at high risk for ovarian cancer (BRCA gene mutation or family history suggesting hereditary cancer syndrome) should undergo genetic counseling to assess their risk and, if appropriate, be offered ovarian cancer screening. Screening with CA-125 and transvaginal ultrasound every six months has been recommended for high-risk patients, but it has not shown to improve survival rates. ACOG recommends offering risk-reducing salpingo-oophorectomy for BRCA1- or BRCA2-positive women by age 40.[9]

Lung cancer

Annual screening for lung cancer with low-dose computed tomography is recommended for adults aged 55 to 80 years who have at least a 30-pack-per-year smoking history and currently smoke or who have quit smoking within the past 15 years. Screenings should stop once a person has not smoked for 15 years or develops a health problem that substantially limits life expectancy or the ability or willingness to have curative lung surgery.[10]

Bone health and osteoporosis

Bone health

Women are five times more likely than men to develop osteoporosis, and women are twice as likely to have a fracture. ACOG recommends discussing bone health early in a woman's life, starting at puberty and adolescence when women are at the peak bone-building stage. Adequate nutrition and regular physical activity are essential for strong bones.[11] Calcium and vitamin D affect bone quality, and adequate quantities should be consumed through diet or supplementation (Table 1-2).[12]

Table 1-2 Calcium and vitamin D recommendations

Nutrient	Age	Recommended daily dietary intake
Calcium	9–18 years	1,300 IU*
	19–50 years	1,000 IU
	>50 years	1,200 IU
Vitamin D	≤70 years	600 IU
	>70 years	800 IU

* International units.
Source: Ross AC, Manson JE, Abrams SA, et al. The 2011 report on dietary reference intakes for calcium and vitamin D from the Institute of Medicine: what clinicians need to know. *J Clin Endocrinol Metab* 2011;96:53–8.

Table 1-3 BMD screening recommendations

Risk factors	Test and frequency
≥65 years	DXA every 2 years; FRAX yearly if osteopenia
<65 years postmenopausal with >1 risk factor*	DXA every 2 years; FRAX yearly if osteopenia
Current smoker	
Alcoholism	
Rheumatoid arthritis	

* Risk factors:
Medical history of a fragility fracture
Body weight less than 127 lbs.
Medical causes of bone loss (medications or diseases)
Parental medical history of hip fracture
Source: American College of Obstetricians and Gynecologists. Osteoporosis. Practice Bulletin No. 129. *Obstet Gynecol* 2012;120: 718–34.

Table 1-4 Interpretation of BMD

Category	T-score*
Normal	≥–1.0
Osteopenia (low bone density)	<–1.0 to >–2.5
Osteoporosis	≤–2.5

* T-score is the number of standard deviations above or below the mean average bone density value for young adult women.
Source: American College of Obstetricians and Gynecologists. Osteoporosis. Practice Bulletin No. 129. *Obstet Gynecol* 2012;120: 718–34.

Table 1-5 Recommendations for osteoporosis treatment

- T-score of –2.5 or less (osteoporosis)
- History of low-trauma fracture
- T-score from –1 to –2.5 (osteopenia) and one of the following:

FRAX score ≥3% for risk of hip fracture
FRAX score ≥20% for risk of a major osteoporotic fracture (forearm, hip, shoulder, or clinical spine fracture)

Source: American College of Obstetricians and Gynecologists. Osteoporosis. Practice Bulletin No. 129. *Obstet Gynecol* 2012;120: 718–34.

Osteoporosis screening

DXA

Bone mineral density (BMD) screening should begin at age 65 for all women. A dual-energy x-ray absorptiometry (DXA) of the lumbar spine and hip is the gold standard for diagnosis. Screening should be done every two years. Postmenopausal women younger than 65 should be screened with DXA only if they have significant risk factors for osteoporosis and/or bone fracture (Tables 1-3 and 1-4).

FRAX

The fracture risk assessment tool, FRAX (www.sheffield.ac.uk/FRAX) determines a patient's probability of developing fracture in the next 10 years. It assesses risk based on BMD at the femoral neck and clinical factors. An annual FRAX score should be calculated to monitor the effect of age on fracture risk when osteopenia is diagnosed by DXA (Table 1-5).

Heart and vascular health

Hypertension

Chronic hypertension is a common and significant health problem predisposing women to increased risks of heart disease, stroke, renal disease, and other vascular diseases. Blood pressure (BP) should be assessed at each visit, and the diagnosis of elevated blood pressure is made if abnormal readings are detected on two separate visits.[13]

It is necessary to be familiar with diagnostic criteria and treatment guidelines (Table 1-6).

Table 1-6 Classification and management of blood pressure*

Classification	Systolic BP	Diastolic BP	Lifestyle modification	Initial drug therapy	
				Without compelling indications	With compelling indications**
Normal	<120	and <80	Encourage	No drug therapy indicated	Drug(s) for compelling indications
Prehypertension	120–139	or 80–89	Yes		
Stage I hypertension	140–159	or 90–99	Yes	Thiazide-type diuretics for most; may consider ACEI, ARB, BB, CCB, or combination	Drug(s) for compelling indications; other antihypertensive medications as needed
Stage II hypertension	≥160	≥100	Yes	Two-drug combination for most (usually thiazide-type diuretic and ACEI or ARB or BB or CCB)	

Drug abbreviations: ACEI – angiotensin converting enzyme inhibitor; ARB – angiotensin receptor blocker; BB – beta blocker; CCB – calcium channel blocker.
* Treatment determined by highest BP category.
** See Table 1-14.
Source: National Heart, Lung, and Blood Institute; National Institutes of Health; US Department of Health and Human Services.

Table 1-7 Basic workup for hypertension

Physical exam	• Fundoscopic eye exam • Auscultation for carotid, abdominal, and femoral bruits • Thyroid palpation • Heart and lung exam • Abdominal exam for enlarged kidneys, masses or abnormal aortic palpation • Lower extremity exam for edema and pulses • Neurological assessment	
Diagnostic tests and labs	Electrocardiogram Lipid profile Blood glucose Creatinine	Serum potassium Calcium Hematocrit Urinalysis

Source: National Heart, Lung, and Blood Institute; National Institutes of Health; US Department of Health and Human Services.

Evaluation

Evaluation for end organ damage (Table 1-7), identifiable causes (Table 1-8), and cardiovascular risk factors should be done once hypertension is diagnosed. Treatment or referral for treatment should also occur.

Treatment

The fundamental goal of treatment is the reduction of cardiovascular and renal morbidity and mortality. The therapeutic BP target is <140/90 mmHg. In hypertensive patients with diabetes or renal disease, the BP goal is <130/80 mmHg. Lifestyles changes (Table 1-9) should be recommended for all patients with hypertension and are first line of treatment unless stage II hypertension or compelling indications exist. Many medications are available for treatment, but typically thiazide-type

Table 1-8 Identifiable causes of hypertension

- Sleep apnea
- Obesity
- Renal diseases
- Endocrine disorders: thyroid, parathyroid, adrenal disorders, primary aldosteronism, pheochromocytoma
- Medications: corticosteroids, adrenal steroids, nonsteroidal anti-inflammatories, oral contraceptives, sympathomimetics (decongestants, anoretics), cyclosporine, tacrolimus, erythropoietin
- Illicit drugs: cocaine, amphetamines, and others
- Herbal medications or dietary supplements: ma huang, ephedra, licorice, bitter orange
- Excessive alcohol intake

Source: National Heart, Lung, and Blood Institute; National Institutes of Health; US Department of Health and Human Services.

Table 1-9 Lifestyle modifications for hypertension management

Modification	Recommendation	Approximate SBP reduction
Weight loss	Maintain normal BMI 18.5–24.9 kg/m^2	5–20 mmHg per 10 kg weight loss
DASH diet	Consume diet rich in fruits, vegetables, and low-fat dairy products with a reduced content of saturated and total fat	8–14 mmHg
Reduce sodium intake	Reduce dietary sodium intake to no more than 2–4 gram sodium or 6 grams of sodium chloride daily	2–8 mmHg
Physical activity	Engage in regular aerobic activity at least 30 minutes per day for most days of the week	4–9 mmHg
Limit alcohol consumption	No more than 1 drink per day in women (2 drinks per day in men)	2–4 mmHg

DASH – dietary approach to stop hypertension.
Source: National Heart, Lung, and Blood Institute; National Institutes of Health; US Department of Health and Human Services.

Table 1-10 Compelling indications and recommended medications

Compelling indication	Recommended drugs*					
	Diuretic	BB	ACEI	ARB	CCB	AldoANT
Chronic kidney disease			X	X		
Diabetes	X	X	X	X	X	
Heart failure	X	X	X	X		X
High coronary disease risk	X	X	X		X	
Postmyocardial infarction		X	X			X
Recurrent stroke prevention	X		X			

Drug abbreviations: ACEI – angiotensin converting enzyme inhibitor; ARB – angiotensin receptor blocker; AldoANT – aldosterone antagonist; BB – beta blocker; CCB – calcium channel blocker.
* Compelling indications for antihypertensive drugs are based on benefits from outcome studies or existing clinical guidelines; the compelling indication is managed in parallel with the hypertension.
Source: National Heart, Lung, and Blood Institute; National Institutes of Health; US Department of Health and Human Services.

diuretics work for most patients (Table 1-10). African Americans respond better to diuretics and calcium channel blockers than the other classes of medications. Certain compelling indications respond better to certain classes of medications (Table 1-10).[14]

Table 1-11 Coronary heart disease risk factors

- Familial hyperlipidemia
- Family history of premature cardiac disease (aged <50 years in men or <60 years in women)
- Personal history of CHD
- Personal or family history of peripheral artery disease
- Personal history of non-coronary atherosclerosis
- Diabetes
- Obesity (BMI >30)
- Hypertension
- Tobacco use

Source: Compiled from American College of Obstetricians and Gynecologists Annual Women's Health Care High Risk Factors (available at www.acog.org/About-ACOG/ACOG-Departments/Annual-Womens-Health-Care/High-Risk-Factors) and USPSTF's Screening for Lipid Disorders in Adults: US Preventive Services Task Force Recommendation Statement, June 2008 (available at (www.uspreventiveservicestaskforce.org/uspstf08/lipid/lipidrs.htm).

Table 1-12 Classification lipid values

	Description	Value (mg/dL)
Total cholesterol	Desirable	<200
	Borderline high	200–239
	High	≥240
LDL cholesterol	Optimal	<100
	Near optimal	100–129
	Borderline high	130–159
	High	160–189
	Very high	≥190
HDL cholesterol	Low	<40
	High	≥60
Triglycerides	Normal	<150
	Borderline high	150–199
	High	200–499
	Very high	≥500

Source: National Heart, Lung, and Blood Institute; National Institutes of Health; US Department of Health and Human Services.

Table 1-13 Therapeutic lifestyle changes for lowering LDL

Essential component	Recommendation
LDL-raising nutrients: Saturated fats Dietary cholesterol	Less than 7% of calories Less than 200 mg/day
Therapeutic options to lower LDL: Plant stanols/sterols Increased viscous (soluble) fiber	2 grams per day 10–25 grams per day
Total calories	Adjust total caloric intake to maintain desirable body weight/prevent weight gain
Physical activity	Include enough moderate exercise to expend at least 200 kcal per day

Source: National Heart, Lung, and Blood Institute; National Institutes of Health; US Department of Health and Human Services.

Lipid screening

ACOG recommends lipid screening women 45 years and older every five years and between the ages of 19 and 45 years based on risk factors (Table 1-11).[3, 15] The National Institutes of Health (NIH) NHLBI recommends lipid screening for all persons age 20 years and older every five years.[16] The USPSTF strongly recommends screening women 45 years and older if they have increased risk of CHD.[17]

Laboratory testing should include total cholesterol, low density lipoprotein (LDL), high density lipoprotein (HDL) and triglycerides (Table 1-12).

A strong relationship exists between LDL-cholesterol level and CHD, therefore LDL is the primary target for treatment. Therapeutic lifestyle changes (Table 1-13) are recommended to lower LDL and minimize other risks factors. Cholesterol lowering drugs should be used when lifestyle modifications fail to reach target LDL levels or when LDL levels are high (≥160) or risk for CHD is high based on cholesterol levels or multiple risk factors. HMG CoA reductase inhibitors (statins) are considered first-line drugs when medications are indicated.[16]

Stroke prevention in women

Aspirin prophylaxis to prevent ischemic stroke in women aged 55 to 79 is recommended by the USPSTF if benefits outweigh the potential harm from gastrointestinal bleeding.[18]

Family planning

In women of reproductive age, including adolescents and women over the age of 40, inquiry into their plans for pregnancy should be made at annual visits.[19]

Pregnancy planning and preconception counseling

Women who desire pregnancy should be encouraged to create a reproductive health plan. This includes timing of pregnancy, spacing, number of children and age-related changes in fertility. Overall health should be optimized. Medical conditions that could impact pregnancy should be identified and treated. Patients should be counseled on unhealthy exposures such as poor nutrition, alcohol, tobacco and other drugs. Folic acid supplementation starting at least one month prior to attempting pregnancy should be recommended. Screening for immunity to rubella, hepatitis, pertussis, and varicella should be done with immunization against these provided if it is indicated. HIV counseling and testing should be done.[19]

Contraception counseling

Women who do not desire pregnancy should be counseled on contraceptive methods. Counseling should be tailored to the patient's needs and lifestyle. It should include various methods, benefits, potential risks, and information on how to decrease contraceptive failures. The patient should be assessed for general health and any medical conditions that could be impacted either by a contraceptive method or by pregnancy. Blood pressure and weight should be measured as these could affect the medical risks or efficacy of certain methods. In women with no health risks, no laboratory testing is needed. Testing for sexually transmitted infections (STIs) is not required prior to prescribing any method. Routine screening for hereditary thrombophilia is not indicated before providing hormonal contraceptives. The ultimate guiding principle in prescribing one method over another should be the patient's choice, barring no contraindications to use of a method. As protection against STIs, the need for barrier methods should always be stressed. Information on when and how to use emergency contraception should be provided. Follow appointments should be made within one to two months of initiating a method, especially in first time users, to assess for side effects and compliance, check blood pressure and address any concerns regarding use.[19]

The CDC provides guidance for contraceptive use in the United States and can be found at www.cdc.gov/mmwr/pdf/rr/rr6205.pdf.[20]

Immunizations

Immunizations are an important part of preventive health care. Indications and ages for administration in the adult population are as follows and are available at www.cdc.gov/vaccines/schedules/hcp/imz/adult.html.

Influenza Administer annually for all ages.

Human papillomavirus (HPV) Offer to all women aged 9 to 26 years.

Tetanus, diphtheria, and pertussis (Td/Tdap) Tdap should be administered for women who have not received Tdap previously or who have unknown status, then Td booster should be given every 10 years. Tdap should be administered in each pregnancy regardless of prior vaccination interval.

Varicella Administer to all without documentation of prior immunization or evidence of immunity.

Zoster Administer one dose to adults 60 years and older regardless of prior episode of herpes zoster.

Measles, mumps, rubella (MMR) Adults born prior to 1957 are considered immune to measles and mumps. Adults born in 1957 or later should have one or more doses of MMR given. Revaccination is recommended in adults if they have nonimmune status, are a student in postsecondary education, work in a health-care facility, or travel internationally. Rubella immunity should be determined for all pregnant women and if nonimmune one dose should be given after delivery prior to discharge from hospital.

Pneumococcal Administer once to all women aged 65 years or older and to adults <65 years of age with one of the following conditions:

- chronic lung disease
- chronic cardiovascular disease
- diabetes
- asplenia
- immune-compromising conditions
- chronic renal failure
- nephrotic syndrome
- chronic liver disease
- resident in nursing home or long-term care facilities
- adults who smoke

One time revaccination is recommended five years after first dose for individuals with asplenia, immune-compromising conditions, chronic renal failure, or nephrotic syndrome.

Meningococcal Administration is recommended for the following persons:

- all adults with asplenia or persistent complement deficiencies
- college students up to age 21 years living in residence hall if not vaccinated at ≥16 years of age
- microbiologists routinely exposed to *Neisseria meningitidis*
- military recruits
- persons at risk during an outbreak
- persons who live in or travel to countries where meningococcal disease is hyperendemic or epidemic

Revaccination every five years is recommended if asplenia, persistent complement deficiencies, or microbiologist routinely exposed to *Neisseria meningitidis.*

Hepatitis A Any person seeking protection from hepatitis A virus or with the following indications:

- chronic liver disease
- persons who receive clotting factor concentrates
- persons traveling or working in countries where hepatitis A is endemic
- unvaccinated persons with close contact to an international adoptee from countries where hepatitis A is endemic

Hepatitis B Any person seeking protection from hepatitis B virus or the following indications:

- sexually active persons with more than one partner in six months
- persons seeking evaluation or treatment for a sexually transmitted disease
- IV drug users
- health-care workers or others exposed to blood or other bodily fluids
- household contacts or sexual partners of persons with hepatitis B
- travelers to countries with intermediate or high prevalence of chronic hepatitis B infection
- clients or staff members of institutions for persons with developmental disabilities
- persons with chronic liver disease
- persons with HIV infection
- persons with end-stage renal disease
- persons with diabetes younger than age 60 or those who are 60 years or older if likelihood of acquiring hepatitis B

Haemophilus influenzae type B Administer to persons with asplenia or sickle cell disease or to those who have had a successful hematopoetic stem cell transplant.

Vaccinations for travel Information on vaccines for travel requirements is available through the CDC at wwwnc.cdc.gov/travel/destinations/list.[21]

Screening for infections

Bacteruria

Asymptomatic bacteruria screening is not recommended in asymptomatic women;[24] however, ACOG recommends screening in women 65 years and older.[3] Pregnant women should be screened at 12 to 16 weeks or at the first prenatal visit if it occurs later.[22]

Chlamydia

All sexually active women ≤25 years of age should be screened annually. Older women should be screened based on risk factors (e.g., new or multiple sex partners).[23]

Gonorrhea

ACOG recommends annual screening for all sexually active women ≤25 years of age.[3] The CDC recommends gonorrhea screening only to those at increased risk for infection (e.g., women with previous gonorrhea infection, other sexually transmitted diseases (STDs), new or multiple sex partners, and inconsistent condom use; those who engage in commercial sex work and drug use; women in certain demographic groups; and those living in communities with a high prevalence of disease).[23]

Hepatitis B virus

Screening for hepatitis B virus (HBV) in nonpregnant women is recommended for individuals with high risk for infection (Table 1-14).[24] All pregnant women should be screened at their first prenatal visit.[25]

Hepatitis C virus

Routine screening for hepatitis C virus (HCV) is not recommended for the general population, including pregnant women. One-time screening for adults born

Table 1-14 High-risk factors for hepatitis B infection

- Household or sexual contacts of HBV infected persons
- Intravenous drug users
- HIV infected persons
- Persons born in a geographic area where prevalence ≥2% (i.e., most of Asia, most of Africa, Australasia with the exception of Australia and New Zealand, and parts of South America)
- Persons not vaccinated as an infant and whose parents were born in geographic area where prevalence ≥8% (i.e., sub-Saharan Africa, central and southeast Asia, and China)
- Persons receiving hemodialysis or cytotoxic or immunosuppressive therapy

Source: USPSTF's Screening for Hepatitis B Virus Infection in Nonpregnant Adolescents and Adults: Final Recommendation Statement, AHRQ Publication No. 12-05172-EF-2, available at www.uspreventiveservicestaskforce.org/uspstf12/hepb/hepbfinalrs.htm.

Table 1-16 Risk factors for HIV infection

- Injection drug users
- Sex partners of injection drug users
- Exchanging of sex for money or drugs
- Sex partners of HIV infected persons
- Sex with men who have sex with men since the most recent HIV test
- More than one sex partner since their most recent HIV test

Source: American College of Obstetricians and Gynecologists. Routine human immunodeficiency virus screening, Committee Opinion No. 596. *Obstet Gynecol* 2014;123:1137–9.

between 1945 and 1965 is recommended. Periodic screening is recommended for persons with a high risk of infection (Table 1-15).[26]

Herpes simplex virus

The USPSTF and CDC do not recommend routine screening for herpes simplex virus (HSV) in asymptomatic patients, even pregnant women.[27] According to the CDC, type-specific HSV serology may be helpful in the following situations:

- recurrent genital symptoms or atypical symptoms with a negative HSV culture

Table 1-15 High-risk factors for hepatitis C infection

- Past or current injection drug use
- Recipient of blood transfusion prior to 1992
- Long-term dialysis
- Born to a mother with HCV infection
- Incarceration
- Intranasal drug use
- Getting an unregulated tattoo
- Percutaneous exposure with HCV infected blood

Source: USPSTF's Screening for Hepatitis C Virus Infection in Adults: Final Recommendation Statement, AHRQ Publication No. 12-05174-EF-2, available at www.uspreventiveservicestaskforce.org/uspstf12/hepc/hepcfinalrs.htm (accessed November 30, 2015).

- clinical diagnosis of HSV without laboratory confirmation
- a partner with genital herpes

For women who are seeking an STD evaluation, HSV serology should be considered if they have multiple sexual partners or have HIV infection.[23]

Human immunodeficiency virus

ACOG recommends screening women aged 13–64 years for human immunodeficiency virus (HIV) at least once in their lifetime and annually thereafter based on risk factors outlined in CDC guidelines (Table 1-16). Physicians should annually review patients' risk factors for HIV and assess the need for retesting. Patients may opt out.[28]

All pregnant women should be screened for HIV as part of their routine prenatal testing.[29]

Syphilis

All pregnant women should be screened and non-pregnant women at increased risk of infection because of high-risk sexual activities including commercial sex workers, persons who exchange sex for drugs, persons in correctional facilities, those with HIV infection, and contacts of persons with active syphilis.[30]

Tuberculosis

Tuberculosis (TB) tests are generally not needed for people with a low risk of infection. Certain people should be tested for TB because they have a higher risk of infection (Table 1-17).[31]

Table 1-17 Risks for TB infection

- Spending time with someone who has TB disease
- HIV infection or another medical problem that weakens the immune system
- Symptoms of TB disease (i.e., fever, night sweats, cough, and weight loss)
- From a country where TB disease is common (i.e., most countries in Latin America, the Caribbean, Africa, Asia, Eastern Europe, and Russia)
- Live or work somewhere in the United States where TB disease is more common (e.g., homeless shelters, prison or jails, some nursing homes)
- Use illegal drugs

Source: Compiled from Centers for Disease Control and Prevention: Testing for Tuberculosis (TB), available at www.cdc.gov/tb/publications/factsheets/testing/TB_testing.htm (accessed June 18 and July 9, 2014).

Injury and violence

Intimate partner violence

Physicians should know the signs and symptoms of abuse and screen all women at routine visits and during pregnancy. Clinician's responsibilities include:

- universal screening
- acknowledge trauma
- assess immediate safety
- help establish a safety plan
- review options (shelters, support groups, legal advocacy, etc.)
- offer educational materials
- offer community and local resources
- provide referrals
- document clinical interactions
- provide ongoing support at subsequent visits [32]

Elderly abuse

ACOG recommends screening all patients 60 years and older for signs and symptoms of elder abuse.[33]

Safe driving practice

ACOG recommends that clinicians counsel all women on the use of seat belts, distracted driving, and driving under the influence of alcohol or drugs. Pregnant women should be counseled on proper seat belt fit during pregnancy and proper use of a car seat for their infant.[3, 34]

Table 1-18 Alcohol use and at-risk drinking in women [37]

Moderate "low risk" drinking	1 drink per day
Binge drinking	>3 drinks per occasion
At-risk alcohol use	>3 drinks per day *or* >7 drinks per week

Source: National Institute on Alcohol Abuse and Alcoholism, Overview of Alcohol Consumption and Alcohol Use Disorders, available at www.niaaa.nih.gov/alcohol-health/overview-alcohol-consumption/alcohol-use-disorders (accessed July 9, 2014).

Prevention of falls

Older patients should be asked about falls during routine health visits. Exercise or physical therapy and vitamin D supplementation are recommended for women 65 years of age and older who are at risk for falls.[35]

Substance abuse and mental health

Alcohol and illicit drug use and abuse

At annual visits women should be directly questioned about their use of alcohol and nonmedical use of illicit or prescription drugs. Brief intervention, patient education, and treatment referral should be provided to those with risky behavior (Table 1-18).[36]

Tobacco use

All clinicians should ask about tobacco use and provide tobacco cessation interventions for those who use tobacco products. The "5 As" intervention model is an evidence-based model successfully used by the busy clinician to address patient smoking. The 5 As are ask, advise, assess, assist, and arrange (Table 1-19).

In addition to counseling, all smokers making a quit attempt should be offered medication to improve quit success and reduce withdrawal symptoms.[38]

Depression

Depression is a common psychiatric illness among women. OB/GYN physicians should be well aware of the symptoms of depression (Table 1-20) and when found make an appropriate plan for treatment or referral. If depression is diagnosed, suicide risk should be assessed.[39]

Table 1-19 "5 As" intervention model for tobacco cessation

- Ask about tobacco use in any form or amount
- Advise patients to quit in a clear, strong, and personalized manner
- Assess the patient's willingness to quit
- Assist with quitting for those who are willing
- Arrange follow-up

Source: American College of Obstetricians and Gynecologists. Tobacco use and women's health. Committee Opinion No. 503. *Obstet Gynecol* 2011;118:746–50.

Table 1-20 Common symptoms of depression

- Loss of interest or pleasure *in normal enjoyable activities*
- Persistent physical symptoms such as headache, digestive disorders, or chronic pain *that do not respond to appropriate treatment.*
- Exaggerated or prolonged depressive symptoms *following life stressors or common reproductive events, conditions or procedures such as miscarriage, childbirth, infertility, hysterectomy, or menopause*
- Multiple somatic problems *including chronic pain, severe premenstrual syndrome or dyspareunia*

Source: American College of Obstetricians and Gynecologists. *Guidelines for Women's Health Care, A Resource Manual*, Third Edition. Washington, DC: American College of Obstetricians and Gynecologists; 2007:288–93.

Metabolic, nutritional, and endocrine disorders

Diabetes

The USPSTF recommends screening for type 2 diabetes in adults with a sustained blood pressure >135/80 mmHg. Evidence shows a reduced incidence of cardiovascular events and mortality in adults with hypertension and diabetes by lowering blood pressure below conventional target values. Screening tests include fasting glucose, two-hour glucose test, or hemoglobin A1c.[40] ACOG recommends screening all women age 45 years and older every three years for diabetes and younger women with the following risk factors: overweight or obese, family history of diabetes, high-risk ethnic group, history of gestational diabetes, hypertension, dyslipidemia, impaired glucose tolerance, or history of vascular disease.[3, 15]

Exercise and fitness

General fitness should be assessed at annual exams and patients should be encouraged to exercise as it improves overall health and reduces the risk of many adverse health outcomes. Inactive persons should gradually increase activity over time to meet recommended activity levels. The benefits of physical activity far outweigh any adverse outcomes. The US Department of Health and Human Services has developed physical activity guidelines for Americans (Table 1-21).[41]

Nutrition

Recommendation for a healthy diet that helps achieve and maintain a healthy weight, promotes health, and prevents disease should be made. The key is to balance calorie intake with physical activity. General recommendations based on the Dietary Guidelines for Americans should be discussed (Table 1-22).[42]

Obesity

Obesity increases the risk of cardiovascular disease, diabetes, hypertension, joint disease, sleep apnea, infertility, gallbladder disease, and some cancers such as breast, colon and uterine. Each annual visit should include an assessment of the patient's weight and body-mass index (BMI) in Table 1–23.

The initial approach for overweight or obese women is weight loss through diet and exercise. FDA-approved weight loss medications may be appropriate for some women who have failed diet and exercise, have a BMI ≥30 or ≥27 with comorbid medical conditions (hypertension, diabetes, dyslipidemia, or cardiovascular disease). Bariatric surgery is an option for women with a BMI of 40 kg/m^2 or higher, or women with a BMI of 35 kg/m^2 or higher and comorbid medical conditions (Table 1-24).[43]

Thyroid disease

Clinicians should be familiar with symptoms of thyroid disease and screen when indicated. ACOG recommends screening women ≥50 years old every five years and younger women if symptoms are present or they are in a high-risk group (strong family history of thyroid disease or history of autoimmune disease).[3, 17]

Table 1-21 Physical activity guidelines for adults

Adults aged 18–64 years

- Some physical activity is better than none. Health benefits can be seen with as little as 60 minutes of moderate intensity aerobic activity per week
- Both aerobic (endurance) and muscle-strengthening (resistance) exercises is beneficial
- 150 minutes of moderate-intensity activity (brisk walking) or 75 minutes of vigorous-intensity activity per week provides major health benefits
- More health benefits occur with 300 minutes of moderate activity or 150 minutes of vigorous-intensity activity per week
- Muscle-strengthening activities should be done a least twice a week

Adults aged 65 years and older

- Any amount of physical activity provides some health benefits
- If physically able, 150 minutes of moderate-intensity activity (or 75 minutes of vigorous-intensity activity) per week is recommended, if unable be as active as physical condition allows
- Walking is shown to provide health benefits with low risk of injury
- Balance exercises are recommended for those at risk of falls

Physical activity intensity

The relative intensity of aerobic activity is related to a person's level of cardiorespiratory fitness.

- Moderate-intensity activity requires a medium level of effort. On a scale of 0 to 10, where sitting is 0 and the greatest effort possible is 10, moderate-intensity activity is a 5 or 6 and produces noticeable increases in breathing rate and heart rate.
- Vigorous-intensity activity is a 7 or 8 on this scale and produces large increases in a person's breathing and heart rate.

Source: Compiled from Office of Disease Prevention and Health Promotion, US Department of Health and Human Services, 2008 Physical Activity Guidelines for Americans, ODPHP Publication No. U0036, October 2008. Available at www.health.gov/paguidelines.

Table 1-22 Summary of dietary guidelines for Americans

- Increase vegetable and fruit intake
- Use fat-free or low-fat milk
- Half of grain intake should be whole grains
- Reduce sodium intake to <2,300 mg daily (1,500 mg daily if >50 years old or has hypertension, diabetes, chronic renal disease or is African American)
- Consume <300 mg cholesterol daily
- Consume <10% of calories from saturated fats
- Reduce calorie intake of solid fats and added sugars
- Consume alcohol in moderation
- Choose a variety of protein foods (e.g., seafood, lean meat, nuts, soy, beans, or peas)
- Replace solid fats with oils
- Choose foods that provide more potassium, calcium, vitamin D, and fiber

Source: US Department of Agriculture and US Department of Health and Human Services. *Dietary Guidelines for Americans, 2010*. Seventh Edition, Washington, DC: US Government Printing Office, December 2010, available at www.dietaryguidelines.gov.

Concluding remarks

Obstetricians and gynecologists have a unique opportunity as leaders in women's health care to provide preventive services and to counsel patients about a healthy lifestyle and minimizing risks. It is important to stay current on guidelines to assist women in maintaining well-being at all stages of their lives.

Table 1-23 BMI and weight classifications

BMI (kg/m²)	Classification
<18.5	Underweight
18.5–24.9	Normal
25.0–29.9	Overweight
30.0–34.9	Obese Class I
35.0–39.9	Obese Class II
≥ 40.0	Obese Class III

Source: National Heart, Lung, and Blood Institute; National Institutes of Health; US Department of Health and Human Services.

Table 1-24 Management of obesity

Recommended therapies	Indications
Weight loss through diet and physical activity and behavior modification	All overweight and obese women BMI ≥25.0
Medications FDA-approved – Orlistat and Sibutramine	BMI ≥30.0 *or* BMI ≥27.0 with comorbid conditions*
Bariatric surgery	BMI ≥40.0 *or* BMI ≥35.0 with comorbid conditions*

* Comorbid conditions include type 2 diabetes, hypertension, dyslipidemia, cardiovascular disease
Source: National Heart, Lung, and Blood Institute; National Institutes of Health; US Department of Health and Human Services.

References

1. American College of Obstetricians and Gynecologists. Well-woman visit. Committee Opinion No. 534. *Obstet Gynecol* 2012;**120**:421–4.
2. US Department of Health and Human Services Health Resources and Services Administration. Women's preventive services guidelines. www.hrsa.gov/womens guidelines (accessed March 26, 2014).
3. American College of Obstetricians and Gynecologists. Well-woman care: assessments and recommendations. www.acog.org/About-ACOG/ACOG-Departments/Annual-Womens-Health-Care/Assessments-and-Recommendations (accessed April 8, 2014).
4. American College of Obstetricians and Gynecologists. Breast cancer screening. Practice Bulletin No. 122. *Obstet Gynecol* 2011;**118**:372–82.
5. Nelson HD, Tyne K, Naik A, et al. Screening for breast cancer: an update for the US Preventive Services Task Force. *Ann Intern Med* 2009;**151**:727–37; W237–42.
6. Nelson HD, Smith MB, Griffin JC, et al. Use of medications to reduce risk for primary breast cancer: a systematic review for the US Preventive Services Task Force. *Ann Intern Med.* 2013;**158**:604–14.
7. American College of Obstetricians and Gynecologists. Screening for cervical cancer. Practice Bulletin No. 131. *Obstet Gynecol* 2012;**120**:1222–38.
8. Rex DK, Johnson DA, Anderson JC, et al. American College of Gastroenterology Guidelines for Colorectal Cancer Screening 2009. *Am J Gastroenterol* 2009 Mar;**104**(3):739–50.
9. American College of Obstetricians and Gynecologists Committee on Gynecologic Practice. Committee Opinion No. 477: the role of the obstetrician-gynecologist in the early detection of epithelial ovarian cancer. *Obstet Gynecol* 2011;**117**: 742–6.
10. Humphrey LL, Deffebach M, Pappas M, et al. Screening for lung cancer with low-dose computed tomography: a systematic review to update the US Preventive Services Task Force recommendation. *Ann Intern Med* 2013;**159**:411–20.
11. American College of Obstetricians and Gynecologists. Osteoporosis. Practice Bulletin No. 129. *Obstet Gynecol* 2012;**120**:718–34.
12. Ross AC, Manson JE, Abrams SA, et al. The 2011 report on dietary reference intakes for calcium and vitamin D from the Institute of Medicine: what clinicians need to know. *J Clin Endocrinol Metab* 2011;**96**:53–8.
13. Guidelines for Women's Health Care: A Resource Manual, Third Edition. Washington, DC: American College of Obstetricians and Gynecologists 2007: 314–19.
14. National Heart, Lung, and Blood Institute. The seventh report of the Joint National Committee on Prevention, Detection, Evaluation, and Treatment of Hypertension. National Institutes of Health Publication No. 03-5233, 2003. www.nhlbi.nih.gov/guidelines/hypertension/express.pdf (accessed June 18, 2014).
15. American College of Obstetricians and Gynecologists. Annual women's health care: high risk factors. www.acog.org/About-ACOG/ACOG-Departments/Annual-Womens-Health-Care/High-Risk-Factors (accessed June 18, 2014).
16. National Heart, Lung, and Blood Institute. Third report of the National Cholesterol Education Program (NCEP) expert panel on detection, evaluation, and treatment of high blood cholesterol in adults (Adult Treatment Panel III). National Institutes of Health

Publication No.01-3670, 2001. www.nhlbi.nih.gov/guidelines/cholesterol/atp3full.pdf (accessed May 9, 2014).

17. US Preventive Services Task Force. Screening for lipid disorders in adults: US Preventive Services Task Force recommendation statement. June 2008. www.uspreventiveservicestaskforce.org/uspstf08/lipid/lipidrs.htm (accessed June 18, 2014).
18. US Preventive Services Task Force. Aspirin for the prevention of cardiovascular disease: US Preventive Services Task Force recommendation statement. *Ann Intern Med* 2009;**150**:396–404.
19. Guidelines for Women's Health Care: A Resource Manual, Third Edition. Washington, DC: American College of Obstetricians and Gynecologists 2007: 174–87.
20. Centers for Disease Control and Prevention. US selected practice recommendations for contraceptive use, 2013. *MMWR* 2013;**62**(5):1–64. www.cdc.gov/mmwr/pdf/rr/rr6205.pdf.
21. Center for Disease Control and Prevention; Advisory Committee on Immunization Practices recommended immunization schedule for adults aged 19 years and older – United States, 2014. *MMWR* 2014;**63**:110–12.
22. US Preventive Services Task Force. Screening for asymptomatic bacteriuria in adults: clinical summary of a US Preventive Services Task Force recommendation statement. AHRQ Publication No. 08-05120-EF-2, July 2008. www.uspreventiveservicestaskforce.org/uspstf08/asymptbact/asbactsum.htm.
23. Centers for Disease Control and Prevention. Sexually Transmitted Diseases Treatment Guidelines, 2010. *MMWR* 2010;**59**(12):14–85. www.cdc.gov/std/treatment/2010/STD-Treatment-2010-RR5912.pdf.
24. US Preventive Services Task Force. Screening for hepatitis B virus infection in nonpregnant adolescents and adults: final recommendation statement. AHRQ Publication No. 12-05172-EF-2. www.uspreventiveservicestaskforce.org/uspstf12/hepb/hepbfinalrs.htm.
25. US Preventive Services Task Force. Screening for hepatitis B virus infection in pregnancy: US Preventive Services Task Force reaffirmation recommendation statement. AHRQ Publication No. 09-05134-EF-1, June 2009. www.uspreventiveservicestaskforce.org/uspstf09/hepb/hepbpgrs.htm.
26. US Preventive Services Task Force. Screening for hepatitis C virus infection in adults: final recommendation statement. AHRQ Publication No. 12-05174-EF-2. www.uspreventiveservicestaskforce.org/uspstf12/hepc/hepcfinalrs.htm.
27. US Preventive Services Task Force. Screening for genital herpes: recommendation statement. AHRQ Publication No. 05-0573-A, March 2005. www.uspreventiveservicestaskforce.org/uspstf05/herpes/herpesrs.htm.
28. American College of Obstetricians and Gynecologists. Routine human immunodeficiency virus screening. Committee Opinion No. 596. *Obstet Gynecol* 2014;**123**: 1137–9.
29. Branson BM, Handsfield HH, Lampe MA, et al. Revised recommendations for HIV testing of adults, adolescents, and pregnant women in health-care settings. Centers for Disease Control and Prevention (CDC). *MMWR* 2006;**55**(RR-14):1–17.
30. US Preventive Services Task Force. Screening for syphilis infection: recommendation statement. July 2004. www.uspreventiveservicestaskforce.org/3rduspstf/syphilis/syphilrs.htm.
31. Centers for Disease Control and Prevention. Testing for tuberculosis (TB). www.cdc.gov/tb/publications/factsheets/testing/TB_testing.htm (accessed June 18 and July 9, 2014).
32. *Guidelines for Women's Health Care: A Resource Manual*, Third Edition, Washington, DC: American College of Obstetricians and Gynecologists 2007: 276–81.
33. American College of Obstetricians and Gynecologists Committee on Health Care for Underserved Women. Elder abuse and women's health. ACOG Committee Opinion 568. *Obstet Gynecol* 2013;**122**:187–91.
34. *Guidelines for Perinatal Care*, Seventh Edition. Washington, DC: American Academy of Pediatricians and the American College of Obstetricians and Gynecologists 2012: 144, 307–12.
35. US Preventive Services Task Force. Prevention of falls in community-dwelling older adults: US Preventive Services Task Force recommendation statement. AHRQ Publication No. 11-05150-EF-2, May 2012. www.uspreventiveservicestaskforce.org/uspstf11/fallsprevention/fallsprevrs.htm.
36. American College of Obstetricians and Gynecologists. At-risk drinking and illicit drug use: ethical issues in obstetric and gynecologic practice. ACOG Committee Opinion No. 422. *Obstet Gynecol* 2008;**112**:1449–60.
37. National Institute on Alcohol Abuse and Alcoholism. Overview of alcohol consumption and alcohol use disorders. www.niaaa.nih.gov/alcohol-health/overview-alcohol-consumption/alcohol-use-disorders (accessed July 9, 2014).
38. American College of Obstetricians and Gynecologists. Tobacco use and women's health. Committee Opinion No. 503. *Obstet Gynecol* 2011;**118**:746–50.
39. *Guidelines for Women's Health Care: A Resource Manual*, Third Edition. Washington, DC: American College of Obstetricians and Gynecologists 2007: 288–93.

40. US Preventive Services Task Force. Screening for type 2 diabetes mellitus in adults, topic page. www.uspreventiveservicestaskforce.org/uspstf/uspsdiab.htm.

41. US Department of Health and Human Services. 2008 physical activity guidelines for Americans; Office of Disease Prevention and Health Promotion. ODPHP Publication No. U0036; October 2008. www.health.gov/paguidelines.

42. US Department of Agriculture and US Department of Health and Human Services. *Dietary Guidelines for Americans, 2010*. Seventh Edition, Washington, DC: US Government Printing Office, December 2010. Available at www.dietaryguidelines.gov (accessed November 30, 2015).

43. National Heart, Blood and Lung Institute Obesity Education Initiative: The Practical Guide to the Identification, Evaluation, and Treatment of Overweight and Obesity in Adults. NIH Publication No. 00-4084, October 2000. www.nhlbi.nih.gov/guidelines/obesity (accessed November 30, 2015).

Chapter 2

Contraception

John Ervin

Introduction and history

Since ancient times, people have attempted to control the size of their families. Many methods of contraception are recorded. Most of the methods from history are barrier or withdrawal methods. The periodic abstinence method taught prior to the 1920s was imparted incorrectly. Soranus, a Greek gynecologist from approximately 200 CE, suggested that women should avoid intercourse during their menses because this was the time women were the most fertile. It was thought that the safest time for a woman was the midpoint of the menstrual cycle.[1] This teaching was overturned in the 1920s with the discovery that ovulation, in fact, occurs at the midpoint of the menstrual cycle. This then became one of the mechanisms of action to target in the development of more modern contraceptive methods.

It was not until 1960 that Enovid, the world's first oral contraceptive pill (OCP) was released by G.D. Searle and Company. The pill was an instant success. After two years, 1.2 million American women were on the pill, and after five years, 6.5 million women were taking the pill, making it the most popular form of birth control in the United States. A current problem with the success of the pill is that modern women have the misconception that a monthly menstrual cycle is normal or needed. For most of human history, a significant portion of most women's lives was spent either pregnant or lactating. Most women of reproductive age prior to the modern era likely had more months without periods than with periods.

Additionally, the number of maternal deaths averted by contraceptive use is high. Worldwide, it is estimated that without contraceptive use, the number of maternal deaths would be almost 266,000 higher per year than the current level. In terms of maternal mortality reduction, this is the equivalent of stating that contraceptive use reduced maternal mortality by almost 44%.[2]

Even with access to contraception, the problem of unintended pregnancy remains. In the United States, approximately half of unintended pregnancies are among women who were not using contraception at the time they became pregnant. However, the other half occurred among women who became pregnant despite reported use of contraception.[3] This is an important distinction and an opportunity to improve the consistent, correct use (CCU) of the chosen method.

How to measure contraceptive effectiveness

There are multiple methods of measuring the efficacy of a contraceptive. The "perfect use" failure rate expresses the number of unintended conceptions that occur when the individual uses the method consistently and correctly for one year. "Typical use" failure rate is the number of conceptions that occur when the individual routinely uses a method in an inconsistent or incorrect manner (i.e., missing medication/pills).

The Pearl Index (PI) is defined as the number of unintended pregnancies per 100 woman-years of method use. The PI is calculated by dividing the number of unintended pregnancies by the total number of woman months or exposure cycles of observation and multiplying by 1,200 (for months) or by 1,200 (for cycles). The PI may underestimate the contraceptive efficacy because it is often based on a lengthy exposure interval, usually one year. Because contraceptive failure rates decline with use, long study intervals may not reflect contraceptive efficacy associated with short-term use.

Contraceptive failure occurs in the first year of typical use for 9% of women using oral contraceptives, patch or ring; 18% of women relying on the male

Office Care of Women, ed. Martin E. Olsen and Botros Rizk. Published by Cambridge University Press.

condom; 3% of women using injectable methods; and 24% using fertility awareness-based methods.[4] Failure rates of sterilization are comparable with those of long-acting reversible contraception methods such as intrauterine devices (IUDs) and the etonegestrel implant. The annual failure rates for the IUD are 0.8% for the copper T380A and 0.2% for the levonogestrel-releasing intrauterine system. The etonogestrel implant has a 0.05% reported failure rate, the lowest of any contraception method.

The U.S. Collaborative Review of Sterilization (CREST) was a prospective, multicenter observational study of 10,685 women conducted in 1996 by the Centers for Disease Control and Prevention (CDC) which showed that sterilization via laparoscopy or minilaparotomy is a highly effective method of contraception.[5] The risk of failure is substantially higher than the initial findings reported. The five-year cumulative failure rate of 13 per 1,000 for aggregated sterilization methods, compared with a five-year cumulative failure rate of 14 per 1,000 procedures for the copper T380A IUD. The five-year rate for the levonorgestrel-releasing IUD ranged from 5 to 11 per 1,000 procedures.[6]

The CREST study did not include Essure®. A summary of Essure experience reported two pregnancies in roughly 130,000 patients with microinsert hysteroscopic sterilization and bilateral occlusion confirmed by HSG (although both cases were the result of perforation/misplacement rather than device failure). If these data could be applied to the CREST data, Essure tubal occlusion with a confirmatory HSG would represent the most effective of all female or male sterilization techniques.[7]

Contraceptive method choice

Many elements should be considered when women, or couples, seek medical care for the purposes of contraception. Some of these elements include safety, effectiveness, availability (which includes accessibility and affordability), and acceptability.

Contraceptive method effectiveness is a critical element to consider, especially among women for whom an unintended pregnancy would pose additional health risks. Effectiveness involves two elements: the inherent effectiveness of the method itself and how it is consistently and correctly used. CCU can vary greatly with patient characteristics such as age, partner selection, income, motivation to prevent or delay pregnancy, and culture. Methods that depend on CCU by patients have a wide range of effectiveness between typical and perfect users. Given the data in the United States that approximately half of unintended pregnancies are among women who became pregnant despite reported use of contraception, there is an increasing trend toward IUDs and implants, which are long-acting reversible contraception (LARCs). These methods are highly effective because they do not depend on regular compliance from the user. LARCs are appropriate for most women, including adolescents and nulliparous women.

In choosing a method of contraception, the risk for HIV and other STDs should also be considered. LARCs and oral contraceptives (OCs) are highly effective at preventing pregnancy; however, they do not protect against STDs and HIV. CCU of the male latex condom reduces the risk for HIV infection and other STDs, including chlamydial infection, gonorrhea, and trichomoniasis.[8]

Availability (which includes accessibility and affordability) of any chosen method will be key to continued use of contraception. Funding of contraception is a public health issue that is worthy of debate.

Confirm nonpregnant state

When starting any form of contraception, a provider must be reasonably certain that the woman is not pregnant at time of initiation. As in other areas of medicine, a detailed history will usually provide the most accurate assessment of pregnancy risk for a woman who is going to initiate a contraceptive method. The following criteria have been found to be highly accurate (i.e., negative predictive value of 99%–100%) in ruling out a pregnancy among women who are not pregnant.[9] If a woman meets any one of the following criteria, then a health-care provider can be reasonably certain that she is not currently pregnant:

1. is ≤7 days after the start of normal menses
2. has not had sexual intercourse since the start of last normal menses
3. has been correctly and consistently using a reliable method of contraception
4. is ≤7 days after spontaneous or induced abortion
5. is within 4 weeks postpartum
6. is fully or nearly fully breastfeeding [exclusively breastfeeding or the vast majority (≥85%) of feeds are breastfeeds], amenorrheic, and <6 months postpartum.

If a woman does not meet any of these criteria, then the health-care provider cannot be reasonably certain that she is not pregnant, even with a negative pregnancy test. Routine pregnancy testing for every woman is not necessary prior to initiation of a contraception method. If a woman has had recent (i.e., within the last five days) unprotected intercourse, consider offering emergency contraception if pregnancy is not desired.

Reversible contraception

Barrier

Barrier methods such as the male and female condom, the diaphragm and cervical cap, as well as the contraceptive sponge, place a physical barrier between sperm and egg and thus prevent fertilization. Male and female sterilization also have the same mechanism of action, but are considered to be permanent.

The male condom is a barrier worn over the penis to prevent semen and sexually transmitted diseases (STDs) from coming into contact with a partner's orifice (i.e., vagina, anus, mouth). Male condoms have been shown to decrease the transmission rate of HIV and other STDs. Step-by-step video instructions on proper condom use are available on the website of Planned Parenthood (www.ppfa.org). The concept of dual method is used to help prevent STDs. Condoms should be used at every sexual encounter, even if the couple is relying on another form of contraception. This additional contraceptive precaution is termed the use of dual methods. Although good in theory, many young women who are at greatest risk for STDs do not follow it.

The diaphragm is a latex rubber or silicone device designed to fit over the cervix and is used with a spermicide. The diaphragm keeps spermicide in close contact with the cervical mucus. Its mechanism of action is to function as a barrier to sperm, and the spermicide acts as a vaginal microbicide to kill sperm. Diaphragms are available only by prescription and must be individually fitted. There is variation between perfect use and typical use, secondary to user placement and motivation. Approximately 6–12 per 100 women per year will become pregnant with this method. The diaphragm must be worn for at least six hours after intercourse, but not more than 24 hours. It does not protect against STDs, and dual method male condom use is encouraged. It is an option for women who desire a nonhormonal method of contraception. Side effects, including increased incidence of urinary tract infections, are possible.

The Today Sponge®, a contraceptive sponge, debuted in the United States in 1983, and withdrawn in 1995 because of manufacturing deficiencies. Sales resumed in April 2005. The FDA never questioned the safety or efficacy of the Today Sponge. The device is moistened with two tablespoons of water and squeezed once. It is then placed high in the vagina covering the cervix. It must be inserted 30 minutes prior to intercourse and left in place for a minimum of 6 hours, and a maximum of 30 hours. One sponge is protective against repeated coital episodes during a 24-hour period. Prolonged sponge use is associated with vaginal infections and possible toxic shock syndrome. Perfect and typical use failure rates are 9% and 16%, respectively, for nulliparous women. In parous women, failure rates are increased to 20% and 32%, respectively. Concomitant male condom use is recommended to protect against STDs.

Hormonal

Oral contraceptive pills

Since the first birth control pill was released in 1960, women in the United States have made OCPs the most popular contraception method, with nearly 12 million US women and more than 100 million women worldwide taking OCPs. Combination OCPs contain estrogen and a progestin. Two estrogen formulations are commonly used. The predominant estrogen in low dose combination OCPs is ethinyl estradiol (EE). Mestranol, an estrogen found in older, high dose combination OCPs, is metabolized to EE. The first OCP Enovid-10 contained 150 μg mestranol and 9.85 mg norethylnodrel. Modern low dose combination OCPs contain between 20 μg and 50 μg of EE for their estrogen component.

The progestin formulation often varies. Combination OCPs are progestin dominant. The progestin is set to oppose the estrogen's effect at the endometrium and prevent the luteinizing hormone (LH) surge in order to inhibit ovulation. There are presently more than 120 different brands of combination OCPs on the market in the United States. Some vary the amount of progesterone by week. Other formulations vary the number of pill-free days. Still others have an extended or continuous dosing.

The contraceptive failure rate for combination OCPs is approximately 0.3% in perfect use and 8.0% in typical use. Multiple variables can lead to decreased contraceptive efficacy, including side effects, general noncompliance (i.e., missing pills), increased body weight, and drug interactions. The side effects are often linked to early OCP discontinuation and subsequent contraceptive failure and unintended pregnancy. With the low dose OCP formulations, consistent timing of ingestion is an important factor in efficacy.

There are multiple contraindications to combination OCPs. Nearly all of the contraindications to combination OCPs are secondary to the pharmacologic level of estrogen. They include (1) prior history of thromboembolism, cerebrovascular disease, or coronary occlusion; (2) severely impaired liver function; (3) known or suspected breast cancer; (4) unexplained vaginal bleeding; (5) known or suspected pregnancy; (6) tobacco smoking in women >35 years; (7) severe hypercholesterolemia or hypertriglyceridemia; (8) uncontrolled hypertension; (9) migraine with aura. Full coverage of all contraindications is beyond the scope of this text; the American College of Obstetricians and Gynecologists (ACOG) has produced a practice bulletin that more completely addresses the use of hormonal contraception in women with coexisting medical conditions.[10] Additionally, the CDC has adapted the WHO recommendations for contraception use to give US Selected Practice Recommendations for Contraceptive Use, 2013.[11] A Google® search for CDC contraceptive guidelines will easily locate these documents free of charge.

Transdermal patch

In response to the need for more consistent dosing, drug developers developed a transdermal approach to medication delivery. Transdermal and transvaginal contraceptive steroid use results in less fluctuation in estrogen and progestin levels than a daily oral medication. They avoid the first-pass effect, with less adverse effect on liver parameters. Disadvantages include visibility of the patch and possible application site reactions. The patch mechanism of action is similar to OCPs. The Ortho Evra® patch is a combination estrogen and progestin transdermal patch that contains 750 μg of ethinyl estradiol and 6.0 mg of norelgestromin (the active metabolite of norgestimate). It delivers 20 μg of EE and 0.150 mg of norelgestromin per day. At three days of patch use, hormone levels achieve a steady state. The effectiveness of the patch was 1.07 per 100 woman-years. Of the 15 failures noted in clinical trials five were in women who weighed >90 kg (>198 lb), who accounted for only 3% of the study population. A similar finding was found in other studies. Women who weigh >90 kg may need to use an additional dual method of contraception.

Contraceptive ring

The Nuvaring® is a combination estrogen and progestin flexible vaginal ring that releases 15 mg of ethinyl estradiol and 0.120 mg of etonogestrel per day. The ring is placed in the vagina by the woman or her partner and left in place for three weeks, even for coitus. It is removed for one week (pill free interval); menses should occur following removal. After one week, a new ring is inserted. Side effects are generally less than that of OCPs with headache (5.8%), vaginitis (5.6%), and leukorrhea (4.8%) the most commonly reported. Efficacy for Nuvaring was 0.65 per 100 woman-years. Improved efficacy is presumably from improved compliance.

Injectable progestin

Depot medroxyprogesterone acetate (DMPA) was approved in 1992 by the FDA for contraception after a World Health Organization (WHO) study found that there was only slight or no increase in risk for breast cancer, an adverse finding that was previously reported in beagle dogs. DMPA is administered at a dose of 150 mg intramuscularly every three months or 13 weeks. With typical use, 6 women out of 100 will become pregnant within the first year of using the injection. DMPA can be used by women soon after childbirth, in women who are breastfeeding, and in women who have a contraindication to estrogen containing contraceptives. Side effects include irregular bleeding during the first six to nine months of use. When used for longer than two years, up to 70% of women no longer have any bleeding, which is why it is also used off label for treatment of dysmenorrhea and menorrhagia. A common side effect is weight gain. More than 60% of women report a weight gain of five pounds during the first year of use. This weight gain is less than occurs with a pregnancy. The FDA added a black box warning regarding the potential for bone loss when used for more than two years. The warning also indicated that it is unknown if use in adolescents will reduce peak bone mass with the potential to increase the risk of osteoporotic fractures later in life. The warning also states that DMPA should not be used as a long-term (longer than two years) contraception unless other methods are considered inadequate. However, additional study of the matter by the

WHO in 2005 concluded that there should be no restriction on the use of DPMA in women aged 19–45 years, including no restriction on the duration of use.[12] Individualized annual reevaluation and counseling is recommended.

Emergency contraception

Emergency contraception (EC) is therapy to prevent pregnancy after an unprotected or inadequately protected act of sexual intercourse. Common indications for EC include contraceptive failure (i.e., condom breakage or missed doses of OCs), failure to use any form of contraception, and sexual assault. The Yuzpe regimen for EC, using a widely available brand of OC, was published in 1974. The first FDA approval for EC was given in 1998. Many women are unaware of the availability of EC, both as a prescription and now available over the counter for most women. Increasing awareness and knowledge of EC are important priorities in the efforts to prevent unintended pregnancy.

Two commonly used over-the-counter regimens for EC exist: the combined estrogen-progestin regimen which consists of two doses – each containing 100 mcg of ethinyl estradiol plus 0.5 mg of levonorgestrel – taken 12 hours apart, and the progestin only regimen. The progestin only regimen is a total of 1.5 mg of levonorgestrel given as a single dose or 0.75 mg levonorgestrel and a second dose 12 hours later. Either is initiated as soon as possible after unprotected intercourse. Both regimens are equally efficacious. A new emergency oral contraceptive, ulipristal acetate, has recently become available. In the United States, ulipristal acetate is available only with a prescription.

Many of the most commonly prescribed OCPs also have an off-label dosing for use as EC listed in drug reference guides, which available on smart phone applications such as Epocrates®, to aid the user in choosing the correct dosing, given the multiple brands and strengths of OCPs on the market currently.

There have been no deaths or serious complications causally linked to EC. However, side effects for EC are common. Short-term side effects include nausea and vomiting in 18% and 4% using levonorgestrel only regimen, and 43% and 16% using the combined regimen.[13] Irregular bleeding (which seems to be in relation to the time of the cycle the EC is taken), breast tenderness, abdominal pain, dizziness, headache, and fatigue have also been reported. Women who require EC may benefit from encouragement to initiate a more consistent method of contraception.

The copper IUD is also recommended for EC. The IUD can be inserted up to five days after unprotected intercourse. Insertion of a copper IUD has the added advantage that it can remain in place for up to 10 years for continued long-acting reversible contraception. There have been no randomized controlled trials comparing IUD insertion with medical regimens for EC. Prospective cohort trials have showed pregnancy rates of 0%–0.1% when the copper IUD was inserted up to five days after unprotected intercourse.[13] The levonorgestrel-releasing intrauterine system is not effective as emergency contraception.[14]

Long-acting reversible contraception

Intrauterine devices and contraceptive implants, also called long-acting reversible contraceptives (LARCs), are the most effective reversible contraceptives. The major advantage is that they do not require an ongoing effort on the part of the user for long-term effective use. Encouraging the use of LARC methods for appropriate candidates may help lower the unintended pregnancy rate. Typical-use pregnancy rates for LARCs are lower, and continuation rates are higher compared to oral contraceptives. In an economic analysis, IUDs were among the least expensive contraceptive methods over a five-year period. Barriers to increased use include high initial cost. When this barrier was removed in the Contraceptive CHOICE project, a prospective cohort of women aged 14–45 years, 67% chose an IUD or the contraceptive implant.[15]

Currently four LARC methods are commonly available in the United States. Three are IUDs: (1) the copper T380A, (2) the levonorgestrel intrauterine system available as a 52 mg system – Mirena®, and (3) the levonorgestrel intrauterine system 13.5 mg – Skyla®. An additional levonorgestrel IUD, Liletta®, was made available in the United States in 2015; it has been used in Europe more extensively. The 52 mg system is indicated for five years of use, and the 13.5 mg system is indicated for three years of use. The final method is the etonogestrel single-rod contraceptive implant that is placed subdermally on the medial aspect of the nondominant upper arm.

The copper T380A is a T-shaped device of polyethelyene wrapped with copper wire around the stem and arms. The FDA has approved the copper IUD for up to 10 continuous years. It has a reported failure rate at one year of 0.8 per 100 women, and a 10-year failure rate similar to female sterilization by tubal interruption by laparoscopy (1.9 per 100 women over 10 years). The most common adverse effects are abnormal bleeding and increased length of menses, both of which are treatable with NSAIDS. The copper T380A is an attractive option for women who do not want a hormonal LARC. The copper T380A is also a good choice for emergency contraception, as noted previously.

The two levonorgestrel intrauterine system are also T-shaped devices containing a polydimethylsiloxane sleeve with 52 mg or 13.5 mg of levonorgestrel on the stem. The one-year failure rate is 0.2 per 100 women.

IUDs are appropriate for nulliparous women and adolescents. IUDs are category 2, for nulliparous and adolescent women, according to the U.S. Medical Eligibility Criteria for Contraceptive Use. The advantages generally outweigh the risks.

Overall, complications with IUDs are uncommon and mainly include expulsion, method failure and perforation. The expulsion rate is between 2% and 10% during the first year. Perforation occurs in 1 per 1,000 insertions or less.[15] The insertion techniques for the copper T380A and the levonorgestrel systems are different. The user should become familiar with the technique prior to attempting any insertion. In difficult cases when the uterus is sharply retroverted or anteverted, or in the case of obesity, simultaneous transabdominal ultrasound can be used to aid proper insertion.

Contraceptive Implants

The Norplant® implant system was a progestin-based contraception medication formulated for five years of continuous use. The implant system consisted of six soft silastic implants, each containing 36 mg of levonorgestrel. The implants were 34 mm long and 2.4 mm in diameter. They were placed in a fan-shaped arrangement into the subcutaneous tissue on the medial aspect of a woman's nondominant upper arm. It was removed from the US market in July 2002. A second generation, Norplant II® (also known as Jadelle®), consists of two small (43 mm × 2.5 mm) silicone rods, each containing 75 mg of levonorgestrel, instead of the original six capsules. The two-rod implant system has not been marketed in the United States but is available in other areas.

The current contraceptive implant system available in the United States consists of a single rod (4 cm in length and 2 mm in diameter) of ethylene vinyl acetate copolymer core containing 68 mg of etonogestrel surrounded by an ethylene vinyl copolymer skin. The device allows for controlled release of etongestrel over a period of three years. Etonogestrel is the active metabolite of desogestrel. It does not contain latex, is not biodegradable, and originally was not radiopaque. It was originally marketed as Implanon®. The insertion device was redesigned and the implant device made radiopaque and renamed Nexplanon®. Implanon was phased out in December 2012; since that date only Nexplanon has been available. The contraceptive implant is the most effective method of reversible contraception, with a typical-use pregnancy rate of 0.05%.[15] The most common side effects are changes in menstrual bleeding pattern including amenorrhea, oligomenorrhea, or prolonged bleeding. The bleeding pattern with contraceptive implant use is unpredictable and is cited as the most common reason for device discontinuation. However, a significant noncontraceptive benefit is a decrease in dysmenorrhea. Other reported adverse effects include gastrointestinal difficulties, headaches, acne, breast pain, vaginitis, and weight gain. According to the package insert, weight gain was reported in only 2.3% of patients who chose to discontinue the implant.

The contraceptive implant is safe to insert anytime in nonbreastfeeding women after childbirth. In breastfeeding women, it is optimal to wait four weeks after childbirth because of theoretic concerns regarding milk production and infant growth and development. A randomized trial compared postpartum insertion of the etonogestrel contraceptive implant at one to three days with standard insertion at four to eight weeks postpartum. No differences were found in breastfeeding outcomes between the groups, including lactogenesis and the risk of lactation failure. An additional nonrandomized comparative study compared milk composition in 80 women using nonhormonal IUD contraception with the etonogestrel implant. Breast milk composition (measured by total protein, fat, and lactose content) did not differ between the groups, nor did the quantity of breast milk. A three-year follow-up also showed no difference in neonatal body length, biparietal head circumference, and body weight. Given the excellent data regarding efficacy and safety for the contraceptive implant, expanded usage could substantially decrease the unintended pregnancy rate.

Insertion of the etonogestrel implant was simplified with the introduction of the Nexplanon® inserter. It is performed with local anesthetic, usually 2 mL of 1% lidocaine. The manufacturer will provide instruction and training to providers free of charge. Removal of a properly placed device is also a simply mastered technique.

Sterilization

Laparoscopic sterilization

Sterilization is a safe and effective method of permanent contraception used by more than 220 million couples worldwide. For married patients, sterilization remains the most commonly used method in the United States. It is used by 47.3% of married couples (tubal occlusion, 30.2%; vasectomy, 17.1%).[6] Female sterilization can be done either before conception or after pregnancy. Timing may affect which of several methods is selected. Postabortion sterilization may be performed immediately after an uncomplicated spontaneous or induced abortion by laparoscopy or minilaparotomy.

Postpartum sterilization can be performed at the time of cesarean delivery or after a vaginal delivery. When performed in conjunction with a cesarean delivery, it can be completed in less than five minutes in most cases when the tubes are easily accessible. When performed after a vaginal delivery, it is usually done through a small (approximately 1.5 cm–3 cm), infraumbilical incision. If epidural anesthesia was used for labor, the catheter can be retained and reused for sterilization the following day. This procedure should be planned (and informed consent obtained) during antepartum care. The Pomeroy and Parkland methods are the most commonly used in the United States, both at the time of cesarean section or with the use of a minilaparotomy incision. When an excisional method is used, the tubal segments should be submitted to pathology to confirm complete tubal transaction.

An interval tubal occlusion is performed via laparoscopy remote from pregnancy. Timing of sterilization in these cases should follow the guidelines listed previously to be reasonably certain that the woman is not pregnant. Laparoscopy does require use of general anesthesia, which slightly increases the risk of procedure, but allows the surgeon to inspect the abdominal and pelvic organs. The procedure is usually done using one or two 5 mm–8 mm incisions. The occlusion may be done using bipolar electrocoagulation, mechanical devices, or tubal excision. When bipolar energy is used, at least 3 cm of the isthmic portion of the tube must be completely coagulated.[6] Available mechanical devices provide compression and destruction of a segment of tube. The Falope Ring® utilizes a silicone rubber band placed over a segment of tube using a specialized applicator device. The Filshie Clip® applies a titanium clip lined with silicone rubber to the tube. The Hulka Clip® uses a spring-loaded silastic clip that is applied to the fallopian tube.

Alternatively, complete or partial salpingectomy may be performed by laparoscopy in order to accomplish sterilization. These techniques may be more technically difficult and require greater surgical skill to perform, but they have advantages in cases of tubal disease such as hydrosalpinx. Advanced surgical devices, such as the harmonic scalpel, or advanced bipolar devices may be used to cut and coagulate the tubes.

Hysteroscopic sterilization

The Essure® hysteroscopic system was approved by the FDA in 2002. Essure is the only hysteroscopic method currently in production. A woman must be at least six weeks postpartum for the procedure to be performed. It consists of a 4 cm long stainless inner coil and nickel titanium outer coil that is placed into each fallopian tube by a disposable delivery catheter. Tubal occlusion occurs by way of an inflammatory reaction and tissue growth in response to polyethylene terphthalate fibers contained within the implant. Essure is usually performed in an office setting with only light sedation (oral medications) and a paracervical block. Hysteroscopy is performed using normal saline as the distention medium. Successful bilateral placement rate approaches 97%.[16] A typical procedure usually takes approximately 15–20 minutes. An alternative method of contraception must be used until a confirmatory hysterosalpingogram (HSG) is performed at three months after implant placement. Many women are attracted to the opportunity to have a sterilization procedure performed in the office with minimal anesthesia and recovery time. Others find the confirmatory HSG three months postprocedure cumbersome. Postprocedure HSG adherence rates are highly variable depending upon the patient population, with follow-up rates of 13%–71%. When the protocol is followed, the Essure procedure is 99.83% effective based on five-year clinical data.[17]

Male vasectomy

Vasectomy can be performed on an outpatient basis with local anesthesia. Male vasectomy is the safest, most effective, most easily verifiable, and least expensive of permanent couples contraception. It does not require general anesthesia. Vasectomy is not immediately effective. A semen analysis should be done to confirm azoospermia; 98%–99% of men are azoospermic at six months after vasectomy. An alternative method of contraception should be used until the confirmatory semen analysis is performed. Some males develop sexual dysfunction after vasectomy. This method is obviously ineffective if the female patient has more than one sexual partner.

Ending contraceptive use

The age at which a woman is no longer at risk of pregnancy is not known. It is uncommon, but spontaneous pregnancies can occur among women aged >44 years. ACOG and the North American Menopause Society recommend that women continue contraceptive use until menopause or age 50–55 years. No reliable laboratory tests are available to confirm definitive loss of fertility in a woman. The assessment of follicle-stimulating hormone levels to determine when a woman is no longer fertile might not be accurate.[18]

The continued use of contraception with each method's inherent risk must be weighed against the risks of pregnancy for women of advanced reproductive age. Advanced maternal age results in higher risk of maternal complications such as hemorrhage, venous thromboembolism, hypertensive disorders, and death. The fetal complications include increased spontaneous abortion, stillbirth, and congenital anomalies, especially Trisomy 21.

Older women have increased risk for chronic conditions such as hypertension, obesity, and thromboembolism; these may become contraindications to a particular method. Continued annual dialog with patients is recommended to determine the appropriate risk level for each individual.

Concluding remarks

The ability to regulate fertility has a profound impact not just on women, but on their offspring and families as measured by infant, child, and maternal mortality and morbidity. Access to reliable contraception increases the education of not only the mother, but of her offspring, leading to improved economic conditions for the family. This is essential for securing the well-being and autonomy of women, while supporting the health, growth, and development of communities.

References

1. Evans ML, A desire to control: contraception throughout the ages. *Historica Medicinae*, 2009;**1**(1): E08.
2. Ahmed S, Li Q, Liu L, Tsui AO. Maternal deaths averted by contraceptive use: an analysis of 172 countries. *Lancet* 2012 Jul 14;**380**(9837):111–25.
3. Finer LB, Henshaw SK. Disparities in rates of unintended pregnancy in the United States 1994 and 2001. *Perspect Sex Reprod Health* 2006;**38**:90–6.
4. Trussell J. Contraceptive failure in the United States. *Contraception* 2011;**83**;397–404. (Level III)
5. Peterson HB, Xia Z, Hughes JM, et al. The risk of pregnancy after tubal sterilization: findings from the US Collaborative Review of Sterilization. *Am J Obstet Gynecol* 1996;**174**:1161–8; discussion 1168–70. (Level II-3)
6. American College of Obstetricians and Gynecologists. Practice Bulletin No. 133: Benefits and risks of sterilization, February 2013.
7. Bartz D, Greenberg JA. Sterilization in the United States. *Rev Obstet Gynecol.* 2008 Winter;**1**(1):23–32.
8. Workowski KA, Bolan GA; Centers for Disease Control and Prevention. Sexually transmitted diseases treatment guidelines. *MMWR Recomm Rep* 2015 Jun 5;**64**(RR-03):1–137.
9. Stamback J, Qureshi Z, Sekadde-Kigondu C, et al. Checklist for ruling out pregnancy among family-planning clients in primary care. *Lancet* 1999;**354**(9178):566.
10. American College of Obstetricians and Gynecologists. Practice Bulletin No. 73: Use of hormonal contraception in women with coexisting medical conditions, June 2006, reaffirmed 2013.
11. Centers for Disease Control and Prevention. US selected practice recommendations for contraceptive use, 2013, adapted from the World Health Organization Selected Practice Recommendations for Contraceptive Use, 2nd Edition, *MMWR* 2013;**62**:1–60.

12. American College of Obstetricians and Gynecologists. Committee Opinion No. 602: Depot medroxyprogesterone acetate and bone effects, June 2014.
13. American College of Obstetricians and Gynecologists. Practice Bulletin No. 112: Emergency contraception, May 2010, reaffirmed 2014.
14. Faculty of Family Planning and Reproductive Health Care in Clinical Effectiveness Unit. FFPRHC Guidance (April 2004). The levonorgestrel-releasing intrauterine system (LGN-IUS) in contraception and reproductive health. *J Fam Plann Reprod Health Care* 2004;**30**(2):99–108: quiz 109 (Level III).
15. American College of Obstetricians and Gynecologists. Practice Bulletin No. 121: Long-acting reversible contraception: implants and intrauterine devices, July 2011, reaffirmed 2013.
16. Basinski CM, A review of clinical data for currently approved hysteroscopic sterilization procedures. *Rev Obstet Gynecol* 2010;**3**:101–10. (Level III)
17. www.fda.gov/medicaldevices/productsandmedicalprocedures/implantsandprosthetics/ucm371014.htm. Accessed June 6, 2014.
18. Hillard PJ, Berek JS, Barss VA, et al. *Guidelines for Women's Health Care: A Resource Manual*, 3rd ed. Washington, DC: American College of Obstetricians and Gynecologists; 2007.

Chapter 3

Lactation

Karen E. Schetzina and Julie Ware

Introduction and background

Introduction

It is recommended that all women exclusively breastfeed their infants, with rare exceptions, for approximately 6 months, followed by continued breastfeeding with the addition of complementary foods for at least the first year of life.[1–5] Although most women desire to breastfeed, many do not continue the recommended length,[6] and about 60% of US mothers do not meet their own breastfeeding goals.[7] Basic breastfeeding support has been described as a standard of care for women's health-care providers; they are uniquely positioned to help women make informed feeding decisions and are a crucial part of the breastfeeding support team.[8, 9]

Breastfeeding rates

Over the past several decades, a number of initiatives and legislation for the promotion, support, and protection of breastfeeding have succeeded in increasing rates of breastfeeding since the post–World War II nadir that occurred, particularly in industrialized countries.[10] The WHO/UNICEF International Code of Marketing of Breast milk Substitutes, endorsed in 1981, provided guidelines recommending no direct marketing or samples of breast milk substitutes to mothers and no promotion of breast milk substitutes in health-care facilities.[11] The Innocenti Declaration [12] and Baby-Friendly Hospital Initiative, developed by the WHO and UNICEF in 1990–1991, called for establishment of national breastfeeding committees, protection of breastfeeding rights for working mothers, the practice of the evidence-based 10 steps to successful breastfeeding (Table 3-1), and the designation as "baby-friendly" for compliant maternity facilities.[13]

The most recent US CDC Breastfeeding Report Card documented that among the 2011 US birth cohort, 79.2% of infants initiated breastfeeding, yet only 49.4% and 26.7% were breastfeeding at 6 and 12 months, respectively. Exclusive breastfeeding occurred in only 40.7% at 3 months and 18.8% of infants at 6 months.[6] These rates have not met US Healthy People 2020 goals.[14] As in many nations, striking disparities in breastfeeding rates exist in the United States, with lower rates among non-Hispanic black mothers, young mothers, and mothers with lower income levels.[15–17] Worldwide, breastfeeding rates are below the WHO/UNICEF recommendations in many countries.[18]

Benefits of breastfeeding and risks of not breastfeeding in developed countries

Based on an extensive review, the Agency for Healthcare Research and Quality (AHRQ) reaffirmed the maternal and infant health risks associated with not breastfeeding and early cessation of breastfeeding in developed countries.[19] The US Surgeon General addressed these excess health risks in her call to action to support breastfeeding (Table 3-2).[8]

Maternal outcomes

Mothers who do not breastfeed experience an increased risk of poor health outcomes including type 2 diabetes mellitus, breast cancer (primarily premenopausal), and ovarian cancer.[19] An inverse relationship has been observed between development of hypertension, hyperlipidemia, cardiovascular disease, and rheumatoid arthritis and the cumulative lifetime duration of breastfeeding.[20, 21]

Bursts of oxytocin during breastfeeding result in uterine contractions, reduced postpartum blood loss, and rapid involution of the uterus. Lactational

Office Care of Women, ed. Martin E. Olsen and Botros Rizk. Published by Cambridge University Press.

Table 3-1 Ten steps to successful breastfeeding: the baby-friendly hospital initiative [12]

Step 1	Have a written breastfeeding policy that is routinely communicated to all health-care staff.
Step 2	Train all health-care staff in the skills necessary to implement this policy.
Step 3	Inform all pregnant women about the benefits and management of breastfeeding.
Step 4	Help mothers initiate breastfeeding within a one hour of birth.
Step 5	Show mothers how to breastfeed and how to maintain lactation, even if they are separated from their infants.
Step 6	Give newborn infants no food or drink other than breast milk unless medically indicated.
Step 7	Practice rooming-in – allow mothers and infants to remain together – 24 hours a day.
Step 8	Encourage breastfeeding on demand.
Step 9	Give no pacifiers or artificial nipples to breastfeeding infants.
Step 10	Foster the establishment of breastfeeding support groups and refer mothers to them on discharge from the hospital or birth center.

Table 3-2 Health risks from not breastfeeding

Outcome	Excess risk% (95% CI)*	Comparison groups
Among full-term infants		
Acute ear infections (otitis media)	100 (56, 233)	EFF vs. EBF for 3 or 6 mos
Eczema (atopic dermatitis)	47 (14, 92)	EBF <3 mos vs. EBF ≥3 mos
Diarrhea and vomiting (gastrointestinal infection)	178 (144, 213)	Never BF vs. ever BF
Hospitalizations for lower respiratory tract infections in the first year	257 (85, 614)	Never BF vs. EBF ≥4 mos
Asthma, with family history	67 (22, 133)	BF <3 mos vs. ≥3 mos
Asthma, with no family history	35 (9, 67)	BF <3 mos vs. ≥3 mos
Childhood obesity	32 (18, 127)	Never BF vs. ever BF
Type 2 diabetes mellitus	64 (18, 127)	Never BF vs. ever BF
Acute lymphocytic anemia	23 (10, 41)	Never BF vs. >6 mos
Acute myelogenous anemia	18 (2, 37)	Never BF vs. >6 mos
Sudden infant death syndrome	56 (23, 96)	Never BF vs. ever BF
Among preterm infants		
Necrotizing entercolitis	138 (22, 240)	Never BF vs. ever BF
Among mothers		
Breast cancer	4 (3, 6)	Never BF vs. ever BF (per year of breastfeeding)
Ovarian cancer	27 (10, 47)	Never BF vs. ever BF

* The excess risk is approximated by using the odds ratio in the studies referenced in the report.
Abbreviations: CI – confidence interval, EFF – exclusive formula feeding, EBF – exclusive breastfeeding, BF – breastfeeding.
Source: Excess Health Risks Associated with Not Breastfeeding. Used with permission from the Department of Health and Human Services.[8]

Table 3-3 Differentiating engorgement, plugged duct, and mastitis

Characteristics	Engorgement	Plugged duct	Mastitis
Onset	Gradual, immediately postpartum	Gradual, after feedings	Sudden, after 10 days
Site	Bilateral	Unilateral	Usually unilateral
Swelling and heat	Generalized	May shift; little or no heat	Localized, red, hot, swollen
Pain	Generalized	Mild, but localized	Intense, but localized
Body temperature	<38.4°C (101°F)	<38.4°C	>38.4°C
Systemic symptoms	Feels well	Fells well	Flulike symptoms

Source: Adapted with permission from *Breastfeeding: A Guide for the Medical Profession*. 6th ed. Lawrence RA, Lawrence RM. Elsevier, Mosby, Philadelphia, PA; 2005:563.[25]

amenorrhea with continued breastfeeding leads to increased child spacing. Postpartum depression has also been associated with not breastfeeding.[19]

Infant outcomes

Dose-response associations between breastfeeding and protection from infant and childhood disease have been well documented.[2, 8, 19] Benefits of human milk among preterm infants include better feeding tolerance, lower rates of necrotizing enterocolitis (NEC), sepsis, and readmissions following NICU discharge, and improved neurodevelopmental outcomes.[2]

In a US extrapolation, current suboptimal breastfeeding rates may be responsible for approximately 5,000 excess cases of breast cancer, 54,000 cases of hypertension, and 14,000 cases of myocardial infarction, totaling more than $730 million in direct medical costs.[22] In addition, if 90% of infants were breastfed exclusively for 6 months, almost 1,000 excess infant deaths would be prevented, along with $2.2 billion per year in excess medical costs.[23] Worldwide, suboptimal breastfeeding is responsible for several thousand deaths per day.[24]

Anatomy and physiology of lactation

The anatomy and physiology of lactation has been described elsewhere extensively.[25] Breast changes during pregnancy include significant lobuloalveolar growth, increased blood flow, and the appearance of superficial veins and Montgomery tubercles on enlarged and darkened areolae. The breast is able to produce milk beginning at 16–20 weeks gestation (lactogenesis stage I); however, production is inhibited by high levels of circulating progesterone.

Two or three days after birth, onset of copius milk production occurs. Lactogenesis is triggered by delivery of the placenta and decrease in progesterone. This occurrence is commonly referred to as milk "coming in." Milk is secreted from epithelial cells lining the alveoli, stored in the alveolar lumen, and then expressed through intralobular ducts and central ducts that exit directly through ductal orifices on the nipple. Colostrum, the first thick, yellow milk produced, is produced in small volumes and contains higher concentrations of protein, immunoglobulins, and other immunoactive components, and lower concentrations of lactose and fat than mature milk. Mature milk is creamier in appearance and produced in larger volumes.

A delay in onset of lactogenesis II (after 72 hours postpartum) is associated with early cessation of breastfeeding, and is more likely to occur in primiparous, obese, or diabetic women and after stressful deliveries.[25] Early lactation failure may occur in the setting of retained placenta, severe postpartum hemorrhage causing pituitary necrosis (Sheehan's syndrome), and primary glandular insufficiency.[25]

Milk production varies in response to the frequency of suckling and degree of breast emptying. Suckling induces periodic rises in prolactin from the anterior pituitary, a hormonal regulator of milk production, and release of oxytocin from the posterior pituitary. Release of oxytocin with milk ejection through contraction of myoepithelial cells surrounding alveoli, or "let down," may also occur in response to other stimuli, such as hearing, smelling, or thinking about the baby, or may be inhibited by maternal stress, fatigue, or pain. Other hormones that support milk synthesis include cortisol, thyroid hormone, insulin, and growth hormone.[26] Subsequently in Lactogenesis III, milk production is regulated primarily by milk removal from the breast. A feedback inhibitor of lactation (FIL) has been described.[25] FIL increases when milk remains in the alveoli/ducts, blocking further milk secretion. Hence milk production is regulated by infant demand. Weaning and subsequent termination of suckling results in decreases in milk production and involution of the mammary gland.

Approach to the patient

Overcoming barriers to breastfeeding: the breastfeeding-friendly office

Women's health-care providers play a significant role in a mother's decision to breastfeed.[27] Creating a breastfeeding-friendly office provides an opportunity to educate, convey positive support for breastfeeding, and link women to community resources. Providing formal breastfeeding education, support from trained health-care providers, and peer support increases breastfeeding initiation, exclusivity, and duration.[28] Preparing mothers to experience each of the 10 steps to successful breastfeeding (Table 3-1), will enable more mothers to breastfeed in a positive dose-response relationship.[29–31]

Patient education

Many new mothers do not have direct, personal knowledge or experience with breastfeeding, and are unaware of the risks of not breastfeeding.[8] Noncommercial educational materials addressing breastfeeding benefits, techniques, common breastfeeding problems, myths, breastfeeding classes, and other resources should be made available in waiting and exam rooms.

Breastfeeding welcomed here

Knowledge about the health benefits of breastfeeding, as well as comfort with breastfeeding in social situations, has been positively correlated with intention to exclusively breastfeed.[32] Embarrassment and the perception that formula feeding is the social norm are barriers to breastfeeding, particularly among certain racial and ethnic populations.[8] Displaying diverse images of breastfeeding families and signs indicating that mothers are welcome to breastfeed in the office help to overcome these barriers. Ensure that your staff is trained in office practices that are consistent with local/national laws providing protection for public breastfeeding. A nursing mothers' area in the office with a comfortable armchair can provide the option for more privacy if desired and a place to conduct breastfeeding assessments. Avoid displaying or distributing infant formula samples as these provide conflicting messages and are associated with decreased rates of breastfeeding.[30]

Provider education and training

Despite published evidence, many health professionals believe that infant formula is nearly equivalent to breast milk in terms of health benefits.[33] All staff should be educated on the importance of breastfeeding and promotion of a supportive environment.[4] Lactation problems are associated with earlier cessation of breastfeeding.[7, 34] Clinicians should receive education and skills training to ensure consistent and effective lactation support and provide referrals as needed to patients. Continuing education conferences, courses, and online modules may be used. Point of care guidelines can help support provider decision making.[29, 31, 35]

Business case for breastfeeding

Mothers planning to work within a year after delivery are less likely to initiate breastfeeding, and maintaining lactation upon returning to work is a barrier for breastfeeding continuation. Providing employees with break time and a space to express milk or breastfeed has been shown to improve employee satisfaction, reduce absences, and lower employer health-care costs.[36] In addition to a comfortable chair and privacy, employers should provide access to an electrical outlet and hand washing supplies, as well as refrigeration if possible. Model these practices in your own office and counsel mothers on how to combine breastfeeding with work or school (discussed later in the chapter). Be familiar with local/national laws for worksite lactation support and communicate these to patients.

Family and social support

Poor family and social support have been identified as barriers to breastfeeding.[37] Therefore, engaging fathers, grandmothers, and other support persons in breastfeeding education and referrals to classes is beneficial for continuation of breastfeeding.[8,30] Counseling and materials must be appropriately based on the socioeconomic, demographic, and cultural characteristics of local patient populations. Mothers will benefit from referrals to breastfeeding peer-support programs.[4]

Contraindications to breastfeeding

Recognized contraindications to breastfeeding are limited and include infants with classic galactosemia and mothers with human T-lymphotropic virus (HTLV) I or II, untreated brucellosis, untreated active tuberculosis (until >2 weeks of treatment and no longer infectious), active herpes breast lesions, and HIV (except in developing countries where benefits outweigh risks). Mothers with peripartum varicella should be separated from their infants, but their expressed milk can be fed to the baby. Even in preterm infants or cases of maternal cytomegalovirus (CMV) seropositivity, the value of human milk feeding typically outweighs the risk of clinical disease.[2]

In mothers with a history of drug abuse who desire to breastfeed, the provider should consider their drug use and substance abuse treatment history, the mother's medical and psychiatric history, the infant's health status, and plans for substance abuse treatment and medical and psychiatric care as well as family/social support after birth. Most illicit drugs do transfer into human milk. Breastfeeding is not recommended in women who are using illicit drugs. However, women in substance abuse treatment who have been abstinent from illicit drug use for at least 90 days with a negative toxin screen at delivery (except for prescribed medications), and without other medical contraindications may breastfeed with close follow-up. Breastfeeding in women with a history of opioid abuse who are stable on methadone or buprenorphine maintenance may reduce the risk of severe neonatal abstinence syndrome (NAS).[38] Alcohol is transmitted into milk and should be avoided while breastfeeding, except for minimal and occasional use. Maternal smoking should be avoided because of its known risks (respiratory illnesses, allergy, and SIDS), but is not contraindicated in breastfeeding mothers.[2]

Maternal medications

The risks of transmitting maternal medications into breast milk must be weighed against the negative consequences of discontinuing breastfeeding for the mother and infant.[4] Prescribers should consult a comprehensive, up-to-date reference for medications and mother's milk, such as *LactMed*, published by the National Library of Medicine, National Institutes of Health.[2, 39] Drugs generally not recommended while nursing include amphetamines, chemotherapeutics, ergotamines, and statins. Diagnostic nuclear medicine agents can enter breast milk, so mothers should be counseled about how long to express and discard their milk, and whether they should be separated from their infants.[40] Conversely, contrast media (iodinated or gadolinium-based) has very low excretion into breast milk and poor oral absorption, so mothers do not need to withhold breastfeeding after these contrast procedures.[41]

Depression screening and treatment of postpartum depression in all mothers is indicated. When selecting or continuing antidepressants, providers should consider maternal response and current known infant risk profile.[39, 40] For instance, sertraline is preferred over fluoxetine because of lower transfer and side effects in the infant; however, it is generally preferable to continue mothers on an antidepressant medication that has shown good response rather than switching medication or discontinuing breastfeeding, so long as the breastfeeding infant is asymptomatic and carefully monitored. Potential infant side effects of antidepressants include irritability, sedation, changes in feeding, and poor weight gain. Side effects are less likely in older (>2 months) infants, and no long-term negative effects in infants have been reported based on limited available data. It is important to encourage the mother to continue breastfeeding while taking medications that are considered safe to take during lactation. The only contraindicated maternal vaccine during breastfeeding is the yellow fever vaccine.[42]

Breastfeeding management

Breastfeeding management for the women's health-care provider

Preconception/interconception

Routine health maintenance and gynecological visits provide an opportunity to normalize, discuss, and recommend breastfeeding to women of childbearing age. Providers may choose to routinely incorporate this discussion with the annual breast examination.[1, 3]

Prenatal management

Patients should be counseled about the benefits of breastfeeding and the risks of not breastfeeding. Prenatal visits may be used to address misconceptions about breastfeeding or previous difficulties, using open-ended questions and motivational interviewing. Asking, "What have you heard about breastfeeding?" is preferable to "Will you breast or bottle feed?" since the latter tends to equate the two feeding methods. Family history of diseases that are reduced when mothers breastfeed should be discussed.[19] Risk factors for breastfeeding difficulties should be elicited, such as maternal obesity, infertility, diabetes, polycystic ovarian disease, and breast surgeries, as well as true or relative contraindications to breastfeeding.[2] Prenatal preparation of mothers should include breastfeeding classes and education about the importance of the ten steps, including step 4, skin-to-skin contact immediately after delivery.[43]

The breast exam provides an opportunity to encourage women that they will likely produce an adequate milk supply for their infant, even in the case of multiple births. Prenatal intervention for inverted and flat nipples is not effective, and a skilled lactation consultant frequently can help the baby latch if problems do occur. Nipple piercings should be removed during breastfeeding; a tract with milk flow may form from the pierced area. Anatomical abnormalities of the breasts rarely affect breastfeeding, except in such cases as tubular breasts or inadequate glandular tissue.[25] (See Figure 3-1.) In cases of breast surgery when milk ducts and/or the afferent nerves of the nipple have been severed, a full milk supply may not be possible, and close follow-up by a lactation professional and the infant's doctor will be important. This is more common with breast reduction surgery, but may be the case in augmentation surgery as well, especially when there is a periareolar incision.[44]

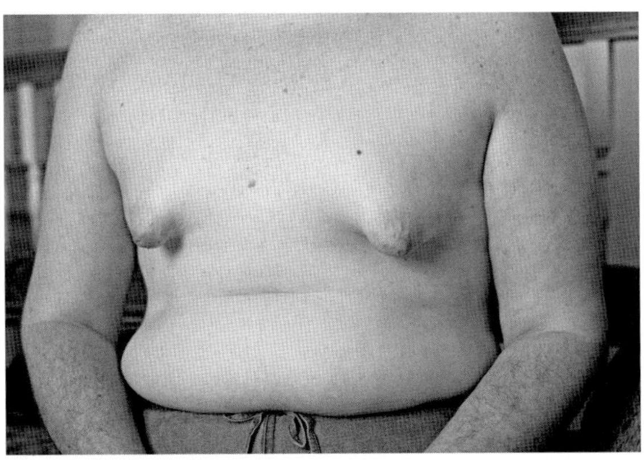

Figure 3-1 Inadequate glandular tissue.
Courtesy of Photograph by Erica.

Peripartum support

Pain management decisions should balance the possible adverse effects on the infant. Meperidine should be avoided, since it has a long neonatal half-life and may accumulate with breastfeeding. Codeine should be avoided because of the rare but serious consequences in the case of an ultra-rapid metabolizer. Morphine, Nalbuphine, and butorphanol have lower transfer into human milk.[45] Effects of epidural anesthesia on breastfeeding are still being studied.

Postpartum support

Providers should continue to encourage successful breastfeeding by identifying any concerns and referring for lactation consultation and or support groups when needed. The infant should be seen by its own healthcare provider within 48 hours after discharge.[2]

Breastfeeding techniques

Proper positioning to keep the baby's head, shoulders, and hips in alignment while facing the mother is important. Effective newborn positions of comfort include the so-called football (or clutch) hold, the cross-cradle hold, and the cradle hold. The side-lying and football positions are preferable after a cesarean delivery.

An important part of proper technique is learning how to achieve a proper latch. An effective latch will not cause pain to the mother, and allows freely flowing colostrum and milk to be transferred to the infant, which in turn leads to development of good milk supply. With nose pointed to nipple, and with a wide open mouth, the baby should take as much areola in the mouth as possible, chin into the breast, with the lips flanged out "like a fish" (Figure 3-2). Once the baby is latched well, suckling begins with bursts of 10–20 sucks before a pause; increased milk volumes yield audible swallows. Typically newborns feed about 15–20 minutes per breast, but watching for signs of continued suckling are more important than watching the clock. When sucks slow to 3–4 sucks before a pause, the baby is likely finishing that breast. Breast compressions to stimulate breast emptying

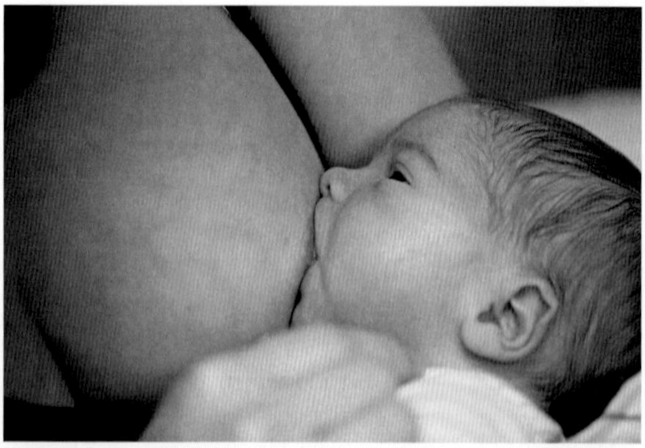

Figure 3-2 "Fish lips."

while babies are well latched can be helpful. A mother should be taught to help the baby release the breast by inserting her finger gently into the corner of the mouth to break the seal if necessary. Newborns eat at least 8–12 times per 24 hours and will sometimes feed in "clusters" with very frequent feeds, followed by a longer break between feedings.[45] Pacifiers should generally be avoided for the first 3–4 weeks until breastfeeding is well established.[2]

Early breastfeeding challenges

If the mother has substantial pain with latching, or the infant is clicking, indenting its cheeks, or not sustaining a latch, help may be needed. Early intervention to correct latch and improve milk transfer can prevent nipple damage, poor infant weight gain, and low milk supply. Mothers with abraded or cracked and bleeding nipples should be seen urgently by a lactation professional. If direct breastfeeding is ineffective or must be interrupted, continued breast emptying is critical.

Nipple pain

Nipple pain is typically due to problems with latch. Pain that persists throughout a feeding, and between feedings should be assessed with an evaluation of mother's breasts and nipples, an oral motor examination of the baby, and observation of a feeding with pre- and post-weight check by a lactation professional. Help with repositioning and latch can prevent further problems, and moisture-retaining occlusive dressings can improve wound healing. A thorough protocol for sore nipples outlining a decision diagnosis tree and treatments is available.[46] If direct breastfeeding is impossible due to severe pain, continued breast emptying is critical to preserve the milk supply until the situation is resolved.[45]

Engorgement

The spectrum of engorgement ranges from physiologic fullness of the breasts, particularly around days 3–5, to severe symptomatic engorgement with firm and painful overfilling and edema. Moderate symptoms of engorgement are experienced by most lactating women.[47] Engorgement must be differentiated from a plugged milk duct and mastitis. Engorgement can occur following an abrupt change in feeding frequency or missed feedings. See Table 3-3 for differential diagnosis of engorgement.

Primary prevention and treatment of engorgement are frequent breastfeeding with effective milk removal. Measures to improve milk removal every 1–3 hours include moist, warm packs or a warm shower 20 minutes before a feeding; breast massage with hand expression to help the baby latch to the full breast; and use of hand expression or electric pump if infant latch is not possible. Comfort measures include a supportive bra and analgesics.[47]

Plugged ducts

Localized areas of milk blockage that commonly present as a painful knot or cord within the breast are possibly plugged ducts; they may decrease in size with nursing or pumping. They can occur when a mother wears tight or constricting clothing, with a change in the feeding pattern, or with inadequate draining of the breast. Mothers with a plugged duct feel well and have no fever or signs of systemic illness. Treatment involves application of heat prior to nursing or pumping, and massage of the affected area before and during feeding. Pointing the infant's nose to the area of blockage during breastfeeding may improve drainage. If a plugged duct does not resolve within 48–72 hours or systemic symptoms develop, the mother should be evaluated.[45]

Mastitis

Affecting 3%–20% of breastfeeding women, mastitis typically occurs in the first six weeks of lactation.[48] Clinical signs and symptoms of mastitis include a single localized and wedge-shaped area that is warm, tender, erythematous, and edematous. Mothers often have myalgias, fever, and flulike symptoms. Predisposing factors include damaged nipples, infrequent or missed feedings, inefficient milk removal, milk oversupply, milk bleb, or maternal stress and fatigue. Treatment involves frequent and effective milk removal from the affected breast by direct breastfeeding, hand expression, and/or pumping. There is no risk to healthy term infants who continue to breastfeed from a breast with mastitis.

Supportive measures for mastitis include maternal rest, appropriate fluid intake, and proper nutrition. Heat application before breastfeeding will encourage milk flow. Ibuprofen effectively reduces inflammation, improves milk flow, and provides analgesia. If symptoms do not resolve within 12–24 hours, antibiotics should be prescribed for presumed infection. The most common pathogen is penicillin-sensitive *S. aureus.* Other causative organisms include *Streptococcus* species, *Escherichia coli, Haemophilus influenzae, Klebsiella pneumoniae*, and *Bacteroides* species. Accordingly, first-line treatment is dicloxicillin, 500 mg four times per day for 10–14 days, or a first-generation cephalosporin. For penicillin-allergic mothers, cephalosporins are usually safe, but clindamycin is recommended for severe penicillin allergy. Methicillin-resistant *S. aureus* (MRSA) is emerging, so local resistance patterns should be determined. Most MRSA strains remain susceptible to vancomycin or trimethoprim/sulfamethoxazole,[48] which are safe with breastfeeding.[39, 40] Inadequately treated mastitis can progress to breast abscess. If mastitis is recurrent or chronic, further investigation is warranted. A midstream clean-catch of expressed milk may be helpful to identify the causative organism and select appropriate antibiotic coverage. Multiple recurrences in the same location warrant investigation to rule out an underlying mass or other abnormality.[48]

Breast abscess

A breast abscess is a walled-off area within the breast containing purulent material. It occurs in 5%–11% of women with mastitis.[45] Symptoms are similar to mastitis, with additional fluctuant mass not responsive to appropriate treatment. Standard therapy includes antibiotics and surgical drainage with culture of the abscess fluid to determine sensitivity of the organism. Breast abscesses may be drained by needle aspiration, but serial aspirations may be required.[48] Breastfeeding should continue on the unaffected breast and may continue on the affected breast providing the infant's mouth does not come into contact with purulent drainage or infected tissue.

Milk fistula

This rare complication follows breast biopsy during pregnancy and lactation or after a nipple piercing. Mothers have continuous leakage from the affected area, and although inconvenient, fistulae usually resolve over time.[44]

Breast masses

The incidence of breast malignancy during pregnancy and lactation ranges from 1:3,000 to 1:10,000 women.[44] Among women diagnosed with breast cancer, 3% will be pregnant or lactating, so a new breast mass warrants careful evaluation. Mammography is safe during lactation, but the breasts should be emptied to allow optimal visualization. Ultrasonography is also safe during lactation to characterize the mass. Fine needle or excisional biopsy can be performed during lactation without prolonged interruption of breastfeeding. Most masses are benign, and 30% have pathology related to lactation, such as lactating adenoma, infarcted fibroadenoma, hypertrophied breast tissue, galactocele, inflammatory lesion, or papilloma.[45]

Bloody nipple discharge

During early lactation, nipple trauma may cause bloody discharge, which typically resolves when the latch is corrected. Sometimes mothers report brownish-red milk ("rusty pipe syndrome") that occurs as milk ducts are distended and capillaries leak. Infants can continue to feed despite bloody nipple discharge if feedings are tolerated. If discharge is persistent and arises from a single duct, further evaluation is warranted, including a thorough breast exam to identify any masses. Most commonly, single duct bloody discharge arises from a benign intraductal papilloma, but intraductal carcinoma can occur.[44, 45]

Breast evaluation during lactation

Women may continue self-breast examinations during lactation, although the exam is challenging due to changes from lactation. Clinical breast exams should be performed at the onset of pregnancy, at the postpartum visit, and at each annual visit.

Maintenance of milk supply

Online instructions are available for increasing milk supply.[50] The best way to ensure a good milk supply is frequent and effective milk removal, preferably by direct breastfeeding, or by hand expression or an electric pump if needed. If the baby is not effectively removing milk, consultation with a lactation consultant can help to improve breastfeeding, and pumping after breastfeeding can ensure complete milk removal. Galactogues are substances or medications used to improve milk supply. Limited evidence for their efficacy exists.[49]

Long-term breastfeeding issues

Maternal nutrition

Women should be counseled to eat a healthy, well-balanced diet (one generally low in fat, sugar, and salt and high in fruits, vegetables, and fiber), with consideration for barriers of food insecurity, cost of healthy foods, and low nutrition literacy. Women who were not at a healthy weight before pregnancy or who experienced nonoptimal weight gain during pregnancy may benefit from dietitian consultation. For obese women, supervised weight loss achieved through healthy eating and physical activity is safe during lactation. Continued supplementation with prenatal vitamins is recommended daily.

Maternal illness

In most cases, mothers may continue to breastfeed in the face of a medical illness; in acute infections breast milk contains protective antibodies against offending organisms. Chronic illnesses offer no contraindication to breastfeeding, unless mothers are taking medications that are unsafe for breastfeeding and no alternative can be substituted. If a mother requires surgery, a suitable anesthetic agent can be used to reduce effects on nursing.

Extended and tandem breastfeeding

Breastfeeding of an older child may continue during a mother's next pregnancy, provided there are no signs of preterm labor because nursing can produce uterine contractions. Pregnancy-associated nipple pain, fatigue, and nausea, as well as declines in milk production at the end of the second trimester may lead to mother- or baby-initiated weaning.

Breastfeeding support while mother and infant are separated

Reasons for maternal-infant separation and/or for inability to directly breastfeed include return to work or school, hospitalization of the mother and illness, prematurity, or congenital anomalies of the infant.

Preparing to return to work or school

Ideally, maternity leave should be maximized as much as is possible to allow time for establishment of breastfeeding, followed by a gradual return to work or school. Mothers may need to be provided with a letter to their employer regarding worksite lactation support laws, benefits, and need.[36, 45] Mothers should practice expressing milk and alternative (i.e., bottle, possibly from someone other than the mother) feeding methods two weeks prior to return to work or school if possible. Adding a pumping session each day allows milk to be stored for later use. When separated, mothers should express milk every three to four hours, or approximate the frequency of usual infant breastfeeding, in order to maintain milk supply.[45] A childcare provider may bring the baby to the mother's worksite for breastfeeding during breaks as another option. Public breastfeeding laws in many communities protect women from indecency charges and help to ensure rights to breastfeed in any public or private location.

Pumping and breastfeeding technology

All mothers should be shown how to hand-express milk.[4] Manual/hand pumps are generally only suitable for occasional use, whereas a double (bilateral) electric pump with automatic cycling is more suitable for regular use due to potential for production of greater milk volume. Mothers who are completely pump-dependent should utilize the most efficient pump available (i.e., hospital grade). Pumps should only be used by one mother unless specifically designed for multiple users (i.e., hospital grade). Women should wash their hands and storage containers with soap and water and clean pump parts according to manufacturer recommendations. Milk storage guidelines are shown in Table 3-4.[25]

Special circumstances

Breastfeeding multiples

Mothers with twins/multiples will have increased caloric requirements estimated 500–600 kcal per baby per day.[45] Twins may be fed simultaneously or separately on-demand, and it is possible for a mother to make enough milk for multiple babies.

Table 3-4 Breast milk storage guidelines

Breast milk	Room temperature	Refrigerator	Freezer
Freshly expressed into closed container	6–8 hour (78°F or lower)	3–5 days (39°F or lower)	2 weeks in freezer compartment inside refrigerator 3–6 months in freezer section of refrigerator with separate door 6–12 months in deep freeze (0°F or lower)
Previously frozen – thawed in refrigerator but not warmed or used	4 hour or less (i.e., next feeding)	Store in refrigerator 24 hour	Do not refreeze
Thawed outside refrigerator in warm water	For completion of feeding	Hold for 4 hour or until next feeding	Do not refreeze
Infant has begun feeding	Only for completion of feeding; then discard	Discard	Discard

Source: Adapted with permission from *Breastfeeding: A Guide for the Medical Profession*. 6th ed. Lawrence RA, Lawrence RM. Elsevier, Mosby, Philadelphia, PA; 2005:563.[25]

Premature infants

Preterm infants should receive human milk, preferably mother's own fresh or frozen milk, or if necessary, pasteurized donor milk from a milk bank. Parental education, close monitoring, and timely support from a trained lactation professional are essential in late preterm infants to overcome potential sleepiness, problems with latch or milk transfer, and lower stamina in the infant, as well as associated maternal risk factors affecting breastfeeding, such as medical conditions, multiple births, or cesarean-section delivery.[51] Very low birth weight infants benefit from early trophic feeds of colostrum via tube feeding and later require fortification of human milk to meet nutrient requirements.[45] Mothers will need support to establish and maintain milk supply, assistance with milk collection and storage, and help with breastfeeding, supplementation, and/or providing non-nutritive sucking as appropriate. Skin-to-skin or "kangaroo" care has been shown to increase milk production and maternal confidence in breastfeeding and improve stability of the infant.[45] Mothers experiencing loss of their infants should be provided with the opportunity to donate any stored breast milk to a milk bank and be assisted in terminating lactation.

Custody issues, adoptive nursing, and relactation

Interruption or termination of breastfeeding should be avoided in custody cases. With sufficient nipple stimulation from suckling or pumping, relactation after cessation of breastfeeding is frequently successful; it may also be possible for a mother of an adopted infant to breastfeed, although this may be more difficult in nulliparous women.[45]

Infant feeding during disasters

Encouraging and supporting mothers to breastfeed during disasters may be lifesaving. Human milk, if available, offers a safe, beneficial source of nutrition for infants in the first year of life and beyond.[52]

Concluding remarks

Breastfeeding is wonderful primary prevention – protecting both the mother and the baby from a variety of short- and long-term poor health outcomes. The women's health-care provider is uniquely positioned to help mothers and families learn about the importance of breastfeeding their babies, for their own health as well as the health and development of the baby. This encouragement during regular, prenatal and postnatal visits makes a difference in a mother's feeding choice, and helps her to reach her breastfeeding goals.

References

1. American Academy of Family Physicians Breastfeeding Advisory Committee, Montgomery A, Dermer A, et al. Breastfeeding, Family Physicians Supporting (Position Paper). [Online] 2014 Available from: www.aafp.org/about/policies/all/breastfeeding-support.html. Accessed on 27 December 2014.
2. American Academy of Pediatrics. Breastfeeding and the use of human milk. *Pediatrics* 2012;**129**(3):e827–41.
3. American College of Obstetrics and Gynecology. Breastfeeding: maternal and infant aspects. ACOG Committee Opinion No. 361. *Obstet Gynecol* 2007;**109**: 479–80.
4. National Institute for Health and Care Excellence (UK). Maternal and Child Nutrition. NICE Public Health Guidance 11; 2008. [Modified 2014]. Available from: guidance.nice.org.uk/ph11.
5. WHO World Health Organization/UNICEF. Global Strategy for Infant and Young Child Feeding. [Online] Geneva, Switzerland: World Health Organization; 2003. Available from: www.who.int/nutrition/topics/infantfeeding_recommendation/en. Accessed on 16 August 2014.
6. Centers for Disease Control for Chronic Disease Prevention and Health Promotion, Division of Nutrition, Physical Activity, and Obesity. Breastfeeding report card, United States/2014. [Online] Atlanta, Georgia: Centers for Disease Control and Prevention; Available from: www.cdc.gov/breastfeeding/pdf/2014breastfeedingreportcard.pdf. Accessed on 15 August 2014.
7. Odum EC, Li R, Scanlon KS, et al. Reasons for earlier than desired cessation of breastfeeding. *Pediatrics* 2013;**131**(3):e726–32.
8. US Department of Health and Human Services. The Surgeon General's Call to Action to Support Breastfeeding. [Online] Washington, DC; 2011. Available from: www.surgeongeneral.gov/topics/breastfeeding. Accessed on 16 August 2014.
9. UNICEF/WHO World Health Organization. Protecting, promoting and supporting breastfeeding: The special role of maternity services, a joint WHO/UNICEF statement. [Online] Geneva, Switzerland: World Health Organization; 1989. Available from: www.who.int/nutrition/publications/infantfeeding/9241561300/en. Accessed on 15 August 2014.
10. Labbok MH. Global baby-friendly hospital initiative monitoring data: update and discussion. *Breastfeed Med* 2012;7(4):210–22.
11. World Health Organization. International code of marketing of breast-milk substitutes. [Online] Geneva, Switzerland: World Health Organization; 1981. Available from: www.who.int/nutrition/publications/code_english.pdf. Accessed on 17 February 2015.
12. WHO/UNICEF. Innocenti declaration on the protection, promotion and support of breastfeeding. [Online] Florence, Italy: WHO/UNICEF (Spedale degli Innocenti); 1990. Available from: www.unicef.org/programme/breastfeeding/innocenti/htm. Accessed on 17 February 2015.
13. WHO/UNICEF. Baby-friendly hospital initiative. Revised, updated and expanded for integrative care. [Online] Geneva, Switzerland: World Health Organization; 2009. Available from: www.who.int/nutrition/publications/infantfeeding/bfhi_trainingcourse_s1/en. Accessed on 1 March 2015.
14. US Department of Health and Human Services. *Healthy People 2020*. [Online] Washington, DC: US DHHS; 2010. Available from: www.healthypeople.gov/2020/topicsobjectives2020/objectiveslist.aspx?topicid=26. Accessed on 17 August 2014.
15. ACOG Committee Opinion. Breastfeeding in underserved women: increasing initiation and continuation of breastfeeding. *Obstet Gynecol* 2013;**122** (2 Pt 1):423–8. Available from: doi:10.1097/01.AOG.0000433008.93971.6a. Accessed on 15 August 2014.
16. Cattaneo A, Burmaz T, Arendt M, et al. Protection, promotion and support of breast-feeding in Europe: progress from 2002 to 2007. *Public Health Nutrition* 2009;**13**(6):751–9.
17. Scanlon KS, Grummer-Strawn L, Li R, et al. Racial and ethnic differences in breastfeeding initiation and duration, by state – national immunization survey, United States, 2004–2008. *MMWR* 2010;**59**:327–34.
18. UNICEF Infant and Young Child Feeding Global Databases, Last update October 2014. [Online] New York, USA: Data and Analytics Section; Division of Data, Research and Policy, UNICEF. Available from: http://data.unicef.org/nutrition/iycf. Accessed on 27 December 2014.
19. Ip S, Chung M, Raman G, et al. Breastfeeding and maternal and infant health outcomes in developed countries. Agency for Healthcare Research and Quality, Evidence Report/Technology Assessment, 2007;153: Publication No. 07-E007.
20. Karlson EW, Mandl LA, Hankinson SE, Grodstein F. Do breast-feeding and other reproductive factors influence future risk of rheumatoid arthritis? Results from the Nurses' Health Study. *Arthritis Rheum* 2004;**50**(11):3458–67.
21. Schwartz EB, Ray RM, Stuebe AM, et al. Duration of lactation and risk factors for maternal cardiovascular disease. *Obstet Gynecol* 2009;**113**(5):974–82.

22. Bartick MC, Stuebe AM, Schwartz EB, et al. Cost analysis of maternal disease associated with suboptimal breastfeeding. *Obstet Gynecol* 2013;**122**:111–19.

23. Bartick M, Reinhold A. The burden of suboptimal breastfeeding in the United States: a pediatric cost analysis. *Pediatrics* 2010;**125**:e1048–56.

24. Hill K, You D, Inoue M, et al. Technical Advisory Group of the United Nations Interagency Group for Child Mortality Estimation: child mortality estimation: accelerated progress in reducing global child mortality, 1990–2010. *PloS Med* 2012;**9**(8):31001313.

25. Lawrence RA, Lawrence RM. Management of the mother-infant nursing couple. In: *Breastfeeding: A Guide for the Medical Profession*, 7th ed. Maryland Heights, MO: Elsevier Mosby, 2011.

26. Stuebe AM. Enabling women to achieve their breastfeeding goals. *Obstet Gynecol* 2014;**123**(3): 643–52.

27. Taveras EM, Li R, Grummer-Strawn L, et al. Opinions and practices of clinicians associated with continuation of exclusive breastfeeding. *Pediatrics* 2004;**113**:e283–90.

28. US Preventive Services Task Force. Primary care interventions to promote breastfeeding: US Preventive Services Task Force Recommendation Statement. *Ann Intern Med* 2008;**149**:560–4.

29. DiGirolamo AM, Grummer-Strawn L, Fein SB. Effect of maternity-care practices on breastfeeding. *Pediatrics* 2008;**122**(Suppl 2):S43–9.

30. Centers for Disease Control and Prevention. *Strategies to Prevent Obesity and Other Chronic Disease: The CDC Guide to Strategies to Support Breastfeeding Mothers and Babies.* Atlanta, GA: Centers for Disease Control and Prevention: US Department of Health and Human Services, 2013.

31. Grawey AE, Marinelli KA, Holmes AV. ABM Clinical Protocol #14. Breastfeeding-friendly physician's office: optimizing care for infants and children, revised 2013. *Breastfeed Med* 2013;**8**:237–42.

32. Stuebe AM, Bonuck K. What predicts intent to breastfeed exclusively? Breastfeeding knowledge, attitudes, and beliefs in a diverse urban population. *Breastfeed Med* 2011;**6**(6):413–20.

33. Li R, Rock VJ, Grummer-Strawn L. Changes in public attitudes toward breastfeeding in the United States, 1999–2003. *J Am Diet Assoc* 2007;**107**:122–7.

34. Wagner EA, Chantry CJ, Dewey DG, Nommsen-Rivers LA. Breastfeeding concerns at 3 and 7 days postpartum and feeding status at 2 months. *Pediatrics* 2013;**132**:e86575.

35. Bunik M. *Breastfeeding telephone triage and advice.* Elk Grove, IL: American Academy of Pediatrics, 2012.

36. Marinelli KA, Moren K, Taylor JS, Academy of Breastfeeding Medicine. Breastfeeding support for mothers in workplace employment or educational settings: summary statement. *Breastfeed Med* 2013;**8** (1):137–42.

37. Wolfberg AJ, Michels KB, Shields W, et al. Dads as breastfeeding advocates: results from a randomized controlled trial of an educational intervention. *Am J Obstet Gynecol* 2004;**191**:708–12.

38. Academy of Breastfeeding Medicine Protocol Committee. ABM Clinical Protocol #21. Guidelines for breastfeeding and the drug-dependent woman. *Breastfeed Med* 2009;**4**(4):225–8.

39. National Library of Medicine. Drugs and Lactation Database (LactMed). 2010. [Online] Available from: http://toxnet.nlm.nih.gov/cgi-bin/sis/htmlgen?LACT. Accessed on 28 December 2014.

40. Hale, T. *Medications and Mother's Milk.* 16th ed. Plano, TX: Hale Publishing, 2014.

41. American College of Radiology Committee on Drugs and Contrast Media. Administration of contrast media to breast-feeding mothers. *ACR Manual on Contrast Media.* [Online] Version 8. 2012:79–80. Available from: www.nxtbook.com/nxtbooks/acr/contrastmedia manual2012/#/82. Accessed on 28 December 2014.

42. Lawrence RM, Circumstances when breastfeeding is contraindicated. *Pediatr Clin North Am* 2013;**60** (1):295–318.

43. Moore ER, Anderson GC, Bergman N, Downswell T. Early skin-to-skin contact for mothers and their healthy newborn infants. *Cochrane Database Syst Rev* 2012;**5**:CD003519.

44. Behrens, PD. Prenatal, intrapartum, and postpartum support of the lactating mother. *Pediatr Clin North Am* 2001;**48**:365–75.

45. American Academy of Pediatrics and American College of Obstetricians and Gynecologists. *Breastfeeding Handbook for Physicians.* 2nd ed. Elk Grove, IL: AAP, 2013.

46. Stuebe A. UNC Protocols, [Online] University of North Carolina School of Medicine, Updated 2012. Available from: http://mombaby.org/PDF/PainProtocols.v3.pdf. Accessed on 28 December 2014.

47. Academy of Breastfeeding Medicine Protocol Committee, Behrens P. ABM Protocol #20. Engorgement. *Breastfeed Med* [Online] 2009;**4**(2): 111–13. Available from: www.bfmed.org/Media/Files/Protocols/Protocol%2020%20-%20Engorgement%206-2009.pdf. Accessed on 14 January 2015.

48. Amir L, Academy of Breastfeeding Medicine Protocol Committee. ABM Protocol #4. Mastitis. (Revised March 2014). *Breastfeed Med* 2014;**9**(5):239–45. Available from: www.bfmed.org/Media/Files/Protocols/2014_Updated_Mastitis6.30.14.pdf. Accessed on 14 January 2015.

49. Academy of Breastfeeding Medicine Protocol Committee. ABM Protocol # 9. Use of galactogues in initiating or augmenting the rate of milk secretion. (First revision January 2011). *Breastfeed Med* 2011;**6** (1):41–9. Available from: www.bfmed.org/Media/Files/Protocols/Protocol%209%20-%20English%201st%20Rev.%20Jan%202011.pdf. Accessed on 22 January 2015.

50. Morton, J. Maximizing Milk Production with Hands On Pumping [video on the internet]. Stanford University School of Medicine; 2015 [cited 2015 Mar 23]. Available from: http://newborns.stanford.edu/Breastfeeding/MaxProduction.html.

51. Academy of Breastfeeding Medicine. ABM Clinical Protocol #10. Breastfeeding the late preterm infant (34 0/7 too 36 6/7 weeks). *Breastfeed Med* 2011;**6**(3):151–5.

52. American Academy of Pediatrics. *Infant Feeding During Disasters*. 2007. Available from: www2.aap.org/breastfeeding/files/pdf/infantnutritiondisaster.pdf. Accessed on 25 January 2015.

Chapter

4 Genetics and cancer screening

Megan Cheney

Introduction

Modern advances in science have allowed early identification of women with an inherited predisposition for gynecologic cancers. The ability to detect these genetic predispositions, also increases the burden on healthcare professionals to understand who to screen, what tests to perform, how to interpret the results, and how to counsel the individual about her risks. This chapter will focus on inherited cancer syndromes that may be encountered in the nonpregnant woman.

Hereditary breast and ovarian cancer syndrome

Breast cancer is the most common cancer in women and the second leading cause of cancer death while ovarian cancer is the fifth most common cause of cancer death in women. In the general population, 12.3% of women will develop breast cancer in their lifetime and 1.3% will develop ovarian cancer.[1] Less than 10% of all breast cancers and less than 15% of ovarian cancers are associated with an inherited genetic mutation.[2] Mutations in breast cancer type 1 and 2 susceptibility genes (*BRCA1* and *BRCA2*) are associated with the majority of hereditary breast and ovarian cancers. Other genes such as *TP53* and *PTEN* associated with Li-Fraumeni and Cowden syndromes, respectively, are less commonly associated with hereditary breast and ovarian cancers (HBOC) and will be discussed briefly. The focus in this chapter will be primarily *BRCA1* and *BRCA2* mutations, testing for the mutations, and the significance of test results.

BRCA1 and *BRCA2*

The general population has a 0.2%–0.3% risk of a *BRCA* mutation, but that risk is increased to 19.8% among women with a family history of breast or ovarian cancer.[2] Certain populations carry an increased risk of a *BRCA* mutation compared to the general population, specifically those founded by a small ancestral group such as Ashkenazi Jews and individuals from Sweden, the Netherlands, Hungary, French Canada, and Iceland. Mutations that are identified more frequently in specific populations are referred to as founder mutations. The three most common founder mutations are the three most commonly associated with the Ashkenazi Jewish population: 185delAG or 5382insC in *BRCA1* and 6174delT in *BRCA2*. Approximately 1 in 40 Ashkenazi Jewish individuals carries one of these three founder mutations.[3]

BRCA1 and *BRCA2* are tumor suppressor genes on chromosomes 17q21 and 13q12-13, respectively, and are involved in repair of double-strand DNA breaks. To date, more than 1,200 mutations have been identified on *BRCA1* and more than 1,300 mutations on *BRCA2*. *BRCA* mutations are inherited in an autosomal dominant fashion with variable penetrance. The second allele must become nonfunctional to lead to tumorigenesis. *BRCA* mutation carriers have a markedly increased risk of breast and ovarian cancers. Overall, they have a lifetime risk of breast cancer of 50%–85% and a 15%–40% risk of ovarian cancer. The risk of ovarian cancer is greater among *BRCA1* carriers (39%–46%) compared to *BRCA2* carriers (11%–20%).[4]

BRCA screening

Screening can be initiated by population-based risk or by family history. When possible, the affected individual should first receive comprehensive sequencing of both *BRCA1* and *BRCA2* and then single-site testing offered to family members. Other options include comprehensive sequencing if the affected family member is unavailable or testing for "founder" mutations in certain populations.

Office Care of Women, ed. Martin E. Olsen and Botros Rizk. Published by Cambridge University Press.

Table 4-1 Populations for whom screening for hereditary breast and ovarian cancer syndromes is recommended

Personal history of:

- Breast *and* ovarian cancer
- Ovarian cancer and a first- or second-degree relative with ovarian cancer or premenopausal breast cancer
- Ovarian cancer and Ashkenazi Jewish descent
- Breast cancer by age 50 and a first- or second-degree relative with ovarian cancer or male breast cancer
- Breast cancer by age 40 and Ashkenazi Jewish descent

Table 4-2 Populations for whom screening for hereditary breast and ovarian cancer syndromes may be considered

- Breast cancer by age 40
- Ovarian cancer of high-grade serous histology
- Bilateral breast cancer
- Breast cancer by age 50 and Ashkenazi Jewish descent
- Breast cancer by age 50 and a close relative with breast cancer by age 50
- Breast cancer at any age and two or more close relatives with breast cancer at any age

A thorough family history assessment includes documentation of the age of diagnosis of a cancer, the site of the tumor, family members with multiple cancers or bilateral disease, and presence or absence of Jewish ancestry. In general, one does not have to verify diagnoses. Exceptions include (1) consideration of risk-reducing surgery when no mutation has been identified or (2) family history of either abdominal malignancies at young ages or sarcomas.[5] The US Preventive Services Task Force (USPSTF) concluded that there is adequate evidence that the net benefit of testing for potentially harmful BRCA mutations is moderate among women whose family history is associated with an increased risk. Testing should only be performed when a woman whose personal or family history suggests an increased risk of an inherited cancer susceptibility, when she has access to a health professional trained in genetic counseling and interpreting test results, and when test results will aid decision making.[6] The USPSTF recommends against routine genetic counseling or *BRCA* testing for women whose family history is not associated with an increased risk of potentially harmful BRCA mutations.

Several organizations have outlined recommendations for genetic screening and identifying at-risk women. For simplicity and the purposes of this chapter, discussion will focus on the recommendations outlined by the American Congress of Obstetricians and Gynecologists (ACOG). *BRCA* testing should be performed on any woman with a known *BRCA* mutation in the family or a risk of 20%–25% as estimated by the clinical criteria in Table 4-1. A woman may want to consider testing if she or a close relative has a personal history of any of the clinical criteria in Table 4-2.

Genetic screening may also be considered if a woman's family history underrepresents female cancers due to adoption, few female relatives, or multiple family members with hysterectomies or oophorectomies at young ages. Family history should be reviewed periodically or at least every 5–10 years. Screening can be initiated as early as the age of consent, although ACOG recommends against screening women under age 21.[7]

Multiple risk stratification tools have been developed to help identify women who would benefit from a referral to genetic counseling. These tools include the Ontario Family History Assessment Tool, Manchester Scoring System, Referral Screening Tool, Pedigree Assessment Tool, and Family History Screen 7. Most of these tools have been found to be greater than 85% sensitive but have not been tested specifically among *BRCA* mutation carriers.[6] Other tools have been developed to predict the risk of deleterious *BRCA* mutations and include the Myriad Genetic Laboratories model, Couch model, Tyrer model, Pen II Risk model, and BRCAPRO. BRCAPRO is currently the most validated tool for assessing such a risk.[8] The USPSTF recommends against using breast cancer risk assessment models based on the Gail model (such as National Cancer Institute Breast Cancer Risk Assessment Tool) because they are not designed to assess which women should receive genetic counseling or *BRCA* testing. If using a risk assessment model, it is important to inform the patient of the uncertainties of estimation.

Several risk thresholds for genetic screening have been suggested but the USPSTF has found insufficient evidence to support a specific risk threshold for referral for genetic counseling or *BRCA* testing. ACOG and the Society of Gynecologic Oncology suggest a threshold of 20%–25%.[7] Women who are eligible for a genetics referral may be offered the option of accessing genetic testing during their initial management or at any time thereafter.[5]

Genetic counseling

Genetic counseling should occur prior to testing and should include pre- and post-test counseling. An important part of the counseling process is identification of affected family members who may be preferred candidates for testing. Other important components of counseling include the following: the natural history of the disorder, the inheritance pattern, options for screening, accuracy of testing, significance of possible results, options for surveillance and risk reduction, psychological and familial implications, cost, and legislation regarding genetic discrimination and privacy. The Genetic Information and Nondiscrimination Act of 2008 has made it illegal for health insurance providers or employers to use genetic information to make decisions about insurance eligibility or terms of employment. It is limited in that it does not apply to life insurance, disability insurance, or long-term care. Women should also be given information about sources of support, lifestyle advice, and any trials or studies. At the end of the visit, health professionals and counselors should send a written summary of a woman's personal risk information and a reminder that her risk will change if her family history changes. Counseling should be performed by a trained provider. The necessary training to provide counseling has yet to be well defined. The National Cancer Institute Cancer Genetics Services Directory has a list of professionals who offer genetic counseling, cancer risk assessment, and genetic susceptibility testing (www.cancer.gov/cancertopics/genetics/directory).

Interpretation of possible results

Possible results of *BRCA* mutation testing are positive, true-negative, uninformative-negative, or variant of uncertain clinical significance (VUS). A positive result means that a potentially harmful mutation has been detected. A true-negative result is the lack of identification of a potentially harmful mutation in a woman with a family history of a known *BRCA* mutation. She can be reassured that her breast cancer risk is generally not increased compared to the general population. An uninformative-negative result is the lack of identification of a potentially harmful mutation in a woman without a known family history of a *BRCA* mutation. The presence of a significant family history of breast or ovarian cancer in a patient who receives a negative result may be explained by the presence of a *BRCA* deletion that the patient did not inherit, an undetectable *BRCA* mutation or other yet unidentified cancer susceptibility gene, or an affected relative with a sporadic cancer and no inherited predisposition in the family. Twelve percent of high-risk families without a *BRCA1* or *BRCA2* coding-region mutation may have other clinically important genomic rearrangements.[9]

The least defined result of *BRCA* testing is a VUS, which is a genetic mutation that has not yet been established as potentially harmful. The rate of identification of a VUS is 2%–13% and the harms associated with the result are not yet known.[10] As genetic research continues, VUS continue to be reclassified and women updated of their risk assessment. In one study, 56% of VUS were reclassified after a median of 39 months, longer than the median time to prophylactic oophorectomy (18.6 months) and prophylactic mastectomy (20.1 months).[11] Due to the lack of understanding of the risk of VUS and the known surgical risk or prophylactic oophorectomy and mastectomy, clinicians should consider managing such women based on their personal and family history.

Surveillance of *BRCA* carriers

Once a *BRCA* mutation is identified, treatment may include intensive surveillance, chemoprevention, or risk-reducing surgery. Evidence is lacking on the effect of intensive screening for *BRCA*-related cancer on clinical outcomes. Breast surveillance is typically initiated at age 25 or sooner depending on family history and includes clinical breast exams every three to six months, annual MRI, and annual mammography. The sensitivity of mammography seems to be lower in *BRCA* mutation carriers than in other high-risk women and may be due to a higher breast density, differences in morphologic features, or more frequent development of interval malignancies.[12] MRI use in breast cancer surveillance increases cancer detection rates in high-risk women. A meta-analysis concluded that combined use of MRI and mammography had higher sensitivity for detecting breast cancer than mammography alone.[13]

Ovarian cancer screening includes annual or semi-annual CA125 and transvaginal ultrasound.[2] ACOG recommends initiation at age 30–35, or 5–10 years earlier than the earliest age of diagnosis of ovarian cancer in the family. There is generally poor compliance with surveillance as rates decline even one year after testing; standardization of care is needed.[14] Compliance was associated with the number of relatives with ovarian cancer, perceived risk of ovarian cancer, and Jewish ancestry.[15] Evidence exists that surveillance does not change the stage of ovarian cancer at the time of diagnosis, reduce the woman's overall mortality, or decrease the number of ovarian cancer deaths. Screening can lead to harm such as complications from major surgical interventions in women who do not have cancer. Fifteen percent of women who underwent surgery for a false positive finding had a serious complication.[16] The USPSTF therefore recommends against ovarian cancer screening of asymptomatic women without a known *BRCA* mutation.

Breast cancer chemoprevention

Women at high or moderate risk of breast cancer with no personal history of breast cancer should be given information regarding the risks and benefits of chemoprevention, the extent of risk reduction, the side effects of medications, and the alternative options. Tamoxifen, raloxifene, and most recently the aromatase inhibitor exemestane have been found to decrease breast cancer incidence among moderate to high-risk women, but so far their effects seem to be limited to hormone-sensitive breast cancers. In a subset analysis of the National Surgical Adjuvant Breast and Bowel Project (NSABP) Breast Cancer Prevention trial (P-1 trial), tamoxifen decreased the risk of breast cancer by 62% in *BRCA2* carriers but not in *BRCA1* carriers.[17] This risk reduction is similar to tamoxifen's effect in estrogen-receptor positive breast cancer patients which correlates with the fact that 65%–79% of tumors in *BRCA2* carriers are estrogen-receptor positive, whereas only 10%–24% of tumors in *BRCA1* carriers are estrogen-receptor positive.[17] Data on the use of breast chemoprevention among *BRCA* mutation carriers is limited and the number of *BRCA* mutation carriers in the P-1 trial is very small.

In summary, the USPSTF found sufficient evidence to recommend offering chemoprevention with tamoxifen for five years to premenopausal women and postmenopausal women with or without a uterus at high risk of breast cancer but no personal history of breast cancer and no history of thromboembolic disease or endometrial cancer.[5] Postmenopausal women with a uterus may also be offered chemoprevention with raloxifene. There is evidence to support considering prescribing chemoprevention to women at moderate risk of breast cancer as well.

Health-care professionals must use chemoprevention with caution due to a proven risk of venous thromboembolism (VTE) and endometrial cancer. Tamoxifen and raloxifene increase the risk of VTEs by four to seven events per 1,000 women over five years.[18] The risk is greater with tamoxifen than raloxifene and greater in older women. Tamoxifen increases the risk for endometrial cancer by four more cases per 1,000 women.[18] Tamoxifen or raloxifene should not be continued beyond five years and women must be informed to stop treatment at least two months before trying to conceive or at least 6 weeks before elective surgery.[5] Women who have a high risk of breast cancer but no personal history of breast cancer and have had a bilateral mastectomy should not be offered chemoprevention.

Use of oral contraceptives for chemoprevention

The use of oral contraceptives seems to be associated with a decreased risk of ovarian cancer. In a meta-analysis of *BRCA1* and *BRCA2* mutation carriers, use of oral contraceptives was associated with a significantly reduced risk of ovarian cancer [summary relative risk (SRR), 0.50, 95% CI 0.33–0.75] and no significantly increased risk of breast cancer (SRR 1.13, 95% CI 0.88–1.45).[19] Nonetheless, oral contraceptive use remains a controversial issue and the USPSTF recommends against the prescription of oral contraceptives solely for the purpose of ovarian cancer prevention. Instead, mutation carriers should receive counseling regarding their individualized risks and expected benefits with oral contraceptive use.

Risk-reducing surgery

Prophylactic mastectomy decreases the risk of breast cancer among patients with an inherited genetic predisposition and has the added benefit of also decreasing the risk of ovarian cancer. It is important, however, to counsel individuals that prophylactic surgery does not completely eliminate their risk given the remote chance that not all at-risk tissue is removed. Prior to surgery, a woman should receive counseling regarding the potential psychosocial and sexual consequences and the possibility of a histologic diagnosis of breast or ovarian cancer. She should be offered access to support groups before making her decision.

Breast cancer risk among *BRCA* mutation carriers can be decreased by as much as 85%–100% with prophylactic mastectomy and by 37%–100% with oophorectomy.[20, 21] In a large, prospective cohort study of *BRCA* mutation carriers, there were no cases of breast cancer during three years follow-up after prophylactic mastectomy. In those women who did not undergo prophylactic mastectomy, 7% were diagnosed with breast cancer during those three years.[22] Bilateral salpingo-oophorectomy (BSO) decreases breast cancer risk by up to 72% [23] Risk reduction is greater among *BRCA1* mutation carriers than *BRCA2* and is more pronounced if a woman is premenopausal at the time of surgery.[23] Short-term hormone therapy after BSO does not diminish the protective effect on breast cancer risk.[24]

If *BRCA* testing has not been performed but a woman is at high risk for breast cancer, bilateral mastectomy should be discussed but may only be appropriate for a small proportion of women and thus should be managed by a multidisciplinary team. In women without an identified inherited mutation, family history should be verified first. If it cannot be verified, the provider should seek agreement by a multidisciplinary team. Women who choose prophylactic mastectomy tend to be younger, have children, and report a greater number of breast and ovarian cancer among family members.[25]

The recommended surgery for maximizing ovarian cancer risk reduction in women with a genetic predisposition is BSO. The rates of risk and mortality reduction vary according to baseline cancer risks among mutation carriers. In one study of 5,783 *BRCA* mutation carriers, prophylactic oophorectomy was associated with an 80% reduction in ovarian, fallopian tube, or peritoneal cancer [hazard ratio (HR) 0.20, 95% CI 0.13–0.30, p <0.001] and a 77% reduction in all-cause mortality to age 70 years (HR 0.23, 95% CI 0.13–0.39, p <0.001).[21] Because there is approximately a 5% risk of histologic detection of ovarian cancer at the time of prophylactic oophorectomy in *BRCA* mutation carriers, it is prudent to routinely collect cytologic washings, peritoneal biopsies, and omental sampling during risk-reduction surgery.[26] Bilateral tubal ligation has also been shown to decrease ovarian cancer risk but not to the same degree as BSO.[2] There is also growing discussion around bilateral salpingectomy with ovarian sparing as a means to decrease risk until an at-risk individual is accepting of oophorectomy, but this approach is not yet supported by SGO as there is still insufficient data to support its use. In women without an identified inherited mutation, family history should be verified first and if it cannot be verified, the provider should seek agreement by a multidisciplinary team before proceeding with BSO.[5]

Risk-reducing BSO is recommended by age 35–40 or after completion of childbearing for women who are *BRCA* carriers or who have a high risk of ovarian cancer as defined by two or more first-degree relatives with ovarian cancer.[2] Despite a relatively low risk of ovarian cancer before age 50 in *BRCA2* carriers (only 3%) compared to the higher risk of 10%–21% in *BRCA1* carriers, timely removal of the ovaries is nevertheless recommended due the protective benefit it confers for breast cancer in this population.[7] Though the majority of *BRCA* carriers (74% in one study) undergo risk-reducing BSO, the majority do not do so by the recommended age of 40.[14] Premenopausal oophorectomy in women with an inherited or increased familial risk of ovarian cancer does not preclude them from participating in hormone therapy. In such women with no personal history of breast cancer, the USPSTF suggests that they should be offered appropriate hormone therapy to continue until the age of natural menopause in line with standard prescribing practices for the general population.

Lifestyle modifications

Women with an increased risk of breast cancer should be informed of lifestyle modifications that may decrease the risk of breast cancer such as breastfeeding, decrease in alcohol consumption, avoidance of tobacco, and maintenance of a healthy weight.

Limitations of *BRCA* testing and future research

BRCA testing continues to be refined but it is currently limited by test sensitivity, ethnic variability in mutation and disease prevalence, genetic heterogeneity, reduced penetrance, and phenotypic variability. Areas for future research include validation of risk stratification tools, characterization of training necessary to perform genetic counseling, improved access to counseling, evaluation of psychosocial consequences of testing, and the effectiveness of intensive surveillance.

Other hereditary breast cancer syndromes

Some of the other hereditary breast cancer syndromes include Li-Fraumeni and Cowden syndromes. Li-Fraumeni syndrome (LFS) is an inherited autosomal dominant disorder linked to germline mutations in the tumor protein p53 gene (*TP53*) on chromosome 17p13.1. Individuals inherit one abnormal copy of the *TP53* gene and then develop a somatic mutation or deletion of the second allele. It is most typically associated with breast cancer, sarcoma, adrenocortical carcinoma, and brain tumors, but to a lesser extent may be related to an increased risk of melanoma, gastric cancer, lymphoma, Wilms tumor, or colorectal cancer. The lifetime risk of cancer among women affected by Li-Fraumeni approaches 100% [27] The median age of breast cancer diagnosis is younger than in the general population, as young as 33 years in one study.[28] Genetic testing only detects up to 75% of individuals with LFS and should be restricted to individuals who satisfy clinical criteria but have no known mutation in the family, women with early-onset breast cancer who test negative for *BRCA1* or *BRCA2*, individuals with either adrenocortical carcinoma or choroid plexus carcinoma, or individuals from a family with a known *TP53* mutation. Also known as multiple hamartoma syndrome, Cowden syndrome is caused by a germline mutation in the *PTEN* gene and is associated with an increased risk of colorectal, breast, endometrial, thyroid, and kidney cancers.

Lynch syndrome

Approximately 20%–30% of colorectal cancers are related to an inherited genetic mutation, the most common of which is an autosomal dominant condition called Lynch syndrome. Lynch syndrome (LS) accounts for 3% of newly diagnosed cases of colorectal cancer, but it is also associated with extracolonic malignancies such as cancers of the endometrium, urinary tract, ovary, stomach, hepatobiliary tract, small bowel, brain, or skin.[29] About 2% of endometrial cancers are associated with LS and have an average age at the time of diagnosis of 50 as opposed to sporadic uterine cancers which have an average age at diagnosis of 60.[30] As many as 20% of LS individuals will have an extracolonic cancer. Women with LS have a 21%–60% risk of endometrial cancer and a 0.3%–20% risk of ovarian cancer.[30]

Lynch syndrome is sometimes referred to as hereditary nonpolyposis colorectal cancer (HNPCC) to differentiate it from other inherited colorectal cancers such as familial adenomatous polyposis. But since some cases of LS have been found to have adenomatous polyps, it is more accurately referred to as Lynch syndrome to specifically refer to individuals with a germline mutation in a DNA mismatch repair gene (such as *MSH2, MLH1, MSH6*, or *PMS2*) or loss of expression of the *MSH2* gene due to deletion in the *EPCAM* gene. The majority of LS, approximately 90%, is caused by a germline mutation in either *MSH2* or *MLH1* which carry a 30%–74% lifetime risk of colorectal cancer.[30] However, other less frequent mutations such as a mutation in *MSH6* carry a lower lifetime risk of colorectal cancer of 10%–22% and a later onset but a higher lifetime risk of endometrial cancer of 71%.[30]

A number of clinical criteria have been proposed to help identify at-risk individuals. The most commonly used criteria are the Amsterdam II criteria and the Revised Bethesda criteria. The Amsterdam criteria can be remembered by the "3-2-1 rule" (three LS-affected members, involving at least two generations, at least one case diagnosed under age 50).[31] The Revised Bethesda criteria has a better sensitivity and specificity compared to the Amsterdam criteria.[32] Models to help calculate an individual's risk for LS seem to have improved prediction capabilities compared to clinical criteria. These models include the $MMR_{predict}$, MMR_{pro}, and $PREMM_{1,2,6}$ and can be found online at hnpccpredict.hgu.mrc.ac.uk, www4ut southwestern.edu/breasthealth/cagene, and premm.dfci.harvard.edu, respectively. The $PREMM_{1,2,6}$ model has the best sensitivity (90%) but worst specificity (67%) compared with the others but has been shown to be cost-effective in determining risk of LS among the general population when a 5% threshold was used to indicate a need for genetic testing.[33] The US Multi-Society Task Force on Colorectal Cancer performed a meta-analysis in 2014 for genetic screening for LS.[30] Table 4-3 summarizes the recommended indications for screening based on history and risk calculators.

Table 4-3 Populations for whom screening for Lynch syndrome is indicated

- Personal history of a tumor with MMR deficiency and no *MLH1* promoter methylation
- Personal history of uterine cancer diagnosed before the age of 50
- Known MMR mutation in the family
- Fulfill Amsterdam I or II criteria
- Fulfill Revised Bethesda criteria
- ≥5% calculated risk by a prediction model

Similar to HBOC syndromes, increased surveillance is recommended for individuals affected with Lynch syndrome or at high risk for Lynch syndrome. In a prospective observational study by Dove-Edwin et al., colonoscopy screening among LS families resulted in a 72% decrease in mortality.[34] The US Multi-Society Task Force concluded that colonoscopy screening in persons affected with LS or first-degree relatives of those affected should occur every one to two years beginning at age 20–25 or two to five years before the youngest age of diagnosis of CRC in the family if diagnosed before the age of 25. They also concluded that women affected by or at risk of LS should be offered endometrial cancer screening with annual pelvic exams and endometrial sampling and ovarian cancer screening with annual transvaginal ultrasound beginning at age 30–35 years. Breast surveillance is not recommended beyond what is advised for the general population.

Although there is no recommendation for prophylactic colectomy for individuals with Lynch syndrome, consideration should be paid to risk-reducing hysterectomy and BSO. In a retrospective analysis of 315 women with MMR mutations, women who underwent risk-reducing surgery had no uterine or ovarian cancers compared with 33% and 5.5% rate, respectively, among women who did not have risk-reducing surgery.[35] A cost-effectiveness analysis found that the optimal balance of screening and surgery was annual screening starting at age 30 followed by risk-reducing surgery at age 40.[36] The US Multi-Society Task Force thus concluded that women affected by LS should be offered hysterectomy and BSO at age 40 or once childbearing is completed.

Familial adenomatous polyposis

Other hereditary syndromes such as familial adenomatous polyposis (FAP) and Peutz-Jeghers are also associated with multiple colorectal adenomatous polyps. FAP accounts for less than 1% of all colorectal cancers.[37] It is an autosomal dominant condition caused by a germline mutation in adenomatous polyposis coli (*APC*), a tumor suppressor gene on chromosome 5q21–q22. Like HBOC and Lynch syndrome, FAP involves a bi-allelic inactivation usually caused by an inherited mutation of the wild-type *APC* allele followed by a "second hit" mutation of the other allele. Genetic testing for an *APC* mutation should be offered to individuals with 10–20 adenomas in their lifetime, first-degree relatives of affected individuals, and second-degree relatives of affected individuals when a first-degree relative is unavailable or has declined testing.[38]

Peutz-Jeghers syndrome

Peutz-Jeghers syndrome (PJS) is a rare autosomal dominant condition with a high penetrance that is caused by a germline mutation in *STK11*, a tumor suppressor gene on chromosome 19p13.3. The syndrome is characterized by multiple hamartomatous polyps in the gastrointestinal tract and pigmented mucocutaneous macules. In addition to risk of colorectal, stomach, small bowel, and pancreatic cancer, women with PJS have a 13%–18% risk of gynecological cancers.[39] The lifetime risk of breast, ovarian, and uterine cancers is 54%, 21%, and 9%, respectively.[40] Not all cases of PJS are associated with a mutation in *STK11* suggesting that other gene locus mutations have yet to be identified. Peutz-Jeghers syndrome, therefore, cannot be excluded in an individual who tests negative for a *STK11* mutation but meets the clinical criteria for PJS and has no known PJS mutation in the family.

Concluding remarks

As the number and availability of genetic tests increases, there is an increasing demand on health providers to understand genetic screening, interpret test results, and recommend appropriate risk-reducing interventions. Family history is important to identify at-risk individuals that will benefit from genetic counseling and testing. *BRCA* mutation risk of 20% or greater and MMR mutation risk of 5% or greater are reasonable thresholds for initiating testing. Pre- and posttest counseling is critical to the screening process. Evidence is lacking for intensive surveillance for ovarian or uterine cancer. Breast and colon cancer screening have been shown to be beneficial for early detection of cancer. Health providers should inform *BRCA* carriers of the benefits of chemoprevention with tamoxifen and oral contraceptives. Cancer risk and all-cause mortality among *BRCA* carriers can be reduced with prophylactic mastectomy and bilateral salpingo-oophorectomy by age 40 or after completion of childbearing. Prophylactic hysterectomy and BSO by age 40 is also recommended for women with Lynch syndrome. Other inherited cancer syndromes may also benefit from similar risk-reduction strategies though less evidence is available in these populations.

References

1. Howlader N, Noone AM, Krapcho M, et al., eds. SEER Cancer Stat Fact Sheets. Bethesda, MD: National Cancer Institute; 2014. Available at: http://seer.cancer.gov/statfacts. Accessed 30 September 2014.
2. Nelson HD, Fu R, Goddard K, et al. Risk Assessment, Genetic Counseling, and Genetic Testing for *BRCA*-Related Cancer: Systematic Review to Update the US Preventive Services Task Force Recommendation. Evidence synthesis no. 101. AHRQ publication no. 12-05164-EF-1. Rockville, MD: Agency for Healthcare Research and Quality; 2013.
3. Struewing JP, Hartge P, Wacholder S, et al. The risk of cancer associated with specific mutations of *BRCA1* and *BRCA2* among Ashkenazi Jews. *N Engl J Med* 1997; **336**:1401–8.
4. Antoniou A, Pharoah PD, Narod S, et al. Average risks of breast and ovarian cancer associated with *BRCA1* and *BRCA2* mutations detected in case series unselected for family history: a combined analysis of 22 studies. *Am J Hum Genet* 2003; **72**:1117–30.
5. National Collaborating Centre for Cancer. Familial breast cancer. In: *Classification and care of people at risk of familial breast cancer and management of breast cancer and related risks in people with a family history of breast cancer.* London (UK): National Institute for Health and Care Excellence (NICE); 2013 Jun, 57 p. (Clinical guideline; no. 164).
6. Moyer V, US Preventive Services Task Force. Risk assessment, genetic counseling, and genetic testing for *BRCA*-related cancer in women: US Preventive Services Task Force Recommendation Statement. *Ann Intern Med* 2014; **160**(4):271–81.
7. American Congress of Obstetricians and Gynecologists. ACOG Practice Bulletin No. 103: Hereditary breast and ovarian cancer syndrome. *Obstet Gynecol* 2009; **113**(4):957–66.
8. Berry DA, Iverson Jr ES, Gudbjartsson DF, et al. BRCAPRO validation, sensitivity of genetic testing of *BRCA1/BRCA2*, and prevalence of other breast cancer susceptibility genes. *J Clin Oncol* 2002; **20**:2701.
9. Unger MA, Nathanson KL, Calzone K, et al. Screening for genomic rearrangements in families with breast and ovarian cancer identifies *BRCA1* mutations previously missed by conformation-sensitive gel electrophoresis or sequencing. *Am J Hum Genet.* 2000; **67**:841–50. [PMID: 10978226]
10. Eggington JM, Bowles KR, Moyes K, et al. A comprehensive laboratory-based program for classification of variants of uncertain significance in hereditary cancer genes. *Clin Genet* 2014; **86**:229.
11. Garcia C, Lyon L, Littell RD, Powell CB. Comparison of risk management strategies between women testing positive for a *BRCA* variant of unknown significance and women with known *BRCA* deleterious mutations. *Genet Med* 2014 May 22. [Epub ahead of print PMID 24854227]
12. Ziv E, Shephard J, Smith-Bindman R, Kerlikowske K. Mammographic breast density and family history of breast cancer. *J Natl Cancer Inst* 2003; **95**(7):556–8.
13. Warner E, Messersmith H, Causer P, et al. Systematic review: using magnetic resonance imaging to screen women at high risk for breast cancer. *Ann Intern Med* 2008; **148**(9):671–9.
14. Garcia C, Wendt J, Lyon L, et al. Risk management options elected by women after testing positive for a *BRCA* mutation. *Gynecol Oncol* 2014 Feb; **132**(2): 428–33.
15. Isaacs C, Peshkin B, Schwartz M, et al. Breast and ovarian cancer screening practices in healthy women with a strong family history of breast or ovarian cancer. *Breast Cancer Res Treat* 2002; **71**:103–12.
16. Buys SS, Partridge E, Black A, et al. Effect of screening on ovarian cancer mortality: the prostate, lung, colorectal and ovarian (PLCO) cancer screening randomized controlled trial. *JAMA* 2011; **305**(22): 2295–303.
17. King MC, Wieand S, Hale K, et al. Tamoxifen and breast cancer incidence among women with inherited mutations in *BRCA1* and *BRCA2*: National Surgical Adjuvant Breast and Bowel Project (NSABP-P1) Breast Cancer Prevention Trial. *JAMA* 2001; **286**:2251.
18. Nelson HD, Smith ME, Griffin JC, Fu R. Use of medications to reduce risk of primary breast cancer: a systematic review for the US Preventive Services Task Force. *Ann Intern Med* 2013; **158**(8)604–14.
19. Iodice S, Barile M, Rotmensz N, et al. Oral contraceptive use and breast or ovarian cancer risk in *BRCA1/2* carriers: a meta-analysis. *Eur J Cancer* 2010; **46**(12):2275–84.
20. Rebbeck TR, Friebel T, Lynch HT, et al. Bilateral prophylactic mastectomy reduces breast cancer risk in *BRCA1* and *BRCA2* mutation carriers: the PROSE Study Group. *J Clin Oncol* 2004; **22**:1055–62.
21. Finch AP, Lubinski J, Moller P, et al. Impact of oophorectomy on cancer incidence and mortality in women with a *BRCA1* or *BRCA2* mutation. *J Clin Oncol* 2014; **32**:1547.
22. Domcheck SM, Friebel TM, Singer CF, et al. Association of risk-reducing surgery in *BRCA1* or *BRCA2* mutation carriers with cancer risk and mortality. *JAMA* 2010; **304**:967.
23. Kauff ND, Domchek SM, Friebel TM, et al. Risk-reducing salpingo-oophorectomy for the prevention of *BRCA1*- and *BRCA2*-associated breast and gynecologic cancer: a multicenter, prospective study. *J Clin Oncol* 2008; **26**:1331–7.
24. Rebbek TR, Friebel T, Wagner T, et al. Effect of short-term hormone replacement therapy on breast

cancer risk reduction after bilateral prophylactic oophorectomy in *BRCA1* and *BRCA2* mutation carriers: the PROSE Study Group. *J Clin Oncol* 2005; **23**(31):7804–10.

25. Lodder LN, Frets PG, Trijsburg RW, et al. One-year follow-up of women opting for presymptomatic testing for *BRCA1* and *BRCA2*: emotional impact of the test outcome and decisions on risk management (surveillance or prophylactic surgery). *Breast Cancer Res Treat* 2002; **73**:97–112.
26. Scheuer L, Kauff N, Robson M, et al. Outcome of preventive surgery and screening for breast and ovarian cancer in *BRCA* mutation carriers. *J Clin Oncol* 2002; **25**:1260–8.
27. Chompret A, Brugieres L, Ronsin M, et al. *P53* germline mutations in childhood cancers and cancer risk for carrier individuals. *Br J Cancer* 2000; **82**:1932.
28. Olivier M, Goldgar DE, Sodha N, et al. Li-Fraumeni and related syndromes: correlation between tumor type, family structure, and *TP53* genotype. *Cancer Res* 2003; **63**:6643.
29. Salovaara R, Loukkola A, Kristo P, et al. Population-based molecular detection of hereditary nonpolyposis colorectal cancer. *J Clin Oncol* 2000; **182**:193–200.
30. Giardiello FM, Allen JI, Axilbund JE, et al. AGA Section Guidelines on genetic evaluation and management of Lynch syndrome: a consensus statement by the US Multi-Society Task Force on colorectal cancer. *Gastroenterology* 2014; **147**:502–26.
31. Vasen HFA, Watson P, Mecklin JP, et al. New criteria for hereditary non-polyposis colorectal cancer (HNPCC, Lynch syndrome) proposed by the International Collaborative Group on HNPCC. *Gastroenterology* 1999; **116**:1453–6.
32. Umar A, Boland CR, Terdiman JP, et al. Revised Bethesda Guidelines for hereditary polyposis colorectal cancer (Lynch syndrome) and microsatellite instability. *J Natl Cancer Inst* 2004; **96**:261–8.
33. Dinh TA, Rosner BI, Atwood JK, et al. Health benefits and cost-effectiveness of primary genetic screening for Lynch syndrome in the general population. *Cancer Prev Res* 2010; **4**:9–22.
34. Dove-Edwin I, Sasieni P, Adams J, et al. Prevention of colorectal cancer by colonoscopy surveillance in individuals with a family history of colorectal cancer: 16 year, prospective, follow-up study. *BMJ* 2005; **331**:1047.
35. Schmeler KM, Lynch HT, Chen LM, et al. Prophylactic surgery to reduce the risk of gynecological cancers in Lynch syndrome. *J Engl J Med* 2006; **354**:261–9.
36. Kwon JS, Sun CC, Peterson SK, et al. Cost-effectiveness analysis of prevention strategies for gynecologic cancers in Lynch syndromes. *Cancer* 2008; **113**:326–35.
37. Wennstrom J, Pierce ER, McKusick VA. Hereditary benign and malignant lesions of the large bowel. *Cancer* 1974; **34**:850.
38. American Gastroenterological Association. American Gastroenterological Association medical position statement: hereditary colorectal cancer and genetic testing. *Gastroenterology* 2001; **121**:195.
39. Van Lier MG, Wagner A, Mathus-Vliegen EM, et al. High cancer risk in Peutz-Jeghers syndrome: a systematic review and surveillance recommendations. *Am J Gastroenterol* 2010; **105**:1258.
40. Giardiello FM, Brensinger JD, Tersmette AC, et al. Very high risk of cancer in familial Peutz-Jeghers syndrome. *Gastroenterology* 2000; **119**:1447.

Chapter 5

Office ultrasound

Norman A. Assad

Introduction

Proper use of ultrasound can greatly enhance the diagnostic acumen of the practicing obstetrician and gynecologist or other practitioner with a strong interest in women's health.

Practitioners determine whether they perform ultrasound themselves, and/or designate other trained personnel to perform the procedures. Some practices may do reference ultrasounds for other physicians. These factors determine selection of equipment.

Selection of the equipment

The decision to purchase or lease an ultrasound unit depends on the clinical practice of the Practitioner. The practitioner must determine if sufficient volume exists to warrant acquiring the equipment and expertise to perform these procedures "in house" versus referring patients to others specializing in these ultrasounds. The practitioner must also decide whether to acquire a basic ultrasound machine or more exotic equipment that includes three-dimensional imaging. This will be determined in large part by the patient mix that the practitioner treats.

Many reliable manufacturers are available but the most important factor in deciding what equipment to purchase is the support offered by that manufacturer. The practitioner must decide whether to include a maintenance contract on the equipment potentially including insurance on the probe. A probe can be quite expensive to repair or replace if dropped or damaged in any way. If a maintenance contract is not purchased then it is strongly advised that the equipment be serviced at least annually by the manufacturer's representative.

Training

Many manufacturers have formalized training programs; most also have application specialists who will spend time in the practitioner's office to provide familiarity with the many features associated with their products.

Training guidelines for physicians who evaluate and interpret diagnostic abdominal, obstetrics and/or gynecologic ultrasound examinations have been established by the American Institute of Ultrasound Medicine (AIUM).[1] Included in these guidelines is a statement addressing training program qualifications: "Completion of an approved residency program, fellowship, or postgraduate training that includes the equivalent of at least 3 months of diagnostic ultrasound training in the area(s) they practice, under the supervision of a qualified physician(s), during which the trainees will have evidence of being involved with the performance, evaluation, and interpretation of at least 300 sonograms."[1] In the absence of formal fellowship or postgraduate training or residency training, documentation of clinical experience could be acceptable providing the following could be demonstrated: (1) evidence of 100 AMA PRA category 1 credits dedicated to diagnostic ultrasound in the area(s) of the physicians practice, and (2) evidence of being involved with the performance, evaluation, and interpretation of the images of at least 300 sonograms within a -three year period.[3] These sonograms should be in the specialty area(s) in which the physicians are practicing. It is expected that in most circumstances, examinations will be under the supervision of a qualified physician(s). The guidelines additionally describe the "maintenance of Competence in Abdominal General Ultrasound," "Maintenance of Competence in Obstetric and/or Gynecologic Ultrasound," and "Containing Medical Education in Obstetrics and/or Gynecologic Ultrasound." The author recommends that the practicing physician be aware of AIUM's "Practice Guidelines" (Table 5-1) as well as "Official Statements."

Office Care of Women, ed. Martin E. Olsen and Botros Rizk. Published by Cambridge University Press.

Table 5-1 AIUM practice guidelines – indications for pelvic sonography[1]

1. Pelvic pain
2. Dysmenorrheal (painful menses)
3. Amenorrhea
4. Menorrhagia (excessive menstrual bleeding)
5. Metrorrhagia (irregular uterine bleeding)
6. Menometrorrhagia (excessive irregular bleeding)
7. Follow-up of a previously detected abnormality
8. Evaluation, monitoring, and/or treatment of infertility patients
9. Delayed menses, precocious puberty, or vaginal bleeding in a prepubertal child
10. Postmenopausal bleeding
11. Abnormal or technically limited pelvic examination
12. Signs or symptoms of pelvic infection
13. Further characterization of a pelvic abnormality noted on another imaging study
14. Evaluation of congenital anomalies
15. Excessive bleeding, pain, or signs of infection after pelvic surgery, delivery, or abortion
16. Localization of an intrauterine device (best done with 3D if available)
17. Screening for malignancy in patients at increased risk
18. Urinary incontinence of pelvic organ prolapsed
19. Guidance for interventional or surgical procedures

Table 5-3 AIUM practice guidelines – indications for the performance of sonohysterography[3]

1. Abnormal uterine bleeding
2. Uterine cavity, especially with regard to uterine myomas, polyps, or synechiae
3. Abnormalities detected on endovaginal sonography, including focal or diffuse endometrial or intracavitary abnormalities
4. Congenital abnormalities of the uterus
5. Infertility
6. Recurrent pregnancy loss

Table 5-2 AIUM practice guidelines – specifications for the performance of first trimester ultrasound examinations[2]

1. Confirmation of the presence of an intrauterine pregnancy
2. Evaluation of a suspected ectopic pregnancy
3. Defining the cause of vaginal bleeding
4. Evaluation of pelvic pain
5. Estimation of gestational (menstrual) age
6. Diagnosis or evaluation of multiple gestations
7. Confirmation of cardiac activity
8. Imaging as an adjunct to chorionic villus sampling, embryo transfer, and localization and removal of an intrauterine device
9. Assessing for certain fetal anomalies, such as anencephaly, in high-risk patients
10. Evaluation of maternal pelvic masses and/or uterine abnormalities
11. Measuring the nuchal translucency (NT) when part of a screening for fetal aneuploidy (special training and/or certification is required by many institutions for the performance of this exam)
12. Evaluation of a suspected hydatiform mole

Performance of ultrasounds

A written or electronic request should be submitted before performing ultrasounds for physicians in the same practice, reference scans for other physicians in the same practice, or reference scans for other physicians. This request should provide sufficient information to allow for the appropriate performance and interpretation of the examination. This request must be originated by a physician or other appropriately licensed health-care providers familiar with the patient's clinical situation and should be consistent with relevant legal and local health-care facility requirements.

To fulfill specifications of the examination, all relevant structures should be identified by a transabdominal and/or transvaginal approach. In some instances, both will be required. A transrectal or transperitoneal approach may be useful in patients who are not candidates for introduction of a vaginal probe and in assessing the patient with pelvic organ prolapse.

Detailed descriptions of mechanisms for imaging the uterus, adnexa including ovaries and fallopian tubes, and cul de sac are detailed in AIUM Enhanced Practice Guidelines. The guidelines also outline equipment specifications, quality control and improvement, safety, infection control, and patient education. The concept "as low as reasonably achievable" principle is also outlined.

Scanning in the first trimester (see Table 5-2 for specifications) may be performed either transabdominally or transvaginally. If a transabdominal examination is not definitive then a transvaginal or transperineal scan should be performed wherever possible.

Guidelines for standard second or third trimester examination also exist but are beyond the scope of this chapter.

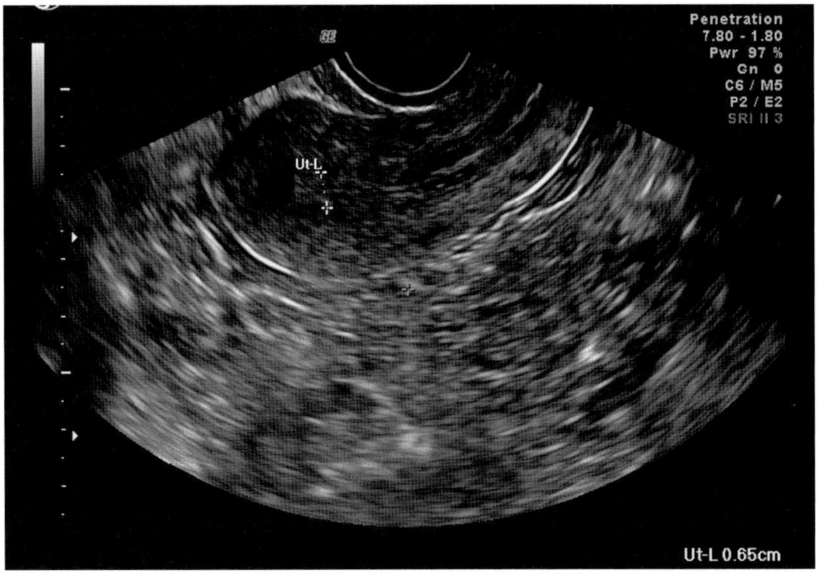

Figure 5-1 Normal uterus.

A detailed description of sonohysteroscopy is outlined in the AIUM guideline, which should be reviewed prior to performance of the procedure.[3] (See Table 5-3 for indications.)

Pelvic organ scanning

It is essential that the physician scanning patients has comprehensive knowledge of the normal pelvic anatomy including normal variants. The physician must have a detailed medical history regarding the patients' complaints, including the dates of the last menstrual period, in order to properly interpret the findings.[4] Figure 5-1 shows a normal uterus.

Uterus

Several uterine conditions can be diagnosed. These include congenital anomalies and submuscosal fibroids.

Congenital anomalies

With proper configuration, the internal contours of the uterus can be visualized. Anomalies include uterus arcuate, septate, bicornuate, or uterus didelphys. Uterine anomalies can result in impaired vascularization of the uterus and the space for an expanding pregnancy; this can increase the rate of miscarriage. Approximately 12%–15% of women with recurrent miscarriage have uterine malformation. Of all of the possible uterine malformations, complete or partial septation of the uterus is the commonest. It occurs about 33% of the time amongst major anomalies, but is the most receptive to treatment. Successful surgery leads to a term delivery rate of about 75% and a live birth rate of 85%.[5] Although these anomalies can be suspected on 2D ultrasounds, 3D ultrasound gives coronal views of the uterus and the depth of the septum can be measured.

Uterine pathology

Polyps, fibroids, and adenomyosis can often be distinguished on ultrasound. Conventional ultrasound will help localize the location of the fibroid and categorized it a pedunculated, subserosal, intramural or submuscosal lesion. It is further possible to distinguish between type 0, type 1 and type 2 submucosal fibroids, although 3D ultrasound is more useful in this regard. Figure 5-2 shows an intramural myoma.

Submuscosal fibroids

Submuscosal fibroids are typically hypoechoic and displace the basalis layer of the endometrium. Evaluation of the amount of extension into the myometrial layer is important in determining the type of surgical procedure to plan.

Polyps have a more homogeneous echogenicity and have a pedunculated attachment to the uterine wall without interruption of the endometrial lining. Color or power Doppler modes are useful to distinguish myomas from polyps or uterine malignancies. Myomas have a typical vascularization pattern of the capsule that forms a circle, whereas endometrial polyps have a vascular pedicle. Malignancies have an abundant irregular vessel distribution.[6] Saline infusion sonohysteroscopy (SIS) increases the specificity of the exam; polyps often show motion with injection of sterile saline. They also have a less round contour and are often elongated in appearance. See Figure 5-3.

Postsurgical evaluation of the endometrium can also be performed with ultrasound. Sagittal and transverse views can be utilized to evaluate the endometrium after removal of polyps or fibroids. SIS can also be used to evaluate an endometrium on a patient receiving tamoxifen therapy as a more detailed view of the endometrial cavity is obtained.

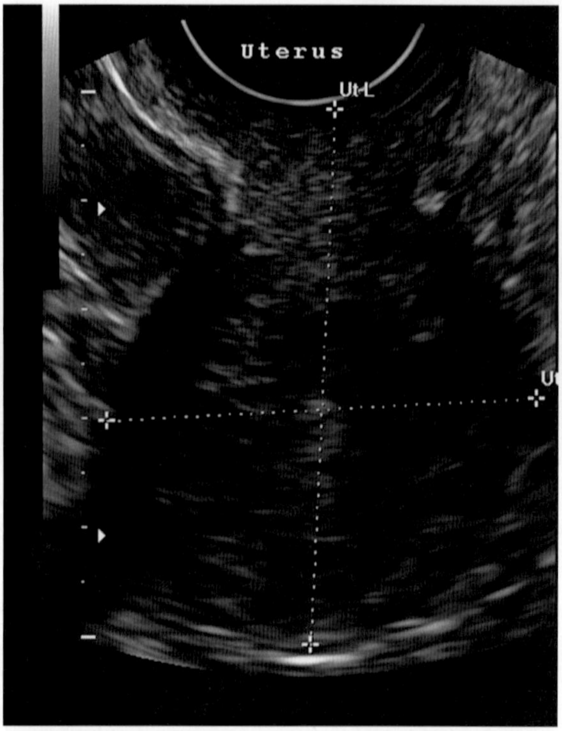

Figure 5-2 Uterine myoma.

An isthmocoele is a fluid filled area in the region of a previous cesarean section. This may be a cause of fluid accumulation in the uterine cavity or be associated with abnormal uterine bleeding and infertility. The persistence of menstrual blood in the cervix might negatively influence cervical mucus quality, obstruct the passage of sperm through the cervical canal, affect sperm quality, or affect implantation of an embryo in the endometrial cavity if fluid is present. Surgical repair of isthmocele may correct bleeding, fluid accumulation and restore fertility. Repair is usually done with the hysteroscope and the area is cauterized.

Nabothian follicles can be visualized within the cervix. These are small sonolucent cysts seen near the region of the cervical canal.

Pregnancy analysis

Ultrasound is a critical modality in the management of intrauterine pregnancy.[8] Before the gestational sac appears, the endometrium is markedly echogenic and the arcuate vessels are somewhat prominent. This appearance, however, is nondiagnostic of pregnancy. Although the blastocyst begins to implant in the endometrium at one-week post conception (or three postmenstrual weeks) the first definitive ultrasound sign of pregnancy is the gestational or chorionic sac. In ultrasound images, the chorionic sac appears as a thick, echogenic rind surrounding a sonolucent center. It appears embedded deep in the thick

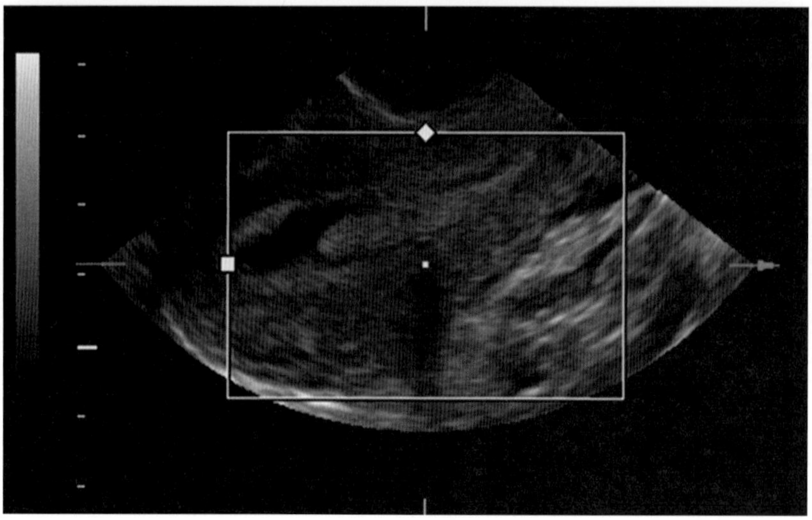

Figure 5-3 Endometrial polyp seen with sonohysteroscopy.

endometrium or decidua on one side of the cavity line, not in the middle of it. The sonolucent center is actually fluid within the chorionic sac. The sac already contains the amnion, a bilaminar embryonic disc, and the yolk sac; these structures are too small to be imaged even with the high magnification of current scanners. The echogenic rind is the result of a trophoblastic decidual reaction. Early in gestation, the entire chorionic sac is surrounded by chorionic villi. These villi are symmetrically located. Some villi will bud and branch into secondary tertiary villi and become chorion frondosum (forerunner of the placenta). Other primary villi will regress and become chorion leave. The appearance of the gestational sac predates the fusion of the decidua parietalis to decidua capsular. One can occasionally image a sonolucent area caused by implantation bleeding that separates the sac from the contralateral decidua. The sac can first be seen at approximately 34.8 days plus or minus two days. The discriminatory level of human chorionic gonadotropin (hCG) has been reported to range from 935 mIU/mL to 2,388 mIU/mL.[7] The presence of fibroids, coexisting intrauterine devices or multiple pregnancies can create exceptions. The chorionic sac grows approximately 1 mm/day in mean diameter in early pregnancy. With further growth, first the yolk sac and later the embryo become visible sonographically inside the chorionic cavity. The yolk sac has a very bright echogenic rim around a sonolucent center. When it first appears at approximately five weeks it may be only 1 mm–2 mm in diameter. Discriminatory size of the yolk sac is reported to range from 8 mm to 13 mm in mean diameter. In abnormal pregnancies, the yolk sac may be enlarged or irregular, or sometimes is described as "floating."

The embryonic period begins at three weeks post conception or five weeks from the last normal menstrual period (LNMP). Before the embryo is 18 mm in length a true "crown" and "rump" do not exist. Therefore, early embryonic size (EES) is measured as the greatest length along the long axis of the embryo. Initially at the somite stage, the embryo is a linear structure 2 mm–3 mm in length. The rostral neuropore closes and develops into the forebrain prominence then the head. The caudal neuropore elongates into a tail. As it grows the embryo is a C-shaped tadpole-like structure. The primitive heart has great prominence, often allowing the sonographer to provide early detection of the cardiac activity pulsations before visualizing an embryo distinct from the adjacent yolk sac. With further development, the tail regresses, the head unfolds from its flexed position, and limb buds develop and are replaced by hands and feet. By 18 mm–22 mm, a recognized crown rump length (CRL) can be measured. By 10 postmenstrual weeks the previous tadpole-like form is now recognizable as a human fetus. The fetal periods begins at 70 days post-LNMP.

In early pregnancy the demonstration of viability may be necessary to exclude ectopic pregnancy, to rule out embryonic demise in cases of vaginal bleeding or abdominal pain, or to clarify uncertain dates. Cardiac activity starts at 21–22 days of embryonic or conceptual age, or approximately 36 days post LNMP. At this stage the embryonic pole is approximately 1 mm–3 mm. Transabdominal sonography can detect cardiac activity by 41–43 days gestation.

A very important clinical question is, "What is the embryonic size without cardiac activity that is diagnostic for pregnancy failure?" Consensus is that the absence of cardiac activity on real-time transvaginal sonography in embryos measuring more than 4 mm is always associated with embryonic demise.[10] Slow embryonic heartbeat of 80–85 or less for a sustained period of time is considered ominous.[13] Rapid embryonic heart rate and arrhythmias in early pregnancy have also been studied.[14] When bradycardia, tachycardia, or arrhythmias are noted the patient should be scheduled for follow-up ultrasounds. The chance of poor outcome is higher if other pathologic ultrasound findings are noted such as growth discrepancy, subchorionic hemorrhages, and abnormalities of the yolk sac or fetal heart rate changes noted earlier.[16]

Assessment of the amnionicity and chronionicity of a multifetal pregnancy is important as these pregnancies have an increase in complications; the number of chorionic sacs can be determined by five postmenstrual weeks. The determination of the number of fetuses occurs at the sixth postmenstrual week, after the onset of cardiac activity when the number of heartbeats can be determined. The number of yolk sacs is not a reliable marker for twin gestation. The detection of the individual amniotic sacs in the case of monochorionic-diamniotic twins becomes possible at 7.15 postmenstrual weeks or immediately thereafter because the amnion separates from the embryo and is easily imaged.

Gestational age assessment is an important role of transvaginal ultrasound. In the past, embryonic crown rump length (CRL) was considered the most accurate method of sonographically dating a pregnancy. With current methods, chorionic sac size expressed as a mean sac diameter can be correlated by the postmenstrual age before visualization of an embryo. Measurements of the sac are taken at the interface of trophoblastic tissue and the fluid filling the sac. Such measurements ideally come from two planes at right angles to each other. One or more tables are usually included in the software of commercially available ultrasound machines.

In dating an early pregnancy, the following are important landmarks. The gestational sac is always present by the fourth week of pregnancy, the yolk sac by the sixth week of pregnancy. The fetal pole with heartbeats by the seventh week of pregnancy, the single brain ventricle in 82% of cases by the seventh week of pregnancy, the falx by the tenth week of pregnancy and midgut herniation by the eighth week of pregnancy.[16]

Assessment of abnormal intrauterine pregnancy

Twenty-five percent of pregnant patients bleed in the embryonic period. Of these, up to 50% will abort. In the author's experience, many "subchorionic bleeds" resolve spontaneously and the pregnancy carries on significantly. In many cases of threatened abortion, no abnormal ultrasound findings are noted.

On ultrasound, a *hydatidiform mole* appears as multiple small sonolucent areas which correspond to the grapelike vesicles seen on pathologic analysis. Sonographically the changes are rarely seen prior to 10 weeks because the trophoblastic proliferation and hydropic changes are not yet present.

When assessing a patient with suspected blighted ovum, it should be realized that in a normal pregnancy, once the mean diameter of the gestational sac on transvaginal ultrasound exceeds 8 mm–13 mm, a yolk sac should become visible.

Embryonic resorption is present more frequently in fertility patients who have undergone superovulation or assisted reproductive technology.

Subchorionic hemorrhage appears as a crescent shaped sonolucent structure outside of the chorionic sac in a patient with threatened abortion. The presence of a fetal heart leads to a better prognosis. Approximately 20% of cases of threatened abortion exhibit this finding.[7]

Ectopic pregnancy

If a patient has a positive pregnancy test and bleeding, she must be evaluated for ectopic pregnancy with or without the presence of pain. The ultrasonographer must be aware that the corpus luteum can mimic an ectopic pregnancy.

Heterotopic pregnancy is the concomitant presence of both an intrauterine and an ectopic pregnancy. The incidence is 1 in 30,000 spontaneous pregnancies and in 1 in 6,000 pregnancies with assisted reproductive technologies (ART).[17] Patients with prior tubal damage seem more susceptible in the latter category. In a normal pregnancy the quantitative HCG will raise a minimum of 66% every 48 hours. Once HCG levels surpass a discriminatory level, it should be possible to image an intrauterine gestation. Absence of a gestational sac at this level either indicates a failing intrauterine or an ectopic pregnancy. If uncertain, the physician may consider performing a dilation and curettage (D&C) for these patients to assess if trophoblastic tissue is present. It is very important from both a clinical and medicolegal perspective to avoid giving methotrexate to an early ongoing intrauterine gestation. The decision to give methotrexate should never be made on evaluation of a single HCG value. A pseudo sac (seen in 20% of women with ectopic pregnancy) can mimic an intrauterine gestation.[16] A true gestational sac is intradecidual whereas a pseudo sac develops within the uterine cavity. Color Doppler with an early intrauterine pregnancy (IUP) can often identify a high-velocity, low resistance trophoblastic arterial flow pattern associated with developing chorionic villi, but this is not a strict diagnostic sign.

A finding of a well-developed sac with decidual casting outside of the uterine cavity is strongly suggestive of an ectopic pregnancy; 15%–28% of ectopic pregnancies develop a yolk sac or cardiac activity. The strictest criterion, with the highest specificity (100%) but the lowest sensitivity (15%–20%) is identifying an extra uterine gestational sac that contains a yolk sac or an embryo. Many of these are in the ampullary portion of the tube where the HCG can continue to double. Free fluid in the pelvis is a suspicious but not diagnostic sign.

Interstitial pregnancy accounts for 2%–4% of ectopic pregnancies. These pregnancies are associated with a higher degree of morbidity and mortality. Diagnosis is suggested when ultrasound images show eccentric implantation of the gestational sac at the superior fundal portion of the uterus. In almost all cases, there is myometrial thinning or absent endometrium around portions of the sac. Rarely visible myometrium has been reported to surround completely a small interstitial ectopic pregnancy. To increase the predicative value of sonography to make this diagnosis, Ackerman and associates described the interstitial line sign.[17] This consists of visualizing a thin, echogenic line that extends from the central uterine cavity echo to about the periphery of the interstitial gestational sac. When used in combination with the ultrasound finding of an incomplete mantle and an eccentric sac, this line may be useful for diagnosing an interstitial pregnancy.

Cervical pregnancy occurs in 0.15% of normal pregnancies, but increases by a factor of 10 with ART. The diagnosis is based on detection of a gestational sac that contains a yolk sac, embryo, or cardiac activity within the cervix.

Diagnosis of abdominal pregnancy is made upon the finding of an empty uterus that is separate from the fetus. It can be confused by a congenital uterine duplication anomaly that consists of one empty uterus and one containing a fetus. Other ultrasound findings include a lack of visualization of surrounding myometrium, extra uterine placental tissue, oligohydramnios and an abnormal fetal lie.

Chapter 11, "Abnormal First Trimester Pregnancy," includes ultrasound images associated with pregnancy assessment.

Fallopian tube

It is easier to detect a pathologic fallopian tube than a normal tube. Prerequisites for imaging an abnormal tube include fluid in the lumen, a thick wall, a tubal ectopic pregnancy, tubal torsion, or involvement in a neoplastic process. One may visualize a convoluted fluid filled structure with incomplete septa with or without cul de sac fluid. Specific processes that may be assessed by ultrasound include torsion of the fallopian tube and tubal cancer.

Torsion of the fallopian tube The tube and ovary may undergo torsion together; in a pure tubal torsion, a normal ovary with normal blood flow visible alongside an engorged tube. There is usually no blood flow within the mass. A paratubal cyst can also undergo torsion.

Tubal cancer This condition is very rare, accounting for only 1% of gynecologic cancers. Ultrasound findings include a distinct adnexal mass, thick walls, solid components, and abundant blood flow.

Ovaries

The optimal way to scan the ovaries is to use a high frequency (4 MHz–8 MHz) ultrasound probe. In general, as the frequency of the probe increases, so does the resolution of the image but the ability of ultrasound to penetrate tissue diminishes. For this reason, an abdominal ultrasound usually uses a 3 MHz probe. In vaginal scanning the author generally uses a 7 MHz probe. For larger women it is often necessary to use the lower value to obtain satisfactory images. The ovaries can usually be distinguished by their relative anechoic sono texture compared to the bowel. The size of the ovaries can be an important indicator of pathology. During the reproductive years the mean volume is 8 mL, whereas in the menopausal years the mean volume is 3.6 mL. The ovaries often assume a position closer to the vagina in the postmenopausal years, whereas in reproductive years are often imaged adjacent to the exterior iliac vein. Figure 5-4 shows a normal ovary. Abnormal findings are seen in Figures 5-5, 5-6, and 5-7.

Polycystic ovarian syndrome (PCOS) assessment criteria was discussed by the 2003, European Society of Human Reproduction and Embrology (ESHRE)

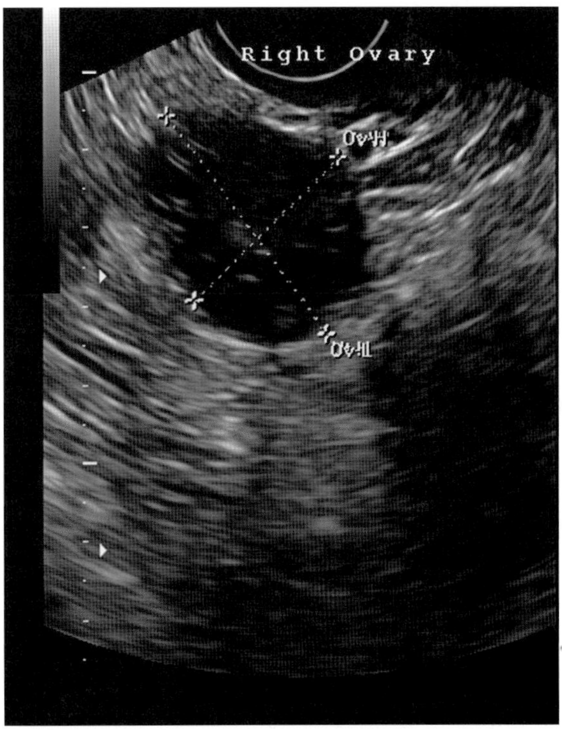

Figure 5-4 Normal ovary.

and American Society of Reproductive Medicine (ASRM) in 2003; these groups co-sponsored Rotterdam polycystic ovary syndrome consensus workshop. This group revised the guidelines for diagnosis and management. To be diagnosed with PCOS by the Rotterdam criteria, a woman must have two of the following three manifestations: irregular or absent ovulation, elevated levels of androgenic hormones, and/or ovaries that met the ultrasound criterion. The Rotterdam consensus defined the polycystic ovary as having 12 or more follicles, measuring between 2 mm and 9 mm, and/or an ovarian volume greater than 10 cc.[18] Lujan and Jarrett give the current ultrasound criteria for PCOS.[18]

An ovary can have a polycystic appearance in other processes such as hyperthyroidism (36% of affected women), hyperprolactinemia (50% of affected women), and hypothalamic hypogonadism (24% of affected women).

Non-neoplastic masses include functional cysts (which are follicles), corpus lutea, and theca lutein cysts. When describing the findings to patients, the word "follicle" should be utilized instead of "cyst" as the word "cyst" can engender anxiety by patients, who may misinterpret normal findings as "pathologic."

Nonfunctional cysts include serous masses and endometriomas. Cystadenofibromas are usually categorized histologically as neoplasms; however, they are very commonly seen on ultrasound.

An essential characteristic of adnexal mass assessment includes wall structure. The thicker the wall, the more likely it is that the mass is malignant. Goldstein and Timor Titsch consider a wall

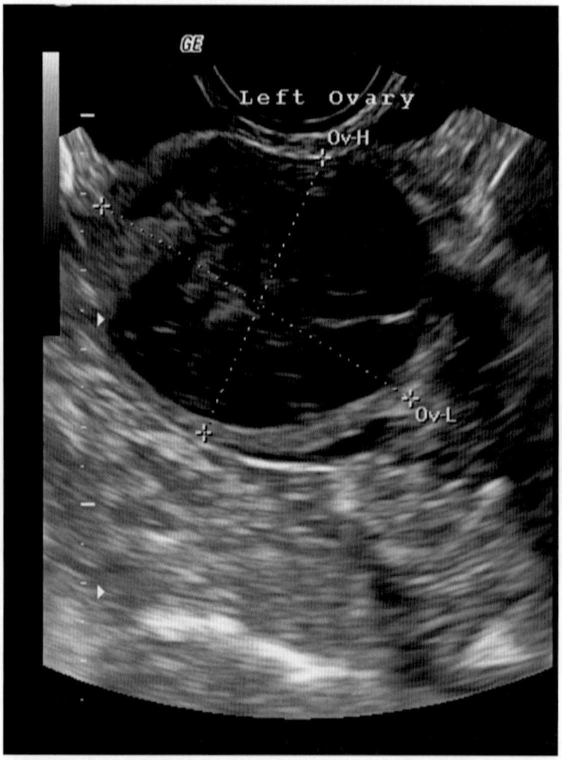

Figure 5-5 Hemorrhagic cyst of ovary.

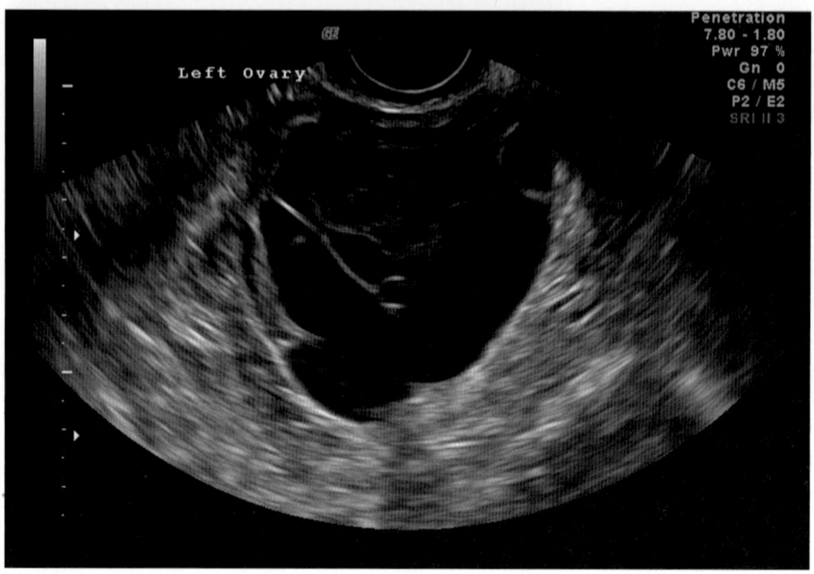

Figure 5-6 Complex ovarian cyst; note the presence of septations, solid components, and cystic components.

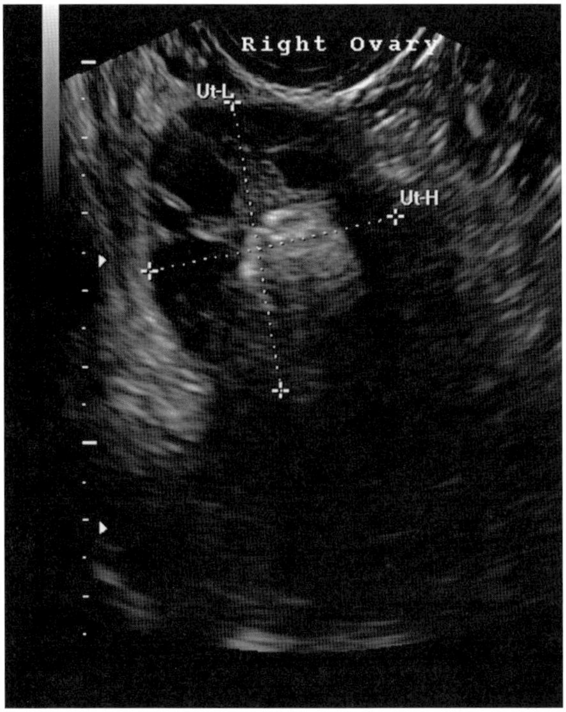

Figure 5-7 Hypoechoic characteristics are seen in this scan of a mature teratoma.

thickness of 4 mm, as suggestive of tumor.[20] Typically a mass is unilocular or multilocular. Multilocularity is more common in tumors of low malignant potential and malignant neoplasms. Papillations are an important feature to assess. Papillarity in an ovarian mass increases its chances of malignancy. Papillae that contain blood vessels with detectable blood flow are more likely to be malignant. Power Doppler is more sensitive and will assess blood flow velocity in the lowest detectable range. Exacoustos et al. found that larger papillae were more likely to be associated with borderline malignancies; papillae as large as 15 mm in height and 10 mm in width (base), were present in 48% of borderline ovarian tumors, but in only 4% of benign and 4% of malignant tumors.[19] However, when the intracystic solid tissue exceeded those dimensions the incidence of invasive cancer increased dramatically.

In addition to wall structure, formal ultrasound assessment of the ovaries also includes internal echo-structure, shadowing, overall appearance, size, ascites, and motion tenderness.

Internal echo-structure should be assessed. A mass can be anechoic, a finding that usually indicates the presence of clear fluid. Mostly solid masses are echogenic. Masses that contain particulate matter such as blood, cellular matter or even mucous materially usually have echogenicity of a low level, often described as a "ground glass" appearance. A mass that has mixed echogenicity, and these are found in teratomas or malignancies.

Shadowing, if present it may suggest the presence of an extremely dense, solid tissue such as bone or calcification. If shadowing is noted in a hyperechoic nodule or mass then one should suspect a benign cystic teratoma or dermoid cyst. Shadowing is rarely present in malignancies.

Overall appearance must be described. On rare occasions, a bizarre shape or "complex" appearance may suggest a malignancy, however this is more likely a teratoma, cystadenoma, or even an atypical corpus luteum.

Size can be misleading, as small ovarian lesions with the appropriate sonographic characteristics may be malignant, and some larger ones without those characteristics may be benign. However, the larger the size of an ovarian lesion, the more likely it is to be malignant.

Ascites, if present should be recorded and investigated further because it may be caused by a malignant intra-abdominal tumor.

Motion tenderness caused by movement of the probe may be a sign of pelvic peritonitis or other inflammatory process.

The provider can add either color or power Doppler to further evaluate characteristics of ovarian mass. Tumors contain a relatively large number of pathologic blood vessels that lack the muscular layer found in normal blood vessels and as a result demonstrate lower resistance to flow. Diastolic flow is high in those vessels, and resistance and pulsatility indices are low. The morphologic appearance of these blood vessels should be assessed.[20] Concern for malignancy is increased when the blood vessels show changes in caliber, anastomoses, vascular lakes or have a tortuous appearance.[21] A centrally located blood vessel is suspicious for malignancy.

Specific ovarian processes that may be assessed via ultrasound include ovarian fibromas, ovarian neoplasms, dermoid cysts, serous cystadenoma, hormone-producing tumors, and other malignant neoplasms.

Ovarian fibromas A fibroma is a slow-growing benign, solid ovarian tumor. It usually has a cystic component and if so is called a cystadenofibroma. The cystic variety is filled with anechoic fluid and has a thin wall. However, the pathognomonic feature is the small (2 mm–3 mm) extremely hyperechoic mural nodules (papillae) present in the majority of cases. No blood vessels are detectable, and the mass is unilocular. It can be recognized in the ovary by the semilunar shape of the tissue surrounding it (crescent sign). Differential diagnosis includes a simple serous cyst. The solid fibroma has a myometricum-like texture, with few or no detectable blood vessels in the stroke. Differential diagnosis includes the Brenner and Krukenberg tumor.

Ovarian neoplasms About 75% of malignant neoplasms are found in postmenopausal women. Ovarian cancers are rare, affecting 50 women per 100,000. Mortality rates are high with a five-year survival rate for all stages of only 50%. If the cancer is detected and treated during stage 1, the five-year survival rate is 95%. Only 25% of cancers are detected while the cancer is still localized. In stages 3 and 4, the five-year survival rate is 28% or less. Earlier detection can have a dramatic effect on survival. The lifetime risk of ovarian cancer in a woman who has no affected relative is 1 in 70 women. When the patient has an affected first-degree relative, the risk rises to 1 in 20 women, and if there are two or more affected relatives, the risk is 1 in 14.

Dermoid cysts These may appear to be solid, cystic, or both. There is shadowing, which may be extreme if the tumor contains a solid, echogenic central mass.

Serous cystadenoma Ultrasound characteristics include multilocularity, multiseptation, with the septae often fanning out from a central, apparently solid structure. Anechoic nature is present when they contain fluid in the serous variety or with low-level echogenicity in mucinous cyst adenoma. Cystadenomas have a paucity of core vessels and normal resistive and pulsatility indices and low peak systolic velocity.

Hormone-producing tumors These tumors are small often residing in an ovary of normal size. They are also vascular, featuring a diagnostic ringlike pattern, much like a corpus luteum. They can also produce androgen like symptoms. An estrogen-secreting tumor is the granulosa cell tumor. It has solid appearing tissue surrounding multiple cyst of different side: it is typically richly supplied with blood vessels.

Other malignant neoplasms These are rare but usually have a complex appearance that includes thick walls (2 mm–4 mm), heterogeneous texture, multilocularity, solid components, and papillary excrescences within the tumor as well as on the outer surface. They exhibit the vascular features described previously.

For a comprehensive review of benign and malignant ovarian findings, see Timor Tritsch and Goldstein.[20]

Infertility

TVS discerns both ovarian and endometrial changes. Follicular growth is a continuous process that is independent of gonadotropin stimulation. It is difficult to discern follicles that are less than 5 mm. Antral or resting follicles can be counted in the early phase of the cycle (cycle days 3–5). The inversion mode on 3D ultrasound can assist in delineating these follicles. Without fertility medications the follicle usually reaches a mean diameter of 18 mm–20 mm. Follicular growth rate is usually 1.5 mm–2 mm daily. A mature follicle is clear in appearance with a well-delineated border. Characteristic ultrasound appearance at ovulation includes diminution in follicle size, blurring of the follicle borders, appearance of intrafollicular echoes, and demonstration of free fluid in the cul de sac. Following ovulation the ultrasound appearance of the corpus luteum appears and is present until the menses, or beyond if the patient is pregnant. The corpus luteum can assume many forms. Cystic corpus lutea can be sonolucent although increasing the gain can reveal more echogenicity than in the preovulatory follicle. The walls appear to be thicker and less regularly shaped than the preovulatory follicle. Many corpus lutea are echogenic and have the speckled appearance associated with blood. Some have a layered appearance secondary to the presence of serum and solid clots.

The endometrium also demonstrates marked changes over the menstrual cycle. This begins with a thin echo at the time of menstruation. Fluid and blood clots can also be seen within the endometrial cavity. The endometrium usually thickens throughout the proliferative phase. It ideally has a trilaminar appearance. After ovulation the rise in progesterone causes an increase in stromal edema and growth of the spiral arteries; this appears as an increase in echogenicity, which is usually maintained until menses.

The follicle is an ellipsoid structure; the two largest diameters are used when assessing follicle maturity. Follicles having a mean diameter of 16 mm–18 mm are considered mature when using gonadotrophin therapy, however with clomiphene the follicles often need to reach a mean diameter of 24 mm–26 mm in order to contain a mature oocyte. Ultrasound changes occurring in stimulation for ART are beyond the scope of this discussion.

Concluding remarks

The office ultrasound practitioner is encouraged to follow the guidelines delineated by the American Institute of Ultrasound in Medicine. Basic training and orientation by the ultrasound manufacturer is essential prior to performing procedures on patients. Transvaginal ultrasound is an extension of the clinician's armentarium, which includes history, physical examination, and laboratory studies. The clinician can extend and improve examination with the appropriate use of ultrasound evaluation.

References

1. American Institute of Ultrasound in Medicine (AIUM). AIUM Practice Guideline for the Performance of Pelvic Ultrasound Examinations. Available at: http://www.aium.org/resources/guidelines/femalepelvis.pdf. Accessed Dec. 9, 2015.
2. American Institute of Ultrasound in Medicine (AIUM). AIUM Practice Guidelines for the Performance of Obstetric Ultrasound Examination: Classification of Fetal Sonographic Examinations. Available at: http://www.aium.org/resources/guidelines/obstetric.pdf. Accessed Dec. 9, 2015.
3. American Institute of Ultrasound in Medicine (AIUM). AIUM Practice Guideline for the Performance of Sonohysteroscopy: Indications/Contraindications. Available at: http://www.aium.org/resources/guidelines/sonohysterography.pdf. Accessed Dec. 9, 2015.
4. Assad NA, Hudson S. Three-dimensional Ultrasound in Gynecology. In: Rizk BRMB, Puscheck EE, eds. *Ultrasonography in Gynecology*. Cambridge: Cambridge University Press; 2015: 1–11.
5. Grimbizis GF, Camus M, Tarlatzis BC, et al. Clinical implications of uterine malformations and hysteroscopic treatment results. *Hum Reprod Update* 2001 Mar–Apr;7(2):161–74.
6. Diagnosing Submuscosal Fibroics (SIS) beyond Hysterectomy: The Contemporary Management of Uterine Fibroids – An International Conference, Phoenix, Arizona; April 11–13, 2003.
7. Timor-Tritsch IE, Goldstein, SR. Early Pregnancy. In: *Ultrasound in Gynecology*, 2nd edition. London: Churchill Livingstone; 2006: 139.
8. Levi CS, Lyons EA, Lindsay DJ. Early diagnosis of nonviable pregnancy with endovaginal US. *Radiology* 1988 May;**167**(2):383–5.
9. Levi CS, Lyons EA, Zheng XH, et al. Endovaginal US: demonstration of cardiac activity in embros of less than 5.0 mm in crown-rump length. *Radiology* 1990 Jul;**176**(1):71–4.
10. Brown DL, Emerson DS, Felker RE, et al. Diagnosis of early embryonic demise by endovaginal sonography. *J Ultrasound Med* 1990 Nov;**9**(11):631–6.
11. Goldstein SR. Significance of cardiac activity on endovaginal ultrasound in very early embryos. *Obstet Gynecol* 1991 Oct;**80**(4):670–2.
12. Schats R, Jansen CA, Qladimiroff JW. Embryonic heart activity: appearance and development in early human pregnancy. *Br J Obstet Gynaecol* 1990 Nov;**97**(11): 989–94.
13. Coubilet PM, Benson CB, Chow JS. Long-term prognosis of pregnancies complicated by slow embryonic heart rates in the early first trimester. *J Ultrasound Med* 1999 Aug;**18** (8):537–41.
14. Coubilet PM, Benson CB, Chow JS. Outcome of pregnancies with rapid embryonic heart rates in the early first trimester. *AJR Am J Roentgenol* 2000 Jul;**175**(1):67–9.
15. Vaccaro H, Amor F, Leyton M, Sepulveda W. Arrhythmia in early pregnancy: a predictor of first-trimester pregnancy loss. *Ultrasound Obstet Gyneccol* 1998 Oct;**12**(4):248–51.
16. Timor-Tritsch IE, Goldstein, SR. Early Pregnancy. In: *Ultrasound in Gynecology*, 2nd edition. London: Churchill Livingstone; 2006: 139–50.
17. Ackerman TE, Levi CS, et al. Interstitial line: sonographic finding in interstitial (corneal) ectopic pregnancy. *Radiology* 1993 Oct;**189**(1):83–7.
18. Lujan ME, Jarrett BY, et al. Updated ultrasound criteria for polycystic ovary syndrome: reliable thresholds for elevated follicle population and ovarian volume. *Hum Reprod* 2013 May;**28**(5): 1361–8.
19. Exacoustos C, Romanini ME, et al. Preoperative sonographic features of borderline ovarian tumors. *Ultrasound Obstet Gynecol* 2005 Jan;**25**(1):50–9.
20. Timor-Tritsch IE, Goldstein SR. The complexity of a "complex mass" and the simplicity of a "simple cyst." *J Ultrasound Med* 2005;**24**(3):255–8.

21. Sladkevicius P, Jokubkiene L, Valentin L. Contribution of morphological assessment of the vessel tree by three-dimensional ultrasound to a correct diagnosis of malignancy in ovarian masses. *Ultrasound Obstet Gynecol* 2007 Nov;**30**(6):874–82.
22. Kudla MJ, Timor-Tritsch IE, Hope JM, et al. Spherical tissue sampling in 3-dinensional power Doppler angiography: a new approach for evaluation of ovarian tumors. *J Ultrasound Med* 2008 Mar;**27**(3):425–33.
23. Alcazar JL, Prka M. Evaluation of two different methods for vaascular sampling by three-dimensional power Doppler angiography in solid and cystic-solid adnexal masses. *Ultrasound Obstet Gynecol* 2009 Mar;**33**(3):349–54.

Chapter 6

Preoperative evaluation

Catherine R. Salva and Onyi Onuoha

Introduction

The obstetrician-gynecologist has special knowledge of the reproductive system and has the expertise as a gynecologic surgeon to offer surgical intervention. It would not be uncommon for an obstetrician-gynecologist to perform a cesarean section, a laparoscopic bilateral tubal ligation, a dilation and curettage (D&C), and a hysterectomy for the same patient as she presents for treatment in various stages of her reproductive life. Although there are numerous options for medical treatment of the various gynecologic disorders, surgery is often warranted after all conservative and medical treatment options have been exhausted. For certain conditions, surgery may be the best option.

The goal of this chapter is to review office preoperative planning and evaluation for the general obstetrician-gynecologist. The authors emphasize that preoperative risk assessment and optimization performed in the office setting can facilitate a smooth and safe intraoperative and postoperative course and improve overall outcomes. Gynecologic surgery is frequently performed for quality-of-life considerations in a generally healthy, low-risk, population. Medicine, however, has become more complex: children with cardiac and pulmonary conditions previously thought lethal are now with medical and surgical intervention surviving into their reproductive years. In addition, there is a projected increase in the population of women aged 65 and older as the baby boomer generation matures and maintains fitness.[1] Thus, women that seek routine and acute gynecologic surgical intervention constitute a population that is diverse, aging, and increasingly complex.

To provide optimal care for this complex female population, we recommend an approach to preoperative evaluation which focuses on (1) risk assessment and (2) identification of characteristics and comorbid conditions that would predispose patients to increased perioperative complications. Risk assessment includes consideration of careful diagnosis, a patient's cardiovascular risk, and risk level of the proposed surgery. The physician must possess knowledge of current evidence-based practice for perioperative management, and be familiar with quality improvement data to identify modifiable risk factors.

History

Before undertaking surgery, every surgeon should reflect on the three basic surgical indications: to save life, to relieve suffering, and to correct deformity.[4]

We begin with careful assessment of the patient, the symptoms, and the choice of surgical intervention. Choosing the appropriate surgical intervention includes consideration of diagnosis, symptom severity, patient expectations and needs for recovery and relief, and physician expertise. Once surgery is contemplated, preoperative medical evaluation provides an opportunity for the generalist to identify previously undiagnosed or incompletely managed medical concerns in order to initiate appropriate treatment. In women with known medical concerns, the physician can identify potential risks for complications, counsel, and plan for appropriate medical optimization and perioperative management.[5] Rarely, serious medical concerns will mandate that alternatives to surgical intervention be explored.

Medical history

The general medical history should address all pertinent systems to assess three major risks: cardiovascular, pulmonary, and thrombotic.[5] This should include discussion of any endocrine disorders including diabetes or thyroid disease, and any history of

Office Care of Women, ed. Martin E. Olsen and Botros Rizk. Published by Cambridge University Press.

hematologic disorders including bleeding diatheses or history of thrombosis. A history of prior surgeries should be noted in detail with special attention to abdominal scars, associated procedures, and any history of complications. Family history may provide important information regarding bleeding risk or potential difficulties with anesthesia. In addition, any family history of breast or other gynecologic cancer could affect the choice of surgical procedure. Identifying a history of tobacco use is a potential area of intervention for the obstetrician-gynecologist. Knowledge of significant alcohol or other substance abuse will help prepare for the possibility of postoperative withdrawal or pain management issues. Allergies and current medications including any herbal supplements are important to note and manage in the perioperative period.[6–8] General health screening should be up to date.

Gynecologic history

A thorough gynecologic history includes age of menarche and menstrual cycle history including date of last menstruation and presence of dysmenorrhea, premenstrual syndrome, or abnormal uterine bleeding and associated treatments. Age of menopause and any history of hormone replacement or postmenopausal bleeding should be noted. History of cervical dysplasia should be considered and could impact choice of surgical procedure. A history of ovarian cysts, fibroids, and any history of sexually transmitted diseases or vaginal infections should be noted. Sexual history, including any history of trauma or dysfunction, must be carefully considered, as a distressingly high number of women that struggle with chronic pelvic pain have a history of abuse.[9] The obstetrician-gynecologist should include a focused comprehensive history addressing the major complaint and current disease for which the procedure is planned.

Obstetric history

An obstetric history details the number of pregnancies and outcomes including full term and preterm births, miscarriages, abortions, and ectopic pregnancies. Mode of delivery (vaginal vs. cesarean) should be considered when planning surgical approach to hysterectomy. The obstetrician-gynecologist should fully explore any past history of infertility and desires for future fertility in order to choose the most appropriate surgical intervention. For the woman of reproductive age, contraception and sexual health through the perioperative period are important issues to discuss.

Review of systems

Finally, the review of systems is most useful to identify undiagnosed or incompletely treated disease, and should be used to assess the functional status of the patient. The comprehensive history including the review of systems defines the extent to which subsequent examinations (physical examination) and diagnostic tests (laboratory and radiologic) are needed to complete the preoperative evaluation.

Physical examination

The general physical examination builds on information gathered during the history, to establish or confirm the physical health status of the patient in view of the preceding history obtained.[6, 7] A thorough gynecologic examination is the main focus for the obstetrician-gynecologist, as it provides more information about the principal complaint or symptom for which surgical intervention is chosen. In most cases, the pelvic examination is repeated under anesthesia at the time of surgery to confirm findings and plans for surgical approach.[8]

General exam

Vital signs including weight and body mass index (BMI) should be recorded. A focused physical examination should include a general assessment of the patient's habitus and physical appearance, cardiovascular examination (heart auscultation for rhythm, rate, murmurs, rales, gallops), pulmonary examination (lung auscultation for upper and lower airway breath sounds and abnormalities such as stridor, inspiratory or expiratory wheezes), gastrointestinal examination (palpation and auscultation of the abdomen for bowel sounds, tenderness, distention, masses, organomegaly) and a focused neurologic examination assessing mental status, and gross function of the cranial nerves and sensorimotor abilities. All surgical scars should be explained and documented. Unexpected abnormal findings on the physical examination should be investigated before elective surgery.[7]

Gynecologic exam

Visual inspection and palpation of external genitalia is customary, with assessment of the introitus and hymenal ring. If indicated by history of pelvic pain, sensory mapping of the vestibule should be done with a cotton-tipped applicator.[9] The bulbocavernosus muscles can be assessed with insertion of one finger into the vagina just past the introitus while asking for contraction and relaxation. The levator muscles can then be palpated at the 4–5 o'clock and 7–8 o'clock positions to assess for uncontrolled contraction and pain. The bladder and urethra are palpated. A bimanual exam is performed to assess the bulk, tenderness, position, and mobility of the cervix and uterus. Palpation of adnexal structures should be performed. A rectovaginal examination with palpation of uterosacral ligaments is a standard part of the pelvic examination and merits particular attention when pelvic pain is the presenting symptom, to detect the presence of posterior cul-de-sac endometriosis.

Both prolapse and urinary incontinence may be observed with the patient supine in heel stirrups, performing a Valsalva maneuver; this may be repeated in standing position if there is concern that the prolapse or incontinence is not being seen at its worst extent.[10] A Graves speculum is inserted into the vagina to visualize the cervix and vaginal mucosa. Any abnormal discharge should be further investigated. To assess for uterine descensus, it is not necessary to apply traction to the cervix with a tenaculum; a Valsalva maneuver should be sufficient to visualize mobility and descent of the apex. A split-speculum examination is then performed to isolate anterior (cystocele) and posterior (rectocele, enterocele) compartment defects. The Baden-Walker system for the evaluation of pelvic prolapse on physical examination has adequate clinical utility for use by the general obstetrician-gynecologist to describe the preoperative gynecologic exam.[10]

Diagnostic risk assessment

Based on the history and physical examination, as well as potential diagnostic tests, the obstetrician-gynecologist may be ready to discuss surgical intervention. Importantly, the physician must perform adequate evaluation to minimize the possibility of undiagnosed malignancy prior to an elective procedure. The advancement of gynecologic subspecialties helps to address the growing needs and increased complexity of the aging female population; the obstetrician-gynecologist who provides comprehensive care must have a good understanding of appropriate specialist referrals to optimize patient outcomes.

Adnexal mass

In the United States, a woman has a 5%–10% lifetime risk of undergoing surgery for a suspected ovarian neoplasm and, within that group, an estimated 13%–21% chance of receiving a diagnosis of ovarian cancer.[11] Ovarian cancer patients have better prognostic outcomes when initial surgery and treatment are performed by a gynecologic oncologist.[12] Thus, it is of critical importance that the generalist, prior to surgery, perform adequate diagnostic testing to distinguish the likely benign mass from likely malignancy. In all asymptomatic women with pelvic masses, transvaginal ultrasound is the imaging modality of choice. In general, the presence of excrescences, ascites, and nodules are highly concerning for malignancy. The American Congress of Obstetrics and Gynecology (ACOG) and the Society of Gynecologic Oncologists (SGO) offer joint referral guidelines recommending that any woman presenting with an adnexal mass be referred to a gynecologic oncologist if she has evidence of metastases or ascites, family history of first-degree relative with breast or ovarian cancer, any elevated CA-125 with postmenopausal status, or marked elevation of CA-125 (>200) with premenopausal status.[11] In addition to CA-125 and pelvic ultrasound, marker HE4, multivariate index assay OVA-1, and the risk of ovarian malignancy algorithm (ROMA) can be useful risk assessment tools.[12]

Abnormal uterine bleeding

The incidence of endometrial cancer increases with age. ACOG recommends that all women older than 45 years who present with suspected anovulatory uterine bleeding be evaluated with endometrial biopsy after excluding pregnancy. Although the incidence of endometrial cancer is very low in women between the ages of 19 years and 39 years, if these women do not respond to medical therapy or have prolonged periods of unopposed estrogen stimulation, they are also candidates for endometrial assessment. Risk factors for endometrial cancer to consider in this younger age group include nulliparity, hypertension, obesity, irregular menstruation, and family history.[13] See Table 6-1.

Morcellation

Power morcellation in gynecologic surgery has come under recent scrutiny because of concern of the risk of

Table 6-1 Effect of age on uterine cancer

Age	Incidence of uterine cancer (per 100,000 women)
Under 20	0.2
20–29	0.3–1.6
30–39	4.0–8.1
40–44	13.6
45–49	24.0
50–54	45.9
55–59	72.6
60–64	89.4
65–9	94.8

Source: From http://seer.cancer.gov/archive/csr/1975_2009_pops09/results_merged/sect_07_corpus_uteri.pdf.[14]

intraperitoneal dissemination of malignant tissue, particularly uterine sarcoma, which is more difficult to diagnose preoperatively than endometrial cancer or cervical cancer. Preoperative evaluation before hysterectomy or myomectomy with morcellation should include current cervical cytology, and may also include pelvic imaging and endometrial sampling. Preoperative risk assessment should include patient age, menopausal status, uterine size and rapid growth, and certain treatments or hereditary conditions.[15]

Additional considerations

Surgical approach

Once the surgeon has completed adequate evaluation to minimize the possibility of undiagnosed malignancy, the type of surgical procedure can be further discussed with the patient. A variety of gynecologic procedures can be performed vaginally, abdominally, or with laparoscopic or robotic assistance. When choosing the route and method for the procedure, the physician should take into consideration how the procedure may be performed most safely and cost-effectively to fulfill the medical needs of the patient.[16] Regarding hysterectomy, specifically, evidence demonstrates that, in general, vaginal hysterectomy is associated with better outcomes and fewer complications.[16, 17] A number of factors may influence the route of hysterectomy, including the size and shape of the vagina and uterus; accessibility to the uterus; surgeon training and experience; extent of disease; available hospital technology, devices and support; and the preference of the informed patient.[16]

Informed consent

The process of obtaining informed consent should be a conversation between the surgeon and patient, about a specific procedure and associated risks, benefits, and alternatives. The patient should be aware of efficacy of the proposed procedure and expectations for symptomatic relief, particularly in the case of procedures with subjective outcomes. Possible complications even when perceived to be unlikely or morbid should be verbalized. A thorough and well-documented consent form delineating details, possible outcomes, and risk both of the surgery and anesthesia should be completed to ensure that the patient's expectations of surgery, recovery, and final outcomes are realistic and appropriate.[18] The patient should be aware of her right to refuse surgical therapy and should not be persuaded to undergo surgery against her own will.[6, 19] The patient should be comprehensively counseled about alternate treatment options. Finally, the physician should confirm that the patient demonstrates comprehension and desires to proceed with surgery. Whether a proposed procedure is low, moderate, or high risk, this is an opportunity to review any living wills, health-care proxies, and health-care directives to ensure that all involved in the procedure understand the wishes of the patient.[19]

Emotional considerations

Gynecologic surgery can evoke a variety of psychological and emotional issues which, in addition to the usual concerns surrounding any surgical procedure (pain, disfigurement, debility, outcome), includes specific issues related to loss of fertility, femininity, sexuality, and attractiveness.[20] With this in mind, the obstetrician-gynecologist should remember that surgical procedures can initiate a complex stress response that can manifest as adverse effects during the perioperative period. Additionally, preoperative identification of women that might react negatively to genital surgical stress would allow for additional preoperative

Table 6-2 Risk factors for poor emotional health after gynecologic surgery*

Gender identity
Previous adverse reactions to stress
Previous depressive episodes
Family history of mental illness
History of multiple physical complaints, especially lower back pain
Numerous hospitalizations or surgeries
Age less than 35 years at time of hysterectomy
Desire for childbearing
Fear of loss of libido
Significant other's negative attitude toward procedure
Marital dissatisfaction or instability
Cultural or religious disapproval
Lack of vocation or hobbies

* Roeske researched 13 factors related to poor prognosis for excellent mental health after hysterectomy. Knowledge of these factors allows a surgeon to be forewarned about which patients are likely to have a more difficult time handling the emotional aspects of gynecologic surgery.[4]

counseling and assessment of readiness.[4] (See Table 6-2.) It follows, then, that decreasing the stress response to surgery is a key factor in improving overall outcome.[7] Gynecologic surgeons must understand the female perspective and use that knowledge to facilitate multidimensional healing.[4] To this end, it can be helpful to refer the patient to established online forums for reliable information and peer support.[21]

Preoperative testing

After informed consent has been obtained and discussion regarding the surgical procedure and the anticipated outcome has been completed, the gynecologic surgeon will often order preoperative testing in preparation for the operating room. Usually these tests are ordered based on age recommendations or institutional policies. Preoperative laboratory analyses often include blood group determination, complete blood count (CBC), bleeding or coagulation studies (prothrombin time – PT; activated partial thromboplastin time – aPTT), and a basic or comprehensive metabolic panel (measuring renal and liver function, electrolytes, blood glucose). A general analysis of the urine and a urine culture may also be performed.[6] The possibility of pregnancy should be excluded with urine HCG. Radiographic studies (mostly electrocardiogram – ECG; chest x-ray – CXR; echocardiogram) when needed are performed to detect significant risks. ECGs in patients with known cardiac disease are useful to the clinician as a baseline tool against which a new study is compared.

Preoperative test selection

Over the past three decades, the notion of "routine" preoperative testing has been challenged. With the current focus on cost-effective and quality health care, there are concerns about the sizable cost of testing, the consequences of false positive tests leading to unnecessary workups or treatments, and the unknown benefit of "routine" testing to patients.[22] "Choosing Wisely" is an ongoing effort by the American Board of Internal Medicine (ABIM) Foundation to promote better stewardship of finite medical resources while optimizing patient safety, improving quality of care and promoting the practice of evidence-based medicine to ensure improved patient outcomes. Today, more than 50 subspecialties and specialties, including the American Society of Anesthesiologists (ASA) and ACOG, have generated evidence-based lists of procedures, or tests that have been shown to have no benefit to patients and, thus, should be avoided for the delivery of optimal care.[23, 24]

With "Choosing Wisely," emphasis is placed on the avoidance of unnecessary preoperative testing, specifically challenging the notion of a battery of "routine" testing.[25, 26] Tests should be ordered only when the history or physical examination indicates the need for testing even if surgery had not been planned.[27] The goal of preoperative testing should be to detect abnormalities that will alter management and ensure better patient outcomes, including mortality, morbidity, cost-savings, and patient satisfaction.[27, 28]

Approach to preoperative testing, in this context, should be done from a risk assessment perspective. The obstetrician-gynecologist needs to consider the risk status of the patient (low, medium, or high) and the risk level of the procedure (low, intermediate, or high), in order to determine what additional information is needed to proceed.

Table 6-3 ASA physical status classification

ASA PS category	Definition
ASA PS 1	A normal healthy patient
ASA PS 2	A patient with mild systemic disease
ASA PS 3	A patient with severe systemic disease
ASA PS 4	A patient with severe systemic disease that is a constant threat to life
ASA PS 5	A moribund patient who is not expected to survive without the operation
ASA PS 6	A declared brain-dead patient whose organs are being removed for donor purposes

* ASA PS – American Society of Anesthesiologists Physical Status.

Table 6-4 Cardiac risk stratification for different types of surgical procedures

High risk (reported cardiac risk* ≥5%)
Emergency major operations, particularly in the elderly
Aortic, and other major vascular
Peripheral vascular surgery
Intermediate risk (reported cardiac risk ≥1%, <5%)
Intraperitoneal and intrathoracic
Carotid endarterectomy
Head and neck surgery
Orthopedic surgery
Prostate surgery
Low risk (reported cardiac risk <1%)**
Endoscopic procedures
Superficial biopsy
Cataract surgery
Breast surgery
Ambulatory surgery

* Combined incidence of cardiac death and nonfatal myocardial infarction.
** Do not generally require further preoperative cardiac testing.
Source: Adapted from ACC/AHA 2007 Guidelines on Perioperative Cardiovascular Evaluation for Noncardiac Surgery.

Functional status

First, the obstetrician-gynecologist should assess the functional status of the patient, easily accomplished during the review of systems. The evaluation of metabolic equivalent of tasks (METs) can be used as a surrogate for functional status. One MET is a unit equal to the metabolic equivalent of oxygen uptake while quietly seated;[5] four METs is equal to walking on a flat surface, climbing a flight of stairs, or light housework. Importantly, a patient is able to proceed to intermediate-risk surgery without further testing if able to perform four METs or greater without cardiac symptoms.[5, 29]

Patient risk status

Regarding the risk status of the patient, anesthesiology uses the ASA physical status classification that includes six categories (see Table 6-3).[6, 19]

Patients assigned ASA 1 or ASA 2 are defined as low risk – healthy and without significant systemic disease or disease that is well controlled. In these patients, routine preoperative testing without any clinical indication rarely changes management and can yield a small percentage of abnormal results that are clinically irrelevant.[28] ASA 3 patients are at higher risk of complications in gynecologic surgery and should be optimized prior to surgery, with strategies for management of systemic disease in the perioperative period planned in collaboration with medical specialists.[3]

Procedure risk

Regarding the risk level of the procedure, the type of surgery has significant implications for perioperative risk. Many gynecologic procedures are associated with a combined morbidity and mortality rate less than 1%, even in high-risk patients.[29–31] Table 6-4 classifies surgery-specific risk into low-, intermediate-, and high-risk categories. Most ambulatory office-based gynecologic procedures are often of short duration with a low risk for intraoperative surgical complications and performed in low-risk patients. A major intraperitoneal gynecologic surgery is considered an intermediate risk

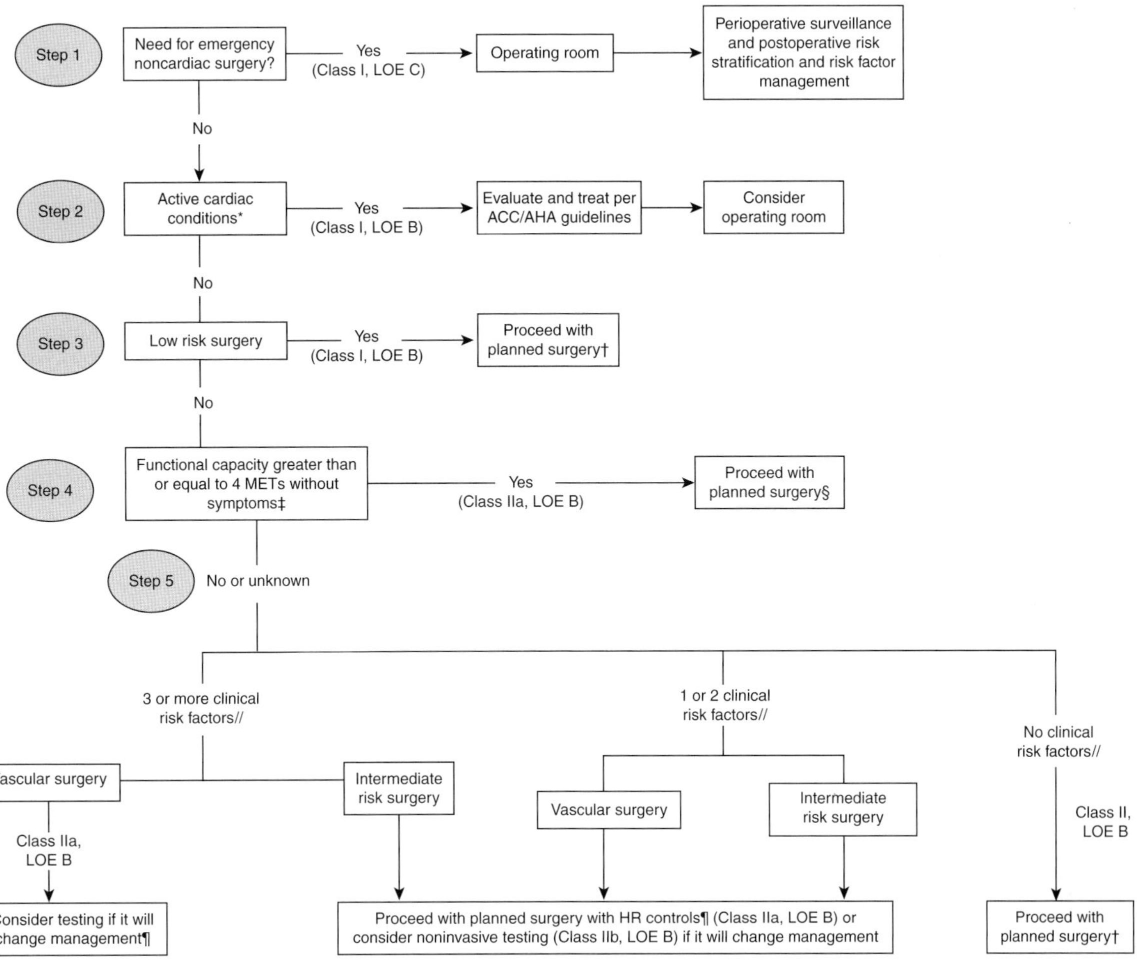

Figure 6-1 Cardiac evaluation and care algorithm for noncardiac surgery based on active clinical conditions, known cardiovascular disease, or cardiac risk factors for patients 50 years of age or greater.

* Active clinical conditions include unstable coronary syndromes, decompensated heart failure – HF (NYHA functional class IV worsening or new-onset HF), significant arrhythmias, and severe valvular disease.
† Class III recommendations for noninvasive stress testing.
‡ Estimated MET level equivalent.
§ Noninvasive testing may be considered before surgery in specific patients with risk factors if it will change management.
// Clinical risk factors include ischemic heart disease, compensated or prior heart failure, diabetes mellitus, renal insufficiency, and cerebrovascular disease.
¶ Consider perioperative beta blockade for populations in which this has been shown to reduce cardiac morbidity/mortality.
Abbreviations: ACC/AHA – American College of Cardiology/American Heart Association; HR eheart rate; LOE alevel of evidence; MET Tmetabolic equivalent.

procedure that has a reported cardiac risk of 1%–5%. Emergency surgery, particularly in the elderly, is associated with a high risk.[29–31] Of note, routine gynecologic surgery would not enter the high-risk category.

Although most patients undergoing elective gynecologic surgery would likely be classified in ASA 1 through ASA 3, it is important to consider the high-risk patient with multiple comorbidities including cardiac disease. As the female population ages, the prevalence of stable cardiovascular disease is bound to increase with the concomitant increase in number of elective gynecologic procedures.[30] In this context, the American College of Cardiology (ACC) and the American Heart Association (AHA) have developed joint guidelines for preoperative cardiovascular evaluation for noncardiac surgery, incorporating clinical predictors and functional status into the preoperative risk-assessment algorithm.[30]

Patients are stratified according to major, intermediate, or minor "clinical predictors" of increased cardiac risk. Those with no risk factors may proceed to surgery without further cardiac evaluation. Patients with one or two risk factors planning for at least intermediate surgery are able to proceed with heart rate control. Noninvasive testing can be considered if results would potentially change management.[30]

To summarize, the obstetrician-gynecologist should choose preoperative testing wisely, with consideration of patient's functional status as assessed during the office visit, risk profile, and risk level of the proposed procedure. Evidence suggests no value of preoperative testing prior to low-risk surgery.[32] For intermediate risk surgery, preoperative testing should be obtained only if the functional status of the patient is questionable. No invasive testing is required for patients with moderate functional capacity (four to seven METs) and intermediate clinical predictors (mild stable angina, prior myocardial infarction, diabetes mellitus, compensated or prior congestive heart failure) with asymptomatic stable disease.[33] Few experts would recommend performing pulmonary function testing in the preoperative assessment of the gynecologic patient. Data also suggests low value from routine preoperative chest x-rays.[5]

Optimization

In a generally low-risk patient population undergoing low to intermediate-risk procedures, surgical risk should be low. In this context, quality improvement processes are imperative for identifying characteristics or comorbidities that predispose women to increased perioperative complications.[2] Outcomes data exists to help the obstetrician-gynecologist with risk stratification and surgical planning.

Modifiable risk

The American College of Surgeons National Surgical Quality Improvement Program (ACS NSQIP), which was started in the Veterans Health Administration in 1991, performs central analysis including additional centers to generate observed/expected ratios for 30-day mortality and morbidity for each of eight major surgical specialties including gynecology. Notably, since the initiation of this program, the 30-day morbidity after major surgery has decreased by 45% and the 30-day mortality has decreased by 31%.[2] This decrease suggests that outcomes data can be used to create a clinical prediction tool to differentiate women at risk. ACS NSQIP data demonstrates complications in gynecologic surgery associated with preoperative anemia, ASA 3 category, smoking, and morbid obesity with BMI greater than 40.[3] The obstetrician-gynecologist largely performs elective surgery in the context of longitudinal and comprehensive care and, thus, is in a unique position to work closely and diligently with patients to improve health and reduce risks in these targeted areas.

In addition, in the perioperative setting, the obstetrician-gynecologist can impact the incidence of known complications of surgical site infection, deep venous thrombosis, and blood transfusion with established evidence-based guidelines.

Surgical site infection prophylaxis

Surgical site infection is the most common surgical complication, occurring in up to 5% of patients undergoing operative procedures. Aseptic technique has been associated with a dramatic decrease in surgical site infection. However, contamination of the operative site with endogenous bacterial flora is inevitable; this includes aerobic gram-positive cocci from the skin, anaerobic bacteria and gram-negative aerobes from the perineum, and mixed aerobes and anaerobes in the vagina. The goal of antimicrobial prophylaxis is to augment natural immune-defense mechanisms, helping to kill bacteria that are inoculated into the wound. Timing of the prophylaxis is essential. To achieve adequate concentrations of the antibiotic given at the beginning and during the procedure, the recommendation is for administration to occur within an hour before incision.[6] For most minor procedures (elective suction curettage abortion is an exception) antibiotic prophylaxis is not indicated. For major procedures where there is contamination of the peritoneal cavity from the vagina (i.e., hysterectomy), one dose is usually sufficient but an additional dose may be recommended either with blood loss greater than 1,500 mL or at intervals of one or two times the half-life of the drug (for cefazolin when the duration of surgery approaches three hours). Morbidly obese patients (BMI over 35) should receive a higher antibiotic dose to achieve adequate tissue concentrations. Guidelines for the prevention of surgical site infection have been outlined by ACOG and by the US Centers for Disease Control and Prevention (CDC).[34, 35] The adequate and appropriate use of prophylactic antibiotics has been shown to reduce the postoperative infection burden as well as morbidity and associated costs.[6]

Bacterial vaginosis is a known risk factor for surgical site infection after hysterectomy. Although ACOG does not offer specific screening guidelines in the preoperative setting, ACOG does recommend that patients found to have preoperative bacterial vaginosis be treated before hysterectomy.[34] In a 2011 cost-comparison study, McElligott et al. suggest that the optimal strategy clinically and economically would be a "treat all" strategy to add metronidazole to standard surgical site prophylaxis before hysterectomy.[36]

Venous thromboprophylaxis

Postoperative venous thromboembolism (VTE) ranges from 15% to 40% in women undergoing major gynecologic surgery without thromboprophylaxis, and about 40% of all deaths after gynecologic surgery are directly associated with pulmonary embolus (PE).[6] The components of Virchow's triad – stasis, endothelial injury, and hypercoagulability – are easily present in gynecologic surgery. Pertinent risk factors for postoperative VTE include age, prior deep venous thrombosis (DVT), varicose veins, infection, malignancy, smoking, obesity, immobility, and trauma associated with extent or prolonged surgery (duration over 300 minutes and blood loss of more than 600 mL).[6]

The strategic plan to avoid VTE in gynecologic surgery should begin in the preoperative period. Patients should be classified into one of four risk categories – (1) low, (2) medium, (3) high, and (4) highest risk – to determine the appropriate thromboprophylaxis regimen.[39] Risk is determined based on procedure type and duration, age, and presence of other risk factors. For patients with history of extensive or recurrent thromobosis, or family history of thrombosis, testing for inherited and acquired thrombophilias should be considered.

Only the patient under 40 years of age with no risk factors, undergoing a short procedure less than 30 minutes in duration, will require no prophylaxis. All others should receive one or a combination of pharmacological and mechanical prophylaxis. Mechanical methods such as graded compression stockings or intermittent pneumatic compression devices reduce venous stasis and promote endogenous fibrinolysis. Low-dose unfractionated heparin and low molecular weight heparin (LMWH) prevent clot formation by disrupting the clotting cascade.[37] All methods have each been shown to effectively reduce development of VTE. Gynecologic surgeons depend on data from the general surgery literature, which suggests that a combined regimen of medical and mechanical prophylaxis may improve efficacy, especially in patients at highest risk of VTE.

Preoperative discontinuation of hormonal contraceptives and hormone replacement is not a routine recommendation in gynecologic surgery. Although the Women's Health Initiative demonstrated an increased risk of VTE with estrogen and progesterone use, no existing trials demonstrate that discontinuation of hormones in the preoperative setting leads to a reduction in postsurgical VTE.[37] General surgery literature often recommends discontinuation of hormones four to six weeks prior to surgery.[5] However, gynecologic surgeons must consider the risks of unintended pregnancy in addition to the therapeutic benefits of hormonal treatments in the perioperative period. Hormonal medications should be considered in risk stratification for VTE prophylaxis.

Blood loss preparation

Patients frequently undergo gynecologic surgery for indications commonly associated with anemia. Importantly, perioperative anemia is associated with a fivefold increased risk of blood transfusion in patients undergoing major gynecologic surgery and has been associated with poor clinical outcome in noncardiac surgery patients.[38] Gynecologic surgeons thus should recognize preoperative anemia as an important and modifiable risk factor for surgery.[39] The preoperative evaluation provides the opportunity to detect and correct anemia prior to elective surgery. Iron deficiency anemia can be corrected with oral or intravenous iron supplementation. Oral iron, inexpensive and highly effective, is considered first line treatment for iron deficiency anemia.[40] Hormonal medications and pharmacologic therapies such as ibuprofen or tranexamic acid to decrease menstrual blood loss in the preoperative period can also be useful either alone or in combination with iron therapy. A Cochrane review on preoperative gonadotropin-releasing hormone (GnRH) analogue therapy before hysterectomy or myomectomy for uterine fibroids concludes that the use for three to four months prior to fibroid surgery is beneficial in the correction of preoperative iron deficiency anemia, and does reduce intraoperative blood loss.[41]

Concluding remarks

Preoperative risk assessment and optimization performed in the office setting can facilitate a smooth and safe intraoperative and postoperative course and improve overall outcomes. A thorough preoperative office evaluation for gynecologic surgery includes a complete history including a review of systems and assessment of functional status, a comprehensive physical examination, and the procurement of more information through laboratory and radiographic studies as indicated, for diagnostic and/or cardiopulmonary risk assessment. In general, the female patient undergoing an elective gynecologic low to intermediate-risk procedure is healthy. However, as the population ages and becomes more complex, it is important for the obstetrician-gynecologist to understand and use the algorithms for cardiac risk stratification for surgery. Preoperative testing should be chosen wisely. Evidence-based practices surrounding the use of thromboprophylaxis and antibiotics and for the treatment of perioperative anemia are followed to minimize surgical morbidity. Finally, the office preoperative evaluation is an opportunity to anticipate postoperative needs and set expectations for healing and recovery. The obstetrician-gynecologist plays a unique role in the longitudinal and comprehensive care of the female patient. Well equipped with knowledge of evidence-based guidelines and outcomes data to choose tests and interventions wisely, the obstetrician-gynecologist can guide the patient safely through the surgical experience.

References

1. Age and Sex Composition: 2010 Census Briefs. [Internet]. 2011 [issued 2011 May, cited 2014 August 31]. Available from: www.census.gov/prod/cen2010/briefs/c2010br-03.pdf.
2. Heisler CA, Aletti GD, Weaver AL, et al. Improving quality of care: development of a risk-adjusted perioperative morbidity model for vaginal hysterectomy. *Am J Obstet Gynecol* 2010; **202**:137.e1–5. doi: 10.1016/j.ajog.2009.06.059. Epub 2009 Aug 18.
3. Erekson EA, Yip SO, Martin DK, et al. Major postoperative complications after benign gynecologic surgery: a clinical prediction model. *Female Pelvic Med Reconstr Surg* 2012; **18**(5):274–80.
4. Rock JA, Thompson JD. *TeLinde's Operative Gynecology*. Philadelphia: Lippincott-Raven Publishers, 1997.
5. Johnson BE, Porter J. Preoperative evaluation of the gynecologic patient: considerations for improved outcomes. *Obstet Gynecol* 2008; **111**(5):1183–94.
6. Lilic G, Zivadinovic R, Petric A, Lilic V. Preoperative preparation of patients for gynecologic surgery. *Scientific Journal of the Faculty of Medicine in Nis* 2011; **28**(2):125–33.
7. Zambouri A. Preoperative evaluation and preparation for anesthesia and surgery. *Hippokratia* 2007; **11** (1):13–21.
8. Mann WJ. Overview of preoperative evaluation and preparation for gynecologic surgery [Internet]. 2013 [updated 2014 Apr 28, cited 2014 Aug 31]. Available from: www.uptodate.com.
9. Steege JF, Siedhoff MT. Clinical expert series: chronic pelvic pin. *Obstet Gynecol* 2014; **124**:616–29.
10. American College of Obstetricians and Gynecologists. Pelvic organ prolapse. ACOG Practice Bulletin No. 85. *Obstet Gynecol* 2007; **110**:717–29.
11. American College of Obstetricians and Gynecologists. Management of adnexal masses. ACOG Practice Bulletin No. 83. *Obstet Gynecol* 2007; **110**:201–14.
12. Moore RG, Miller MC, Disilvestro P, et al. Evaluation of the diagnostic accuracy of the risk of ovarian malignancy algorithm in women with a pelvic mass. *Obstet Gynecol* 2011; **118**(2):280–8.
13. American College of Obstetricians and Gynecologists. Management of abnormal uterine bleeding associated with ovulatory dysfunction. ACOG Practice Bulletin No. 136. *Obstet Gynecol* 2013; **122**:176–85.
14. Howlader N, Noone AM, Krapcho M, et al., editors. SEER Cancer Statistics Review, 1975–2009 (vintage 2009 populations), National Cancer Institute. Bethesda (MD) [Internet]. 2012 [updated 2012 Aug 20, cited 2014 Aug 31]. Available from: http://seer.cancer.gov/csr/1975_2009_pops09.
15. American College of Obstetricians and Gynecologists. Power morcellation and occult malignancy in gynecologic surgery: a special report [Internet]. 2014 May [updated 2014 May; cited 2014 Aug 31]. Available from: www.acog.org/~/media/Task%20Force%20and%20Work%20Group%20Reports/MorecellationSpecialReport.pdf.
16. American College of Obstetricians and Gynecologists. Choosing the route of hysterectomy for benign disease. ACOG Committee Opinion No. 444. *Obstet Gynecol* 2009; **144**:1156–8.

17. Nieboer TE, Johnson N, Lethaby A, et al. Surgical approach to hysterectomy for benign gynaecological disease. *Cochrane Database Syst Rev*. 2009 Jul 8; **3**: CD003677. doi: 10.1002/14651858.DC003677.pub4.

18. ACOG Committee on Ethics. Informed consent. ACOG Committee Opinion No. 439. *Obstet Gynecol* 2009; **114**:401.

19. Barash, PG, Cullen BF, Stoelting RK, et al. *Clinical Anesthesia*, 6th ed. Philadelphia: Lippincott Williams & Wilkins, 2009.

20. Dresner N, Kurzman AR. Preoperative evaluation and preparation of the gynecologic patient. *Glob Libr Women's Med* (ISSN 1756–2228) 2008; doi: 10.3843/GLOWM.10423.

21. Bunde M, Suls J, Martin R, Barnett K. Hystersisters online: social support and social comparison among hysterectomy patients on the internet. *Ann Behav Med* 2006; **31**(3):271–8.

22. Kumar A, Srivastava U. Role of routine laboratory investigations in preoperative evaluation. *J Anaesthesiol Clin Pharmacol* 2011; **27**(2):174–9.

23. Choosing Wisely: an initiative of the ABIM Foundation [Internet]. 2014 [updated 2014, cited 2012 Jul 30]. Available from: www.choosingwisely.org.

24. American College of Obstetricians and Gynecologists: Five things physicians and patients should question. Choosing Wisely: an initiative of the ABIM Foundation [Internet]. 2013 [updated 2013 Feb 21, cited 2014 Aug 31]. Available from: www.choosingwisely.org/doctor-patient-lists/american-college-of-obstetricians-and-gynecologists.

25. American Society of Anesthesiologists: Five things physicians and patients should question. Choosing Wisely: an initiative of the ABIM Foundation [Internet]. 2013 [updated 2013, cited 2014 Aug 31]. Available from: www.choosingwisely.org/doctor-patient-lists/american-society-of-anesthesiologists.

26. Onuoha OC, Arkoosh VA, Fleisher LA. Choosing Wisely in anesthesiology: the gap between evidence and practice. *JAMA Intern Med* 2014 Jun 16. doi: 10.1001/jamainternmed.2014.2309. [Epub ahead of print].

27. Schein OD, Katz J, Bass EB, et al. The value of routine preoperative medical testing before cataract surgery. *N Engl J Med* 2000; **342**:168–75.

28. Benarroch-Gampel J, Sheffield KM, Duncan CB, et al. Preoperative laboratory testing in patients undergoing elective, low-risk ambulatory surgery. *Ann Surg* 2012; **256**(3):518–28.

29. Lee TH, Marcantonio, ER, Mangione CM, et al. Derivation and prospective validation of a simple index for prediction of cardiac risk of major noncardiac surgery. *Circulation* 1999; **100**: 1043–9.

30. Fleisher LA, Beckman JA, Brown KA, et al. ACC/AHA 2007 guidelines on perioperative cardiovascular evaluation and care for noncardiac surgery: a report of the American College of Cardiology/American Heart Association Task Force on practice guidelines (writing committee to revise the 2002 Guidelines on Perioperative Cardiovascular Evaluation for Noncardiac Surgery). *Circulation* 2007; **116**:e418–500.

31. Karnath B. Preoperative cardiac risk assessment. *Am Fam Physician* 2002; **66**(10):1889–97.

32. Sheffield KM, McAdams PS, Benarroch-Gampel J, et al. Overuse of preoperative cardiac stress testing in medicare patients undergoing elective noncardiac surgery. *Ann Surg* 2013; **257**(1):73–80.

33. Raymond R. Anesthetic management of the elderly patient. 53rd ASA Annual Meeting Refresher Course Lectures #321. 2002; p1–7.

34. American College of Obstetricians and Gynecologists. Antibiotic prophylaxis for gynecologic procedures. ACOG Practice Bulletin No. 104. *Obstet Gynecol* 2009; **113**:1180–9.

35. Mangram AJ, Horan TC, Pearson ML, et al. Guideline for prevention of surgical site infection [Internet]. 1999 [updated, cited 2014 Aug 31]. Accessible from: www.cdc.gov/ncidod/dhqp/gl_surgicalsite.html.

36. McElligott KA, Havrilesky LJ, Myers ER. Preoperative screening strategies for bacterial vaginosis prior to elective hysterectomy: a cost comparison study. *Am J Obstet Gynecol* 2011; **205**:500.e1–7.

37. American College of Obstetricians and Gynecologists. Prevention of deep vein thrombosis and pulmonary embolism. ACOG Practice Bulletin No. 84. *Obstet Gynecol* 2007; **110**:429–40.

38. Browning RM, Trentino K, Nathan EA, Hashemi N, Western Australian Patient Blood Management Program. Preoperative anaemia is common in patients undergoing major gynaecological surgery and is associated with a fivefold increased risk of transfusion. *Aust N Z J Obstet Gynaecol* 2012; **52**(5):455–9. doi: 10.1111/j.1479-828X.2012.01478.x. Epub 2012 Sept 7.

39. Baron DM, Hochrieser H, Posch M, et al. Preoperative anaemia is associated with poor clinical outcome in non-cardiac surgery patients. *Br J Anaesth* 2014; **113**(3):416–23. doi: 10.1093/bja/aeu098. Epub 2014 May 14.

40. Schrier SI, Mentzer WC. Treatment of the adult with iron deficiency anemia [Internet]. 2014 [updated 2014 Aug 5, cited 2014 Aug 31]. Available from: www.uptodate.com.

41. Lethaby A, Vollenhoven B, Sowter MC. Pre-operative GnRH analogue therapy before hysterectomy or myomectomy for uterine fibroids. *Cochrane Database Syst Rev* 2001; **2**:CD000547.

Chapter 7

Office procedures

Eric Swisher, Christinne Canela, and Patrice M. Weiss

Introduction

Recent trends in health-care delivery have dramatically increased the frequency of office based surgical procedures. Office procedures have quickly become more accessible and prevalent as technology, physician comfort, and reimbursement have reinforced this paradigm shift. Surgical procedures such as dilation and curettage, hysteroscopy, loop electrosurgical excision procedures, and global endometrial ablation are particularly well suited to an office setting provided the surgeon's skill set and patient selection are considered. Patient preference, medical history, pain tolerance, anatomy and anxiety among other factors must be evaluated in selecting patients for surgical management in the office. For some patients, the office may provide a more comfortable and less intimidating setting while limiting cost and reducing exposure to hospital acquired infections. Time management, logistics, and administrative burdens may also be more favorable both for patients and providers in the office versus a hospital surgical suite. Despite the migration of some procedures out of a more formal surgical setting, attention to quality of care, physician competency, and patient safety remains paramount and must be equivalent irrespective of the chosen setting.[1]

Several aspects of safe surgical care are universal irrespective of the facility in which such care is delivered. Although not historically implemented in the office environment, credentialing and privileging of providers for surgical procedures should be part of a culture of safety in offices providing invasive care.[1] Although the office setting may allow for less paperwork, a detailed patient history and physical including attention to allergies, medications, bleeding dyscrasias, and surgical risk factors are still required preparations.[1] Informed consent is a universal standard and must not be approached more casually for office based surgical procedures. Consent is a process and requires more than a signed form to ensure the patient is fully prepared for the proposed surgery. The surgeon must ensure that patients are aware of and agree with the procedure, its possible complications, the anticipated level of discomfort, the potential for aborting *in medias res*, and the option for choosing a hospital or surgery center instead of the office. Though the tenets of care are similar, a patient planning for surgery in the office must understand the limitations and nuances of office care. Ambulatory Care National Patient Safety Goals (NPSG) established by the Joint Commission provides an excellent framework for surgical safety in the office setting. Fundamental elements of the NPSG are patient identification, attention to medication safety, patient history and documentation, a preoperative verification process, and the intraoperative time out.[2] Perioperative patient identification and confirmation of surgical plans should follow well established operating room protocols and practices. A reliable mechanism for specimen management and result tracking must be in place. Checklists are very useful adjuncts to safe patient care, verification of preparation, and compliance with office procedures.[1]

D&C/Hysteroscopy

Hysteroscopy is an outpatient surgical procedure particularly amenable to safe and convenient delivery in the office setting. Such procedures may offer prompt diagnostic, and in some cases, therapeutic benefits such as the identification and removal of endometrial polyps. Patients suspected to have submucosal myomas would typically be less ideal candidates for office surgery unless resection was not intended. Office hysteroscopy also provides the option of transcervical tubal sterilization procedures – currently the Essure®

Office Care of Women, ed. Martin E. Olsen and Botros Rizk. Published by Cambridge University Press.

Table 7-1 Sample medication algorithm

- PM preop: Cytotec 100 mcg–200 mcg (4–5 PM)
- 1 hour preop:

Hydrocodone or oxycodone 1–2 tablets PO
Promethazine 25 mg PO or ondansetron 8 mg PO
Ketorolac 60 mg IM

- Postop:

Ibuprofen or another NSAID
Hydrocodone or oxycodone prn

Table 7-2 Typical equipment list

- Hysteroscope camera and monitor and fluid/tubing
- Paracervical block (2 × 10 cc 1% lidocaine)
- D&C tray (speculum, ring forceps, tenaculum, dilators, curette)
- Drape
- Sterile gown and sterile gloves
- Betadine or hibiclens
- Large Q-tips
- 4 × 4 sponges
- Specimen cup and fixative
- Endometrial sampling device (curette)
- Global endometrial ablation equipment if ablation planned

. Dilation and curettage (D&C) for missed abortion is also easily provided in the office. In many practices, office based D&C offers the additional benefit of readily available sonography for guidance of the cannula or curette, which avoids perforation and ensures complete evacuation or lesion retrieval. Global endometrial ablation by several methods lends itself to satisfactory delivery in the office. The authors prefer to pair hysteroscopy with all office endometrial ablations, which may add some degree of safety to the "blind" methods for the global endometrial ablation commonly in use. A sample medication algorithm for hysteroscopy and similar procedures is listed in Table 7-1. A typical equipment list for such procedures follows in Table 7-2.

Careful patient selection is prudent, and while postmenopausal and nulliparous patients may be safely evaluated by hysteroscopy in the office, a severely stenotic cervix or highly anxious patient should give the surgeon pause in the planning process. If the patient does not want her case in the office, the surgeon does not want her case in the office. Likewise, morbidly obese patients may be better served with a hospital procedure if medical complications are a concern or hyperflexion of the thighs is required to adequately access the cervix. Patients with cardiac or pulmonary disease and those with a complicated medical history should be carefully considered before offering surgical procedures in the office setting.

In the absence of plans for sedation, patients are not generally *nil per os* (NPO) and intravenous access is typically optional in most clinical situations. However, patients may be managed with more or less aggressive anesthesia protocols on an individual basis. In these authors' experience, the "awake" patient may provide some degree of protection against the risk of perforation versus the patient under heavy sedation or general anesthesia where the surgeon's tactile sense may be the only preventive measure. Pulse oximetry is an excellent monitoring device for instantaneous patient assessment throughout the surgical process. Some offices may utilize an anesthesia provider for sedation, thus making for a more outpatient surgery center experience. This approach is beyond the perspective of this chapter and does require a more rigorous medical screening process and more conservative perioperative management (NPO, IV access, supervised recovery).

Preoperative cervical ripening with misoprostol 12–24 hours prior to transcervical surgery often facilitates or eliminates the cervical dilation portion of the procedure. Patients are dosed with analgesics 30–60 minutes preoperatively. Oral oxycodone or hydrocodone, oral promethazine or ondansetron, and IM ketorolac in our practice are typical, although protocols vary considerably. Anxiolytics may be beneficial in some cases with use tailored to the individual patient. As with any surgical procedure, a time out is completed and the patient's antiseptic preparation will vary by surgeon preference. We use betadine or chlorhexidine to cleanse the cervix and vagina for hysteroscopy or D&C with drapes limited to either side of the vulva. Some providers may opt to include antiseptic cleansing of the vulva and thighs followed by a more formal draping process, but infection rates are low with either approach. In fact, the rates of infection are so low that many surgeons do not administer prophylactic antibiotics as a routine for office hysteroscopy.[3] Oral doxycycline or clindamycin may be administered if prophylaxis is desired. A cervical or paracervical block is a useful adjuvant, typically using 10 cc–15 cc of 1% xylocaine. While the block is evolving, the previously inspected and assembled surgical instruments are readied for use.

Office dilation and curettage can be very useful for both expedient management and patient convenience. As noted earlier, preoperative cervical ripening with misoprostol the day prior to surgery eases the cervical dilation portion of the procedure. In the case of a missed abortion, this ripening may cause undesirable cramping and bleeding. As previously mentioned, patients' may be dosed with analgesics 30–60 minutes preoperatively. Oral oxycodone or hydrocodone, oral promethazine or zofran, and IM ketorolac are commonly utilized. Anxiolytics may useful depending upon the patient. The D&C is performed in the usual manner following placement of a paracervical block using 10 cc–15 cc 1% xylocaine. The cervix is secured with a single tooth tenaculum and the os (opening) is dilated if necessary to accommodate a sharp currette or suction cannula. A 6 mm–7 mm suction cannula directed by sonography provides a safe and effective means of accomplishing surgical evacuation of most incomplete or missed abortions while minimizing risk of perforation or retained gestational tissue. Sharp curettage may be similarly utilized though often with greater patient discomfort. Several passes may be required, but the advantage of ultrasound guidance for the procedure is verification of complete evacuation without excessive endometrial trauma or risk of perforation. Perioperative hemorrhage is uncommon, but may be effectively treated with fluid resuscitation and 0.2 mg IM methylergonovine or 400 mcg–800 mcg misoprostol rectally. Intrauterine balloon via Foley or Bakri™ device may be an effective management of hemorrhage in extreme cases.

For simple diagnostic hysteroscopy, premedication and preparation are completed as previously detailed, and the hysteroscope is readied for insertion by priming the irrigation fluid though the tubing and completing a white balance for the camera. A single tooth tenaculum is placed on the anterior or posterior ectocervix. The cervix is then gently dilated to accommodate the hysteroscope as necessary. Preoperative misoprostol ripening may obviate the need for cervical dilation, especially in the parous patient. In fact, some patients may require use of the tenaculum to buckle the cervix around the hysteroscope to adequately seal the scope for uterine distension. The hysteroscope is advanced into the endometrial cavity under direct and hysteroscopic visualization. The findings may be documented by photography or by videography. Once the procedure is accomplished and the hysteroscope withdrawn, endocervical and endometrial tissue samples for histology may be obtained as clinically indicated. A repeat hysteroscopy may be performed following curettage to confirm adequate sampling of the endometrium or sampling of a particular lesion targeted for the procedure. Upon completion, the tenaculum and speculum are withdrawn and the patient is gradually returned to a supine and then sitting position.

Endometrial ablation

A global endometrial ablation in the office follows a similar preparation and implementation as described for hysteroscopy. If well screened for tolerance, motivation, and medical risk factors, the office ablation can be a very satisfying approach for clinician and patient. Preparing patients emotionally for the experience is critical. Once the patient has been dosed with preoperative narcotic, antiemetic, and NSAID as detailed earlier, the procedure is initiated with visualization of the cervix and paracervical block placement. The cervix is dilated to accommodate the hysteroscope if a cavity assessment was planned prior to the ablation. A preablation and postablation hysteroscopy is helpful in our opinion to evaluate the anatomy, confirm the trajectory for safe entry into the endometrial cavity, verify cavity dimensions, and to confirm a thorough ablative result upon completion. Endometrial sampling is accomplished if not previously performed. The ablation is then completed with the surgeon's preferred device (balloon, radiofrequency, cryoablation). Due to the potential for vagal hypotension and bradycardia, continuous pulse oximetry is a prudent choice during such a procedure. Such patients may require intramuscular atropine in severe cases.

Hysteroscopic sterilization

Essure and Adiana for tubal sterilization were developed with the expectation of in-office placement for most patients desiring this contraceptive approach. The Adiana is no longer marketed or available, but the Essure is a very effective and well-tolerated office sterilization procedure. It is so well tolerated that in our experience, some may only require a paracervical block in patients motivated to avoid all other perioperative medications for personal reasons. It is a safe

Table 7-3 Key components in counseling patients on hysteroscopic sterilization [6]

1. Sterilization is considered permanent and not meant for reversal.
2. The details of the procedure, including the risks and benefits of the procedure itself and of analgesia should be reviewed with the patient.
   Some of the risks associated with hysteroscopy and Essure® include fluid overload, infection, cervical injury, uterine or tubal perforation, insert expulsion, cramping, pain, nausea, vomiting, dizziness, light-headedness, vasovagal response, vaginal bleeding/ spotting.
3. Five-year failure rate for Essure is 1.64 pregnancies per 1,000 procedures, including the possibility of ectopic pregnancies.
4. The risk of regret, which is higher in women who are younger than 30 years, regardless of parity or marital status, should be discussed.
5. Alternative methods of contraception such as long-acting reversible methods and vasectomy should be reviewed.
6. Sterilization does not protect against sexually transmitted infections; therefore, condom use should be encouraged.
7. The patient needs to use an alternative method of contraception until tubal occlusion can be confirmed by hysterosalpingogram, typically three months after the procedure.
8. Regulations mandating time interval from consent to procedure, if applicable.

and viable option for women who have completed childbearing. Advantages include the ability to safely perform the procedure in the office setting with minimal or no anesthesia, avoidance of intra-abdominal entry, and the avoidance of incisions. Appropriate patient selection and counseling is mandatory prior to the procedure (Table 7-3). Complications of Essure placement include tubal perforation (1%–3% in the Essure clinical trials), improper coil placement (intraperitoneal placement in 0.5%–3% and other improper placements in 0.5%) and expulsion of the occlusion device (in 0.4%–2.2%). A retrospective study of 4, 306 office-based Essure placements demonstrated its efficacy and safety with 98.5% of patients having successful bilateral coil placement and a low overall complication rate of 2.7%, the most common of which was vasovagal syncope.[4, 5] Patients should be counseled on the possibility that bilateral coil placement may not be achievable for each patient, therefore, contingency plans should be reviewed in the event that bilateral placement is not achieved. Known contraindications to the procedure should also be identified prior to the procedure (Table 7-4).[6]

Table 7-4 Contraindications for hysteroscopic sterilization

- Pregnancy
- Less than six weeks postpartum or post abortion
- Uncertainty about sterilization
- Active or recent pelvic infection
- Abnormal uterine or tubal anatomy that precludes access to the tubal ostia
- Prior tubal surgery (e.g., prior tubal ligation, surgery for tubal pregnancy or tuboplasty)
- Those who can only have one tubal insert placed (e.g., suspected unicornuate uterus, contralateral proximal tubal occlusion)
- History of hydrosalpinx
- Known allergy to contrast media

Ideally, the patient is scheduled during the early proliferative phase of her menstrual cycle to ensure a thin endometrium. Alternatively, she may be pretreated with combined oral contraceptives or progestins. If indicated, she may be provided with a single dose of misoprostol 200 mcg–400 mcg the night prior to the procedure for cervical preparation. A negative pregnancy test is required. The patient is given NSAIDs (e.g., IM ketorolac) one hour prior to the procedure. An anxiolytic may be provided 30 minutes prior to the procedure. IV sedation may also be provided if desired. The patient is prepped for hysteroscopy as described previously. The uterine cavity is distended with prewarmed saline at a minimum infusion pressure to visualize both tubal ostia and prevent tubal spasm. The procedure should be aborted if the tubal ostium is not visible or accessible or if either ostium does not appear to be patent. For cost containment, it is prudent to delay opening the Essure packaging until visualization of both tubal ostia is confirmed. The speculum may be removed following introduction of the hysteroscope into the uterine cavity. The introducer is inserted through the sealing cap on operating channel of the hysteroscope. The delivery catheter is then inserted through the introducer and under direct visualization; the catheter is advanced through the operating channel into the proximal fallopian tube with gentle, constant forward movement to prevent tubal spasm. If excessive resistance is encountered, the procedure should be terminated to avoid uterine perforation or placement into a false passage. The proximal end of the black positioning marker is aligned with the ostium. The delivery system is stabilized against the hysteroscope to prevent inadvertent forward movement. The thumbwheel is rotated on the handle toward the surgeon until the wheel no longer rotates. The delivery catheter and the black positioning marker will move away from the tubal ostium and disappear into the operating channel. The gold marker should be just outside the ostium and the distal tip of the green release catheter should be easily visualized. If more than 1 cm of the insert is visible in the uterus, the insert can be repositioned by moving the entire system further into the tube. The button on the purple handle is pressed, thus enabling one to rotate the thumbwheel further for insert deployment. When the thumbwheel cannot be rotated any further and the expanded outer coils are visible, the delivery system may be removed. The same procedure is performed on the opposite tube. Ideally, three to eight expanded outer coils should be trailing into the uterus. The number of visible coils should be recorded. The patient is advised to call for fevers, excessive vaginal bleeding, or severe or persistent pain. It is imperative that a hysterosalpingogram (HSG) be performed three months after placement to confirm tubal occlusion and that back-up contraception is used until then.[7]

LEEP

The loop electrosurgical excision procedure (LEEP) is another procedure that may readily be performed in the office setting. It involves removal of the transformation zone of the cervix and is currently the most common method for the treatment of cervical intraepithelial neoplasia CIN 2,3. It is typically performed in the office under local anesthesia. It is well tolerated by patients and offers the advantage of less bleeding and smaller volume of tissue loss compared to cold knife conization.[8]

Counseling the patient adequately on the risks associated with the procedure such as bleeding, infection, discomfort, potential cervical stenosis, implications for future pregnancies including the risk of preterm birth is necessary. The potential for positive margins requiring repeat excision should also be reviewed with the patient.

An insulated speculum with suction via intravaginal tubing is placed in the vagina ensuring good visualization of the cervix. The cervix is cleansed and acetic acid or Lugol's solution is placed on the cervix to better identify the lesion(s) for excision. A paracervical block using 1% lidocaine with or without epinephrine is injected circumferentially into the cervix. Studies performed to evaluate pain relief for women undergoing loop excisions found that intracervical injection of local anesthetic with a vasoconstrictor appears to provide optimum analgesia for treatment.[9] The patient is grounded appropriately. An appropriately sized wire loop is chosen and attached to the cautery instrument that provides a cutting current. The appropriate settings are chosen and set into the electrosurgical generator. Some providers use a blended current, which mixes cutting and coagulating currents (one can set the generator at 30 W–40 W on blend 1). It is important to note that the higher the blend, the more the coagulating current and the greater the thermal damage. Some providers use a pure cutting current at 80 W. Normal saline can be applied to the exocervix to rehydrate the tissue and decrease the risk of the loop electrode sticking to the tissue. The loop is then carefully passed around and under the transformation zone, thus excising it fully. Care should be taken to move the loop along the tissue properly to obtain an appropriate specimen. If the loop is passed too quickly through the cervix, the loop can drag, bend, or adhere to the tissue, which may result in a shallower excision than intended. If the loop is passed too slowly through the tissues, there may be excess thermal damage to the specimen. If the lesion extends into the endocervical canal, additional tissue may be excised using a smaller diameter rectangular loop or a top hat. Once the specimen is obtained, it is carefully removed in the correct orientation. A suture placed at the 12 o'clock position on the excised specimen will better orient the specimen for histopathologic examination.

Hemostasis of the LEEP bed typically requires coagulation using the 5 mm ball electrode on a coagulating setting. Use of Monsel's (ferric subsulfate) paste/solution will also aid in hemostasis. If bleeding continues despite these measures, one can place a suture at the 3 o'clock and 9 o'clock positions at the distal point of the cervix to decrease the pulse pressure from the cervical arteries. Gelfoam® may also be placed at the base and a suture tied across the front of the cervix to keep the Gelfoam in place.[8, 10, 11]

After the procedure, the patient is then advised to avoid intercourse and observe pelvic rest for two to four weeks. The patient is typically seen in the office six weeks after the procedure. The patient is also advised of signs to watch for including: abnormal looking vaginal discharge and excessive vaginal bleeding.

Vulvar biopsy

The investigation of a vulvar lesion or persistent irritation will often include a biopsy. This is typically an office procedure in all but the most hesitant of patients or in the case of a very extensive lesion. Vascular lesions may also be better served in a better equipped surgical setting. Any lesion of uncertain etiology, irritation that has failed medical or expectant therapy, abnormal pigmentation, or tissue suspicious for atypia warrants a biopsy for histologic evaluation. Targeting biopsies when atypia is suspected may improve with the application of 5% acetic acid and magnification via a colposcope.

Vulvar tissue samples may be obtained as a punch biopsy (Keyes punch), shave biopsy, or elliptical excisional biopsy. Location may dictate the diagnostic approach and anesthetic options. Topical xylocaine-prilocaine may provide adequate anesthesia for some patients, but the typical biopsy is performed with local subcutaneous xylocaine anesthesia. Take care during injection to avoid distorting the targeted tissue with an excessive volume of anesthetic. A deeper subcutaneous injection of xylocaine may elevate the lesion to improve access for a shave biopsy. Excessive infiltration may obscure the targeted tissues and compromise accurate sampling.

Once a antimicrobial preparation has been preformed and adequate local anesthesia is established, a punch biopsy is obtained by stabilizing the skin between the thumb and forefinger while cutting tissue perpendicularly into the skin with a Keyes punch or with a cervical biopsy instrument such as a Kevorkian or Tischler cervical biopsy punch. When using a cervical punch biopsy device on the vulva, avoid skimming the epidermis when closing the jaws by applying pressure against the targeted tissue prior to closing the device to obtain a more substantial biopsy. A Keyes punch cuts a cylindrical biopsy using a simple twisting motion – clockwise and counterclockwise perpendicular to the vulvar surface. The cored specimen may require forceps to retrieve and scissors or a scalpel to divide at the base. A localized lesion highly suspicious for atypia or malignancy should be excised with peripheral margins of normal tissue if possible. This may require an elliptical excision if the lesion is larger than a few millimeters. Using a scalpel and stabilizing the vulvar skin in the linear direction of the incision, an elliptical incision around the lesion may allow for full exision, but will likely require suture closure for approximation and hemostasis.

Direct pressure may accomplish adequate hemostasis for small biopsy sites, but the vascularity of the vulva typically results in a magnitude of bleeding which may exceed expectations even in the most minimal of excisions. Silver nitrate or ferrous subsulfate (Monsel's solution) applied to the biopsy site followed by direct pressure will achieve hemostasis in most cases. If bleeding persists, place simple interrupted or figure-eight stitches using fine (3–0 or 4–0) catgut or polyglactin suture. Application of a folded gauze or sanitary pad to be held in place by the patient's underwear may avoid subsequent bleeding or soiled clothing.

Nexplanon

The Nexplanon® device is a long-term reversible contraceptive method that is implanted subdermally in the upper arm. It is easily placed and removed in the office setting. It consists of a single 4 cm radio-opaque rod that contains 68 mg of etonorgestrel that is slowly released over a three-year period. Careful counseling prior to placement is important and should include the risks of infection, scarring, hematoma, irregular/breakthrough bleeding, failure, migration, expulsion, and risks of deep insertion including difficult removal requiring removal in the operating room and the risk of neurovascular injury. Prior to placement, one should ensure that there are no contraindications to progesterone use and that pregnancy is excluded.

When placing the Nexplanon device, the patient is laid in supine position with the nondominant arm flexed at the elbow and externally rotated with the wrist parallel to the ear and the hand next to the patient's head. The insertion site is identified and marked. This is located on the inner side of the nondominant upper arm about 8 cm–10 cm or 3 in–4 in above the medial epicondyle of the humerus in the sulcus between the biceps and the triceps. A second mark is made several centimeters proximal to the initial mark to serve as a guide during the insertion process. The insertion site is cleansed with an antiseptic solution such as Betadine. Local anesthesia such as 1% lidocaine is injected along the intended track. The protection cap on the Nexplanon applicator should be easy to remove and the presence of the device can be confirmed by visualizing the white-colored implant by looking into the tip of the needle. The skin at the insertion site is stretched with one's free hand. The skin is then punctured with the tip of the needle angled about 30 degrees. The applicator is then lowered to a horizontal position and the entire needle is inserted along the track. It is important to lift the skin as the needle is inserted into the track to ensure subdermal placement. A seated position and looking at the applicator from the side is the best position to see the movement of the needle. With the applicator in place and stabilized, the purple slider is pushed and slid back fully until it stops to deploy the device. The implant will now be in place and can be palpated in its subdermal position. It is important not to touch the purple slider until this point. The implant should be palpated by the physician and the patient. Steri-Strips and Mastisol should then be applied to the puncture site; this can be removed in three to five days. A pressure bandage using sterile gauze is then applied to minimize bruising, the patient is instructed to remove this in 24 hours.

To remove the Nexplanon device, it is important to know the exact location of the implant on the arm, as verified by palpation. The distal end of the implant (closest to the elbow) is marked and cleaned with an antiseptic solution. The incision site is anesthesized with local anesthesia, the anesthetic is injected under the implant to keep the implant close to the skin. A longitudinal incision toward the elbow is made with the scalpel on the distal end of the implant. The implant is gently pushed toward the incision site until the tip is visible. The implant is then grasped with forceps and removed. If it is encapsulated, an incision can be made into the tissue sheath and the implant removed with forceps. If the implant is not visible, forceps could be inserted into the incision and a second pair forceps can be used to dissect the tissue around the implant and grasp the implant for removal. Once removed, the implant is measured (should be 4 cm) to ensure complete removal of the device. If a new implant is desired, it may be placed immediately after the old implant is removed using the same incision. The incision is then closed with Steri-Strips and Mastisol, which may be removed in three to five days. A pressure bandage using gauze is applied to minimize bruising and the patient is instructed to remove this in 24 hours.

If the implant is not immediately palpable, efforts to locate the implant such as two-dimensional x-ray, x-ray computer tomography (CT), ultrasound scanning with a high-frequency linear array transducer (10 MHz or higher), or magnetic resonance imaging (MRI) should be undertaken. If this fails to identify the implant, the company should be called at 1-877-467-5266 to determine etonorgestrel levels. After confirming the location of the implant, removal can be undertaken with ultrasound guidance. Exploratory surgery is not recommended until the exact location of the implant is known. If an implant is deeply inserted, removal should be performed by a health-care provider familiar with anatomy of the arm to avoid injury to deeper neurovascular structures.

Ultrasound utilization

Ultrasound guidance is an invaluable adjunct to office procedures. Specifically, sonography may contribute to the ease and safety of IUD placement, IUD retrieval, endometrial polypectomy, endometrial sampling by directed curettage, and suction evacuation of early pregnancy loss. For difficult IUD insertions (e.g., nulliparous patients or those with a malpositioned uterus), one may consider the use of 400 mcg of intravaginal or oral misoprostol administered 12 hours prior to insertion. Data on the use of intravaginal misoprostol for cervical preparation in IUD candidates have been conflicting. A double blind randomized trial using 400 mcg of intravaginal misoprostol administered three hours prior to IUD insertion showed no difference in patient perception of pain and provider ease of IUD placement.[13] Conversely, a randomized controlled trial using administration of 400 mcg sublingual misoprostol was associated with easier insertion as perceived by the provider and no difference in patient perception.[14] A paracervical or intracervical block using 10 cc–15 cc of 1% lidocaine may also improve patient tolerance.[15] Sonography during or following a difficult IUD insertion may assist with appropriate placement or confirmation of appropriate placement within the uterine cavity. During retrieval of an IUD when the strings are not visible, sonography often makes recovery a simple and easy process. This obviates the need for retrieval by operative hysteroscopy. IUD forceps or Randall stone forceps combined with transabdominal imaging allows for real time visualization of an IUD or polyp for the safest possible entry into the uterus and efficient recovery of the target. A paracervical block is typically helpful for patient tolerance of the procedure and oral or intramuscular analgesia may be appropriate for some patients. Patients with a missed or incomplete abortion may benefit from ultrasound guided suction curettage. A sonogram guided D&C provides the additional benefit of confirmatory imaging immediately preoperatively. This verification is especially helpful for the potential doubt of a patient suffering a miscarriage and in other patients to reassess the location and size of endometrial polyps or pathology. In the author's experience, the addition of sonography improves efficiency of the evacuation and reduces the risk of perforation by real-time visualization of the cannula or curette throughout the procedure.

Concluding remarks

Surgical care in the office introduces a variety of logistical and safety issues beyond those typical of routine office care. The additional risk of a perioperative complication requires emergency preparedness, which should include staff training, resuscitation equipment, and mock drills. There should be one standard of care for procedures whether in the hospital or ambulatory surgical setting or the office. It is expected that office procedures will only increase over the next few years, and strict attention and diligence to protocols is paramount. This chapter sought to present a few such protocols and safety standards to ensure that patients having procedures in the office for convenience are not compromising safety. Finally, it is the providers' responsibility to assure that the patient is an appropriate candidate for an office procedure as well as assuring that all office personnel are trained and educated in emergency preparedness if complications arise.

References

1. American College of Obstetricians and Gynecologists. Report of the Presidential Task Force on Patient Safety in the Office Setting. In: *Quality and Safety in Women's Health Care*, 2nd edition. Washington, DC: American College of Obstetricians and Gynecologists; 2010: 91–8.
2. Ambulatory Health Care: 2011 National Patient Safety Goals, effective July 1, 2011. Available at: www.jointcommission.org.
3. Nezhat C, Nezhat F, Nezhat C. *Nezhat's Operative Gynecologic Laparoscopy and Hysteroscopy*. London: Cambridge University Press; 2008: 98–100.
4. Basinski CM. A review of clinical data for currently approved hysteroscopic sterilization procedures. *Rev Obstet Gynecol* 2010; **3**:101–10.
5. Povedano B, Arjona JE, Velasco E, Monserrat JA, Lorente J, Castelo-Branco C. Complications of hysteroscopic Essure® sterilisation: report on 4306 procedures performed in a single centre. *BJOG* 2012; **119**:795–9.
6. American College of Obstetricians and Gynecologists. Benefits and risks of sterilization. ACOG Practice Bulletin No. 133. *Obstet Gynecol* 2013; **121**:392–404.
7. Essure®. Instructions for use. Available at: www.essuremd.com/App_Themes/BaseTheme/PDFs/Link%20Essure%20IFU.pdf. Accessed Jun 3, 2014.
8. Noller KL. Intraepithelial neoplasia of the lower genital tract (cervix, vulva): etiology, screening, diagnostic techniques, management. In: Lentz GM, Lobo RA, Gershenson DM, Katz VL, editors. *Comprehensive Gynecology*, 6th edition. Philadelphia: Elsevier Mosby; 2012: 653–65.
9. Gajjar K, Martin-Hirsch PP, Bryant A. Pain relief for women with cervical intraepithelial neoplasia undergoing colposcopy treatment. *Cochrane Database Syst Rev*. 2012 Oct 17; **10**:CD006120.
10. Damewood DD, Keye WR, Coddington III CC. Office gynecology and surgical procedures. In: Gibbs RS, Karlan BY, Haney AF, Nygaard IE, editors. *Danforth's Obstetrics and Gynecology*, 10th edition. Philadelphia: Lippincott Williams & Wilkins; 2008: 514–39.
11. Fuh K, Blumenthal PD. Loop electrosurgical excision procedure (LEEP). In: *A Practical Guide to Office Gynecologic Procedures*. Philadelphia: Lippincott Williams & Wilkins; 2013: 80–6.
12. www.merck.com/product/usa/pi_circulars/n/nexplanon/nexplanon_pi.pdf. Accessed Oct 30, 2014.
13. Heikinheimo O, Inki P, Kunz M, et al. Double-blind randomized placebo-controlled study on the effect of misoprostol on ease of consecutive insertion of the levonorgestrel-releasing intrauterine system. *Contraception* 2010; **81**:481–6.
14. Sääv I, Aronsson A, Marions L, et al. Cervical priming with sublingual misoprostol prior to insertion of an intrauterine device in nulliparous women: a randomized controlled trial. *Hum Reprod* 2007; **22**: 2647–52.
15. Vickery Z, Madden T. Difficult intrauterine contraception insertion in a nulligravid patient. *Obstetrics & Gynecology* 2011 Feb; **117**(2 Pt 1):391–5.

Chapter 8

Office management of cervical intraepithelial neoplasia

Sheri Holmes and Martin E. Olsen

Introduction

Cervical intraepithelial neoplasia (CIN) can be a precursor for malignancy of the uterine cervix.[1] Health-care providers screen and diagnose CIN, and if indicated will treat CIN, in order to prevent cervical cancer. Pathologically, CIN is characterized by cellular changes including increased cellularity, nuclear abnormalities, and increased nuclear to cytoplasmic ratio. There is a progressive polarized loss of squamous differentiation. To remain within the category of preinvasive disease, the abnormality must not penetrate the basement membrane; if it does so, the abnormality is defined as cervical cancer.

Squamous epithelial abnormalities are referred to as CIN when they involve the ectocervix; abnormalities involving the endocervix are referred to as glandular cell abnormalities and include adenocarcinoma and adenocarcinoma in situ. Box 8-1 shows a list of terms associated with the description and management of CIN.

Previously, premalignant abnormalities of the cervix were labeled dysplasia and stratified as mild, moderate, or severe. The Bethesda terminology system of reporting was developed in 1988 and has under gone two revisions since that time, the last being in 2001. In the Bethesda system, cervical intraepithelial neoplasia also has three degrees of severity. CIN 1 is considered a low-grade lesion with mildly atypical cellular changes in the lower third of the epithelium. These changes are often human papillomavirus (HPV) mediated with koilocytotic changes. The cellular changes with CIN 2 are confined to the basal two-thirds of the epithelium. CIN 2 is considered a high-grade lesion with a fair degree of intraobservational variability.

CIN 3 refers to cellular changes involving greater than two-thirds of the epithelial thickness and is also a high-grade lesion.[2] Figure 8-1 shows a schematic representation of the spectrum of CIN 3 to normal.

In an effort to streamline terminology, in 2012 the Lower Anogenital Squamous Terminology (LAST) project of the American Society for Colposcopy and Cervical Pathology (ASCCP) and the American College of Pathology released findings and subsequently developed a system, which combines histologic cervical abnormalities with the same terminology as cytologic findings.[3]

In this system, CIN 1 is referred to as low-grade squamous cell intraepithelial lesion (LSIL). CIN 2 has poor reproducibility and is thought to be a mixture of lesions that could be CIN 1 and/or CIN 3. CIN 3 is

BOX 8-1 Abbreviations, acronyms, and terms

AIS – adenocarcinoma in situ

ASCCP – American Society for Colposcopy and Cervical Pathology

ASCUS – atypical squamous cells of undermined significance

ASC-H – atypical squamous cells: cannot rule out high-grade squamous intraepithelial lesion

AGC – atypical glandular cells

CIN – cervical intraepithelial neoplasia

Co-test – perform both cytology (Pap test) plus HPV test

EC/TZ – endocervical/transformation zone

HPV – human papillomavirus

HSIL – high-grade squamous intraepithelial lesion

LAST – Lower Anogenital Squamous Terminology

Lesser abnormalities – include ASCUS, LSIL, HPV 16+ on 18+, persistent HPV

LSIL – low-grade squamous intraepithelial lesion

NILM – negative for intraepithelial lesion or malignancy

NOS – not otherwise specified

Office Care of Women, ed. Martin E. Olsen and Botros Rizk. Published by Cambridge University Press.

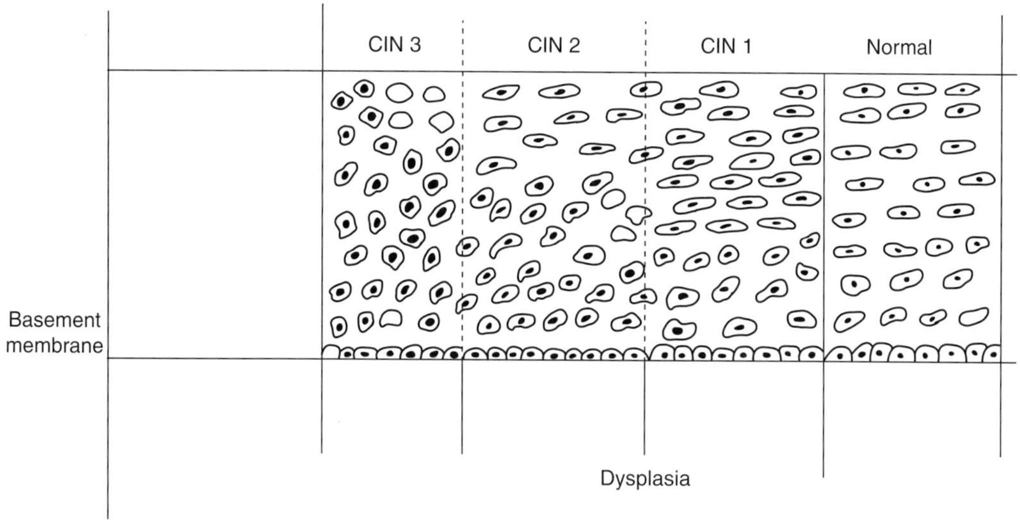

Figure 8-1 Schematic of cervical intraepithelial neoplasia.

categorized as high-grade squamous intraepithelial lesion (HSIL). An immunohistochemical marker used in gynecologic pathology and associated with high-risk HPV viral subtypes is p16. A lesion that is p16 negative is categorized as LSIL, whereas a lesion that is p16 positive is categorized as HSIL.

Scope of the problem

Both the incidence and mortality from cervical cancer in the United States has decreased by more than 50% in the past 40 years. This improvement is largely due to widespread screening with cervical cytology. The incidence of cervical cancer in 1975 was approximately 14.8 per 100,000 women and with increased screening had been reduced to 6.6 per 100,000 women in 2008.[4]

Similarly, in 1975 the mortality rate was 5.5 per 100,000 women with a decrease to 2.38 per 100,000 women in 2008. In 2011, 4,092 women in the United States died as a result of cervical cancer.[5]

Additionally, a diagnosis of cytologic abnormality or HPV infection creates concerns and anxieties in many patients. This can result in a negative impact on a woman's psychologic well-being in addition to the risk of progression to cervical cancer.[6]

Natural history of cervical intraepithelial neoplasia

HPV is the causative agent for both CIN and cervical cancer. Contraction of HPV by the patient results in either transient or persistent infection.[7] Most infections are transient and pose little risk of progression to CIN or cancer.

HPV types are classified as either low-risk (nononcogenic) or high-risk (oncogenic). The majority of invasive cervical cancers have been found to have an HPV infection etiology. While there are over hundred HPV subtypes only a small percentage of those directly involve the anogenital region. Low-risk subtypes such as HPV 6 and 11 are considered to be nononcogenic. These cause low-grade lesions such as benign condyloma or genital warts.[8] See Table 8-1 for a list of risk factors associated with the development of cervical dysplasia.

High-risk subtypes, primarily recognized as HPV 16 and 18, but also including 33, 35, 45, 51, 52, 56, and 58 have been found to be involved in the genesis of CIN. Infection with these subtypes does not, however, automatically translate into cervical disease; a large percentage of these infections are transient in nature. Only a small percentage of these infections have continued persistence. Persistence at one and two years is predictive of development of CIN 3, regardless of age.[9] HPV 16 is recognized as having the highest carcinogenic potential and it accounts for approximately 60% of all cervical cancer cases worldwide. HPV 18 is the next most common accounting for 10%–15% of cervical cancer cases. More than 50% of new HPV infections will resolve spontaneously in 6–18 months; approximately 90% resolve within two to five years.[10] As the majority of these HPV infections

Table 8-1 Recognized risk factors for the development of cervical dysplasia

- Coitus during puberty (during time of peak metaplasia)
- Diethylstilbestrol (DES) exposure in utero
- Multiple sexual partners
- Exposure to sexually transmitted diseases
- HIV
- Substance abuse
- High-risk male partner
- Depressed social economic status
- Lack of access to care
- Tobacco use
- HPV infection

resolve without treatment, expectant management is prudent in many cases. Even with persistent HPV infection, however, most cervical neoplasia will have slow progression. The average development to invasive cervical cancer from CIN 3 may take anywhere from three to seven years. For patients with untreated CIN 3, the cumulative incidence of invasive cancer has been found to be approximately 30% at 30 years. This indicates that the presence of CIN 3 is a significant risk for progression to cancer.[11]

High-risk cervical HPV is also associated with high-risk anal HPV and subsequent abnormal anal cytology.[12]

Prevention of cervical intraepithelial neoplasia

The primary prevention for CIN and subsequent development of cervical cancer is administration of vaccines that target HPV 16 and HPV 18. Two vaccine types have been available in the United States for approximately 10 years, the first of which is bivalent and the second of which is quadrivalent. Both types cover HPV 16 and HPV 18, whereas the quadrivalent provides additional coverage against the low-risk types HPV 6 and HPV 11. Release of a nonavalent vaccine became available in 2015; it covers nine HPV subtypes. The American Congress of Obstetrics and Gynecology (ACOG) and the Centers for Disease Control and Prevention (CDC) recommend that the vaccine be administered to females between 9 and 26 years of age. For the vaccine to be most efficacious, it should be provided prior to viral exposure to increase the vaccine efficacy.[13]

It is surmised that a significant reduction in the incidence in cervical cancer will not be observed until approximately 20 years after widespread vaccination is utilized. Cervical cancer has been reported in women who have previously been immunized, so continued cervical surveillance is definitely indicated after vaccination.[14, 15]

Screening for cervical intraepithelial neoplasia

The majority of cervical cancers occur in women who were inadequately or never screened.[16, 17] Only a small percentage of women infected with HPV will develop CIN or cancer of the cervix. Cervical cytology screening techniques include the traditional method where exfoliated cells are collected from the transformation zone of the cervix and transferred directly to a slide or a liquid-based method where the cells are transferred to a vial of liquid preservative. Both methods are acceptable for screening.[18] In the United States, cytologic test results reported using the Bethesda system (see Table 8-2).

HPV screening has two indications:[18]

1. Reflex testing helps determine the need for colposcopy in women with an atypical squamous cells of undetermined significance (ASCUS) cytology result.
2. Co-testing, the use of HPV typing with cytology, can be done in women aged 30 years and older as an adjunct to cytology alone.

Testing is done only to detect high-risk HPV; there is no role for the screening of low-risk genotypes.

Women aged 21–29 should be tested with cytology alone every three years.[19] Co-testing every five years is the recommended screening for women aged 30–65 years by ACOG. Alternatively, conventional or liquid-based cytology alone could be performed every three years in the 30–65 age group. It must be remembered that these recommendations are for the general population of patients. Patients with a history of treatment for CIN may benefit from more frequent screening. HIV-positive patients, women who are immunocompromised, and women exposed to diethylstilbestrol in utero may require more frequent screening. Screening may be discontinued after age 65 in women with negative prior screening results and no history of CIN 2 or higher. Women who have had a hysterectomy with removal of the cervix, and are without a history of CIN 2 or higher, also no longer require screening.

Table 8-2 Bethesda system of cervical cytologic test reporting and descriptive terms (abbreviated)

Specimen type
Conventional Pap test or liquid-based preparation
Specimen adequacy
Satisfactory for evaluation
Unsatisfactory for evaluation: (a) specimen rejected or not processed, (b) specimen processed and examined but was unsatisfactory for evaluation because of a specified reason
General categorization
Negative for intraepithelial lesion or malignancy
Other findings
Epithelial cell abnormality (specify squamous or glandular if appropriate)
Interpretation/result
Negative for intraepithelial lesion or malignancy
Organisms (list organisms visualized or changes associated with the presence of fungal bacterial and viral infections)
Other nonneoplastic findings
Epithelial cell abnormalities including ASC, ASC US, ASC-H, LSIL, HSIL, squamous cell carcinoma
Glandular cell abnormalities
Endocervical adenocarcinoma in situ (AIS)
Adenocarcinoma
Other malignant neoplasms

Women with prior high-grade cervical intraepithelial lesions continue to require screening after hysterectomy.

Colposcopy

Colposcopy is an accepted diagnostic standard for women with abnormal cytologic testing and positive high-risk HPV results.[20] A colposcope is used to magnify and visually assess the cervix for abnormalities. Colposcopically directed biopsies can then be performed in any abnormal areas; colposcopic expertise requires significant training and is beyond the scope of this chapter. Biopsies of all visual lesions are warranted.[21]

At the time of colposcopy, sampling of the endocervix can be performed with endocervical curettage or vigorous endocervical brush sampling. [21] Pregnant patients should *not* receive endocervical sampling. Sampling should be performed if the colposcopy is inadequate or if ablative therapy (discussed later in the chapter) is planned. Endocervical sampling is optional for patients with ASCUS or LSIL.[21]

For some patients, follow-up is sub-optimal at times. Some of these patients will have biopsy proven CIN 2 or higher and be lost to follow-up. For this reason, some patients have been offered a "see and treat" approach such that a loop electrical excision procedure (LEEP, discussed later in the chapter) is performed on selected patients at the time of colposcopy. This approach may be preferable for some patients but does result in overtreatment.[22] LEEP has long-term complications such as preterm labor and increased miscarriage.[23, 24] Younger patients are therefore best treated with a two-step approach. [22, 23] Young in this case applies to women who have plans for future conception.

Management

Modern management of CIN is tailored to the population served as well as the specific lesion involved. Consensus is strong that lesions at the level of CIN 1 should be observed. These lesions will usually regress as the patient's immune system confronts the HPV virus. The management of higher grade lesions will be discussed later in the following sections and in the accompanying tables. Many portions of the reported data are compiled from publications by the ASCCP and ACOG.[25, 26]

Mobile applications such as ASCCP mobile are purchased by many practitioners to access guidelines and algorithms since recent management guidelines have become complex and are probably not amenable to memorization

Adolescents

Current guidelines recommend against cervical screening for patients under the age of 21. Isolated cases of cervical cancer in adolescents have been reported, [27–29] but the consensus is strong that the risk–benefit ratio favors delay in screening until age 21. When screening occurs earlier than recommended, increased anxiety, morbidity, and expense are found

Table 8-3 Ages 21–24, ASCUS or LSIL

- Repeat cytology at 12 months preferred; reflex HPV testing acceptable for ASCUS only
- If ASCUS, HPV negative, resume routine screening
- If ASCUS, HPV positive, repeat cytology at 12 months (immediate colposcopy or repeat HPV *not recommended*)
- On 12-month repeat cytology:
  - If negative, ASCUS, or LSIL – again repeat in 12 months – if negative ×2, resume routine screening
  - If ASC-H, AGC, HSIL – proceed to colposcopy
- If LSIL, repeat cytology in 12 months (colposcopy not recommended)

Table 8-5 Ages 21–24, with no lesion or CIN 1 after

a) **ASC US or LSIL**

- 21–24 years old with CIN 1 – treatment is *unacceptable*; may repeat cytology at 12 months intervals, but HPV testing *unacceptable*
- If 12 months repeat <ASC-H or HSIL, repeat cytology at 12 months; if >ASC-H or HSIL perform colposcopy

b) **ASC-H or HSIL – perform colposcopy**

- If colposcopy inadequate, proceed to diagnostic excision procedure
- If colposcopy adequate, observation with colposcopy and cytology 6-month intervals for 1 year

with overuse of follow-up procedures.[18] Pediatric sexual assault may be an independent risk factor for the development of cervical cancer, [30, 31] but to the authors' knowledge this population has not been studied.

Specific recommendations for women aged 21–24

When this group of patients has ASCUS, reflex HPV testing is acceptable, whereas repeat cytology in 12 months is also acceptable. See Table 8-3. If cytology reveals atypical squamous cells cannot rule out high-grade squamous intraepithelial lesion (ASC-H) or HSIL, colposcopy is recommended (see Table 8-4). Table 8-5 describes the management of these younger patients

Table 8-4 Ages 21–24, ASC-H or HSIL

- Immediate LEEP or excisional procedure *unacceptable*
- Colposcopy indicated
- If CIN 2, 3 noted – proceed with excisional procedure
- If no CIN 2, 3 (must have adequate colposcopy plus endocervical sampling negative or CIN 1) – observation with colposcopy and cytology at 6-month intervals up to 24 months
- If HSIL persists 24 months, proceed with excisional procedure

Table 8-6 Age ≥30, cytology negative, HPV positive

- May either co-test in 1 year vs. HPV DNA typing
- If co-test in 1 year and cytology and HPV negative, repeat co-test at 3 years
- If co-test in 1 year and >ASC or HPV positive, proceed to colposcopy
- If HPV DNA typing positive 16 or 18, proceed to colposcopy
- If HPV DNA typing negative 16 and 18, repeat co-test in 1 year

Table 8-7 Unsatisfactory cytology

- Consider that some tests may lack control for epithelial cellularity, so HPV may be falsely negative
- Unsatisfactory tests should be less than 1% across all types HPV
- May need to treat atrophy or infection
- If HPV unknown, negative or positive, repeat cytology after 2–4 months
- If HPV positive, is acceptable to proceed to colposcopy

with no lesion or CIN 1 after ASCUS/LSIL or ASC-H/HSIL.

Specific recommendations for women aged 30 and older

For this group, either co-testing in one year or HPV DNA typing is appropriate. See Table 8-6.

Suboptimal cytology results

Cytology results may be reported as undiagnostic. Table 8-7 describes a plan for the management of unsatisfactory cytology, and Table 8-8 describes

Table 8-8 Cytology negative but EC/TZ absent

- Ages 21–29, is *unacceptable* to test for HPV; only need routine screening
- Ages ≥30, HPV testing preferred; if HPV positive, may either genotype or co-test in 1 year; if genotype is positive 16/18, colposcopy recommended; if genotype negative 16/18, repeat co-test 12 months

Table 8-10 LSIL

(a) **LSIL with negative HPV**

- Preferred repeat co-test at 1 year; colposcopy acceptable
- If repeat co-test negative cytology and negative, HPV – repeat co-test at 3 years
- If repeat co-test >ASC or HPV positive, proceed to colposcopy

(b) **LSIL with no HPV test**

- Proceed to colposcopy
- If inadequate examination or no lesion identified, endocervical sampling preferred
- If lesion identified and colposcopy adequate, biopsy lesion; endocervical sampling acceptable

(c) **LSIL with positive HPV Test**

- Proceed to colposcopy
- If inadequate examination or no lesion identified, endocervical sampling preferred
- If lesion identified and colposcopy adequate, biopsy lesion; endocervical sampling acceptable

(d) **Postmenopausal, LSIL with no HPV test**

- May choose reflex HPV; repeat cytology at 6 and 12 months or colposcopy
- If reflex HPV negative, repeat cytology at 12 months recommended
- If reflex HPV positive or >ASCUS, colposcopy recommended

Table 8-9 ASCUS

- Most common Pap abnormality; 70% are not HPV associated
- HPV testing preferred; repeat cytology in 1 year acceptable
- Repeat cytology in 1 year: if negative, routine screening; if >ASCUS, colposcopy preferred
- HPV testing performed: if negative, repeat co-testing at 3 years; if positive, colposcopy preferred, with endocervical sampling if acceptable; if colposcopy negative, co-test at 12 months
- If postmenopausal, ASCUS with negative HPV is considered abnormal; co-test at 1 year preferred, cytology only acceptable
- If pregnant, may manage same as nonpregnant except endocervical sampling contraindicated; is acceptable to defer colposcopy until 6 weeks postpartum

Table 8-11 Pregnant with LSIL

- Colposcopy preferred; it is acceptable to defer colposcopy until at least 6 weeks postpartum
- On colposcopy, if no CIN 2,3, then postpartum follow-up (additional cytology, colposcopy *unacceptable*)
- Endocervical sampling *unacceptable* in pregnant patients

a plan for negative cytology but the sampling lacks the transformation zone.

Abnormal cytology results, less than high-grade

These tests require follow-up, but treatment will only be necessary if the dysplasia is discovered to be worse than expected on further evaluation. Table 8-9 discusses ASCUS, Tables 8-10 LSIL, and 8-11 LSIL in the pregnant patient.

Findings of no lesion or CIN I on colposcopy

Women with cytologic findings of ASCUS, LSIL, and positive or persistent HPV 16 or 18 frequently are found to have no lesion or CIN 1 on colposcopic evaluation. Management of these patients is described in Table 8-12. Patients whose evaluation included higher grade cytologic findings are managed via the description in Table 8-13.

CIN 2 or CIN 3 on biopsy

These patients require treatment (see Table 8-14). For young women in special circumstances, see Table 8-20.

Table 8-12 Women with no lesion or CIN 1, preceded by lesser abnormalities

- Lesser abnormalities include ASC US or LSIL cytology, HPV 16 or 18, and persistent HPV
- Should co-test at 12 months:
  - If co-test negative/negative, may proceed to age-appropriate retesting
  - If co-test >ASC or HPV positive, perform colposcopy; if CIN 1 and persists at least 2 years, may proceed to ablation or excision; if CIN 2,3, may proceed to ablation or excision
- CIN 1 – high-rate regression and progression to CIN 2 uncommon; hysterectomy *unacceptable* as primary treatment
- Pregnant with CIN 1 – treatment is *unacceptable*
- CIN 1 on endocervical sampling – no longer proceed directly to excision; repeat endocervical sampling in 12 months
- CIN 3 five-year risk:
  - After LSIL, ASC US with positive HPV approximately 3%–8%
  - After HSIL, approximately 15%

Table 8-13 Women with no lesion or CIN 1, preceded by ASC-H or HSIL cytology

- Any one of these three are acceptable:
  - Diagnostic excision procedure or
  - Review of cytologic and histologic, colposcopic findings or
  - Co-testing at 12 and 24 months – if HSIL, proceed to excisional procedure; if HPV positive or any cytology except HSIL, perform colposcopy; if both HPV negative and cytology negative at both visits, perform age-specific testing in 3 years
- Reflects more aggressive approach to ASC-H, HSIL even with no lesion or CIN 1

Table 8-14 Biopsy confirmed CIN 2,3

- If adequate colposcopy was performed, proceed to either excision or ablation of transformation zone; then co-test at 12 and 24 months; if negative results ×2, repeat co-testing in 3 years
- If inadequate colposcopy or recurrent CIN 2,3, or endocervical CIN 2,3 –perform diagnostic excisional procedure (ablation is *unacceptable*); then co-test at 12 and 24 months; if any co-test abnormal, perform colposcopy with endocervical sampling
- If positive margins after excision, or if positive endocervical curettage, repeat cytology with endocervical sampling at 4–6 months; repeat excision is feasible and hysterectomy is acceptable if repeat excision not feasible
- Hysterectomy is *unacceptable* as primary management
- Continue post-treatment screening for at least 20 years, even if this extends beyond 65 years old
- Unambiguous CIN 3 is immediate precursor to invasive cancer and should not be observed, regardless of age or concerns of fertility

Atypical glandular cells

Patients with this finding are at risk for both cervical and/ or endometrial abnormalities. See Tables 8-15 and 8-16 for management description.

High-grade lesions

These patients are at significant risk for cervical cancer; they require close follow-up. Table 8-17 describes the management of ASC-H, Table 8-18 describes the management of HSIL, and Table 8-19 describes the management plan for a patient found to have adenocarcinoma in situ (AIS) through an excisional procedure

Young women

Young women are defined as those who have not completed childbearing. Special circumstances for these patients are described in Table 8-20.

HIV and cervical intraepithelial neoplasia

Women living with human immunodeficiency virus (HIV) and acquired immunodeficiency syndrome (AIDS) have faster progression of CIN, higher rates of cervical cancer, and increased rates of HPV infection. Cervical cancer is listed as an AIDS-defining illness.[32] The risk of progression increases as the immunosuppression, defined by CD4 (cluster of differentiation) counts, becomes more severe.[33] It is therefore felt that the increased risk of cervical lesion development in women living with HIV/AIDS is secondary to an altered immune response and also a change in the natural history of cervical cancer in these women.[34] Although it has been postulated that a reduction in progression of cervical lesions may be seen with antiretroviral therapy (ART), more

Table 8-15 AGC – initial workup

- All subcategories – colposcopy with endometrial sampling
- Atypical endometrial cells – endometrial and endocervical sampling preferred; colposcopy acceptable
- AGC age >30 years – risk CIN 2 = 9–38%, risk cancer 3%–17%
- AGC more common with squamous lesions (50% AIS may have CIN)
- Benign endometrial cells are rarely associated with malignancy; however, in postmenopausal women, 5% have clinically significant pathology, including endometrial cancer. Therefore all warrant endometrial evaluation. For post-hysterectomy patients with benign glandular cells, no further evaluation is recommended.

Table 8-17 ASC-H

- Colposcopy regardless of HPV status
- Reflex HPV unsuitable due to high rate positivity; even if HPV negative, risk of cancer as high as 2%, which is too high for observation
- If colposcopy, biopsy negative, repeat co-testing at 12 and 24 months
- If colposcopy, biopsy positive CIN 2,3, manage per ASCCP guidelines

Table 8-19 AIS diagnosed with excisional procedure

- Hysterectomy preferred (due to possibility of "skip lesions")
- Conservative management is acceptable if future fertility desired; if margins are negative, reevaluate in 6 months with co-testing, colposcopy, and endocervical sampling; if margins are positive or if endocervical curettage positive, re-excision is recommended, then 6 month follow-up

data is needed in this area. The relationship between ART and progression of CIN is incompletely understood at present.[34, 35]

The management of CIN in HIV-positive patients may be quite different in high resource environments with excellent screening programs and access to ART as compared to low resource environments. In a low resource environment, a recurrence rate of 12.8 per 100 woman-years was reported along with an invasive cancer rate of 1.3 per 100 women years after LEEP.[36] Currently, in high resource environments, many

Table 8-16 AGC – subsequent management

- AGC – not otherwise specified (NOS); if no CIN 2+, AIS, or cancer, co-test at 12 and 24 months; if any abnormality on co-test, perform colposcopy; if co-test negative, may advance co-test to 3 years
- AGC (favor neoplasia) or AIS – if no invasive disease on workup, proceed to diagnostic excisional procedure
- Aged 21–24 – proceed with same management
- Pregnant – proceed with same management except endocervical sampling and endometrial biopsy *unacceptable*
- Premenopause, with benign glandular cells, no symptoms – no further workup necessary
- Postmenopause, with benign glandular cells – endometrial assessment is recommended
- Post-hysterectomy with benign glandular cells – no further workup needed

Table 8-18 HSIL

- Immediate excisional procedure vs. colposcopy with endocervical sampling
- HPV testing or repeat cytology *unacceptable*
- If HSIL positive, HPV negative, 5-year risk of CIN 3 is 29% and risk of cancer is 7% – these risks preclude HPV triage
- If colposcopy, biopsy negative or CIN 1, repeat co-testing at 12 and 24 months
- If biopsy CIN 2,3, proceed to excisional procedure

Table 8-20 Biopsy confirmed CIN 2,3 – young women in special circumstances

- If colposcopy is adequate, either treatment or observation is acceptable
- If CIN 2 is specified, observation is preferred
- If CIN 3 is specified, treatment is preferred
- If observation, perform colposcopy and cytology at 6-month intervals for 12 months
- During observation, if colposcopy worsens or HSIL persists for 1 year, repeat colposcopy and biopsy; if CIN 2,3 persists another 24 months, or if biopsy CIN 2,3, then treatment recommended
- During observation if cytology negative ×2 and colposcopy normal, co-test in 1 year; if co-test negative, repeat co-test in 3 years
- In early pregnancy and no invasion, repeat cytology and colposcopy in approximately 12 weeks; repeat biopsy only if worsens or cytology now indicates invasion; is acceptable to defer follow-up to 6 weeks postpartum

practitioners perform Pap tests annually after two negative results. Guidelines may change in the future for HIV-positive women with consistent care, good CD4 counts and persistently negative Pap tests. Such women may be candidates for longer follow-up intervals.[33, 35]

Treatment

As noted earlier, CIN for many patients is managed with close observation; spontaneous regression will occur. For those patients who require treatment, options include ablative treatment, such as cryotherapy and laser vaporization, or excisional therapy such as LEEP, laser conization and cold knife conization (CKC). Combinations of laser ablation and excision are also available.

Operator experience, available equipment, and lesion size are factors in the decision on which treatment is best for a particular patient. Invasive cancer must have been excluded before an ablative therapy is selected; inadequate colposcopy, CIN in the endocervical assessment, cytology or colposcopy suspicious for cancer, and history of prior therapy should all exclude ablative therapy.[26] Lesion extension onto the vagina may in some cases be best treated with laser ablation. When comparing the excision therapies, LEEP can be easily done in the office setting while CKC and laser conization are best done in an operating room setting. Both LEEP and laser conization require careful attention to avoid cautery artifact which may affect ability to assess specimen margins. Although many practitioners prefer CKC to avoid cautery artifact, this is not a guideline, and a CKC has higher blood loss than LEEP.[26] CKC is usually performed in an operating room instead of a more cost-effective office environment. It may therefore be reasonable to reserve CKC for patients with suspected microinvasive cancer or AIS where significant need for accurate margin assessment exists.

Concluding remarks

The proper management of CIN is a major component of comprehensive women's health. Cervical screening is frequently a component of a patient's first contact with a women's health specialist. Many patients experience anxiety about the cervical screening process, and it is incumbent on health-care providers to manage this process competently, compassionately, and knowledgeably. Complexity of management has increased as the process has focused on the needs of specific patient groups. It is therefore appropriate for the clinician to refer to tables, algorithms, or mobile applications to ensure patients receive the most recent recommended management plan.

References

1. Montz FJ. Management of high-grade cervical intraepithelial neoplasia and low-grade squamous intraepithelial lesion and potential complications. *Clin Obstet Gynecol* 2000 Jun; **43**(2): 394–409.
2. Solomon D, Davey D, Kurman R, et al. The 2001 Bethesda System: terminology for reporting results of cervical cytology. *JAMA* 2002; Apr 24; **287**(16): 2114–19.
3. Waxman AG, Chelmow D, Darragh TM, et al. Revised terminology for cervical histopathology and its implications for management of high-grade squamous intraepithelial lesions of the cervix. *Obstet Gynecol* 2012; **120**: 1465–71.
4. National Cancer Institute. Surveillance, Epidemiology, and End results Program. SEER Cancer Statistics Review, 1975–2009.
5. Center for Disease Control and Prevention. *United States Cancer Statistics: 1999–2011 Incidence and Mortality Web-based Report*. Atlanta, GA: Department of Health and Human Services, Centers for Disease Control and Prevention, and National Cancer Institute; 2014. Available at: http://apps.nccd.cdc.gov/uscs. Accessed 2 Feb 2015.
6. Cendejas BR, Smith-McCune KK, Khan MJ. Does treatment for cervical and vulvar dysplasia impact women's sexual health? *Am J Obstet Gynecol* 2015 Mar; **212**(3): 291–7.
7. Wright TC, Schiffman M. Adding a test for human papillomavirus DNA to cervical cancer screening. *N Engl J Med* 2003 Feb 6; **348**(6): 489–90.
8. Muñoz N, Bosch FX, de Sanjosé S, et al. Epidemiologic classification of human papillomavirus types associated with cervical cancer. *N Engl J Med* 2003; **348**: 518.
9. Kjaer SK, Frederiksen K, Munk C, Iftner T. Long-term absolute risk of cervical intraepithelial neoplasia grade 3 or worse following human papillomavirus infection: role of persistence. *J Natl Cancer Inst* 2010 Oct 6; **102**(9): 1478–88.
10. Kjaer SK, van den Brule AJ, Paull G, et al. Type specific persistence of high risk human papillomavirus (HPV) as indicator of high grade cervical squamous intraepithelial lesions in young women: population based prospective follow up study. *BMJ* 2002; **325**: 572.
11. McCredie MRE, Sharples KJ, Paul C, et al. Natural history of cervical neoplasia and risk of invasive cancer in women with cervical intraepithelial neoplasia 3:

a retrospective cohort study. *Lancet Oncol* 2008 May; **9**: 425–34.

12. Lammé J, Pattaratornkosohn T, Mercado-Abadie J, et al. Concurrent anal human papillomavirus and abnormal anal cytology in women with known cervical dysplasia. *Obstet Gynecol* Aug; 124(2 pt.1): 242–8.
13. ACOG Committee on Adolescent Health Care. Committee Opinion No. 588: human papillomavirus vaccination. *Obstet Gynecol* 2014 Mar; **123**: 712–18.
14. Beller U, Abu-Rustum NR. Cervical cancers after human papillomavirus vaccination. *Obstet Gynecol* 2009 Feb; **113**(2 pt 2): 550–2. doi: 10.1097/AOG.0b013e318191a54a.
15. Teixeira JC, Derchain SFM, Oliveira ERZ, et al. Microinvasive adenocarcinoma of the cervix in a young woman vaccinated against human papillomavirus: the screening must be continued. *J Lower Genit Tract Dis* 2014; **18**(2): E50–4.
16. Sung HY, Kearney KA, Miller M, et al. Papanicolaou smear history and diagnosis of invasive cervical carcinoma among members of a large prepaid health plan. *Cancer* 2000 May 15; **88**(10): 2284–9.
17. Leyden WA, Manos MM, Geiger AM, et al. Cervical cancer in women with comprehensive health care access: attributable factors in the screening process. *J National Can Instit* 2005 May; **97**(9): 675–83.
18. American College of Obstetricians and Gynecologists. ACOG Practice Bulletin No. 109: screening for cervical cancer. *Obstet Gynecol* 2009 Dec; **109:** 1–18.
19. Committee Opinion No. 534: Guidelines for women's healthcare. A resource manual. 4th ed. *Obstet Gynecol* 2012; **120**: 421–4.
20. Huh WK, Sidri M, Stoler M, et al. Relevance of random biopsy at the transformation zone when colposcopy is negative. *Obstet Gynecol* 2014 Oct; **124**(4): 670–8.
21. American College of Obstetricians and Gynecologists. ACOG Practice Bulletin No. 99: management of abnormal cervical cytology and histology. *Obstet Gynecol* 2008 Dec; **112**(6): 1419–44. doi: 10.1097/AOG.0b013e318192497c.
22. Bosgraaf RP, Mast PP, Struik-van der Zanden PHTH, et al. Overtreatment in a see-and-treat approach to cervical intraepithelial lesions. *Obstet Gynecol* 2013 Jun; **121**(6): 1209–16.
23. Long S, Leeman L. Treatment options for high-grade squamous intraepithelial lesions. *Obstet Gynecol Clin North Am* 2013 Jun; **40**(2): 291–316.
24. Ciavattini A, Clemente N, Delli Carpini G, et al. Loop electrosurgical excision procedure and risk of miscarriage. *Fertil Steril* 2015 Apr; **103**(4): 1043–8.
25. Massad LS, Einstein MH, Huh WK, et al. 2012 updated consensus guidelines for the management of abnormal cervical cancer screening tests and cancer precursors. *J Lower Genit Tract Dis* 2013; **17**(5): S1–27.
26. American College of Obstetricians and Gynecologists. ACOG Practice Bulletin No. 140: management of abnormal cervical cancer screening test results and cervical cancer precursors. *Obstet Gynecol* 2013; **122**: 1338–67. (Replaces Practice Bulletin No. 99, Dec 2008.)
27. Roberts OA, Owonikoko KM, Abdus-Salam AA, Ogun O. Advanced carcinoma of the cervix in a 17-year-old girl. *J Obstet Gynaecol* 2013 Oct; **33**(7): 747–8. doi: 10.3109;01443615.2013.813911.
28. Guo Y, Song L, Liu H. Cervical clear cell adenocarcinoma infected with human papillomavirus type 18 in an adolescent. *J Pediatr Adolesc Gynecol* 2014 Feb; **27** (1): e1–3. doi: 10.1016/j.jpag.2013.04.007. Epub 2013 Jul 10.
29. Goncalves CV, Quintana SM, Marcolin AC, et al. Microinvasive carcinoma of the uterine cervix in a 14-year-old adolescent: case report and literature review. *São Paulo Med J* 2009 May; **127**(2): 105–7.
30. Costa MJ, Tadros T, Tackett E, Naib Z. Vaginocervical cytology in victims of sexual assault. *Diagn Cytopathol* 1991; 7(4): 337–40.
31. Coker AL, Hopenhayn C, DeSimone CP, et al. Violence against women raises risk of cervical cancer. *J Womens Health (Larchmt)* 2009 Aug; **18**(8): 1179–85. doi:10.1089/jwh.2008.1048.
32. Centers for Disease Control and Prevention. 1993 revised classification system HIV infection and expanded surveillance case definition for AIDS among adolescents and adults. *MMWR* 1992; **41**: 1–19.
33. Massad LS, Xie X, D'Souza G, et al. Incidence of cervical precancers among HIV-seropositive women. *Am J Obstet Gynecol* 2015 May; **212**(5): 606.e1–8. Epub 2014 Dec 10.
34. Denslow SA, Rositch AF, Firnhaber C, et al. Incidence and progression of cervical lesions in women with HIV: a systematic global review. *In J STD AIDS* 2014 Mar; **25**(3): 163–77. doi:10.1177/0956462413491735.
35. Lofgren S, Tadros T, Herring-Bailey G, et al. Progression and regression of cervical pap test lesions in an urban AIDS clinic in the combined antiretroviral therapy era: a longitudinal, retrospective study. *AIDS Res Hum Retroviruses* 2015 Feb; **19**: 1–20.
36. Huchko MJ, Leslie H, Maloba M, et al. Outcomes up to twelve months after treatment with loop electrosurgical excision procedure for cervical intraepithelial neoplasia among HIV-infected women. *J Acquir Immune Defic Syndr* 2015 Feb; **2**: 1–19.

Chapter 9

Office emergencies

Felicity Plaat and Sarah Griffiths

Introduction

Gynecology offices are often self-contained units lacking same site access to an emergency department or the infrastructure of a large hospital. As a result, patients suffering significant surgical complications or requiring other emergency medical treatment will usually require transfer to another medical facility. It is important, however, that all office clinicians be familiar with common medical emergencies which they may encounter in their practices, and that they are able to instigate initial treatment (Table 9-1). These first-treatment measures may be lifesaving.

The presentation and initial management of common office emergencies are discussed in further detail in this chapter. Office emergencies may be broadly divided into those which could occur at any time and may perhaps be associated with underlying patient comorbidities, and those which are more likely to occur in conjunction with office gynecological procedures.

Table 9-1 Common office emergencies

General office emergencies	Cardiac arrest Acute coronary syndrome Acute asthma Seizures
Procedure-related emergencies	Hemorrhage Anaphylaxis Gas or air embolism Local anesthetic toxicity Water intoxication syndrome

General planning for office emergencies

Emergencies can arise at any time and by definition are unexpected. The general principles developed for management in the hospital setting should be adapted for office based practice.[1] The equivalent of the crash cart should contain, in addition to an automated external defibrillator (AED), equipment and drugs required for the initial management of the emergencies. It is essential that the contents are regularly and systematically checked by staff trained to do so and that this is documented. Used or out-of-date equipment and drugs must be replaced immediately. The contents should be kept to a minimum to avoid confusion. For example it is recommended that only one concentration of any drug be kept. Pre-prepared syringes should be used whenever available. The contents of an emergency trolley are listed in Table 9-2. The exact list will depend on local facilities and activity.

Airway management, requires bag-valve-mask devices with adjuncts such as oropharyngeal and nasal pharyngeal airways in a limited range of sizes. A source of oxygen and suction must be available. As an alternative to tracheal intubation, a supraglottic airway device such as a second-generation laryngeal mask airway, provides limited protection against aspiration. Such devices are disposable; a range of sizes should be kept. It is recommended that the simplest version is chosen. An example is the i-gel®, which does not require inflation of the cuff (Figure 9-1).

The 2010 American Heart Association (AHA) guidelines on cardiopulmonary resuscitation suggest that continuous monitoring of expired carbon dioxide is mandatory if the patient is being ventilated via an endotracheal tube or supraglottic airway (Figure 9-2).[2]

In addition to capnography, monitoring should include pulse oximetry, ECG, and noninvasive blood pressure measurement.

Staff must be trained and regularly updated in the management of emergencies and the use of drugs,

Office Care of Women, ed. Martin E. Olsen and Botros Rizk. Published by Cambridge University Press.

Table 9-2 Contents of emergency trolley

System	Equipment & drugs	Monitoring
Airway & breathing	Source of oxygen – able to deliver 10–25 L/min Oxygen tubing & masks Suction & suckers Bag-valve-mask Oropharyngeal airways Supraglottic airways	Continuous capnography Pulse oximetry
Circulation	IV cannulae dressings, giving sets, IV fluids (balanced salt solution, dextrose) *Drugs:* adrenaline, amiodarone, aspirin, clopidogrel, chlorpheniramine, glyceryl trinitrate hydrocortisone, Intralipid±; orazepam/ midazolam Magnesium	Automated defibrillation device (AED) ECG Noninvasive blood pressure
Other	Warming blanket	Temperature measurement Glucometer

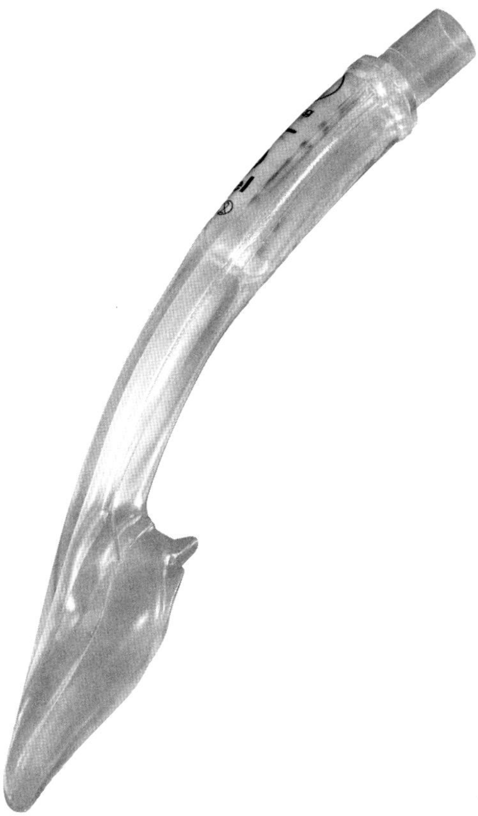

Figure 9-1 I-gel® spraglottic device (with permission from Intersurgical Ltd, Wokingham, Berkshire, United Kingdom).

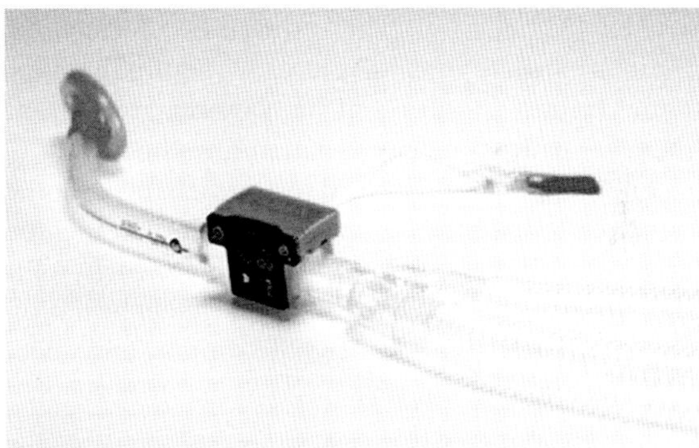

Figure 9-2 CO_2 detector.

equipment and monitoring required. The use of protocol based drills enables health-care providers to become proficient in the skills required. Teamwork practice in the actual work environment is important. The evidence that higher fidelity simulation training in the management of emergencies improves patient outcomes does not yet exist. As emergencies are rare, easily accessible checklists and algorithms of care are recommended and have been shown to impact patient outcome.[3]

Finally it is crucial that there is a validated transfer protocol in place. The likely time for transfer, the means by which it occurs, the destination and the staff who will be involved should be determined in advance. Protocols, documentation, and equipment must be agreed upon by transferring and receiving parties. The unexpected emergency department arrival of a patient suffering a complication from an office based procedure, without prior communication and planning, should be viewed as a failure of care.

Cardiac arrest

Introduction

Ischemic heart disease is the leading cause of death among women in the United States and is associated with increasing levels of obesity, smoking, hypertension, diabetes, and hypercholesterolemia;[4] 60% of deaths from ischemic heart disease are due to sudden cardiac arrest. Many of the complications discussed in this chapter may lead to cardiac arrest. The more rapidly a return of spontaneous circulation occurs, the more likely the outcome will be good; up to 30%–40% survival is thought to be possible with prompt cardiopulmonary resuscitation (CPR).

Survival after out-of-hospital cardiac arrest is poor with only 50% victims receiving bystander CPR. Survival in the office setting should approach that of hospital in-patients. The American Society of Anesthesiologists guidelines already require that personnel trained in advanced life support are present whenever patients receive sedation/anesthesia.[5]

The components that lead to a successful outcome have been termed the "chain of survival" and include early recognition and summoning help, early CPR with effective chest compressions, early defibrillation if indicated, effective advanced life support and effective post-resuscitation care.

Presentation

Prompt recognition is vital. The patient is unresponsive since cardiac arrest leads to unconsciousness within 15–30 seconds. Pulses are absent and abnormal gasping respiration or apnea is present. The pupils will usually be dilated. Seizures may occur. The 2010 AHA guidelines recommend summoning help and beginning CPR on an unresponsive patient who is breathing abnormally or apneic, as time can be wasted trying to palpate for a pulse. The advice to "look, listen, feel" has been withdrawn.

Initial management

Initial management follows the AHA basic life support algorithm (Figure 9-3).[6] Chest compressions should start *before* airway maneuvers or rescue breaths. The emphasis is on effective compressions with minimal interruptions. The ratio of compressions to breaths is 30:2 with a rate of 100 compressions per minute. Compression only resuscitation is an option for adults not suffering drowning. As long as the airway is patent, air will be drawn into the lung and the oxygen (21%) will be sufficient to address hypoxemia.

Securing the airway allows the patient to be ventilated without having to halt compressions. Attempts to secure the airway, however, must not lead to compression interruption. As soon as possible, an AED should be attached. If a shockable rhythm is detected the 2010 guidelines suggest a single shock immediately followed by compressions. Compressions should cease only once the pads have been attached to the chest and the machine charged to further minimize interruption to compressions.

Intravenous access should be secured as early as possible in order to administer epinephrine 1 mg every 3–5 minutes as per the advanced life support (ALS) algorithm (Figure 9-4). If ventricular fibrillation persists after three shocks amiodarone 300 mg should be administered. Atropine is no longer recommended. If intravenous access is impossible the interosseous route can be used. The tibial and humeral sites are usually accessible and fluids as well as drugs can be administered by this route when the equipment is available (Figure 9-5). Reversible causes of cardiac arrest that may arise and can be treated in the office setting include hypoxia, hypovolemia (hemorrhage), and toxins (e.g., local anesthetic toxicity).

Compressions and defibrillation should be continued during transfer and compressions should not cease until there are clear signs of return of spontaneous circulation.

Investigations

As mentioned previously, continuous waveform capnography is recommended in ventilated patients. Return of spontaneous circulation will be indicated by an increase in expired CO_2. Blood pressure should be measure and oxygen saturations measured. A 12-lead ECG should be performed, and blood taken for biochemistry and full blood count.

Acute coronary syndrome

Introduction

Acute coronary syndrome (ACS) refers to a diagnosis of myocardial infarction or unstable

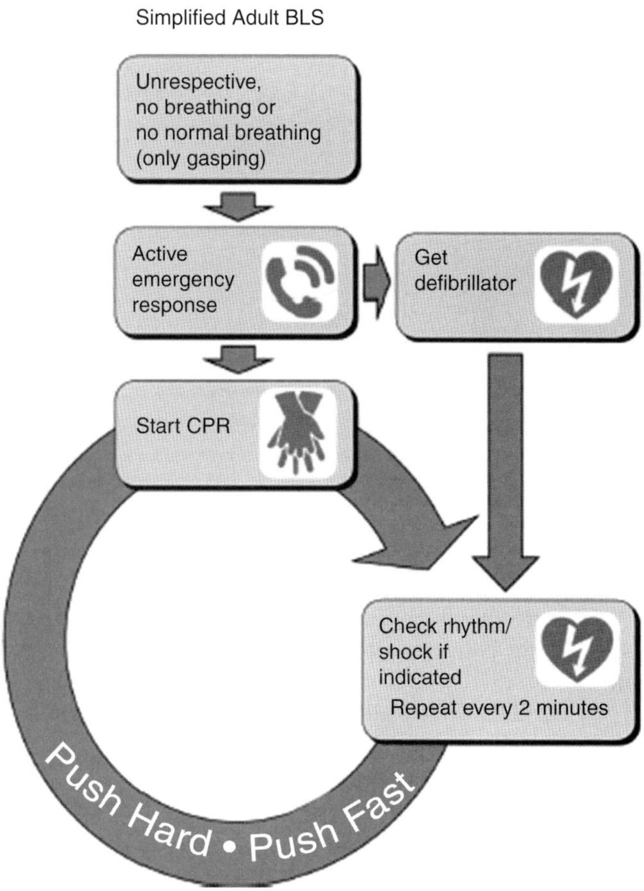

Figure 9-3 American Heart Association basic life support algorithm.

angina. Myocardial infarction (MI) may be further subdivided into ST elevation MI (STEMI) and non-ST elevation MI (NSTEMI). NSTEMI and unstable angina occur as a result of the development of thrombus on an atheromatous plaque. In contrast to STEMI, the thrombus is nonocclusive, but distal vasospasm or embolization may lead to subsequent myocardial necrosis.[7]

It is estimated that MI goes unnoticed or unreported in women in approximately one third of cases as symptoms may be more subtle than in men.[8] Furthermore, there is now a rising population of young women in their third and fourth decades of life who have undetected but significant coronary artery atheroma. Consequently, clinicians working in the office environment need to be alert to the possibility of ACS occurring in women of any age group, particularly when underlying cardiac disease may be exacerbated by anxiety and stress in the perioperative period.

Presentation

Acute coronary syndrome presents classically with severe central chest pain which is crushing or squeezing in character and may be referred to the left arm or shoulder. There may be associated symptoms of sweating, dyspnea, nausea, or vomiting. In women with ACS, these symptoms may be more prominent than the pain itself. Pain secondary to MI will often last several hours with no respite. In unstable angina, pain usually occurs at rest due to critical myocardial perfusion. This pain will often resolve after 20–30 minutes, either due to spontaneous clot lysis and restoration of a patent coronary artery lumen, or due to relaxation of coronary artery spasm.[7]

Initial management

In the acute setting, it may be difficult for the clinician to differentiate between MI and unstable angina since

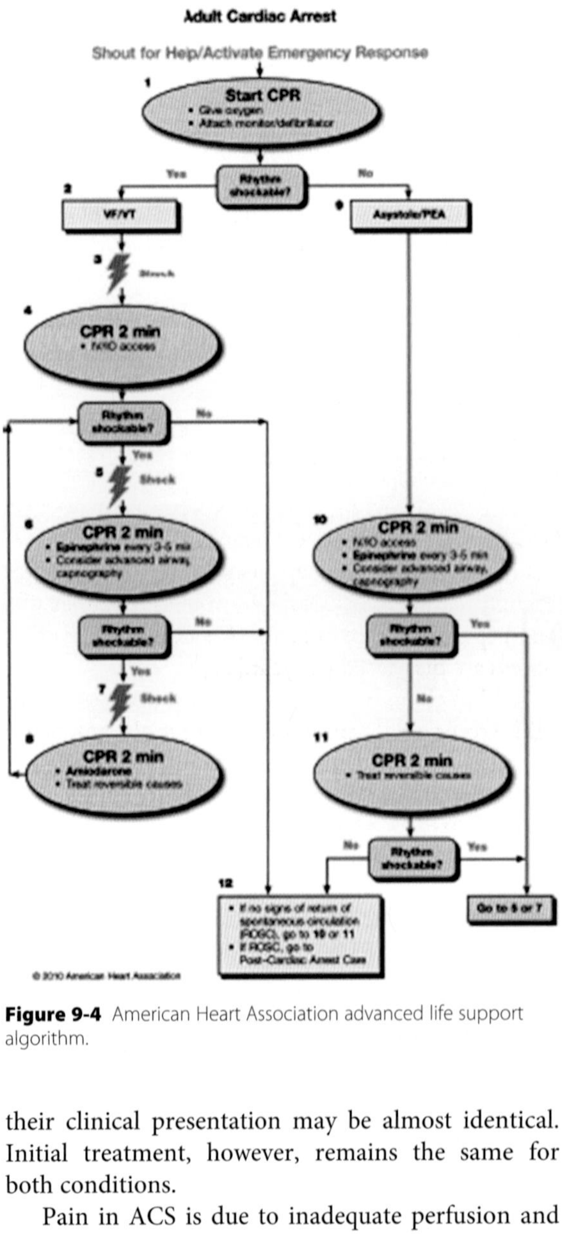

Figure 9-4 American Heart Association advanced life support algorithm.

their clinical presentation may be almost identical. Initial treatment, however, remains the same for both conditions.

Pain in ACS is due to inadequate perfusion and a lack of oxygen delivery to the cardiac muscle. The initial management should therefore aim to maximize the availability of oxygen to the heart and to restore coronary artery patency. High-flow oxygen should be administered via a face mask at 10 L–15 L/minute. The patient should be asked to chew aspirin 300 mg, or to take clopidogrel 300 mg if there is a hypersensitivity to aspirin or major gastrointestinal intolerance.[9, 10]

Sublingual administration of glyceryl trinitrate spray (400 mcg) or administration of an oral nitrate will also help to promote vasodilatation and increase coronary artery perfusion. Nitrates should be avoided if the patient is already hypotensive. The pain of ACS is severe, and intravenous morphine should be titrated to help with this in addition to the administration of an antiemetic.

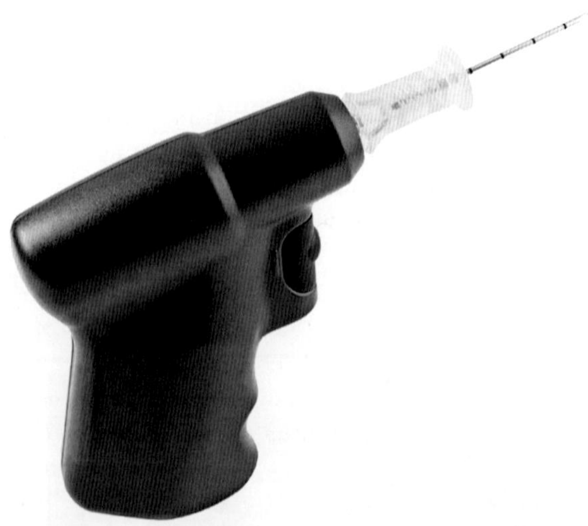

Figure 9-5 Ezio interosseous drill.

Investigations

A 12-lead ECG should be performed as early as possible to look for ST segment elevation, T wave inversion or new left bundle branch block. It should be noted, however, that a normal ECG does not rule out ACS since NSTEMI is more common than STEMI. Cardiac-specific troponins (Troponin I or T) are gold standard diagnostic tests. Troponin level may be normal initially, but usually rises within 2–12 hours and peaks at 12–24 hours post-MI. In an office setting and with a normal ECG, the diagnosis of ACS remains a clinical one, and immediate transfer to a center with percutaneous coronary intervention (PCI) capabilities is indicated, regardless of ECG findings.

Acute asthma

Introduction

Acute asthma remains a major cause of death among young adults. In the United States there are 5,000–6,000 deaths per year, a good proportion being pre-hospital.

Acute attacks account for 2 million visits to emergency departments every year, with one in 4 leading to admission. Up to one in five inpatients need intensive care with a third of these requiring mechanical ventilation.

Death is most commonly due to asphyxia as a result of a combination of bronchospasm, airway inflammation, and mucous plugging. Other potentially fatal complications include tension pneumothorax, pulmonary edema, pneumonia, and atelectasis.[11]

Presentation

The patient may give a history of a respiratory tract infection or worsening of previously well-controlled asthma. She may not be able to complete sentences. Although wheeze is common, the severity is not related to the degree of airway compromise: a silent chest indicates almost complete obstruction. The respiratory rate is raised and greater than 25 per minute indicates acute severe asthma, as does a pulse rate greater than 110 bpm. The condition is life threatening when the patient becomes exhausted, has altered level of consciousness, or becomes cyanosed with a silent chest. Arrhythmia and hypotension may intervene.

Initial management

Treatment should be started immediately even if transfer time is short, as patients can become critically ill very rapidly. Initial treatment includes oxygen, inhaled β_2 agonists, and steroids. Intravenous access should be obtained. All patients should be given high-flow oxygen, regardless of whether their oxygenation is within the normal range as it may decrease with treatment (see later in the chapter).

Inhaled β_2 agonists such as albuteral are potent bronchodilators with a dose-dependent effect and minimal side effects. There is no evidence that nebulizers are more effective than metered dose inhalers; if one method produces no improvement it is sensible to try the alternative. Bronchodilation may result in a decrease in oxygenation due to an increase in ventilation perfusion mismatch. The addition of an anticholinergic agent such as ipratropium bromide has been shown to produce a modest improvement over Inhaled β_2 agonists alone.

Because steroids take up to 12 hours to exert their anti-inflammatory effect they should be given early. Dexamethasone 10 mg or methylprednisolone 125 mg should both be given intravenously.

Magnesium sulfate relaxes bronchial smooth muscle and has been shown to be effective in severe acute asthma. The dose is 2 g given over 20 minutes, intravenously.

Investigations/monitoring

Any asthmatic patient suffering an attack severe enough to prevent her from finishing sentences, who is tachypnoeic, tachycardic, or showing signs of exhaustion should have continuous pulse oximetry and not be left alone. Baseline spirometry for FEV_1 (forced expiratory volume in one second) or peak expiratory flow should be measured and repeated at 30 minute intervals.

Seizures

Introduction

Seizures occurring in the office environment are most likely to be secondary to known seizure disorder or a first presentation of epilepsy in a patient. In the United States alone, nearly 2.2 million people suffer from epilepsy; approximately 150,000 new cases of the illness are diagnosed per year.[12]

Although many seizures occur unprovoked, some of the commonest causes of seizures in the absence of primary head trauma include electrolyte disturbance (hypoglycemia is the most common precipitant, particularly in diabetic patients), an intracranial lesion or spontaneous hemorrhage, noncompliance with anti-epileptic medication or sub-therapeutic dosage, stress or anxiety, and use of drugs and/or alcohol.

Iatrogenic causes of seizures which may be directly associated with the performance of certain office gynecological procedures include local anesthetic toxicity and endoscopic fluid resorption leading to water intoxication syndrome.

Initial management

Most seizures are self-terminating, but in some cases a seizure may persist or there may be seizure recurrence. Status epilepticus is defined as a seizure that lasts longer than five minutes or recurrence of seizures without an intervening return of consciousness.[13]

The incidence of permanent brain damage increases with seizure duration.[14] Consequently, in status epilepticus, drug treatment to terminate the seizure state is required as a matter of urgency.

Regardless of the cause of the seizure, the primary goals of treatment in all cases are the same: the protection of the patient's airway, the prevention of physical injury secondary to convulsions and the rapid termination of the seizure itself. If possible, a patient who is suffering from a seizure should be turned into the left lateral or recovery position to help prevent the aspiration of any regurgitated gastric contents. If the patient is on the operating table, a degree of head-down tilt may also be used to facilitate the drainage of gastric fluid away from the lungs.

High-flow oxygen at 10 L–15 L/minute should be administered via a face mask, vital signs monitored and a patent airway maintained. This can be achieved by simple airway opening maneuvres such as a chin lift or jaw thrust that will prevent the patient's tongue from falling backward and obstructing the oropharynx. Suction of the oropharynx may be necessary if gastric regurgitation occurs, but this should be performed carefully and under direct vision to avoid causing trauma to friable tissues or a vagal response. In the post-ictal phase, the patient will still need to be monitored closely due to the risk of repeat seizures. Airway opening maneuvres may also still be required at this stage, since airway obstruction can occur secondary to a reduced level of consciousness in the post-ictal state.

If the seizure has not resolved after five minutes, then pharmacologic therapy will be required. First-line drug treatment that can be undertaken in the office environment should be the administration of a benzodiazepine such as lorazepam, diazepam, or midazolam. Intravenous lorazepam (0.1 mg/kg adult dose) is the drug of choice; however, buccal, intramuscular, or rectal benzodiazepines may be quicker to administer in cases where an intravenous cannula is not already in place or where cannulation is difficult. One further dose of the same or a different benzodiazepine should be administered five minutes after the first dose if the seizure is still ongoing.

If no seizure resolution occurs following two doses of benzodiazepine, then the patient will need to be transferred to a definitive care facility for ongoing treatment. The patient is likely to require endotracheal intubation for definitive airway protection prior to transfer, and so urgent and early anesthetic assistance should be sought.

Investigations

As part of the initial office management of the patient with a seizure, a finger-stick blood glucose should be checked urgently. If this is found to be low (<3 mmol/L or 50 mg/dL), an intravenous infusion of dextrose should be commenced immediately. If there is on site access to a blood gas analyzer, then a venous or arterial blood gas sample may be taken to allow detection and correction of any other abnormal electrolyte levels.

Hemorrhage

Introduction

Most procedures undertaken in an office setting are not associated with a high risk of hemorrhage. Occasionally large loop excision of transition zone is associated with significant blood loss. Should there be an undetected coagulopathy (pathological or iatrogenic and undeclared), however, the risk of significant hemorrhage from office procedures is significant.

Presentation

The patient may complain of an unusual amount of pain for the procedure. Early signs of acute hypovolemia include increased respiratory rate and pulse rate. The patient on beta blockers, however, will not mount a tachycardia. Occasionally there is a paradoxical bradycardia. The patient may complain of feeling faint, dizzy, feeling generally unwell, and/or become agitated or confused. Her skin may become cold and clammy. Capillary refill will be delayed.* Pulse pressure (the difference between systolic and diastolic) may be narrowed: The diastolic is increased. Especially in the pregnant patient, a falling systolic blood pressure is a late sign; it would be a mistake to wait for this sign before initiating treatment.[15]

In pregnancy, the signs of hypovolemia are hidden until a much greater amount of blood is lost from the circulation (see Figure 9-6). Small women have smaller blood volumes and will decompensate earlier.

Initial management

Intravenous access with as wide bore cannula (two are preferable) should be achieved as early as possible. High-flow supplementary oxygen should be given. If the bleeding point is accessible compression should be applied. Crystalloid or colloid, warmed if possible, should be rapidly infused to achieve a rise

* To test capillary refill the nail bed should be pressed for five seconds. Capillary refill time (CRT) is normal if color returns within two seconds of the compression being released.

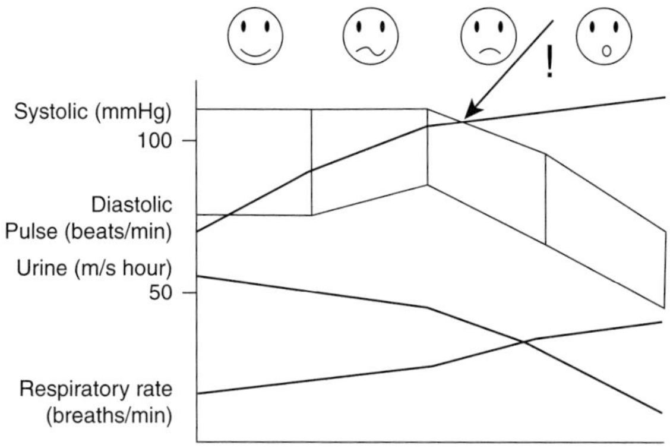

Figure 9-6 Clinical parameters following increasing blood loss in the pregnant woman.

in blood pressure/fall in pulse rate/improvement in mental state. There is little advantage to colloid over crystalloid although a slightly smaller volume of the former may initially produce a response. Given the choice, a balanced salt solution is preferable to normal saline as large quantities of the latter produce a hyperchloremic acidosis. From mid trimester it is vital to minimize aortocaval compression that will further compromise tissue perfusion in the pregnant patient. This is most effectively achieved by placing the patient in the left lateral position. As a temporizing measure if the blood pressure is significantly low and there are signs of vital organ underperfusion (e.g., deteriorating conscious level), the legs can be raised. Small boluses of a vasoconstrictor may also be used (consider ephedrine 5 mg/metaraminol 0.5 mg–1 mg/phenylephrine 25 mcg–50 mcg). Monitoring the patient suspected of hemorrhage should include frequently repeated pulse rate and blood pressure assessment. Oxygen saturation monitoring is desirable. If possible the patient should be catheterized so that urine output – a sensitive indicator of hypovolemia – can be measured.

Investigations and subsequent management

Early transfer to a unit with imaging to detect site of blood loss, and appropriate facilities should surgery be required, should not be delayed. The patient will require close monitoring during transfer and the receiving facility will need to be given up to date clinical details. The severity of hemorrhage is frequently underestimated and delayed resuscitation and surgical control of bleeding were sited as contributory factors leading to a fatal outcome in a recent report on maternal mortality in the UK.[16]

Anaphylaxis

Introduction

Anaphylaxis is defined as a severe, life-threatening, generalized or systemic hypersensitivity reactions.[17]

It may be subdivided into "allergic" anaphylaxis, which is usually an IgE-mediated reaction, and "nonallergic anaphylaxis," which is not immunologically mediated. In the office setting, anaphylaxis is most likely to be triggered by exposure to drugs (especially β-lactam-based antibiotics such as penicillins and cephalosporins,[18] latex, antiseptic cleaning solutions, or intravenous colloid.

Presentation

Signs and symptoms of anaphylaxis may be evident immediately after exposure to the allergenic agent, but they often develop between 30 minutes and one hour post exposure. The most common manifestation of an anaphylactic reaction is severe hypotension that may lead rapidly to cardiac arrest. Wheeze secondary to bronchoconstriction may also be an early presenting feature. It is a common misconception that anaphylaxis is always associated with an urticarial rash. This may be the initial presenting feature in as few as 4% of cases or may be a late sign.[19] Consequently, clinicians must retain a high index of suspicion for anaphylaxis in all situations of cardiovascular collapse, even in the absence of a cutaneous reaction.

Initial management

The immediate management of a suspected anaphylactic reaction is focussed on the removal of any suspected triggers, restoration of cardiac output, and provision of adequate oxygenation. If the patient is in cardiac arrest, cardiopulmonary resuscitation must be commenced immediately according to standard life support algorithms.

High-flow oxygen at 10 L–15 L/minute should be administered immediately via a face mask in a conscious patient. Airway edema may develop rapidly and may be heralded by worsening cough, wheeze or voice changes. In such cases it is vital for the airway to be secured rapidly via endotracheal intubation and an anesthetist should be called immediately. In the unconscious patient, administer oxygen via a bag-valve-mask device while waiting for anesthetic assistance.

The key treatment step in the management of anaphylaxis is the administration of intramuscular epinephrine (0.5 mg/kg; 0.5 mL of 1:1,000 solution for an adult). Epinephrine is used in preference to other drugs as it has both alpha and beta adrenergic effects. The alpha adrenergic effects of the drug help to restore the blood pressure by reversing the widespread vasodilatory response to the allergen. The beta adrenergic effects of epinephrine promote relaxation of smooth muscle spasm thus reducing bronchoconstriction. They also attenuate the leakage of capillary fluid that helps to reduce edema, and counteract the negative inotropic effects on the heart which are induced by circulating inflammatory mediators.[20]

Since the effects of epinephrine are short-lived, repeated doses of the drug may be required at five-minute intervals if symptoms are severe.

A liter of crystalloid solution (e.g., Ringer's lactate) should be given through a large bore cannula and the patient's legs elevated above the level of the heart. These measures will assist in the restoration of blood pressure and cardiac output by optimizing preload. If colloid is suspected to have been the trigger for the anaphylactic reaction then ensure that the entire giving set and cannula are changed before the administration of crystalloid solution.

Secondary management of an anaphylactic reaction includes the administration of chlorpheniramine (10 mg IV adult dose) and hydrocortisone (200 mg IV adult dose). Chlorpheniramine will help to prevent further mast cell degranulation, whereas the administration of hydrocortisone helps to dampen down the inflammatory response over the following hours. All patients who have suffered an anaphylactic reaction should be transferred to the nearest emergency department as soon as possible. Even those patients who appear to have recovered well following initial treatment have a propensity to develop recurrent symptoms up to six hours after the initial reaction (biphasic response).

Investigations

Mast cell tryptase levels are elevated in most but not all patients who have had an anaphylactic reaction. Levels should be taken at one hour, six hours, and 24 hours post reaction provided that this does not interfere with treatment and stabilization of the patient. Since patients who suffer an anaphylactic reaction in the office will be transferred elsewhere for ongoing management, it is unlikely that the office clinician will have to perform these blood tests on site.

Embolic complications

Introduction

Pregnancy and gynecologic cancers are associated with an increased risk of thromboembolic complications. Additionally, thrombosis and thromboembolism is now the leading obstetric cause of maternal mortality in the latest UK report.[21] In nononcology gynecological patients the risks are increased with rising BMI, increasing age, and certain comorbidities. Young patient who have recently undertaken long-haul flights are also at increased risk.

Gas emboli have classically been linked to laser ablation procedures but can occur during any hysteroscopic or laparoscopic procedures.[22] Carbon dioxide as a distending medium has the advantage of being highly soluble, allowing relatively large amounts to dissolve in the circulation without the formation of bubbles. This, however, leads to acidosis and hypercarbia and subsequent cardiac arrhythmias. Eventually bubbles will form. Air emboli are potentially much more dangerous as air is highly insoluble, so even very small amounts in the circulation can be fatal. Air embolization occurs if air is allowed to enter the distension tubing, usually when bags of irrigation fluid are being changed.

The venous side of the circulation can accommodate relatively large volumes of gas. Conversely even tiny bubbles can cause havoc on the arterial side. The pulmonary capillaries should protect the latter by trapping small bubbles. However this is bypassed in the 20%–35% of the healthy population who have a patent foramen ovale allowing a direct right to left shunt.

Initial presentation

Although pulmonary embolism can present as a major life-threatening event, the presentation is often insidious and easily missed. There may be a combination of symptoms including cough, hemptysis, dyspnea, pleuritic chest pain and low-grade fever. The patient may be tachypneic and/or tachycardic. only a couple of these may be present initially.

Signs of right heart failure, such as raised internal jugular pressure, liver distension, and ECG changes are unlikely unless the patient is in extremis. Massive pulmonary embolism may present with marked dyspnea and cyanosis. There may be chest pain due to right ventricular myocardial ischemia, hypotension and circulatory collapse and pulseless electrical activity cardiac arrest.

Gas embolism may present with tachypnea and tachyarthymias. The most sensitive indicator of gas in the pulmonary circulation is a sudden fall in expired CO_2 associated with a fall in oxygen saturation indicating interrupted gas exchange. Gas in the cerebral circulation will cause convulsions, paralysis, and sudden death. Intracardiac gas can mechanically obstruct the circulation and cause myocardial ischemia through coronary artery occlusion. The typical "mill wheel" cardiac murmur is not always heard. Pulmonary edema is common.

Initial management

The procedure should be terminated and if gas embolism is suspected the patient should be placed head down in the left lateral position to minimize gas transit to the brain. Regardless of the etiology, high-flow (preferably 100%) oxygen should be administered and intravenous access secured. Cardiopulmonary resuscitation should be initiated without delay if required, and the patient rapidly transferred for investigation and further management.

Monitoring should include ECG, blood pressure, oxygen saturations, and if feasible end-expired CO_2 concentrations.

Investigations

Once transferred, arterial blood gas analysis, complete blood count, electrolyte analysis and liver functions tests should be sent. Other investigations such as chest x-ray, ventilation/perfusion lung scan, or computed tomography pulmonary angiogram and echocardiology may be indicated. Doppler ultrasound is the most sensitive detector of gas in the precordium.

Local anesthetic toxicity

Introduction

Local anesthetics are routinely used to provide analgesia and anesthesia for a variety of office gynecological procedures. Toxicity may occur following excessive dosage and absorption or secondary to inadvertent intravascular injection. Clinicians should be alert to the possibility of local anesthetic toxicity in their patients and take steps to reduce the risk of development. These include the use of the smallest effective clinical dose of local anesthetic, careful aspiration, and use of a test dose to help ascertain correct needle placement, slow and incremental injection, and adequate monitoring of patient vital signs and mental state. Early detection of this complication is important.

Presentation

The signs and symptoms of local anesthetic toxicity may be neurological or cardiovascular. Neurological effects tend to occur first; the conscious patient may develop peri-oral numbness or tingling, a metallic taste in the mouth, tinnitus, lightheadedness, agitation, and/or disorientation. Seizures may occur in severe cases. Cardiovascular effects tend to occur with higher blood levels of local anesthetic. These signs include the development of arrhythmias, chest pain, hypotension, and cardiac arrest. Of the local anesthetics in common use, bupivacaine in particular is very cardiotoxic. It adheres strongly to sodium channels in the myocardium and inhibits oxidative phosphorylation.

Initial management

The American Society of Regional Anesthesia and Pain Medicine (ASRA) has published an algorithm for the management of local anesthetic toxicity which is available on its website.[23]

It is recommended that this algorithm is prominently displayed in all office environments where local anesthetics are in common use.

Since hypoxia and acidosis can exacerbate the toxic effects of local anesthetic, the initial management of local anesthetic toxicity involves the administration of high-flow oxygen via face mask at 10 L–15 L/minute. If seizures are present, a small dose of a benzodiazepine should be given to try to terminate the seizures in addition to taking measures to protect the patient from aspiration and to ensure a patent airway is maintained.

The use of a 20% lipid emulsion, such as Intralipid®, is now recommended as first-line treatment of local anesthetic toxicity. The lipid acts as a "sink" for circulating local anesthetic and prevents it from binding to cardiac muscle. It can also reverse neurological signs and symptoms including seizures and altered mental state, and thus is useful even when cardiovascular symptoms are absent.[24]

The initial intravenous bolus dose for an adult is 1.5 mL/kg lean body mass administered over one minute (~100 mL), and this should be followed immediately by a continuous infusion of 0.25 mL/kg/minute (~ 18 mL/minute).

Persistent cardiovascular collapse may require repeated bolus doses of lipid emulsion every five minutes (maximum of two repeated doses). The lipid infusion rate may be doubled to 0.5 mL/kg/minute at any point after five minutes if cardiovascular instability or hypotension persists. Treatment with lipid emulsion should be in conjunction with standard cardiac advanced life support measures if cardiorespiratory arrest occurs. Good quality cardiac compressions are vital in ensuring that lipid reaches the coronary circulation. Recovery from cardiac arrest secondary to local anesthetic toxicity may require prolonged cardiopulmonary resuscitation (>1 hour).

Any patient who develops severe local anesthetic toxicity should be transferred to a site where she can be fully monitored for further complications. A potential exists for a recurrence of cardiovascular depression up to 12 hours after the initial injection of local anesthetic.[13] Use of lipid emulsion should be reported to the international registry at www.lipidregistry.org and cases of local anesthetic toxicity recorded at www.lipidrescue.org.

Investigations

To date, there have been no serious side effects reported in relation to the use of lipid emulsion for resuscitation in local anesthetic toxicity. It is recommended, however, that the total dose of lipid emulsion be limited to approximately 10 mL–12 mL/kg over 30 minutes (~1,000 mL).[24] In addition, amylase levels should be monitored in a place of definitive care, since there may be the potential for hyperlipidemic pancreatitis to develop when large lipid volumes are used.

Vasovagal reactions

Introduction

The vagus forms the major part of the parasympathetic nervous system. Vagal reflexes can cause bronchospasm, laryngospasm, and bradycardia. The latter can be associated with complete heart block and even asystole. Stimulation through dilatation of the cervix is a particularly potent vagal stimulant associated with both bradycardia and bronchospasm (the Brewer-Lickhardt reflex). Stimulation of mesentery, uterus, bladder, urethra can also initiate such reflexes.

Presentation

The patient may give a history of inability to tolerate gynecologic procedures such cervical screening. The conscious patient will complain of feeling dizzy, faint, and unwell and become cool and clammy with a slow pulse and hypotension. She may lose consciousness, suffer a seizure, or even decrease cardiac output. In the anesthetized patient, bradycardia is a fairly common response to cervical manipulation as is distension of the abdomen during laparascopy. Brochospasm or laryngospasm will cause a rise in inflation pressures and problems with ventilation.

Immediate management

Frequently all that is required is for the stimulus to be stopped. To prevent recurrence an anticholinergic such as atropine or glycopyrronium should be given. Glycopyrronium has the advantage that it does not cross the blood brain barrier. A dose of 200 mcg–600 mcg intravenously should be sufficient to bock further vagal reflexes.

Water intoxication syndrome

Introduction

Endometrial ablation, transcervical resection of the endometrium (TCRE), and other hysteroscopic procedures performed in the office setting often require the use of fluid for irrigation, distention of the uterine cavity, and optimal visualization of the surgical field. The most commonly used fluids for these purposes are saline or glycine 1.5% since they are relatively inexpensive, have good optical properties, and lack significant allergic side effects. Alternative fluids that are sometimes used include mannitol, dextran, and sorbitol solutions. Fluid overload complicates 0.1%–0.2% of hysteroscopic gynecologic procedures, although some procedures such as resection of uterine septa and myomectomy are associated with a greater risk.[25]

Fluid overload can result in dilutional coagulopathy, pulmonary and cerebral edema, and heart failure;

these can be fatal. Hyponatremia and hyposmolarity result from fluid overload with electrolyte free, low viscosity fluids. Premenopausal women are 25 times more likely to die or suffer permanent neurological damage from cerebral edema caused by hyponatremia than the postmenopausal or male population due to inhibition of the NA-K adenosine pump by estrogens. Fluid overload with metabolic complications can, however, also occur with the use of isotonic solutions. Normal saline overload has been associated with dilutional coagulopathy and hyperchloremic acidosis.[26]

The driving force for fluid absorption into the circulation is the pressure of the fluid itself. When the fluid pressure exceeds the venous pressure of ~1.5 kPa, fluid is forced into open veins which have been severed during surgery. The volume absorbed increases significantly with the length of time at which the fluid pressure exceeds the venous pressure.[27]

Presentation

The syndrome may manifest itself either intraoperatively or postoperatively (often 30–45 minutes post procedure) with a mixture of circulatory and neurological signs and symptoms. These will be dependent on both the volume of fluid absorbed and the type of fluid used. Symptoms may occur with as little as 500 mL of fluid absorption and are due to a combination of intravascular volume overload, intracellular edema and hyponatremia, with or without complications directly related to the choice of irrigation fluid.

The most consistent signs of water intoxication syndrome are bradycardia and arterial hypotension.[28]

Chest pain, pulmonary edema, and oliguria may also occur. Conscious patients may become agitated or confused and experience nausea and vomiting or headache. Glycine is an inhibitory neurotransmitter that has particularly marked effects on the transmission of retinal impulses to the central nervous system; it is metabolized to ammonia by the liver. Transient visual disturbances occur in approximately 10% of patients who absorb an excess of 500 mL of glycine. Cerebral edema has been reported after the absorption of >1 L of glycine during TCRE. In the most severe cases, water intoxication syndrome may be associated with seizures (serum sodium < 120 mmol/L), loss of consciousness, and cardiorespiratory arrest.

Initial management

The prevention of water intoxication syndrome should be the main aim. There is growing evidence to suggest that preoperative treatment with gonadotropin-releasing hormone (GnRH) agonists both reduces the amount of fluid absorbed and minimizes the effects of hyponatremic hypo-osmolar encephalopathy by reversing the estrogen inhibition of the Na-K adenosine triphosphatase pump. Simple preventative measures include ensuring that the patient has a normal serum sodium concentration and is euvolemic prior to undertaking surgery. There should also be careful monitoring of the amount of fluid being used and absorbed intraoperatively in all cases.

If water intoxication syndrome does occur or is suspected, then the treatment is mainly supportive. There should be a predetermined volume of absorption; after this level, electrolytes should be measured and diuretics given. Furosemide should not be given when hypotonic fluid is implicated as it may worsen the hyponatremia. The maximum fluid deficit tolerated without terminating the procedure will depend on the fluid used and presence of comorbidities. A maximum deficit of 1,000 mL has been recommended when hypotonic solutions are used in the healthy patient, (although complications of hyponatremia have been associated with as little as 200 mL deficit). Up to 2,500 mL is suggested when isotonic solutions are used.[29] Obviously the procedure should be halted earlier should there be clinical signs of overload.

Investigations

Serum sodium and serum osmolality should be measured. The administration of hypertonic saline may be indicated after transfer to higher level care if there is evidence of cerebral edema or the serum sodium level falls below 120 mmol/L. Correction of serum sodium should not occur at a rate exceeding 1 mmol/L/hour due to the risk of cerebral pontine myelinolysis.[28]

Concluding remarks

In order to minimize the likelihood of an office emergency occurring, it is important that careful patient selection occurs prior to surgery, particularly with reference to underlying comorbidities and general patient health. When dealing with an office emergency, staff must follow relevant and current guidelines and these must be readily available for review.

Frequent multidisciplinary training and simulation in emergency scenarios should be undertaken to ensure that staff are fully prepared, and emergency equipment and drugs should be regularly checked and kept up to date. Clear protocols must be in place to allow the rapid transfer of a patient to a definitive care facility once initial emergency treatment has been instigated.

References

1. American College of Obstetricians and Gynecologists. Preparing for clinical emergencies in obstetrics and gynecology. Committee Opinion No. 487. *Obstet Gynecol* 2011; **117**: 1032–4.
2. Neumar RW, Otto CW, Link MS, et al. Part 8: adult advanced cardiovascular life support: 2010 American Heart Association guidelines for cardiopulmonary resuscitation and emergency cardiovascular care. *Circulation* 2010: **122**[Suppl 3]: S729–67.
3. Rosenberg NM, Urman RD, Gallagher S, et al. Effect of an office based surgical safety system on patient outcomes. *Eplasty* 2012; 12: e59.
4. National Center for Health Statistics (US). *Health, United States, 2013*. Hyattsville (MD). May 2014. Report No: 2014–32.
5. American Society of Anesthesiologists. Guidelines for office-based anesthesia. Available at: asatest.asahq.org/publicationsAndServices/standards/12.pdf. Accessed October 19, 2014.
6. Berg RA, Hemphill R, Abella BS, et al. Adult basic life support: 2010 American Heart Association guidelines for cardiopulmonary resuscitation and emergency cardiovascular care. *Circulation* 2010: **122**[Suppl 3]: S685–705.
7. Sheppard LP, Channer KS. Acute coronary syndromes. *CEACCP* 2004; **4** (6): 175–80.
8. American Congress of Obstetricians and Gynecologists. Women's Health, 2011: Stats and Facts. Available at: www.acog.org/-/media/NewsRoom/MediaKit.pdf.
9. Anderson JL, Adams CD, Antman EM, et al. 2011 ACCF/AHA focused update incorporated into the ACC/AHA 2007 guidelines for the management of patients with unstable angina/non ST-elevation myocardial infarction: a report of the American College of Cardiology Foundation/American Heart Association Task Force on Practice Guidelines. *Circulation* 2011; **123**: e426–579.
10. O'Gara PT, Kushner FG, Ascheim DD, et al. 2013 ACCF/AHA Guideline for the Management of ST-Elevation Myocardial Infarction: a report of the American College of Cardiology Foundation/American Heart Association Task Force on Practice Guidelines. *J Am Coll Cardiol* 2013; **61**(4): e78–140.
11. Vanden Hoek TL, Morrison LJ, Shuster M, et al. Part 12: cardiac arrest in special situations 2010 American Heart Association guidelines for cardiopulmonary resuscitation and emergency cardiovascular care. *Circulation* 2010: **122**(Suppl 3): S829–61.
12. Institute of Medicine (US) Committee on the Public Health Dimensions of the Epilepsies. *Epilepsy across the spectrum: promoting health and understanding.* England MJ, Liverman CT, Schultz AM, Strawbridge LM (Eds.). Washington, DC: National Academies Press (US), 2012.
13. Brophy GM, Bell R, Claassen J, et al. Guidelines for the evaluation and management of status epilepticus. *Neurocrit Care* 2012; **17**(1): 3–23.
14. Sutula TP, Hagen J, Pitkänen, A. Do epileptic seizures damage the brain? *Curr Opin Neurol* 2003; **16**(2): 189–95.
15. Paterson-Brown S, Howell C. (Eds.) *Managing obstetric emergencies & trauma: the MOET course manual*, 3rd Edition. Cambridge: Cambridge University Press, 2014.
16. Paterson-Brown S, Bamber J. Prevention and treatment of haemorrhage. In: Knight M, Kenyon S, Brocklehurst P, et al. (Eds.) on behalf of MBRRACE-UK. *Saving lives, improving mothers' care – lessons learned to inform future maternity care from the UK and Ireland confidential enquiries into maternal deaths and morbidity 2009–12*. Oxford: National Perinatal Epidemiology Unit, University of Oxford, 2014.
17. Johansson SO, Bieber T, Dahl R, et al. A revised nomenclature for allergy for global use: Report of the nomenclature review committee of the World Allergy Organization. *J Allergy Clin Immunol* 2004; **113** (5): 832–6.
18. Ebo DG, Fisher MM, Hagendorens MM, et al. Anaphylaxis during anaesthesia: diagnostic approach. *Allergy* 2007; **62** (5): 471–87.
19. Whittington T, Fisher MM. Anaphylactic and anaphylactoid reactions. *Baillière's Clin Anaesthesiol* 1998; **12**; 301–23.
20. McLean-Tooke AC, Bethune CA, Fay AC, et al. Adrenaline in the treatment of anaphylaxis: what is the evidence? *BMJ* 2003; **327**: 1332–5.
21. Knight M, Nair M, Shah A, et al. Maternal mortality and morbidity in the UK 2009–12: surveillance and epidemiology. In: Knight M, Kenyon S, Brocklehurst P, et al. (Eds.) *on behalf of MBRRACE-UK.* Saving lives, improving mothers' care – lessons learned to inform future maternity care from the UK and Ireland confidential enquiries into maternal deaths and

morbidity 2009–12. Oxford: National Perinatal Epidemiology Unit. University of Oxford, 2014.

22. Mushkat Y, Luxman D, Nachum Z, et al. Gas embolism complicating obstetric and gynecologic procedures. Cases reports and review of the literature. *Eur J Obstetrics and Gynecology & Reproductive Medicine* 1995; **63**: 97–103.
23. American Society of Regional Anesthesia and Pain Medicine. Checklist for treatment of local anesthetic systemic toxicity. Available at: www.asra.com. Accessed July 31, 2014.
24. Weinberg GL. Lipid emulsion infusion: resuscitation for local anesthetic and other drug overdose. *Anesthesiology* 2012; **117** (1): 180–7.
25. Propst AM, Liberman RF, Harlow BL, et al. Complications of hysteroscopic surgery: predicting patients at risk. *Obstetrics & Gynecology* 2000; **96**(4): 517–20.
26. Schafer M, Von Ungern-Sternberg BS, Wight E, Schneider MC. Isotonic fluid absorption during hysteroscopy resulting in severe hyperchloraemic acidosis. *Anesthesiol* 2005; **103**(1): 203–4.
27. Hahn RG. Fluid absorption in endoscopic surgery. *Br J Anaesth* 2006; **96** (1): 8–20.
28. Ayus JC, Arieff AI. Glycine-induced hypo-osmolar hyponatremia. *Arch Intern Med* 1997; **157** (2): 223–6.
29. AAGL Practice Report: practice guidelines for the management of hysteroscopic distending media. *Journal of Minimally Invasive Gynecology* 2013; **20**(2): 137–48.

Chapter 10

Preconception evaluation

Susanne Bathgate and Nancy Gaba

Scope of the problem

Preconception counseling affords the opportunity to identify, educate about, and modify risk factors for poor pregnancy outcome for both the woman and the child. In the United States, only about 50% of pregnancies are planned;[1] therefore, preconception counseling should be considered even if that is not the expressed purpose of the health-care encounter. Preconception counseling is not just for those with identified personal or family medical conditions, but also for "healthy women." The thought "every woman, every time" for preconception counseling has been articulated and is a useful concept to keep in mind.[2] Pregnancy planning should also be incorporated into prenatal and postpartum health care, as well as visits for acute and chronic health conditions.

The concept of a reproductive life plan has been offered to help women make life and contraceptive decisions to optimize reproductive outcomes.[3] A woman should be encouraged to consider the timing, spacing, and number of children she plans, as well as barriers to this plan, such as age-related fertility changes. A woman should be encouraged to consider her readiness for pregnancy and her contraceptive options, if appropriate.

Planning for pregnancy may be a time of particular motivation for lifestyle and health choice changes. Some women may be motivated to make changes that were previously postponed or overlooked. Planning for pregnancy may also be a time to reassess family medical history issues that were previously considered intrusive or superfluous.

Including the partner in the preconception process can be helpful. Information about the partner's family history may allow targeted genetic screening. Counseling the partner about pregnancy planning and lifestyle interventions such as smoking cessation and decreasing exposure to toxic substances may improve pregnancy outcomes. Vaccinating the partner and other newborn caregivers against influenza and pertussis reduces the rate of transmission of these diseases to the newborn.[4]

History

A preconception counseling visit may involve both the woman and her partner and may be facilitated by the use of questionnaires followed by questions to elicit a thorough history.

Menstrual history

An irregular or long menstrual cycle may indicate hypothyroidism, hyperprolactinemia, or polycystic ovarian syndrome. In the case of regular menstrual cycles, many couples appreciate a review of the menstrual cycle and ovulation to help plan timing of intercourse for conception. In general, ovulation proceeds the next menstrual cycle by 14 days. The most fertile time is thought to be the day of ovulation and the five prior days; however, this timing can be quite variable.[5] Advising a woman to maintain a menstrual diary can be very helpful in providing targeting counseling about maximizing chances of conception.

Past medical history

Assessment of preexisting medical conditions affords the opportunity to counsel patients about the implications of these disorders and to optimize these conditions prior to pregnancy thereby mitigating potential risks. Indeed, some conditions are especially associated with adverse outcomes of unintended or unplanned pregnancies (Table 10-1).

Specific disorders

Diabetes mellitus

Women with diabetes should be counseled about optimum preconception and periconception blood glucose

Office Care of Women, ed. Martin E. Olsen and Botros Rizk. Published by Cambridge University Press.

Table 10-1 Conditions associated with increased risk for adverse health events as a result of unintended pregnancy

- Breast cancer
- Complicated valvular heart disease
- Diabetes: insulin-dependent; with nephropathy/retinopathy/neuropathy or other vascular disease; or of >20 years' duration
- Endometrial or ovarian cancer
- Epilepsy
- Hypertension (systolic >160 mmHg or diastolic >100 mmHg)
- History of bariatric surgery within the past 2 years
- HIV/AIDS
- Ischemic heart disease
- Malignant gestational trophoblastic disease
- Malignant liver tumors (hepatoma) and hepatocellular carcinoma of the liver
- Peripartum cardiomyopathy
- Severe cirrhosis
- Sickle cell disease
- Solid organ transplantation within the past 2 years
- Stroke
- Systemic lupus erythematosus
- Thrombogenic mutations
- Tuberculosis[1]

Source: Adapted from US Medical Eligibility Criteria for Contraceptive Use, 2010.

control. For instance, a hemoglobin A1c in the normal range is associated with a rate of congenital anomalies comparable to the nondiabetic population. However, a hemoglobin A1c of 10% is associated with a rate of congenital anomalies of about 20%, most commonly neural tube defects and congenital heart defects. Similarly, miscarriage is more common for women with poorly controlled glucose levels in early pregnancy. Controlling glucose levels before conception and in the early pregnancy period can reduce the number of birth defects and decrease the rate of spontaneous abortion.[6, 7] The preconception period is an optimal time for encouraging weight loss and lifestyle modifications for these women. For many women, converting to insulin instead of oral hypoglycemic agents is recommended prior to pregnancy. Education about the additional challenges of changing glucose metabolism due to the antagonistic effects of pregnancy hormones such as human placental lactogen (HPL) may help prepare the diabetic woman for the additional vigilance necessary in pregnancy. Diabetic women should be screened for coexistent renal and/or cardiac involvement. Women with pre-pregnancy diabetic nephropathy have a higher rate of preeclampsia.[8] Women with pre-pregnancy coronary artery disease have a higher rate of morbidity and mortality from pregnancy.[9]

Hypertension

Women with mild chronic hypertension are at increased maternal and fetal risks including perinatal mortality, placental abruption, and impaired fetal growth.[10] Women with hypertension for five years or more, or those who also have diabetes should have renal and cardiovascular function assessed.[11] Women with organ dysfunction or prior cerebrovascular accident, ventricular failure or myocardial infarction are at significantly increased risk for worsening during pregnancy or recurrence. Serum creatinine more than 1.4 mg/dL increases the risk of fetal loss and acceleration of renal disease.[12]

Consideration should also be given to underlying disease processes related to hypertension, for example, control of systemic lupus erythematosus. Women on angiotensin converting enzyme (ACE) or angiotensin receptor blocker (ARB) medications should be counseled on the risks of those medications in pregnancy and alternative medications should be prescribed. Optimization of factors that contribute to hypertension, including body mass index (BMI), glucose control if diabetic, nutrition, and activity, should be encouraged.

HIV/AIDS

If human immunodeficiency virus (HIV) infection is detected prior to conception, antiretroviral therapy and reduction of HIV viral load can be achieved prior to conception and the likelihood of transmission to the fetus/neonate can be thus reduced. Couples should be counseled about the risks of vertical transmission and the decreased rates of transmission with low or undetectable viral loads during pregnancy. For couples discordant for HIV infection, methods of conception to reduce transmission from one partner to the other should be discussed. The antiretroviral medications being used should be reviewed and altered if efavirenz is part of the regimen, as this drug may slightly increase the incidence of neural tube defects.[13] Screening and treatment of concurrent infections is recommended.

Epilepsy

Women with seizure disorders on medication prior to conception should be maintained at the lowest effective dose of the fewest medications prior to pregnancy,[14] especially if the last seizure was two or more years ago.[15] A number of anticonvulsant medications have teratogenic potential; for instance, the incidence of neural tube defects in the offspring of women taking valproic acid is 1%.[16] A woman should be made aware of this potential and the decision whether to continue or change medications is best be made prior to conception in consultation with the provider caring for her seizure disorder. Folic acid supplementation is recommended for all women prior to conception, but especially for those taking anticonvulsant medications.

Mental health disorders

For women on medical therapy for psychiatric disorders, the medication itself should be reviewed and the risks of unmedicated psychiatric disease compared to the risk of the specific medication. In the case of some medications, such as lithium, an alternate medication may be chosen. In other cases, the risk to that woman of stopping the medication may be substantial and the medication may be continued.[17]

Women with a history of depression, anxiety, and/or body image disorders may find pregnancy and the postpartum period a time of particular vulnerability to recurrence or worsening of these disorders. The couple should be given resources and counseled ahead of time to have support systems in place. Collaboration with the patient's mental health provider prior to conception can reduce the likelihood of difficulty during pregnancy.

Systemic lupus erythematosus

Pregnancy outcomes such as preeclampsia and preterm delivery are generally reduced if lupus has been inactive or well controlled for six months or more prior to conception. The disease activity of lupus in pregnancy varies with the activity of the lupus prior to pregnancy, with 7%–33% of women with quiet disease in the six months prior to pregnancy having exacerbation or active disease compared to 61%–67% of those with active disease at the beginning of pregnancy.[18, 19] Methotrexate should be discontinued one month or more prior to conception due to its teratogenicity.[20]

Asthma

Unless asthma is severe, pregnancy outcomes for women with asthma are generally excellent.[21] Therapy and lifestyle changes to optimize pulmonary function should be started prior to conception, including objective evaluation of lung function, optimization of pharmacologic therapy, patient education, and avoidance of triggers. The woman should be encouraged to continue asthma therapy once pregnant.[22] Women should be reassured that there is no adverse safety data regarding use of albuterol, budesonide, or intranasal corticosteroids in pregnancy.[23]

Anemia

If iron deficiency anemia is found, iron supplementation should be started to replete iron stores prior to pregnancy. Iron deficiency anemia in pregnancy increases the chance of preterm labor, low birth weight babies, and the potential need for transfusion with delivery. If microcytic anemia is found, evaluation with hemoglobin electrophoresis to identify sickle cell or beta thalassemia or hemoglobin C carriers is recommended. Sickle cell testing alone will not identify carriers of these other hemoglobinopathies.

Cancer

Depending on the timing and the type of therapy for the cancer, fertility preserving options may be available, such as embryo cryopreservation, oocyte cryopreservation, ovarian cryopreservation, or pre-radiotherapy ovarian transposition.[24] The woman should be counseled on the potential impact of cancer therapy on her fertility since fertility may be diminished after radiation or chemotherapy.[25] Also, depending on the nature and prognosis of the cancer, the woman should be counseled on the potential impact of the pregnancy on her disease. Breast cancer survivors are typically advised to wait two years after completion of therapy to conceive after the highest risk of recurrence has passed; however, for women with localized disease, conception before this time has not been shown to adversely affect survival.[26] Similarly, women with previous melanoma may be advised to wait two years to conceive to have a better estimate of their chance of recurrence.[27]

Thyroid disease

Women with overt hypothyroidism often have difficulty conceiving. Screening for thyroid disease in women with a family history, obesity, type 1 diabetes mellitus, age over 35, or other risk factors followed by subsequent treatment with thyroid hormone replacement may facilitate conception. Untreated hypothyroidism is associated with an increase in pre-eclampsia and prematurity.[28, 29] Severe maternal hypothyroxinemia is associated with cognitive delay in early childhood.[30]

Obesity/low body weight

Women who are obese have more problems with infertility. Once pregnant, they are more prone to miscarriage, birth defects, gestational diabetes, hypertensive disorders of pregnancy, and stillbirth. Shoulder dystocia and cesarean deliveries are more common in obese women as are postpartum wound infection, hemorrhage, and thromboembolic disease. Trial of labor after prior cesarean is less likely to result in successful vaginal birth in obese women.[31] Preconception weight loss can reverse these tendencies. Obese women should be screened for diabetes and hypothyroidism. Offspring of obese women are more likely to have meconium aspiration, be large for gestational age, be admitted to the neonatal intensive care unit (NICU), and have childhood obesity, diabetes and heart disease later in life. Women who have previously undergone bariatric surgery should be screened for vitamin deficiencies such as B12, folate, and D and additionally supplemented for these vitamins.[32]

An underweight status prior to pregnancy increases a woman's rate of infertility. Women who are underweight at the time of conception have higher incidences of pregnancy complications, such as low birth weight and preterm delivery. Babies born prematurely and/or small for gestation may have long-term development issues.

Cardiac disease

The prevalence of cardiovascular disease among women of childbearing age is increasing and can dramatically impact pregnancy outcome. Women with risk factors for cardiovascular disease, such as obesity, smoking, sedentary lifestyle, increasing maternal age, and comorbidities such diabetes, hypertension, and hyperlipidemia are at relatively higher risk of myocardial infarction in pregnancy and may benefit from assessment of cardiac function prior to pregnancy, although the absolute risk of myocardial infarction in pregnancy is low.

Some maternal cardiac conditions have a significant chance of worsening during pregnancy or of causing maternal mortality. For instance, women with Marfan's syndrome and a dilated aortic root have a substantial risk of obstetric complications and death in pregnancy that may be lower in women with prior aortic root replacement. Women at especially high risk include those with New York Heart Association (NYHA) class III and IV disease. Pulmonary hypertension and cyanotic heart disease confer high risks of mortality during pregnancy. Women with prior mechanical cardiac valve replacement require anticoagulation during pregnancy. Women with a previously identified structural or functional cardiac defect may benefit from consultation with either a maternal fetal medicine specialist and/or cardiologist prior to pregnancy.[33]

Renal disease

Renal insufficiency confers increased risks of pre-eclampsia, low birth weight and preterm birth, and possibly further deterioration of renal function. Women with renal insufficiency should have optimal blood pressure management prior to conception.[34] Women with mild renal disease (creatinine 0.9 mL/dL–1.4 mL/dL) and normal blood pressure experience successful pregnancy outcome 90% of the time and have a low risk of progression of renal disease. Women with moderate (creatinine 1.4 mg/dL–2.5 mg/dL) or severe renal disease (creatinine >2.5 mg/dL) are at risk for worsening renal function during pregnancy.[35] Women on ACE or ARB medications should be counseled on the risks of those medications in pregnancy and alternative medications should be prescribed.

Phenylketonuria

Adults with phenylketonuria may have stopped dietary restrictions. The fetus of a patient with untreated phenylketonuria may demonstrate impaired brain development. Women who were diagnosed with phenylketonuria as infants can reduce their chances of delivering an impaired infant by following a reduced phenylalanine diet at least three months before and during pregnancy to reduce the circulating levels of phenylalanine, which can harm the developing fetus. Because many some women may not know that they were ever diagnosed with phenylketonuria, all women should be asked if they were ever placed on a special diet during childhood.[36]

Thromboembolic disease

For a personal or strong family history of thromboembolic disease, the woman should be counseled on the increased risk of venous thromboembolism during pregnancy. A personal history of thromboembolism, especially in the absence of risk factors such as immobilization, surgery, long-distance air travel or use of estrogens should prompt investigation of inherited thrombophilia. Similarly, a family history of recurrent thrombosis or sudden death due to pulmonary embolism should also prompt such testing.[37]

In some patients, anticoagulation may be recommended for pregnancy. Warfarin should be avoided due to its teratogenicity.

Myotonic dystrophy

Certain disorders, such as myotonic dystrophy, are transmitted to offspring with potentially increasing severity in subsequent generations. Although the parent may be only mildly affected, the children may be more profoundly disabled.[38]

Past obstetric history

Women with a history of preterm birth are at increased risk of having another premature delivery.[39] Gathering history about causes or contributing factors to prior preterm birth affords the opportunity address modifiable risk factors such as under- or overweight status, anemia, poorly controlled hypothyroidism or diabetes. Supplemental progesterone and/or cervical length monitoring in the next pregnancy can be offered to women with a history of preterm birth due to preterm rupture of membranes or preterm labor.

If a prior pregnancy was complicated by preeclampsia at less than 34 weeks gestation, or if preeclampsia was experienced in more than one pregnancy, treatment with low dose aspirin in a future pregnancy beginning late in the first trimester may reduce the chance of recurrent preeclampsia.[40]

For prior pregnancy complicated by stillbirth, an attempt should be made to learn the cause of that stillbirth. The woman should be counseled to make modifications to any amenable risk factors, such as smoking cessation, normalizing body weight, and controlling diabetes. Testing for antiphospholipid antibodies, lupus anticoagulant, anticardiolipin antibodies and beta 2 microglobin, should be performed, and if found, treatment with low dose aspirin and heparin for the next pregnancy should be offered.[41]

Prior unexplained recurrent pregnancy loss should prompt an investigation of uterine anomalies and parental karyotypes.

Interconception intervals of less than 18 months or more than 59 months are significantly associated with adverse pregnancy outcomes.[42] Short interpregnancy intervals of less than six months are associated with increased risks of low birth weight babies and preterm birth, compared to intervals of more than 18 months. Interconception intervals of 18 months or greater are associated with fewer uterine ruptures during trial of labor after previous cesarean delivery. Interconception intervals greater than 59 months are associated with higher rates of preeclampsia.

Family history/ethnicity

Family history of congenital anomalies

The family history of both the woman and the male partner should be obtained. In this way, there is the opportunity to counsel about inherited diseases. For instance, if the partner has a family history of neural tube defect, the woman should be advised to increase her folic acid intake to 4 mg daily. There is some evidence that folic acid may help reduce the incidence of other multifactoral birth defects such as orofacial clefts and congenital heart disease. The couple should be screened for consanguinity. A convenient tool for the couple to use to record family history is www.hhs.gov/familyhistory.[43]

Women with premature ovarian insufficiency or family history of predominantly male delayed development, mental retardation, or autism should have screening for fragile X premutation and be referred to a genetic counselor.

Some recessive genetic traits are prevalent in specific populations, and screening before conception for these traits can offer couples the chance to make informed decisions about conception. Some couples may choose to conceive and have diagnostic testing for these conditions once pregnant. Others may choose reproductive technologies that allow for embryo biopsy and transfer of only unaffected embryos. Some couples may choose not to conceive at all if they learn that they are both carriers. Preconception education allows all to understand their chances for an affected child.

Cystic fibrosis is prevalent among many populations, more so for those of Northern European ancestry. Cystic fibrosis screening should be offered to all women of Caucasian ancestry and made available to those of all genetic backgrounds. If there is a family history of cystic fibrosis, documentation of the particular mutations involved is helpful, as not all mutations are included in the current commercially available panels.

Beta thalassemia is prevalent in those of Mediterranean ancestry. Sickle cell trait is found in those of African and Latin American ancestry. Alpha thalassemia is found in the Asian population.

The Ashkenazi Jewish population carries genetic mutations for several recessive diseases with a carrier rate for Tay-Sachs disease of 1/30, Canavan disease 1/40, Gaucher disease 1/15, cystic fibrosis 1/29, Bloom syndrome 1/100, and so on. Several commercially available panels are available for detecting these mutations. French Canadian and Cajun populations have a prevalence of Tay-Sachs disease mutations of 1/30.[44]

Medications

One in 25 prescriptions written for women aged 15–45 is for a potentially teratogenic medication.[45] Ideally, all women of reproductive age should receive pregnancy counseling about the medications that they are prescribed at the time they initiate those medications, and medications with high likelihood of teratogenicity are best to only be prescribed to women with very low likelihood of conception, such as those using long-acting reversible contraception (LARC) or dual methods of contraception. Such medications would include isotretinoin (Acutane), lithium, trenotoin (Retin A), thalidomide, methotrexate, warfarin, ACE inhibitors, and ARBs. Other medications of lower teratogenicity that should also be avoided include the tetracyclines, which can cause discoloration of teeth when used after 25 weeks gestation. The decision to continue or change medications should involve a risk-benefit analysis of the medication and its alternative or absence on the medical condition being treated.

Maternal and paternal age

Pregnancy at a later maternal age confers increased risks for trisomies, especially trisomy 21, such that the rate of clinically significant aneuploidies at delivery is 5 per 1,000 for age 35 years, 15 per 1,000 at age 40 years, and 50 per 1,000 at age 45 years.[46] Pregnancy complications such as multiple gestation, hypertension, and diabetes also increase with advancing maternal age. Pregnancy after age 35 compared to before age 35 is more often complicated by outcomes such as maternal near miss morbidity, maternal death, preterm birth, stillbirth, low birth weight, perinatal mortality, and NICU admission.[47] Miscarriage is more common as maternal age increases.[48]

Later paternal age confers increased risks for single gene mutation, autosomal dominant disorders such as achondroplasia, and neurofibromatosis, although the incidence of these disorders is still low. Some studies have linked paternal age over 50 years to increased development of schizophrenia in offspring compared to paternal age less than 25 years.[49] Other studies have linked older paternal age more than 50 years to an increased risk of autism in offspring.[50]

Nutrition, wellness, lifestyle, environmental exposures

Nutrition

An assessment of the woman's dietary intake should be made. Simple questions, such as "How many servings of fruits and vegetables do you eat daily?" and "Do you exclude any kinds of foods?" can be helpful. In particular, women should be educated to eat food sources of folic acid, iron, calcium, docosahexaenoic acid (DHA), and protein prior to and during pregnancy. Women with special circumstances, such as adherence to a vegan diet or after bariatric surgery, should have blood tests for vitamin B12 and assessment of iron stores. Nutrition education resources are available through the US Department of Agriculture (USDA) www.ChooseMyPlate.gov. Women can be educated about food safety such as avoiding seafood higher in environmental contaminants, and sources of Listeria including unpasteurized cheeses.[51]

Supplements

Folic acid supplementation prior to pregnancy and continuation of this supplementation in the first trimester reduces the occurrence of neural tube defects and should be recommended. Most prenatal vitamins contain at least 400 mcg–800 mcg of folic acid. For women who have had a prior pregnancy complicated by neural tube defect, consumption of 4 mg of folic acid is recommended to reduce recurrence.[52] Women should be questioned about their use of nutritional supplements, as, for instance, excessive supplementation of vitamin A can be teratogenic.[53]

Similarly, women should be asked about whether they use herbal supplements. Herbal supplements are not regulated by the Federal Drug Administration (FDA), so their ingredients and strength is not certain, nor are herbal supplements subjected to the same testing as are FDA-approved substances so information about outcomes when taken in pregnancy is limited. For these reasons, it seems reasonable to recommend that women avoid herbal supplements during pregnancy.

Exercise

Most women who exercise before pregnancy can continue to exercise during pregnancy, sometimes with modifications, such as avoiding activities more likely to result in contact. An exercise routine can be part of maintaining a healthy weight and bone density, and continuation of exercise during can reduce the likelihood of gestational hypertension and diabetes. Some studies show that women who exercise in pregnancy have higher rates of vaginal delivery.[54] Exercise is part of health maintenance and should be encouraged.

Dental health

Periodontal disease in pregnancy has been linked to preterm birth;[55] however, efforts to improve outcome by treatment during pregnancy have not been successful.[56] Newer research efforts are focused on good dental health prior to pregnancy and across the lifespan to reduce related poor health outcomes, such as cardiovascular disease and diabetes, in addition to pregnancy problems.

Intimate partner violence

Pregnancy is a particularly vulnerable time for domestic violence. Violence against women occurs in an estimated 4%–8% of pregnancies. Nonjudgmental screening, education, and provision of resources prior to pregnancy is recommended.[57] In some instances it may be appropriate for a woman to postpone pregnancy.

Environmental exposures

Alcohol

Consumption of alcohol is not safe at any time during pregnancy. No minimum amount of alcohol has been identified that has not been linked to fetal alcohol syndrome. Women should be encouraged to stop drinking alcohol before pregnancy. Screening for alcohol abuse is recommended for all women.

Tobacco

Preterm birth, low birth weight, and sudden infant death syndrome are all neonatal outcomes more likely in infants born to women who smoke. Tobacco cessation before pregnancy reduces the risks of these conditions. Women who are in the process of quitting should be advised to postpone pregnancy until they are no longer using tobacco or tobacco cessation aids such as nicotine replacement or medications including varenicline (Chantix) or bupropion (Zyban).

Drugs of abuse

Illicit substance use complicates 16.2% of teen pregnancies and 7.4% of pregnancies in women aged 18–25 years.[58] Neonates exposed in utero, most commonly to opiates in dependent women, but also to benzodiazapenes, cocaine, or even selective serotonin reuptake inhibitors (SSRIs), may experience neonatal abstinence syndrome manifested by increased irritability, hypertonia, tremors, feeding intolerance, and respiratory distress. In utero opiate dependence in pregnancy is also associated with an increased risk of low birth weight (<2,500 gm) and mortality.[59] Referral for cessation treatment prior to pregnancy offers the opportunity to reduce pregnancy exposures.

Infectious agents

Cytomegalovirus (CMV) infection is common in young children. Women who work in childcare such as day care workers or elementary school teachers should be cautioned to avoid body fluids from children in general, especially sick children, as CMV infection in utero can cause diminution of mental capacity in children. Similarly, new maternal *Toxoplasma gondii* infection can be transmitted to the fetus, which can cause in utero intracranial calcifications, hydrocephalus, and chorioretinitis, often with neonatal seizures. Precautions against handling cat litter infected by toxoplasmosis spores and against eating rare or raw meats or unwashed vegetables should be advised for women without toxoplasmosis immunity. Women can be screened for toxoplasmosis prior to pregnancy to determine if they have Toxoplasma IgG, which is protective against in utero infection. Assessment of past history of chicken pox (varicella) and German measles (rubella) disease or vaccination offers the opportunity to vaccinate prior to pregnancy to prevent the pregnancy-associated complications associated with new infections in pregnancy. Couples discordant for herpes simplex virus (HSV) infection, specifically where the woman does not have HSV antibodies, are at risk for new HSV infection in pregnancy and should be advised to avoid intercourse while the male partner has an outbreak of HSV to limit new transmission to the woman during pregnancy.

Environmental contaminants

Preconception and prenatal exposure to environmental contaminants, such as lead, mercury, pesticides and endocrine disrupting chemicals has been linked to birth defects and impaired mental development of offspring. Identifying and screening women at risk for these exposures allows time for intervention and reduction of risk.[60]

Prenatal exposure to lead has long been known to be neurotoxic to the developing fetus. Maternal risk factors including pica practices, the use of lead-glazed pottery, renovating or remodeling a home built prior to 1970, and water contamination from wells or solder in pipes in older homes. Women with risk factors should have lead blood levels tested. Mercury exposure during pregnancy can cause adverse neurodevelopmental outcomes such as lower IQ and poor language and motor development. Mercury sources include consuming recreationally caught fish, occupational exposure such as working with dental amalgams and use of skin-lightening creams sold outside the United States. Eating fish is an excellent way to consume omega-3 fatty acids, which has been shown to improve visual acuity and scores on the Denver Developmental Screen and may possibly prolong gestation. Women prior to conception, while pregnant or while breastfeeding, should follow US Environmental Protection Agency and state-specific fish consumption guidelines.

Pesticide exposure during preconception and pregnancy has been associated with lower IQ and performance on other neurodevelopmental tests, possibly childhood leukemia, congenital anomalies, intrauterine growth restriction and low birth weight in populations exposed to agricultural and inner city environments. Pesticide exposure in the home can come from eating produce and using pesticides in the home or on pets. Exposure can be minimized by consuming organic produce or avoiding foods high in pesticide contamination as published by the Environmental Working Group (www.ewg.org/foodnews),[61] washing all fruits and vegetables before eating and removing shoes at the door.

Endocrine disrupting chemicals (EDCs) are chemicals that either mimic or antagonize the effects of endogenous hormones in the endocrine system and consequently can cause adverse health effects that can be passed on to future generations.[62] Diethlystilbesterol is the EDC most commonly known to medical personnel. Examples such as parabens, phthalates, bisphenol-A (BPA), and polybromnated diphenyl ethers (PBDEs) are found in plastics (phthalates and bisphenol-A), upholstery foam produced prior to 2005, and carpet padding (polybrominated diethyl ethers). Bisphenol-A is used in a wide variety of products that include hard polycarbonate plastics, canned food linings, and cash register receipts.[63]

Women who have occupational exposure to ionizing radiation should take precautions to minimize that exposure to prevent fetal effects. Dose monitoring is recommended if a pregnant woman may be significantly exposed.

Physical examination

The physical examination for preconception care should include assessment of weight and height for calculation of BMI, blood pressure, dental health, evidence of androgenization, thyroid enlargement, breast examination, heart and lungs, external genitalia, uterus, and ovaries.

Laboratory tests

Routine laboratory testing should be guided by the couple's history and current conditions. Testing for immunity to toxoplasmosis, parvovirus B19, varicella, and rubella should be offered, depending on suspected exposures, and prior disease and vaccination history. Sexually transmitted infection screening should be offered to all couples not previously tested, including HIV, hepatitis B, hepatitis C, syphilis, gonorrhea, and chlamydia testing. In particular, the Centers for Disease Control and Prevention (CDC) recommends testing for HIV infections in routine health-care settings for patients aged 13–64 where the prevalence of HIV is ≥1 per 1,000 or the prevalence is unknown, on an opt-out basis.[64] Testing for HIV should be performed for patients diagnosed with TB and at each visit for a new complaint of a sexually transmitted infection. Patients at high risk for HIV infection should be retested at least annually.

Cystic fibrosis carrier testing should be offered to all couples, and based on ethnicity, sickle cell and thalassemia testing, and Jewish panel testing should be offered. If a family history of developmental delay or mental retardation is elicited, fragile X premutation carrier screening should be performed.

Testing for antiphospholipid antibodies is recommended for women with prior unexplained stillbirth or recurrent first trimester pregnancy loss. For suspected environmental exposures, blood lead and mercury levels can be tested. See Table 10-2 for a complete list of recommended tests for preconception evaluation.

Women with hypertension and/or renal disease should have an assessment of current renal function performed by testing creatinine levels and proteinuria. Screening for vitamin B12 deficiency should be performed in women with prior bariatric surgery or restrictive nutritional intake such as vegan diet. Women with current thyroid disease, a history of thyroid disease, or symptoms suggestive of thyroid disease should have thyroid function testing performed. Women with pregestational diabetes should undergo hemoglobin A1c level assessment, and women with risk factors for type 2 diabetes mellitus should have diagnostic testing for diabetes prior to pregnancy (Table 10-3).

Preconception interventions

The mainstay of treatment for preconception is identification of risk factors for adverse pregnancy outcome, modification of those risk factors amenable to change, and counseling about all risk factors, including lifestyle and medical therapy options to improve pregnancy outcome. In some cases, treatment will involve referral to specialists to optimize current health conditions, such as diabetes or inflammatory bowel disease, or referral to a reproductive endocrinologist for assisted reproductive therapy.

Folic acid supplementation

Folic acid supplementation prior to pregnancy and in early pregnancy has led to decreased rates of neural tube defects. In addition to dietary sources, supplemental folic acid 400 mcg daily, alone or in a multivitamin, is recommended to decrease the risk of neural tube defects, such as spina bifida and anencephaly, by as much as two-thirds. Such supplementation may also reduce the risk of congenital heart defects. To prevent recurrence of pregnancy affected by neural tube defects, consumption of 4 mg of folic acid daily is recommended.[65]

Vaccination

Vaccination should be part of routine health maintenance and a preconception visit is another time to revisit adequacy of immunizations.[66] Some vaccines protect against teratogenic effects of some viral infections during pregnancy. Specifically, Rubella and Varicella infections may cause fetal malformations if those occur for the first time during pregnancy; these fetal effects can be prevented by preconception administration of these vaccines. Although there are no known teratogenic effects of rubella or varicella vaccination during pregnancy, women should be advised to delay conception one month after vaccination. Vaccination against hepatitis B prevents infection of the fetus and/or newborn. If a woman is unvaccinated against hepatitis A or B, she can begin and/or complete the series while pregnant. Although there are no known adverse effects of completing the HPV vaccination series during pregnancy, women are generally advised to wait until the postpartum period to do so. Pneumococcal vaccination is recommended for women with chronic conditions such as diabetes or connective tissue diseases as well as those who have decreased spleen function like women with sickle cell disease. Women should be up to date on their tetanus-diphtheria-acelluar pertussis (Tdap) vaccinations before conception and a Tdap booster should be given during 27 to 36 weeks gestation of subsequent pregnancies to prevent neonatal pertussis.[67] Tdap vaccine should also be given to those who anticipate contact with infants less than 12 months old (the cocoon strategy or cocooning) such as partners, grandparents, and other caregivers for children.[68]

Preconception prevention also includes raising awareness of potentially harmful exposures, whether through lifestyle choices or through inadvertent environmental exposure, and counseling women on avoidance of these risks.

Table 10-2 Preconception laboratory tests

Condition	Test	Candidates for test
Sexually transmitted infection	HIV, hepatitis B, hepatitis C, syphilis, gonorrhea, chlamydia	Offered to all
Cystic fibrosis carrier testing	Cystic fibrosis mutation panel	Offered to all, especially those with Northern European ancestry
Sickle cell anemia, thalassmemia, and other hemoglobinopathy carrier testing	Complete blood count, hemoglobin electrophoresis	African American, Mediterranean, Southeast Asian
Tay Sachs carrier testing	Tay-Sachs	Ashkenazi Jewish ancestry, French Canadian, Cajun
Ashkenazi Jewish panel	Cystic fibrosis, Tay-Sachs, familial dysautonomia, canavan, Gaucher disease type 1, mucolipidosis type IV, Fanconia anemia group C, Neimann-Pick type A, Bloom syndrome	Ashkenazi Jewish ancestry
Fragile X carrier testing	Fragile X mental retardation 1 (FMR 1) gene premutation assessment	Premature ovarian insufficiency or family history of autism or predominantly male delayed development or mental retardation
Vitamin B12 sufficiency	Vitamin B12 level	Prior bariatric surgery, vegan diet, pernicious anemia
Assessment of glucose control	Hemoglobin A1c	Pregestational diabetes, polycystic ovarian syndrome
Immunity testing	Toxoplasma IgG, parvovirus B19 IgG, varicella, rubella	As indicated by history
Environmental exposure	Lead, mercury	As indicated by history
Antiphospholipid antibody testing	Lupus anticoagulant, anticardiolipin antibody, beta 2 microglobulin	Recurrent pregnancy loss or unexplained stillbirth
Renal function	Urine protein, serum creatinine	History of hypertension, renal disease, or diabetes
Iron deficiency anemia	Complete blood count	History of previous anemia, heavy menses, vegetarian or vegan diet
Hypothyroidism	Thyroid-stimulating hormone	History of thyroid disease or current symptoms of thyroid disease
Thrombophilia	Antithrombin and protein C functional assays, free protein S level, prothrombin gene mutation DNA test, factor V Leiden mutation, lupus anticoagulant, anticardiolipin antibody, beta 2 microglobulin	Personal history of thromboembolic event, especially with recurrent thrombosis, at less than age 45, without risk factors or family history of with two or more first-degree relatives with thrombosis.

Table 10-3 Risk factors for type 2 diabetes mellitus

- Age 45 or older
- Overweight or obese
- First-degree relative with diabetes
- Polycystic ovarian syndrome
- Ethnic predisposition: African Americans, Native Indians/Alaska Natives, Asian Americans, Hispanics/Latinas, Native Hawaiians/Pacific Islanders
- Past pregnancy performance: prior gestational diabetes, infant large for gestational age, stillbirth

Concluding remarks

Preconception care offers the opportunity for prospective parents to plan for pregnancy, to make lifestyle choices, to reduce or avoid risks and to improve pregnancy and health outcomes. Preconception counseling should be considered at every health-care encounter of a reproductive age woman, "every woman, every time." Ideally, preconception counseling should include the partner. A comprehensive preconception visit should include a careful history of both the patient and her partner, including current medical conditions, medications and supplements, past medical history, past reproductive history, family history, environmental and occupational exposure, and mental health conditions. When examining the woman, the provider should be alert to signs that may indicate conditions potentially hazardous in pregnancy. Preconception planning should include targeted laboratory screening for sexually transmitted infections, medical conditions, and recessive genetic conditions.

References

1. Finer L, Henshaw S. Disparities in rates of unintended pregnancy in the United States, 1994 and 2001. *Perspect Sex Reprod Health.* 2006 Jun;**38**(2):90–6.
2. Cullum AS. Changing provider practices to enhance preconception wellness. *J Obstet Gynecol Neonatal Nurs.* 2003 Jul 1;**32**(4):543–9.
3. Johnson K, Posner SF, Biermann J, et al.; CDC/ATSDR Preconception Care Work Group. Select Panel on Preconception Care. Recommendations to improve preconception health and health care – United States. *MMWR Recomm Rep.* 2006;**55**(RR-6):1–23.
4. Frey KA, Navarro SM, Kotelchuck M, Lu MD. The clinical content of preconception care: preconception care for men. *Am J Obstet Gynecol* 2008 Dec;**199**(6 Suppl 2):S389–95.
5. Wilcox AJ, Dunson D, Baird DD. The timing of the "fertile window" in the menstrual cycle: day specific estimates from a prospective study. *BMJ* 2000 Nov 18;**321**(7271):1259–62.
6. Ylinen K, Stenman UH, Kesaniemi-Kuokkanen T, Teramo K. Risk of minor and major fetal malformations in diabetics with high haemoglobin A1c values in early pregnancy. *Br Med J (Clin Res Ed).* 1984 Aug 11;**289**(6441):345–6.
7. Wender-Ozegowska E, Wroblewska K, Zwiejska A, et al. Threshold values of maternal glucose in early diabetic pregnancy – prediction of fetal malformations. *Acta Obstet Gyneol Scand.* 2005 Jan;**84**(1):17–25.
8. Sibai BM, Caritis S, Hauth J, et al. Risks of preeclampsia and adverse neonatal outcomes among women with pregestational diabetes mellitus. *Am J Obstet Gynecol* 2000 Feb;**182**(2): 364–9.
9. James AH, Jamison MG, Biswas MS, et al. Acute myocardial infarction in pregnancy: a United States population-based study. *Circulation* 2006;**113**: 1564–71.
10. Ferrer RL, Sibai BM, Mulrow CD, et al. Management of mild chronic hypertension during pregnancy: a review. *Obstetrics and Gynecology* 2000;**96**(5, Part 2): S849–60.
11. August P, Jeyabalan A, Roberts JM. Chronic hypertension in pregnancy. In: Taylor RN, Roberts JM, Cunningham FG (eds.). *Chesley's Hypertensive Disorders in Pregnancy.* Amsterdam: Academic Press, 2014.
12. Working Group report on high blood pressure in pregnancy: report of the National High Blood Pressure Education Program Working Group on High Blood Pressure in Pregnancy. *Am J Obstet Gynecol* 2000;**183**: S1–22.
13. Antiretroviral Pregnancy Registry Steering Committee. Antiretroviral Pregnancy Registry international interim report for 1 Jan 1989–31 July 2013. 2013. Available at www.APRegistry.com. Accessed December 15, 2014.
14. American Academy of Neurology. Practice parameter: management issues for women with epilepsy (summary statement): report of the Quality Standards Subcommittee of the American Academy of Neurology. *Neurology* 1998;**41**:994–98.
15. Randomized study of antiepileptic drug withdrawal in patients in remission. *Lancet* 1991; **337**:1175–80.
16. Morrell MJ. Guidelines for the care of women with epilepsy. *Neurology* 1998;**51**:S21–7.
17. Frieder A, Dunlop AL, Culpepper L, Bernstein PS. The clinical content of preconception care: women with psychiatric conditions. *Am J Obstet Gynecol* 2008;**199**(6 Suppl 2):S328–32.

18. Hayslett JP. Maternal and fetal complications in pregnant women with systemic lupus erythematosus. *Am J Kidney Dis* 1991;**17**(2):123.

19. Bobrie G, Liote F, Houillier P, Grünfeld JP, Jungers P. Pregnancy in lupus nephritis and related disorders. *Am J Kidney Dis* 1987;**9**(4):339.

20. Weber-Schoendorfer C, Chambers C, Wacker E, et al. Pregnancy outcome after methotrexate treatment for rheumatic disease prior to or during early pregnancy: a prospective multicenter cohort study. *Arthritis Rheumatol* 2014 May;**66**(5):1101–10.

21. Dombrowski MP. Asthma and pregnancy. *Obstet Gynecol* 2006 Dec;**108**(6):1556.

22. National Asthma Education and Prevention Program (National Heart, Lung, and Blood Institute). Working Group on Asthma and Pregnancy. Working Group report on managing asthma during pregnancy: recommendations for pharmacologic treatment. *NIH publication 04-5236*. Bethesda, MD: National Institutes of Health; 2005.

23. National Heart, Lung, and Blood Institute. *National Asthma Education and Prevention Program Expert Panel Report 3: guidelines for the diagnosis and management of asthma*. Bethesda, MD: National Institutes of Health; 2007.

24. Woodruff TK. The Oncofertilty Consortium – addressing fertility in young people with cancer. *Nat Rev Clin Oncol* 2010 7(8):466.

25. American Society for Reproductive Medicine. Fertility preservation and reproduction in patients facing gonodotoxic therapies: a committee opinion. *Fertil Steril* 2013 Nov;**100**(5):1224–31.

26. Ives A, Saunder C, Bulsara M, Semmens J. Pregnancy after breast cancer: population based study. *BMJ* 2007;**334**:194.

27. Lens M, Bataille V. Melanoma in relation to reproductive and hormonal factors in women: current review on controversial issues. *Cancer Causes Control.* 2008 Jun;**19**(5):437–42. doi: 10.1007/s10552-008-9110-4. Epub 2008 Jan 16.

28. Leung AS, Millar LK, Koonings PP, et al. Perinatal outcome in hypothyroid pregnancies. *Obstet Gynecol* 1993;**81**:349–53.

29. Davis LE, Leveno KJ, Cunningham FG. Hypothyroidism complicating pregnancy. *Obstet Gynecol* 1988;**72**:108–12.

30. Henrichs J, Bongers-Schokking JJ, Schenk JJ, et al. Maternal thyroid function during early pregnancy and cognitive functioning in early childhood: the generation R study. *J Clin Endocrinol Metab.* 2010 Sep;**95**(9):4227–3.

31. Callegari LS, Sterling LA, Zelek ST, Hawes SE, Reed SD. Interpregnancy body mass index change and of term vaginal birth after cesarean delivery. *Obstet Gynecol* 2014;**210**:330e1–7.

32. Landsberger EJ, Gurewitsch ED. Reproductive implications of bariatric surgery: pre- and postoperative considerations for extremely obese women of childbearing age. *Curr Diab Rep* 2007;7(4):281–8.

33. Zollner J, Curry R, Johnson M. The contribution of heart disease to maternal mortality. *Curr Opin Obstet Gynecol* 2013;**25**:91–7.

34. Jungers P, Chauveau D, Choukroun G, et al. Pregnancy in women with impaired renal function. *Clin Nephrol* 1997;**47**:281–8.

35. Lindheimer MD, Katz AI. Gestation in women with kidney disease: prognosis and management. *Baillieres Clin Obstet Gynaecol* 1994;**8**:387–404.

36. American College of Obstetricians and Gynecologists. Maternal phenylketonuria. ACOG Committee Opinion No. 449. *Obstet Gynecol* 2009;**114**:1432–3.

37. Anderson JA, Weitz JI. Hypercoagulable states. *Crit Care Clin* 2011;**27**:933.

38. Frazer KL, Porter S, Goss C. The genetics and implications of neuromuscular disease in pregnancy. *J Perinat Neonat Nurs* 2013;**27**(3):205–14.

39. Spong CY. Prediction and prevention of recurrent spontaneous preterm birth. *Obstetrics and Gynecology* 2007;**110**:405–15.

40. Duley L, Henderson-Smart DJ, Meher S, King JF. Antiplatelet agents for preventing pre-eclampsia and its complications. *Cochrane Database Syst Rev* 2007 Apr 18;**2**:CD004659.

41. Empson M, Lassere M, Craig JC, Scott JR. Recurrent pregnancy loss with antiphospholipid antibody: a systematic review of therapeutic trials. *Obstet Gynecol* 2002;**99**:135–44.

42. Conde-Agudelo A, Rosas-Bermúdez A, Kafury-Goeta AC, et al. Birth spacing and adverse pregnancy outcomes. *JAMA* 2006;**295**(15):1809–23.

43. US Department of Health & Human Services. www.hhs.gov/familyhistory. Accessed Jan 25, 2015.

44. American College of Obstetricians and Gynecologists. Preconception and prenatal carrier screening for genetic diseases in individuals of Eastern European Jewish descent. ACOG Committee Opinion No. 442. *Obstet Gynecol* 2009;**114**:950–3.

45. Bimla Schwarz E, Postlewaite DA, Hung YY. Documentation of contraception and pregnancy when prescribing potentially teratogenic medications for reproductive-age women. *Ann Int Med* 2007;**147**(6): 370–6.

46. Hook EB, Cross PK, Schreinemacher D. Chromosomal abnormality rates at amniocentesis and in live-born infants. *JAMA* 1983;**249**(15):2034–8.

47. Laopaiboon M, Lumbiganon P, Intarut N, et al. Advanced maternal age and pregnancy outcomes: a multicountry assessment. *BJOG* 2014 Mar;**121**(Suppl 1):49–56.

48. Hansen J. Older maternal age and pregnancy outcome: a review of the literature. *Obstet & Gynecol Surv* 1986 Nov;**41**(11):726–42.

49. Sipos A, Rasmussen F, Harrison G, et al. Paternal age and schizophrenia: a population based cohort study. *BMJ* 2004;**329**(7474):1070.

50. Hultman CM, Sandin S, Levine SZ, et al. Advancing paternal age and risk of autism: new evidence from a population-based study and a meta-analysis of epidemiological studies. *Molecular Psychiatry* 2011;**16**:1203–12. doi:10.1038/mp.2010.121. Epub 2010 Nov 30.

51. United States Department of Agriculture. www.choosemyplate.gov/pregnancy-breastfeeding.html. Accessed Jan 21, 2015.

52. American College of Obstetricians and Gynecologists. Neural tube defects. ACOG Practice Bulletin No. 44. *Obstet Gynecol* 2003;**102**:203–13. Reaffirmed 2014.

53. Rothman KJ, Moore LL, Singer MR, et al. Teratogenicity of high vitamin A intake. *N Engl J Med* 1995 Nov 23;**333**(21):1369–73.

54. Beckman CR, Beckman CA. Effect of a structured antepartum exercise program on pregnancy and labor outcome in primaparas. *J Reprod Med* 1990;**35**:704–9.

55. Stamilio DM, Chang JJ, Macones GA: Periodontal disease and preterm birth: do the data have enough teeth to recommend screening and preventive treatment? *Am J Obstet Gynecol* 2007;**196**:93–4.

56. Michalowicz BS, Hodges JS, DiAngelis AJ, et al. Treatment of periodontal disease and the risk of preterm birth. *N Engl J Med* 2006 Nov 2;**355**:1885–94.

57. Gazmararian JA, Petersen R, Spitz AM, et al. Violence and reproductive health: current knowledge and future research directions. *Matern Child Health J* 2000;**4**(2):79–84.

58. Substance Abuse and Mental Health Services Administration. *Results from the 2010 National Survey on Drug Use and Health: Summary of National Findings*, NSDUH Series H-41, HHS Publication No. (SMA) 11–4658. Rockville, MD: Substance Abuse and Mental Health Services Administration, 2011.

59. Patric SW, Schumacher RE, Benneyworth BD, et al. Neonatal abstinence syndrome and associated health care expenditures United States, 2000–2009. *JAMA* 2012;**307**(18):doi:10.1001/jama.2012.3951.

60. McDiarmid MA, Gehle K. Preconception brief: occupational/environmental exposures. *Matern Child Health J* 2006;**10**(5 Suppl):S123–8.

61. Environmental Working Group, Washington, DC. www.ewg.org/foodnew. Accessed Jan 25, 2015.

62. Gore A. *Endocrine Disrupting Chemicals*. Totowa, NJ: Humana Press, 2007.

63. Diamanti-Kandarakis E, Bourguignon JP, Giudice LC, et al. Endocrine-disrupting chemicals: an Endocrine Society scientific statement. *Endocrine Reviews* 2013;**30**(4):293–342.

64. CDC. Revised guidelines for HIV counseling, testing, and referral. *MMWR* 2001;**50**(RR-19):1–62.

65. Grosse SD, Collins JS. Folic acid supplementation and neural tube defect recurrence prevention. *Birth Defects Res A Clin Mol Teratol* 2007 Nov;**79**(11):787–42.

66. Coonrod DV, Jack BW, Boggess KA, et al. The clinical content of preconception care: immunizations as part of preconception care. *Am J Obstet Gynecol* 2008;199(6 Suppl 2):S290–5.

67. Advisory Committee on Immunization Practices (ACIP). Updated recommendations for use of tetanus toxoid, diphtheria toxoid and acelluar pertussis vaccine (Tdap) in pregnant women. *MMWR* 2013 Feb 22;**62**(7):131–5.

68. Advisory Committee on Immunization Practices (ACIP). Updated recommendations for use of tetanus toxoid, reduced diphtheria toxoid and acellular pertussis vaccine (Tdap) in pregnant women and persons who have or anticipate having close contact with an infant aged <12 months. *MMWR* 2011 Oct 21;**60**(41):1424–6.

Chapter 11

Abnormal first trimester pregnancy

Lisa M. Keder and Wing Kay Fok

Introduction

Women with early pregnancies may present for routine care or with specific symptoms such as bleeding or pain. Office evaluation of early pregnancy is important to establish the location of the pregnancy, determine gestational age, and evaluate for abnormal development. Blighted ovum, fetal demise, ectopic pregnancy, molar pregnancy, and pregnancy of undetermined location comprise potential diagnoses. Accurate evaluation of a symptomatic first trimester pregnancy is important to women's health and emotional well-being. Moreover, diagnosis of abnormal pregnancy facilitates appropriate treatment, while correct identification of normal pregnancy is equally important to initiate prenatal care and alleviate anxiety.

Scope of the problem

Abnormal pregnancies can be either intrauterine or extrauterine. Abnormal intrauterine pregnancies include: blighted ova in which a gestational sac develops without a visible fetal pole; embryonic/fetal demise in which a fetus develops, but has no cardiac activity; and molar pregnancies. A spontaneous abortion (SAB) or miscarriage is defined as an intrauterine pregnancy loss prior to 20 weeks' gestation. Each year in the United States, over one million SABs occur. Data from the US National Survey of Family Growth suggest that 17% of recognized pregnancies are lost, but this rate is likely low due to underreporting and under detection.[1] Wilcox et al. evaluated early pregnancy loss by daily urine hCG measurement in women attempting pregnancy. They found that 22% of pregnancies were miscarried before being clinically recognized, and the total rate of pregnancy loss after implantation was 31%.[2] Several risk factors have been linked to spontaneous abortions, including advanced maternal age, obesity, underweight, a short inter-pregnancy interval (pregnancies less than three to six months apart), history of prior spontaneous abortion, maternal diabetes mellitus, and maternal smoking. Molar pregnancy occurs in approximately one in a thousand pregnancies is the United States. The rate is higher in women of advanced maternal age and of Asian descent. Therefore, trends in US demographics may increase the expected incidence.[3]

Abnormal first trimester pregnancies also include those that are in a location outside the normal uterine cavity, specifically ectopic pregnancies (EP). In the United States, it is estimated that 1%–3% of all pregnancies are ectopic. Ectopic pregnancies are the leading cause of maternal death in the first trimester.[4] They may occur not only in any portion of the fallopian tube, but also in the abdomen or on the ovary. Pregnancies are also considered ectopic if they implant within a cesarean section scar or in the cervix of the uterus. The former has become increasingly common, as the rate of cesarean section has risen.[5]

Approach to the symptomatic patient

History

A detailed history may help distinguish between a normal intrauterine versus an abnormal pregnancy. Interpretation of ultrasound findings can then be made in the context of expected milestones. A general obstetric and gynecologic history with attention to prior ectopic pregnancy, gynecologic surgery and infections should be collected.[6, 7] Table 11-1 outlines risk factors for ectopic pregnancy. The health-care provider should obtain the date of the last menstrual period (LMP) including whether it was normal and if it arrived at the expected time. Additionally the patient should be asked what the normal cycle length is and if there was any immediate antecedent hormonal contraceptive use; these factors may affect the timing of ovulation.

Office Care of Women, ed. Martin E. Olsen and Botros Rizk. Published by Cambridge University Press.

Table 11-1 Risk factors for ectopic pregnancy

- Prior ectopic pregnancy
- Prior history of pelvic infection
- Prior tubal surgery
- Infertility
- Pregnancy conceived while IUD in place
- Smoking

Table 11-3 Normal pregnancy

Ultrasound milestones	Weeks from LMP
Gestational sac	4.5–5
Yolk sac	5–5.5
Fetal pole	6
Cardiac activity	6.5

Table 11-2 reviews gestational dating criteria. Patients can also sometimes identify a specific date or range of dates of conception, especially if they have been seeking pregnancy. The date of the first positive pregnancy test, whether it was clearly or weakly positive, and if there were any preceding negative tests, can be helpful information. A history of bleeding since the LMP, with its duration and quantity, should also be elicited. Finally, if the patient is having pain, the location, duration, quality, and intensity should be described.

Physical exam

Vital signs should be obtained including orthostatics if the patient gives symptoms that suggest intra-abdominal bleeding. The physical examination should include an abdominal exam with attention to of the lower abdomen to determine if the uterus is palpable. Tenderness with or without rebound and guarding should be noted. The pelvic examination should include inspection of the vagina to see if bleeding is present. The cervix should be examined to see if it is open or closed and if there is active bleeding. Bimanual examination allows evaluation for cervical motion tenderness, assessment of uterine size and position, and palpation for adnexal masses or pain.

Laboratory analysis

Although over-the-counter tests are advertised as being able to diagnose pregnancy before a missed menstrual period, their accuracy has not been consistent in comparative trials.[8] Confirmation of pregnancy can generally be achieved with a urine pregnancy test in the office. However, if the test is negative in a patient who has had a positive home test, a serum beta human chorionic gonadotropin (β-hCG) should be obtained. A blood type and hemoglobin or hematocrit should be obtained in any patient who has been experiencing bleeding or has signs concerning for ectopic pregnancy. In the setting of a pregnancy of undetermined location, a trend in the quantitative β-hCG may be needed to clarify a diagnosis. If the patient is at risk, screening for sexually transmitted infections including gonorrhea and chlamydia should be obtained.

Table 11-2 Pregnancy dating

- Date of last menstrual period
- Typical cycle length
- Date of first positive pregnancy test
- Estimated date of conception

Imaging

Ultrasound evaluation of a symptomatic patient in early pregnancy requires not only careful examination of uterine contents, but also of the adnexa. Ultrasound interpretation is based on the predictable sequence of anticipated developmental events.[9] A gestational sac is first seen at approximately five weeks gestational age. The gestational sac is described by the mean sac diameter (the average of sagittal, transverse, and anteroposterior diameters of the sac). A yolk sac, a circular structure about 3 mm –5 mm in diameter, is visible at around 5.5 weeks gestation. The embryo is seen at 6 weeks, with fetal cardiac activity detectable as a flicker.[10] Table 11-3 describes normal developmental milestones.

The sensitivity of ultrasound in detecting ectopic pregnancy is dependent upon the skill of the sonographer. Its positive predictive value will depend on the underlying likelihood of ectopic in the population being studied. A recent study reported one center's experience using transvaginal ultrasound performed by obstetrics and gynecology residents. In patients presenting with symptoms, who were eventually diagnosed as having ectopic pregnancies, 62% had a non-diagnostic ultrasound.[11] In contrast, in an early pregnancy unit an initial ultrasound was able to detect 75% of ectopic pregnancies with 99% specificity.[12] Endometrial thickness cannot differentiate ectopic pregnancy from either viable or non viable intrauterine pregnancy.[13] The presence of free fluid in the posterior cul de sac is also not diagnostic of ectopic

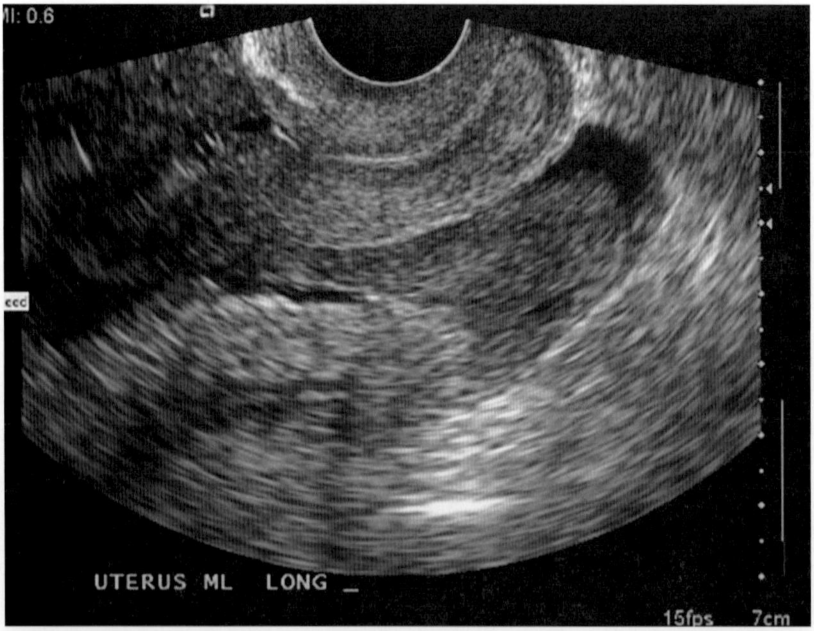

Figure 11-1 Complex fluid collection in the cul de sac.

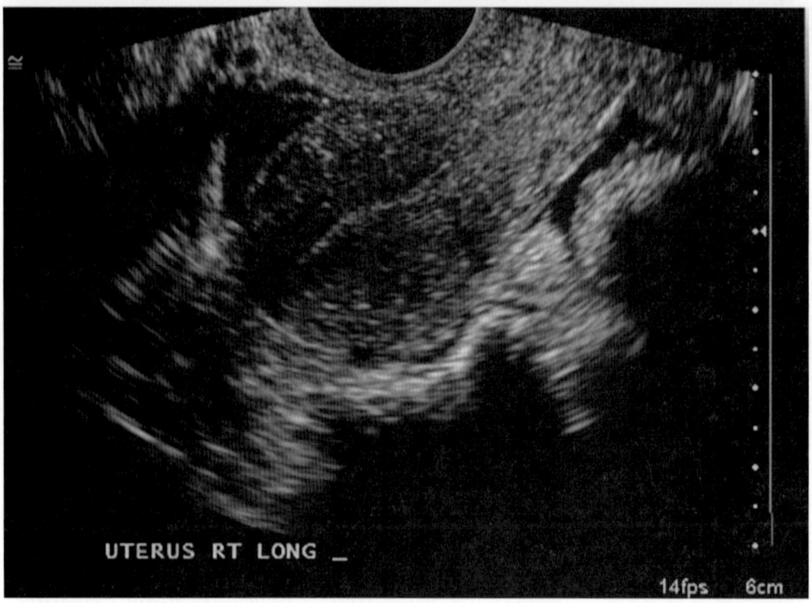

Figure 11-2 Large amount of fluid in the pelvis.

pregnancy. However, it may raise suspicion of intra-abdominal bleeding. A subjective assessment of the amount of fluid and whether it appears clear or echogenic, can help evaluate the likelihood that it represents hemoperitoneum. Figure 11-1 demonstrates echogenic fluid in the cul de sac, consistent with blood. Figure 11-2 shows an atypical, large amount of free fluid within the pelvis, tracking both in front of and behind the uterine body.

Diagnosis and treatment

Early IUP/threatened abortion

A patient presenting to the office for evaluation of early pregnancy symptoms may have the diagnosis of definite intrauterine pregnancy made when a yolk sac or an embryo is identified within an intrauterine gestational sac. Clarification regarding

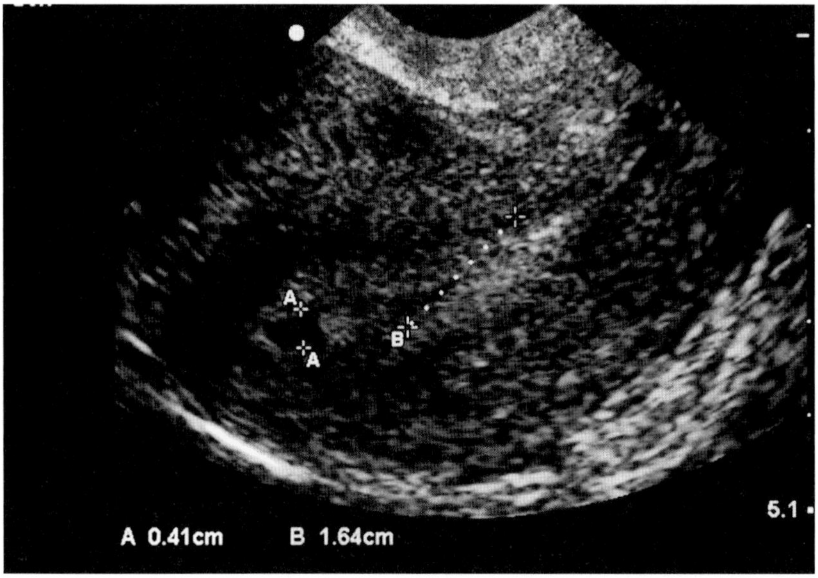

Figure 11-3 Fluid collection in the uterine cavity mimicking early pregnancy.

whether an intrauterine pregnancy is normal or abnormal depends upon an accurate history, careful evaluation with ultrasound, and occasionally use of serial β-hCG measurements. Skilled ultrasonographers may identify an early gestational sac by the fact that an ovoid lucency is present, implanted eccentric from the midline endometrial echo, and surrounded by a decidual reaction that is brighter than the endometrium itself. However, care should be taken not to mistake an intrauterine fluid collection for a gestational sac. A fluid collection will often have a "beak sign," which is a visible tapering point to the fluid at its distal end. Additionally fluid within the endometrial cavity appears midline and lacks a decidual halo. Figure 11-3 demonstrates a fluid collection or pseudo sac. Figure 11-4 shows an early intrauterine pregnancy with gestational sac located off the midline at the fundus of the uterus. In a patient with a desired pregnancy, identification of an early gestational sac should be followed up in an appropriate time to confirm the development of a yolk sac and eventually a fetal pole. If the pregnancy is aborted, confirmation of products of conception should be confirmed by gross inspection or pathologic exam to confirm the diagnosis and avoid missing an ectopic pregnancy.

Blighted ovum/missed abortion

An anembryonic pregnancy or blighted ovum is diagnosed by the presence of an empty gestational sac on ultrasound. An abnormal pregnancy may be suspected based on a sure last menstrual period with lagging ultrasound findings, but a definitive diagnosis should be confirmed by meeting a minimum sac size without embryonic tissue or by failure of development on serial ultrasound.

The criteria most often used to diagnose pregnancy failure are the absence of cardiac activity by the time the embryo has reached a specified crown rump length, the absence of a visible embryo by the time the gestational sac has grown to a certain size, or the absence of a visible embryo by a certain point in time.[14] A single ultrasound showing a gestational sac diameter of 25 mm with no visible embryo yields a specificity and positive predictive value of 100% for an anembryonic gestation. Additionally recent studies have shown that a cutoff of 7 mm for crown rump length with no fetal cardiac activity is diagnostic of a failed pregnancy with specificity and positive predictive value of 100%.[15] The findings on ultrasound must be evaluated in the clinical context of the certainty of historical dating factors. Additionally, the patient's desire to continue her pregnancy should be considered in situations where a definitive diagnosis of a failed pregnancy cannot be made on initial evaluation. A repeat ultrasound in 7–10 days will clarify the diagnosis in almost all situations. Table 11-4 includes guidelines for the diagnosis of pregnancy failure in the first trimester.[14]

Table 11-4 Guidelines for TVUS diagnosis of pregnancy failure in a woman with an intrauterine pregnancy of uncertain viability [16]

Findings diagnostic of pregnancy failure	Findings suspicious for pregnancy failure
CRL ≥7 mm and no heartbeat	CRL <7 mm and no heartbeat
MSD ≥25 mm and no embryo	MSD 16 mm–24 mm and no embryo
Absence of embryo with heartbeat ≥2 weeks after a scan that showed a gestational sac without a yolk sac	Absence of embryo with heartbeat 7–13 days after a scan that showed a gestational sac without a yolk sac
Absence of embryo with heartbeat ≥11 days after a scan that showed a gestational sac with a yolk sac.	Absence of embryo with heartbeat 7–10 days after a scan that showed a gestational sac with a yolk sac
	Absence of embryo ≥6 weeks after LMP
	Empty amnion (amnion seen adjacent to yolk sac, with no visible embryo)
	Enlarged yolk sac (>7 mm)
	Small gestational sac in relation to the size of the embryo (<5 mm difference between MSD and CRL)

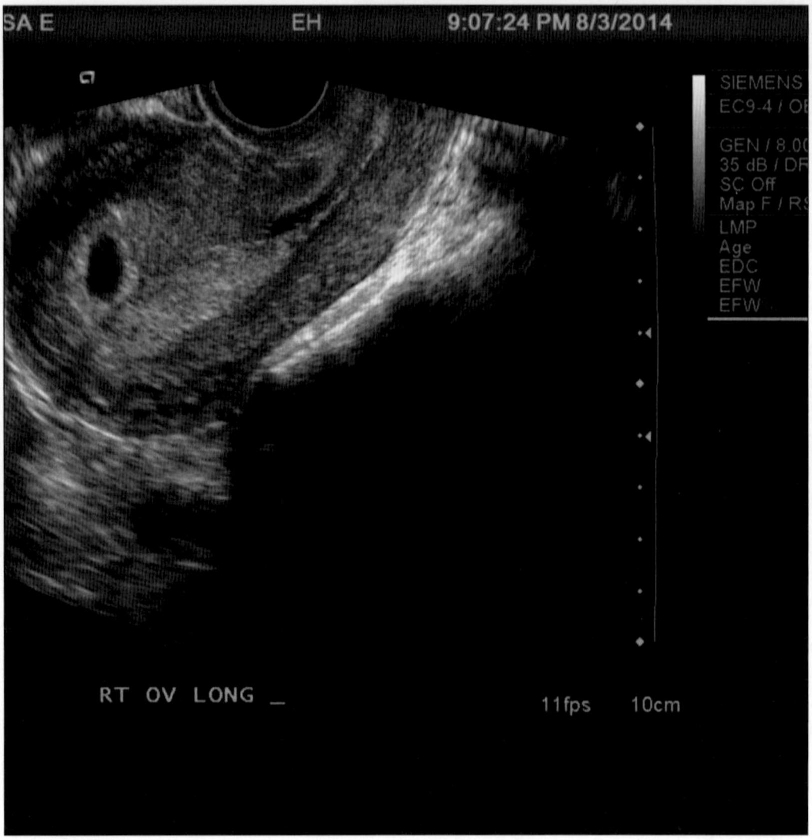

Figure 11-4 Gestational sac in the endometrial cavity at the fundus.

Once a diagnosis of a failed intrauterine pregnancy is made three options should be considered: expectant observation, medication administration, and surgical treatment. Observation without intervention may appeal as a more "natural" approach to some women, while others will not want a delay in treatment or the uncertainty of knowing when the miscarriage will occur. A Cochrane review evaluated seven trials of expectant management. It found that expectant management was associated with higher rates of incomplete abortion at two weeks, blood transfusion, and unplanned surgical intervention. Rates of infection, levels of pain, and measures of psychological impact were similar. Costs incurred were lower with expectant care. The rate of surgical intervention for those who were managed expectantly was 28%.[16] Medical management of first trimester miscarriage has also been summarized in a Cochrane review. Of the studies evaluated, three compared misoprostol to expectant management and found no difference in rates of complete abortion or need for surgery. Twelve studies compared medical to surgical management. There was a lower incidence of complete miscarriage and more unplanned procedures with misoprostol.[17] Surgical evacuation of the uterus can be performed in the office setting with electric vacuum aspiration or manual vacuum aspiration, with a paracervical block and oral analgesia, with or without sedation. Complication rates associated with surgical intervention are low. The majority of studies evaluating the risk of dilatation and curettage in early pregnancy come from the literature reviewing elective abortion. The complications most commonly encountered are: infection (~1%), hematometra (<1%); incomplete abortion (1%–2%).[18]

Follow-up of patients with failed early intrauterine pregnancies depends upon the management chosen. Patients who elect expectant management should be seen for a return appointment in one to two weeks. Additionally, the clinician should provide information regarding the amount of pain and bleeding to expect as well as reasons to seek emergent care. A narcotic prescription can be provided for women in advance. For women using misoprostol for medical management, an antiemetic may be needed as well. Patients treated medically are generally followed up within the week after medication use. It is expected that the gestational sac would be expelled at that time, but the endometrial stripe may still be thick. Women undergoing surgical management may be followed up within two to four weeks. Pelvic exam is not indicated unless ongoing bleeding or signs of infection are present. However, future pregnancy planning and need for contraception should be addressed at that time.

Molar pregnancy

The classic presentation of a molar pregnancy includes vaginal bleeding, passage of vesicles per vagina, uterine enlargement greater than expected for gestational age, and abnormally high levels of β-hCG. However, in one study 40% of molar pregnancies were asymptomatic, 60% presented with vaginal bleeding and 2% with hyperemesis symptoms.[19] Due to availability of present day ultrasound technology, many molar pregnancies are identified early in gestation as abnormal intrauterine pregnancies, and the diagnosis is confirmed later by pathology. On ultrasound, the typical "snowstorm" appearance is less likely to be seen in the first trimester. More commonly, an anembryonic pregnancy is detected. Only 40% of women with confirmed hydatidiform mole had a preevacuation ultrasound diagnosis suggesting molar pregnancy. The sensitivity, specificity, and positive and negative predictive values for routine pre-evacuation ultrasound examination for hydatidiform mole are 44%, 74%, 88%, and 23%, respectively.[20, 21] Molar pregnancy is often diagnosed after treatment of a failed pregnancy. However, if it is suspected preoperatively, suction dilatation and curettage is the preferred route of uterine evacuation to ensure complete removal and to allow pathologic evaluation of the tissue.[22] A quantitative β-hCG level, complete blood count, and chest x-ray should be obtained preoperatively. Additional laboratory tests may be indicated if there are signs of hyperthyroidism or preeclampsia.

Surgical evacuation in the operating room is recommend for uterine size greater than 16 weeks, due to the increased risk of hemorrhage. Hysterectomy can be considered for women who have completed childbearing.[23] Following uterine evacuation, the quantitative β-hCG level should be followed every one to two weeks until negative and then monthly for an additional six months. A plateau or rise in the β-hCG should trigger evaluation for a new conception, and if excluded, prompt referral for treatment of gestational trophoblastic disease. Women diagnosed with molar pregnancy should use an effective method of contraception during the six-month follow-up period.

Ectopic pregnancy

The classic, clinical presentation of ectopic pregnancy includes vaginal bleeding, abdominal pain, and a positive pregnancy test. In such a patient, if an ultrasound examination reveals a gestational sac with yolk sac or fetus visible in the adnexal area, the diagnosis of ectopic pregnancy is simple. Figure 11-5

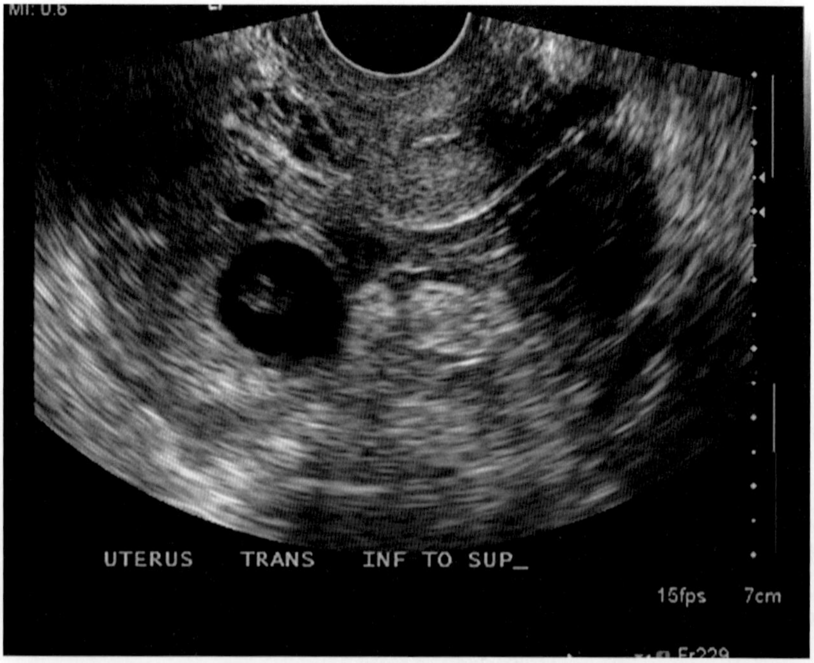

Figure 11-5 Gestational sac with yolk sac in the adnexa.

demonstrates a gestational sac visible within the adnexal area. Likewise, an implantation in a cesarean section scar or in the cervix can be made by imaging alone; although it needs to be distinguished from a spontaneous abortion in progress. More commonly, ectopic pregnancies are originally diagnosed as pregnancies of undetermined location (PUL) and a final diagnosis made with additional follow-up over time. The diagnosis of ectopic pregnancy is often clinically challenging and may involve serial β-hCG follow-up or diagnostic surgery including dilation and curettage or laparoscopy. It is incumbent upon the clinician to avoid potentially harmful intervention with methotrexate in an early normal pregnancy and to establish a correct diagnosis for the individual patient.[24]

The concept of a discriminatory level of β-hCG has been utilized for ectopic evaluation. This refers to the value above which an ultrasound should be diagnostic of an intrauterine pregnancy. The discriminatory value is both user and equipment dependent. It should be considered a relative concept.[25] Uterine malposition or malformation, the presence of fibroids, and patient obesity can all affect the quality of imaging. Most algorithms in use suggest that, if a normal intrauterine pregnancy is present, it would be detected on ultrasound when the β-hCG level is 2,000 or more.[26] This assumes a singleton IUP. In multiple gestations the β-hCG will be higher at any particular point in gestation. Additionally, a recently published analysis of one center's experience described a patient with β-hCG of 2317 with no IUP visualized, who went on to develop a normal, singleton pregnancy. The authors modeled the association of β-hCG and visualization of the gestational sac. They found that the probability of detecting a sac would be 99% at a level of 3,510, suggesting that the discriminatory value in their institution may be higher, and the concept should be used cautiously.[27] An accurate assessment of gestational age based on dates is better predictive of ultrasound landmarks than is a single measurement of β-hCG. In the stable patient, with a level below the discriminatory value, serial β-hCG follow-up may be useful in evaluation PUL.

Initial work by Kadar suggested that a rise of 66% should be expected over a 48 hour period of time.[28] Subsequent studies have identified a somewhat lower rate of rise, 53%, as being compatible with normal pregnancy.[29] If such a rise does not occur, then the pregnancy is abnormal, but not necessarily extrauterine. Uterine evacuation with pathology evaluation can be diagnostic of a failed IUP if chorionic villi are found. Alternatively, it may be suggestive of an ectopic pregnancy if no villi are identified and the β-hCG fails to drop appropriately postoperatively. If an

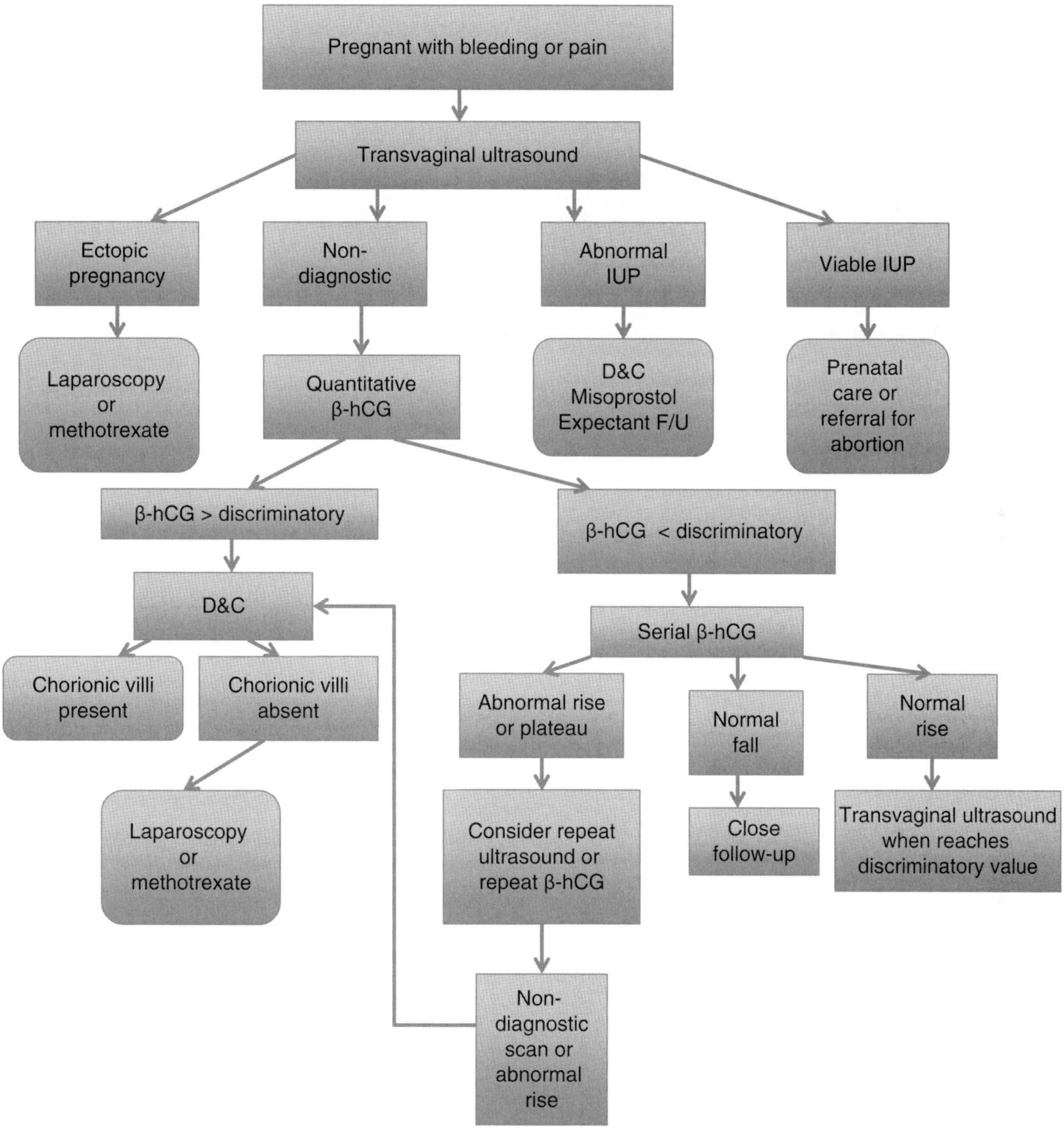

Figure 11-6 Algorithm for the evaluation of symptomatic early pregnancy.

appropriate rise occurs it could still be ectopic. The patient should be followed closely and undergo repeat ultrasound examination when the β-hCG reaches the discriminatory zone. Published algorithms are useful in assisting the clinician to come to a timely diagnosis.[26] Figure 11-6 shows that currently in use at our institution.

In a patient with an unruptured ectopic pregnancy, medical or expectant management can be considered. It is imperative that a thorough evaluation has been made to ensure that methotrexate is not inappropriately administered to a woman a normal early pregnancy, such as an early IUP with a β-hCG below the discriminatory zone or an early pregnancy with β-hCG rise on the border of normal. Medical management with methotrexate was first introduced in the 1980s base on experience with treatment of gestational trophoblastic disease. It is now widely used. The American College of Obstetrics and Gynecology (ACOG) reviewed the use of methotrexate in a 2008 practice bulletin, which was reaffirmed in 2012.[30] In these guidelines, a gestational sac greater than 3.5 cm in size or the presence of fetal cardiac activity are considered relative contraindications to methotrexate. Studies have also demonstrated that a high pretreatment β-hCG level is a marker for potential failure.[31] ACOG suggests that multi-dose regimens be considered for women with β-hCG above 5,000.

Expectant management is sometimes appropriate in asymptomatic women. ACOG suggests this can be considered in women with initial low and dropping β-hCG levels. A recent randomized trial compared expectant management to single dose methotrexate in women with ectopic pregnancies defined as an ultrasound diagnosis with plateaued β-hCG less than 1,500 or a PUL with plateaued β-hCG less than 2,000.[32] Sixty percent of women in the expectant management group and 76% of those in the methotrexate group required no additional treatment. Two percent of the methotrexate group and 13% of the expectant management group required surgery. Another, less rigorously designed trial evaluated a cohort of women treated for ectopic pregnancy.[33] In that study, 49% of women managed expectantly did not require other treatment.

Should the diagnosis of a ruptured ectopic pregnancy be suspected in the office setting, emergent transport should be initiated if there are signs of intra-abdominal bleeding based on ultrasound, clinical exam, or vital signs. In the case of rupture, surgical intervention is warranted using laparoscopy, except in cases of hemodynamic instability, which might require laparotomy. The decision to perform salpingectomy or salpingostomy is first based on feasibility of the more conservative approach. If the tube is badly damaged or has been the site of a prior ectopic, it should be removed. If unruptured, as in this case, salpingostomy can be considered. Expert opinion suggests that in the presence of a diseased, or absent contralateral tube, salpingotomy is the preferred approach to maximize future fertility. Controversy has surrounded the choice between salpingotomy and salpingectomy in the patient with a contralateral normal tube. This debate centers on future reproductive outcome including both fertility as well as risk of recurrent ectopic pregnancy. A recent population-based study examined prospectively the cumulative rates of intrauterine pregnancy for women who had undergone ectopic treatment.[34] In multivariate analysis there was no difference in fertility among women who underwent salpingectomy, salpingostomy, or medical treatment. Moreover, the rate of repeat ectopic pregnancy did not differ. However, a subgroup of women 35 or older, with a history of infertility or tubal disease, seemed to benefit from conservative surgery. Prior research has also failed to clearly favor one approach over the other.[35] The disadvantage of salpingostomy is the risk of persistent ectopic tissue; 10%–15% of patients will require additional medical or surgical treatment. The treatment of cervical and cesarean section scar pregnancies often requires both medical and surgical therapies.

Patients treated with salpingostomy, methotrexate, or expectant management are all in need of careful follow-up due to the potential for persistent growth of trophoblastic tissue and risk of tubal rupture. The β-hCG is expected to drop by 15% between days 4 and 7 post-administration. It is then followed weekly until resolution, as is the same for women who have undergone salpingostomy. Surveillance for those managed expectantly is generally performed more frequently in the initial week by repeating the β-hCG every two to four days and then weekly. In recommending treatment options, the need for this rigorous follow-up should be considered. Two reports in the literature examined compliance with β-hCG follow-up in inner city populations. One found that only 10% of patients completely complied and 15% were completely lost to follow-up despite rigorous attempts to reach them. The other study had an 11% complete loss to follow-up and only 45% were followed to the point of a negative β-hCG.[36, 37]

Concluding remarks

Early pregnancy failure pregnancy is common. Women presenting with symptoms of bleeding or pain in early pregnancy should be evaluated in a comprehensive fashion using historical gestational dating to guide use of imaging and laboratory studies. Abnormal first trimester pregnancies that are intrauterine, can be managed expectantly, medically, or surgically except in the case of suspected molar pregnancy in which case surgical evacuation is warranted. Ectopic pregnancy is a potentially life-threatening condition. A high index of suspicion and systematic evaluation will allow the clinician to make a timely diagnosis and choose an appropriate treatment plan.

References

1. Curtin SC, Abma JC, Ventura SJ, Henshaw SK. Pregnancy rates for US women continue to drop. *NCHS Data Brief* 2013;**136**:1–8.

2. Wilcox AJ, Weinberg, CR, O'Connor JF, et al. Incidence of early loss of pregnancy. *N Engl J Med* 1988;**319**:189–94.
3. Di Cintio E, Parazzini F, Rosa C, et al. The epidemiology of gestational trophoblastic disease. *Gen Diagn Pathol* 1997;**143**:103–8.
4. Centers for Disease Control and Prevention. Ectopic pregnancy mortality – Florida, 2009–2010. *MMWR.* 2012;**61**:106–9.
5. Fuchs N, Manoucheri E, Verbaan M, Einarsson JI. Laparoscopic management of extrauterine pregnancy in caesarean section scar: description of surgical technique and review of the literature. *BJOG* 2014; doi: 10.1111/1471-0528.13060. [Epub ahead of print]
6. Ankum WM, Mol BW, Van der Veen F, Bossuyt PM. Risk factors for ectopic pregnancy: a meta-analysis. *Fertil Steril* 1996;**65**:1093–9.
7. Li C, Meng CX, Zhao WH, et al. Risk factors for ectopic pregnancy in women with planned pregnancy: a case-control study. *Eur J Obstet Gynecol Reprod Biol* 2014;**181**:176–82.
8. Cole LA, Khanlian SA, Sutton JM, et al. Accuracy of home pregnancy tests at the time of missed menses. *Am J Obstet Gynecol.* 2004;**190**:100–5.
9. Bree RL, Edwards M, Bohm-Velez M, et al. Transvaginal sonography in the evaluation of normal early pregnancy: correlation with hCG level. *Am J Roentgenol* 1989;**153**:75–9.
10. Goldstein I, Zimmer EA, Tamir A, et al. Evaluation of normal gestational sac growth: appearance of embryonic heartbeat and embryo body movements using transvaginal technique. *Obstet Gynecol* 1991;**77**:885–8.
11. Chung K, Chandavarkar U, Opper N, Barnhart K. Reevaluating the role of dilation and curettage in the diagnosis of pregnancy of unknown location. *Fert Steril* 2011;**96**:659–62.
12. Kirk E, Papageorghiou AT, Conous G, et al. The diagnostic effectiveness of an intial transvaginal scan in detecting ectopic pregnancy. *Hum. Reprod* 2007;**22**: 2824–8.
13. Kirk E. Ultrasound in the diagnosis of ectopic pregnancy. *Clinical Obstet Gynecol* 2012;**55**:395–401.
14. Doubilet PM, Benson CB, Bourne T, Blaivas M. Diagnostic criteria for nonviable pregnancy early in the first trimester. *N Engl J Med* 2013;**369**:1443–51.
15. Pexsters A, Luts J, Van Schoubroeck D, et al. Clinical implications of intra- and interobserver reproducibility of transvaginal sonographic measurement of gestational sac and crown-rump length at 6–9 weeks' gestation. *Ultrasound Obstet Gynecol* 2011;**38**:510–15.
16. Nanda K, Lopea LM, Grimes DA, et al. Expectant care versus surgical treatment for miscarriage. *Cochran Database Syst Rev* 2012. doi: 10.1002/14651858 .CD003518.pub3.
17. Neilson JP, Gyte GML, Hickey M, et al. Medical treatments for incomplete miscarriage. *Cochran Database Syst Rev* 2013. doi: 10.1002/14651858 .CD007223.pub3.
18. Yonke N, Leeman LM. First-trimester surgical abortion technique. *Obst Gynecol Clin North Am* 2013;**40**:647–70.
19. Gemer O, Segal S, Kpomar A, Sassoon E. The current clinical presentation of complete molar pregnancy. *Arch Gynecol Obstet* 2000;**264**:33–4.
20. Sebire NJ, Makrydimas G, Agnantis NJ, et al. Updated diagnostic criteria for partial and complete hydatidiform moles in early pregnancy. *Anticancer Res* 2003;**23**:1723–8.
21. Fowler DJ, Lindsay I, Seckl MJ, Sebire NJ. Histomorphometric features of hydatidiform moles in early pregnancy: relationship to detectability by ultrasound examination. *Ultrasound Obstet Gynecol* 2007;**29**:76–80.
22. Doll KM[1], Soper JT. The role of surgery in the management of gestational trophoblastic neoplasia. *Obstet Gynecol Surv* 2013;**68**:533–42. doi: 10.1097/ OGX.0b013e31829a82df.
23. Lurain JR. Gestational trophoblastic disease I: epidemiology, pathology, clinical presentation and diagnosis of gestational trophoblastic disease, and management of hydatidiform mole. *Am J Obstet Gynecol.* 2010;**203**:531–9.
24. Nurmohamed L, Moretti ME, Schechter T, et al. Outcome following high-dose methotrexate in pregnancies misdiagnosed as ectopic. *Am J Obstet Gynecol* 2011;**205**:533.e1–3.
25. Condous G, Kirk E, Van Huffel S, et al. Diagnostic accuracy of varying discriminatory zones for the prediction of ectopic pregnancy in women with pregnancy of unknown location. *Ultrasound Obstet Gynecol* 2005;**26**:770–5.
26. Van Mello NM, Mol F, Ankum WM, et al. Ectopic pregnancy: how the diagnostic and therapeutic management has changed. *Fertil Steril* 2012;**98**: 1066–73.
27. Connolly AM, Ryan DH, Stuebe AM, Wolfe HM. Reevaluation of discriminatory and threshold levels for serum β-hCG in early pregnancy. *Obstet Gynecol.* 2013;**121**:65–70.
28. Kadar N, Caldwell BV, Romero R. A method of screening for ectopic pregnancy and its indications. *Obstet Gynecol* 1981;**58**:162–6.
29. Barnhart K. Early pregnancy failure: beware the pitfalls of modern management. *Fertil Steril* 2012;**98**: 1061–5.

30. American College of Obstetricians and Gynecologists. ACOG Practice Bulletin No. 94: Medical management of ectopic pregnancy. *Obstet Gynecol* 2008;**111**:1479–85.
31. Bachman EA, Barnhart K. Medical management of ectopic pregnancy: a comparison of regimens. *Clinc Obstetr Gynecol* 2012;**55**:440–7.
32. Van Mello NM, Mol F, Verhoeve HR, et al. Methotrexate or expectant management in women with an ectopic pregnancy or pregnancy of unknown location and low serum hCG concentrations? A randomized comparison. *Human Reproduction* 2013;**28**: 60–7.
33. Rodriques SP, de Burlet KJ, Hiemstra E, et al. Ectopic pregnancy: when is expectant management safe? *Gynecol Surg* 2012;**9**:421–6.
34. De Bennetot M, Rabischong B, Aulet-Cuvelier B, et al. Fertility after tubal ectopic pregnancy: results of a population based study. *Fertil Steril* 2012;**98**:1271–6.
35. Juneau C, Bates GW. Reproductive outcomes after medical and surgical management of ectopic pregnancy. *Clinical Obstet Gynecol* 2012;**55**:455–60.
36. Jaspan D, Giraldo-Isaza M, Dandolu V, Cohen AW. Compliance with methotrexate therapy for presumed ectopic in an inner-city population. *Fertil Steril* 2010;**94**:1122–4.
37. Dueñas-Garcia OF, Young C, Mikhail M, Salafia C. Compliance with follow-up in an inner-city population treated with intramuscular methotrexate for suspected ectopic pregnancy. *Int J Gynecol Obstet* 2012 Mar;**120** (3):254–6.

Chapter 12

Prenatal care

Brian Brocato and David Lewis

Maternal mortality

The Centers for Disease Control and Prevention (CDC) defines maternal mortality as the death of a woman while pregnant or within one year of termination of pregnancy, irrespective of the duration and sight of the pregnancy, from any cause related to or aggravated by the pregnancy or its management but not from accidental or incidental causes.[1] It is reported as a ratio of deaths to 100,000 live births. The US maternal mortality rate in 1950 was reported as 83 deaths/100,000 live births. This rate fell to a low of 7.2 deaths/100,000 live births in 1997. Since 2007, the United States has seen an increase in maternal mortality, which last reported by the CDC in 2009 was 17.8 deaths/100,000 live births.[1, 2] When broken down by race, the maternal mortality ratio for white women, black women, and women of other races are 11.7, 35.6, and 17.6 deaths/100,000 live births, respectively.[1, 3]

Although peripartum hemorrhage remains a leading cause of maternal mortality in nondeveloped countries, cardiovascular diseases are the leading cause of maternal mortality in the United States. This is followed by infection, noncardiovascular disease, cardiomyopathy, hemorrhage, hypertensive disorders of pregnancy, venous thromboembolism, cerebrovascular accidents, amniotic fluid embolism, and anesthesia related complications.[1]

Comprehensive pregnancy care includes preconception, prenatal and postpartum care. Although the focus of prenatal care is to promote the health of the pregnant women and developing fetus, the health of the entire family can be affected during this time period.[4] The goal of prenatal care is to achieve a healthy outcome for the mother and her baby by ensuring availability of resources and delivering treatments that improve the outcome of the pregnancy.[5]

The success of prenatal care in ensuring a healthy outcome for both the mother and her baby is not solely dependent on the provider or mother but must be a cooperative approach. Improving access to care is considered an integral step in the goal of improving pregnancy outcomes. The US Department of Health and Human Services launched the program Healthy People 2020 with the goal of raising the proportion of pregnant women who receive early and adequate prenatal care from a baseline goal of 70% in 2012 to 77% by 2020.[6] Access to care in the United States continues to vary significantly among different racial, ethnic and socioeconomic groups.[7]

Although there have not been randomized controlled trials comparing prenatal care to no prenatal care, several trials have demonstrated the benefits of assessment of maternal and fetal conditions. Examples include the benefit of early ultrasound to detect multiple pregnancy, accurate dating and congenital anomalies, as well as HIV screening of women to improve maternal and neonatal outcomes.[8, 9]

Medical assessment

To achieve the best possible outcome for pregnancy, a thorough history should be obtained to identify conditions that may affect or be affected by pregnancy. Chronic medical disease may improve or be exacerbated by pregnancy, while some will remain unaffected. Chronic conditions may pose a threat to normal pregnancy while others will have no impact on the pregnancy. Many times, it is not the disease itself but the treatment that must be addressed in pregnancy; some medications such as angiotensin-converting enzyme inhibitors are considered contraindicated in pregnancy, whereas other medications pose no additional risk. It is imperative that any chronic conditions are addressed as early in pregnancy as possible.

Office Care of Women, ed. Martin E. Olsen and Botros Rizk. Published by Cambridge University Press.

First trimester

Establishing gestational age

Gestational age in modern obstetrics is first established by knowledge of the last menstrual period (LMP). Using the first day of the LMP through delivery, pregnancy has a duration of 280 days. Traditionally, Naegele's rule has been used estimate a date of delivery (EDD) by subtracting three months and adding one week from the first day of the LMP.[4] Because of the possible variation of menstrual cycle days and to avoid reliance on maternal recall of the LMP, many clinicians use a combination of Naegele's rule and fetal biometry measurements to establish as accurate an EDD as possible. When there is discrepancy between the EDDs of the LMP and fetal biometry, ultrasound dating should be used. The American College of Obstetricians and Gynecologists (ACOG), American Institute of Ultrasound in Medicine and the Society of Maternal-Fetal Medicine have recommended a protocol to follow when dating by LMP and ultrasound do not agree.[15] When there is discrepancy between ultrasound dating and LMP dating in the third trimester, caution should be used in reassigning EDD. Some centers use a three-week discrepancy to reassign dates. In these cases, a follow-up ultrasound to assess interval growth is often performed to detect cases of fetal growth restriction.[4]

Prior obstetric outcome

Prior fetal demise

Although stillbirth does not have a uniform definition among all jurisdictions, fetal deaths after 20 weeks' gestation are reported by the CDC. The fetal mortality rate in 2006 was reported as 6.05 deaths at 20 weeks of gestation or more per 1,000 live births and fetal deaths.[16] In women with a prior unexplained stillbirth, the risk of recurrence has been cited to be between 7 and 10 per 1,000, if growth was present, the risk of recurrence is much greater, up to 21 per 1,000.[12] If not already completed, a workup for the etiology of the prior stillbirth is indicated; evaluation for conditions such as antiphospholipid antibody syndrome, tobacco use, and diabetes should be completed as these will impact the management of future pregnancies.

Antenatal testing with non-stress test or biophysical profile can be considered at 32–34 weeks' gestation. Delivery timing of subsequent pregnancies should not take place before 39 weeks' gestation in the absence of other indications. Delivery before 39 weeks' gestation for the history of prior stillbirth should only be done after documenting fetal lung maturity by amniocentesis.[12]

History of spontaneous preterm delivery

All pregnant women are at risk of spontaneous preterm delivery (SPTD). Demographic factors such as African American or black race, low socioeconomic status, and less education increase a woman's risk of SPTD. Pregnancy characteristics such as multiple gestation, assisted reproductive technology, shortened cervical length, and tobacco use are also associated with a higher rate of SPTD.[4, 17] One of the strongest risk factors for SPTD is a history of SPTD in a prior pregnancy. The earlier the gestational age of delivery in the prior affected pregnancy, the greater the risk of recurrence in future pregnancies. The risk also appears to increase according to the number of prior pregnancies complicated by SPTD. Using baseline population-specific risks for non-Hispanic white women and non-Hispanic black women, an estimated recurrence risk for SPTD can be calculated. Using the baseline risk for non-Hispanic white women of 11%, a factor of 1.5 for each prior SPTD can be used to calculate recurrence risk.[18] For a non-Hispanic white woman with one prior SPTD, her recurrence risk would be 17% (11% × 1.5).

Women with a history of SPTD can benefit from several interventions to reduce the risk of recurrence. Smoking cessation, progestational agents, and cerclage are all potential interventions depending on the obstetric history and current pregnancy risk factors. Use of 17-alpha-hydroxyprogesterone caproate in pregnancies complicated by prior SPTD between 20 and 36 weeks' gestation has been shown to reduce the risk of recurrence PTD and should be offered to this population.[19] The weekly intramuscular injection of 17 alpha-hydroxyprogesterone caproate (250 mg) is started between 16 and 20 weeks' gestation and continued through 36 weeks' gestation.[19] Women with a history of SPTD between 17 and 34 weeks' gestation who have a sonographically demonstrated shortened cervix in the current pregnancy (less than 25 mm between 16 and 23 weeks' gestation) have been shown to benefit from placement of a cerclage to reduce the risk of recurrent preterm delivery.[20] Women with a history of SPTD benefit from preconception consultation and/or maternal-fetal medicine consultation early in pregnancy to evaluate for appropriate screening modalities and potential treatment with cerclage or progestational agents.

Prior congenital malformation

Women who have had prior pregnancies complicated by fetal congenital anomaly are best served with preconception consultation as potential preventative efforts may need to begin prior to or very early in subsequent pregnancies. Two populations where prevention is possible is with pregnancies complicated by a fetal neural tube defect (NTD) and congenital anomalies in the setting of poorly controlled diabetes evident by an elevated glycosylated hemoglobin (HbA1 C). For all women capable of becoming pregnant, 0.4 mg/day of folic acid supplementation is recommended. In women with a prior pregnancy complicated by a NTD, the recommended folic acid supplementation is 4 mg beginning 1 month prior to conception carried throughout the first trimester.[17]

Women whose pregnancies are complicated by pregestational diabetes are at risk for fetal congenital anomalies greater than the general population. Approximately 6%–12% of infants of diabetic women will have a congenital anomaly.[10] Women should attempt to bring the HbA1 C below 6.1% as a HbA1 C greater than 10% is associated with a significant increase in the risk for congenital anomalies.[21]

History of severe preeclampsia

In women with a history of preeclampsia/ecclampsia in a prior pregnancy are indeed at risk for developing preeclampsia/ecclampsia in future pregnancies. Recurrence rates have been reported between 11%–70% for recurrence of preeclampsia. Recurrence of eclampsia has been reported at 5%.[17] In women with a history of early onset severe preeclampsia with subsequent delivery less than 34 weeks' gestation, low-dose aspirin beginning in the late first trimester is recommended to reduce the risk of recurrence.[22] Women with multiple pregnancies complicated by preeclampsia may benefit from low-dose aspirin therapy as well.[22]

Initial visit

History and physical

Once pregnancy has been documented, prenatal care is begun with a history and physical examination. This is accompanied by laboratory testing to screen for various comorbidities that will affect the care of the pregnant women.

A medical, surgical, and family history including genetic history is obtained. Medications, allergies, drug use, and substance abuse screening should be carried out as well.

It is important to review prior pregnancies regardless if the pregnancy resulted in a live birth. The circumstances surrounding prior pregnancies should be documented, including if the onset of labor was spontaneous, the mode of delivery, the weight of the newborn(s), location of delivery and any complications that occurred in the antepartum, during the time of delivery or postpartum periods. It is important to note details of the delivery such as the need for assisted-vaginal delivery, the presence of shoulder dystocia or the occurrence of postpartum hemorrhage.

The gynecologic history including menstrual details, prior results of Pap smears and any history of sexually transmitted infections should be obtained. Gynecologic surgeries or procedures should be noted such as colposcopies, loop electrosurgical excision procedure (LEEP), tubal ligations, or surgery for adnexal pathologies.

A good social history is important. The family dynamics such as occupation or schooling, partner status, contact with animals, living conditions and relationships with others that may live or spend time in the home should be elicited. This is an appropriate time to screen for intimate partner violence (IPV). IPV affects more than 300,000 pregnant women annually; screening of women at the initial prenatal visit and each trimester including postpartum visits is recommended.[23]

Laboratory evolution

Infection screening

Sexually transmitted infections can cause significant morbidity and at times mortality in women. Infections in pregnancy may result in fetal or neonatal infections, maternal infection, and may contribute to pregnancy morbidity including preterm delivery.

It is important to screen all pregnant women for sexually transmitted infections; positive results must be promptly treated. The CDC recommends that all pregnant women undergo screening for *Chlamydia trachomatis* at the first prenatal visit. Treatment should prompt rescreening three to six months later or during the third trimester. High-risk populations should undergo rescreening in the third trimester regardless of negative results during initial screening. High-risk populations should be screened for *N. gonorrheae*. Treatment, if positive, is followed by retesting at three to six months.[24]

HIV

HIV testing in pregnancy should follow a provider-initiated approach and be done as early in the pregnancy as possible. Women should be informed that an HIV test is considered routine for all pregnant women and should be given the option to opt out of testing.[25] Populations that are considered high risk should be retested in the third trimester.[24]

Hepatitis B

Hepatitis B screening should be carried out in all pregnant women as early as possible in the pregnancy regardless of vaccination history. Initial screening should test for hepatitis B surface antigen (HbSAg).[24] Susceptible women should be offered vaccination as pregnancy is not a contraindication.[26]

In the event that HbSAg is detected, further testing is necessary to identify evidence of an acute or chronic infection and active viral replication via hepatitis B core antibodies (IgG and IgM) and hepatitis "e" antigen. Immunity is evident if hepatitis surface antibody (IgG) is present.

Syphilis

All pregnant women should be screened with serologic testing for syphilis; tests include rapid plasma reagin (RPR) or Venereal Disease Research Laboratories (VDRL) studies.[24] False positive results are seen in other health conditions, so reactive tests should be confirmed with *Treponema pallidum* (MHA-TP) or fluorescent terponemal antibody absorbed (FTA-ABS) testing.[4] In high-risk populations, rescreening at 28–32 weeks' gestation is appropriate. Some states may require testing at the time of delivery. Infants should not be sent home from the hospital without evidence of maternal testing for syphilis.[5]

Cervical cancer screening

Women should undergo cervical cancer screening beginning at age 21 and pregnancy does not alter this recommendation. An exception to screening initiation is women with HIV under the age of 21; screening of this population should begin when HIV is diagnosed.[27] The goal of cervical cancer screening in pregnancy is to identify invasive disease. Colposcopy and biopsy is appropriate if indicated, although endocervical curettage or endometrial biopsy should not be done. Once invasive cancer is ruled out, it is appropriate to reevaluate postpartum. Cervical intraepithelial neoplasm 2 or 3 are unlikely to progress to invasive disease during pregnancy.[28] Management of abnormal cervical cytology should follow guidelines published by ACOG.[28]

Complete blood count

A complete blood count (CBC) should be obtained early in pregnancy. Not only are baseline values established, but many diseases are screened for via the CBC. The CBC screens for anemia and thrombocytopenia and provides clues to hemogloblinopathies. Pregnancy is associated with a dilutional anemia secondary to increased plasma volume; this effect is greatest after 30 weeks' gestation.[4] Microcytic anemia is often the result of iron deficiency anemia. If treatment with iron supplementation does not improve the red cell indices, further studies should take place to investigate the cause of the anemia. In African-American, Asian, and Mediterranean women, screening for hemoglobinopathies with a hemoglobin electrophoresis should accompany a baseline CBC.

Screening for asymptomatic bacteruria

Urinalysis may give clues to underlying urinary system pathologies including urolithiasis and infection. Pregnancy is associated with an increased risk for asymptomatic bacteruria that may result in pyelonephritis. To prevent pyelonephritis and the associated comorbidities, urinalysis and culture is recommended in early pregnancy for all women.[29]

Physical examination

A full examination should be completed at the first prenatal visit. The purpose of the examination is to screen for any pathology such as poor dentition, breast masses, cardiac/respiratory abnormalities, adnexal masses, and uterine or cervical pathologies. Normal physiologic changes of pregnancy can be appreciated as well and should not be considered pathologic. Examples of these changes in the cardiovascular system include lateral displacement of the left ventricular apex, mild tachycardia, exaggerated splitting of the first and second heart sounds and a mid-systolic ejection murmur.[4] Although a clinically enlarged goiter should be evaluated further, the thyroid is normally mildly enlarged in pregnancy.[4] The gravid uterine fundus can be palpated easily after 12–13 weeks' gestation as it grows above the pelvic brim. The cervix may appear bluish in pregnancy due to the increased vascularization; this is known as "Chadwick's sign." Although normal changes to the maternal anatomy are often appreciated, any suspected pathology must be addressed. Diagnosis must not be delayed due to pregnancy.

Second trimester

Visits during the second trimester will increase as the pregnancy approaches term. Many important tests should be performed during this period. These include aneuploidy screening, ultrasound for fetal abnormalities, evaluation for the development of gestational diabetes, and immunoprophylaxis for prevention of Rh isoimmunization in Rh negative mothers.

Aneuploidy screening

This topic has become very complicated over the last 30 years since a low MSAFP was found to predict fetuses with trisomy 21.[30] Currently several tests and screening protocols are available. This topic has even become more complicated with the introduction of free cell fetal DNA detection from maternal plasma of pregnant women.

Second trimester quad screening became the primary test used for many years in the United States.[31] This is usually performed between 15 and 21 weeks of gestational age. This test includes the analysis of MSAFP, HCG, inhibin A, unconjugated estriol. The identification rate for Down's syndrome using a 5% positive rate is 81%.[32] Some companies have added other analytes such as free beta sub unit of HCG but this only increases the detection rate slightly.[33] Recently, a first trimester test has been added.[34] This has the advantage of earlier detection and therefore the potential for earlier intervention for confirmed cases of aneuploidy. The test includes the measurement of the nuchal translucency, plus PAPP-A along with free or total beta HCG. This test has an identification rate of 82%–87%.[35] First and second trimester testing can be combined in a variety of ways to further increase the detection rate. Use of the test in a step wise sequential manner may offer a detection rate as high as 95% using a 5% positive screening rate.[36]

Invasive procedures to determine karyotype or presence of genetic syndrome

Over the years several invasive procedures have stood the test of time for diagnosing fetal aneuploidy and genetic syndromes. Chorionic villus sampling is a procedure that is performed either transcervically or transabdominally between 10 and 14 weeks of gestational age. The advantage of this procedure is earlier detection. Conversely, some experts feel the loss rates are higher than traditional amniocentesis.[37] The loss rate does appear to be related to the number of procedures the performing physician has done.[38]

The second and more common procedure is a genetic amniocentesis. This procedure is usually performed between 15 and 20 weeks of gestational age. The benefit of the procedure is the ease of performance and the fact that the procedure does not have the same requirements requiring large numbers of procedures to be performed to decrease complications. The technique involves a 22-gauge needle that is passed transabdominally under continuous ultrasound guidance into the intra-amniotic cavity utilizing sterile technique. Some centers have reported very low loss rates.[39] Other complications of the procedure include infection, leaking of amniotic fluid, and maternal cramping.

Noninvasive prenatal testing for fetal aneuploidy

Recently free fetal DNA has been isolated from the maternal plasma. This test has been shown to have a high detection rate for some chromosomal abnormalities and certain genetic disorders; for Down's syndrome the detection rate is approximately 98%. False positive and false negative tests do occur, though the rate is low.[40] ACOG has not currently recommended routine screening with this test but states that it is reasonable to offer it to patients who have advanced maternal age, abnormal serum screening, abnormal ultrasounds, or a history of aneuploidy in a previous pregnancy.[41] This test is not considered to give definitive information but is only considered to be a screening test which requires an invasive procedure for confirmation.

Ultrasound for fetal anatomic survey and detection of aneuploidy

Ultrasound offers physicians the ability to diagnose and ultimately treat many disorders in utero. This is important as 2% of all pregnancies are complicated by congenital malformations.

Many advocate using ultrasound to diagnose these defects. This is best accomplished between 18 and 22 weeks. Ultrasound is by no means 100% accurate. The RADIUS trial demonstrated this point and reinforced how inaccurate ultrasound may be.[42] This tool can pick up many defects; this can prepare patients and obstetricians for deliveries which may include transfer of care to a higher level center.

The quality and detection rate of these defects is very dependent on the type of equipment and the skill of the sonographer and interpreting physician. Many other variables cannot be controlled by physicians or equipment. These include size of maternal habitus, history of previous abdominal surgery, amount of amniotic fluid, and the position of the fetus at the time of the examination. These should all be considered when determining when to best perform the procedure in order to achieve the maximum benefit. Over the last 30 years many "soft findings" have been found to predict aneuploidy in certain patients. The finding of one of these soft finders is by no means diagnostic of aneuploidy but should alert the caregiver to refer the patient out for targeted evaluation.[43]

Screening for gestational diabetes

Placentas secrete hormones such as human placental lactogen that promote glucose intolerance in pregnancy. Screening is recommended during pregnancy particularly if risk factors exist. Many centers screen all patients. If risk factors exist many will screen patients early in the second trimester and again at the traditional time between 26 and 28 weeks of gestation.[44] The screening test currently recommended is a 50-gram glucose load ingested with a serum glucose level drawn in one hour. Experts have argued over the appropriate cut off abnormal values for many years. Traditionally the range of abnormal value requiring further evaluation is 130 mg/dL–140 mg/dL.[45] If the patient's test is above the cut-off value, a second test – a 100-gram glucose load glucose tolerance test (GTT) – is administered. If there are two or more abnormal values on the GTT, the patient should be instructed on appropriate diet and serial glucose monitoring. If after initiating the diet glucose remains elevated, then insulin or oral agents such as glyburide should be initiated.

Cervical lengths

Prematurity continues to be a major problem in obstetrics today. Iams and colleagues demonstrated in the mid-1980s that cervical shortening predicted preterm delivery.[46] Recently, several large trials have shown vaginally administered progesterone decreases preterm delivery in these high-risk patients. Many authorities have recommended universal screening during the second trimester of pregnancy.[47] Cost analysis have shown benefit to universal screening.[48] At this time, however, ACOG has *not* recommended universal screening. In high-risk patients such as those with a history of preterm delivery screening is recommended.

Rh immunoprophylaxes

Approximately 10% of women are Rh negative in the United States.[49] Administration of RhoGAM, has made isoimmunization a rare event in developed countries. Usually RhoGAM is administered between 24 and 28 weeks of gestational age. If bleeding, abdominal trauma, or invasive procedures are performed, it is administered also at the time of the event. Although utilization of this immunoprophylaxes does not totally eliminate the occurrence of Rh-sensitized pregnancies, following this protocol makes the occurrence very rare.

Third trimester

Infection screening

Several infections should be assessed or reassessed in the third trimester. Patience with risk factors should be rescreened for HIV and syphilis during the third trimester. Risk factors include a history of sexually transmitted diseases, multiple sexual partners, and history of drug abuse.[5] Some authors advocate repeat cervical assessment for both gonorrhea and chlamydia for these patients.

Late third trimester is an appropriate time to evaluate patients for the presence of group B streptococcus (GBS). Detailed protocols have been developed.[50] Currently ACOG advocates screening from 35 to 37 weeks' gestational age. This culture should be obtained starting at the cervix. The culture is continued throughout the length of the vagina, the vulva and finally the anal area should be swabbed. This culture must be transferred in a specific transport media and cultured in a specific media for accurate results to be obtained.[50] Sensitivity should be obtained particularly in penicillin-allergic patients if cultures are positive. Recently, resistant organisms have become much more common. Penicillin remains the treatment of choice, but clindomycin and vancomycin have been more commonly used in patients requiring prophylaxis for resistant strains. Data shows that delayed rupture membranes until at least one dose of antibiotics has been administered is beneficial in preventing neonatal infections. Patients undergoing elective cesarean section without labor do not require prophylaxis.[50] Protocols established by ACOG and the American Academy of Pediatrics have not totally eliminated group B strep sepsis; however, the incidence has markedly decreased since these protocols have been established.[5]

Antenatal testing

A complete review of antenatal testing is beyond the scope of this chapter. In high-risk pregnancies, antenatal testing appears to decrease stillbirth rates based on anecdotal information. No prospective randomized trial has been performed.[51] The widespread use of antenatal testing in obstetrics and high-risk patients has, however, occurred at the same time as a marked decrease in the incidence of stillbirth. But false positive results do occur leading to early deliveries of some patients. Therefore, low-risk patients should not be tested because of this risk as well as the cost of the test.[51]

Several tests exist including the non-stress test, contraction stress test, biophysical profile and umbilical artery Doppler velocimetry. The non-stress test and biophysical profile are currently the most commonly used tests. Umbilical artery Doppler and contraction stress test are used in specific situations. Indications for antenatal testing are listed in Table 12-1. Initiation of the test is indication specific with variation for patients whose clinical conditions are worsening.[51]

Fetal movement assessment

Fetal movement assessment can be used in all patients. Studies in both high-risk and low-risk patients have shown lower stillbirth rates in patients routinely performing this test. Several protocols exist with no data showing superiority of one technique over another. Patients must understand that pregnancies not meeting the minimal number of movements require immediate evaluation regardless of the time of day. Fetal movement assessment should be considered for all patients but are particularly important for patients with high-risk conditions.

Table 12-1 Indicators for antepartum testing

- Preeclampsia
- Chronic hypertension
- Diabetes mellitus
- Anemia
- Rh isoimmunization
- Maternal pulmonary or disease
- Thrombophilia
- Uncontrolled hypothyroidism
- Intrauterine growth restriction
- Oligohydramnios
- Renal disease
- Post-term pregnancy
- Collagen vascular disease
- Hemoglobinopathies
- Decreased fetal movement
- Growth discordance in multiple gestations
- Monochoronic twins
- Fetal anomally

Timing of delivery

Elective delivery has become common placed in obstetrics. This practice has come at a price. Elective induction particularly with an unfavorable cervix leads to an increase in the incidence of primary cesarean section with associated increased morbidity and cost.[52] Patient demand has been a major driver. Unfortunately, this has led to earlier deliveries. To combat this trend, ACOG has strongly recommended no elective delivery until the patient is greater than 39 weeks in a well-dated pregnancy.[52] This approach has decreased the number of NICU admissions in the less than 39 week group.

Delivery timing for high-risk pregnancies has also changed. For many years, fetal lung maturity assessment via amniocentesis was commonplace; early delivery was performed once fetal lung maturity was documented. This led to many early deliveries. Recently ACOG has established time frames for delivery of pregnancies without the use of amniocentesis for fetal lung maturity assessment.[53] Some authors have questioned this protocol,[54] but amniocentesis for fetal lung maturity has markedly decreased. Certain conditions may warrant early delivery; see Table 12-2. Another recent development is the adoption of the elective cesarean section on maternal requests. This practice, though discouraged by

Table 12-2 Conditions that may lead to early delivery

- Fetal anomalies
- Growth restriction
- Abruption
- Previa
- Suspected accretia
- Preterm premature rupture of membranes
- Isoimmunization
- Diabetes mellitus
- Multiple gestations
- Prior classical cesarean section
- Prior myomectomy
- Oligohydramnios
- Preeclampsia
- Gestation hypertension
- Chronic hypertension
- Cholestasis of pregnancy

ACOG, must be acknowledged as an option for certain women, but it has certain requirements. Explanation of the risks for future pregnancies is required in counseling these patients prior to performing these procedures.[55]

Postterm pregnancy management

Management of postterm pregnancies has changed. If allowed to continue up to 10% of all pregnancies go beyond 42 weeks of gestational age. Prenatal morbidity and mortality increase after 41 weeks. Most authorities advocate delivery after 41 weeks.[56] If a pregnancy is to be continued after 41 weeks, close antepartum testing is indicated with specific attention paid to the amount of amniotic fluid. The use of cervical opening agents such as prostaglandin derivatives has made the management of these pregnancies much easier with many centers preceding with induction of labor at 41 weeks despite cervical status.[56]

References

1. Centers for Disease Control and Prevention. *Pregnancy mortality surveillance system*; 2013. Available from: www.cdc.gov/reproductivehealth/maternalinfan thealth/pmss.html. Accessed December 5, 2015.
2. US Department of Health and Human Services, Health Resources and Services Administration, Maternal and Child Health Bureau. *Women's health USA 2010*. Rockville, MD: US Department of Health and Human Services; 2010. Available from: http://mchb.hrsa.gov/whusa10/hstat/mh/pages/237mm.html#footnote1. Accessed December 5, 2015.
3. Edwards JE, Hanke JC. An update on maternal mortality and morbidity in the United States. *Nursing for women's health*. 2013;**17**(5):376–88.
4. Gabbe SG. *Obstetrics: Normal and Problem Pregnancies*. 6th ed. Philadelphia: Elsevier/Saunders; 2012: xvii, 1, 291.
5. American Academy of Pediatrics, American College of Obstetricians and Gynecologists. *Guidelines for perinatal care*. 7th ed. Elk Grove Village, IL and Washington, DC: American Academy of Pediatrics; American College of Obstetricians and Gynecologists; 2012: xiv, 580.
6. www.healthypeople.gov/2020/topicsobjectives2020/objectiveslist.aspx?topicId=26#376463. Accessed December 5, 2015.
7. Phillippi JC. Women's perceptions of access to prenatal care in the United States: a literature review. *Journal of midwifery & women's health*. 2009;**54**(3):219–25.
8. Whitworth M, Bricker L, Neilson JP, Dowswell T. Ultrasound for fetal assessment in early pregnancy. *Cochrane database of systematic reviews*. 2010;**4**: CD007058.
9. Hardy LM, Institute of Medicine (US), Committee on Prenatal and Newborn Screening for HIV Infection. *HIV screening of pregnant women and newborns*. Washington, DC: National Academy Press; 1991: 146.
10. ACOG Practice Bulletin No. 60: Pregestational diabetes mellitus. *Obstetrics and gynecology*. 2005; **105**(3):675–85.
11. Dunne F, Brydon P, Smith K, Gee H. Pregnancy in women with type 2 diabetes: 12 years outcome data 1990–2002. *Diabetic medicine: a journal of the British Diabetic Association*. 2003;**20**(9):734–8.
12. ACOG Practice Bulletin No. 102: Management of stillbirth. *Obstetrics and gynecology*. 2009;**113**(3):748–61.
13. Preboth M. ACOG guidelines on antepartum fetal surveillance. American College of Obstetricians and Gynecologists. *American family physician*. 2000;**62** (5):1184, 7–8.
14. Sokol RJ, Blackwell SC, American College of Obstetricians and Gynecologists. Committee on Practice B-G. ACOG practice bulletin: Shoulder dystocia. Number 40, November 2002. (Replaces practice pattern number 7, October 1997). *International journal of gynaecology and obstetrics: the official organ of the International Federation of Gynaecology and Obstetrics*. 2003;**80**(1):87–92.
15. ACOG Committee Opinion No. 597: Committee on Obstetric Practice: Labor induction or augmentation and autism. *Obstetrics and gynecology*. 2014;**123**(5): 1140–2.
16. MacDorman MF, Kirmeyer SE, Wilson EC. Fetal and perinatal mortality, United States, 2006. *National vital*

statistics reports: from the Centers for Disease Control and Prevention, National Center for Health Statistics, National Vital Statistics System. 2012;**60**(8):1–22.

17. Creasy RK, Resnik R, Greene MF, et al. *Creasy and Resnik's maternal-fetal medicine: principles and practice.* 7th ed. Philadelphia, PA: Elsevier/Saunders; 2014.
18. Berghella V. *Preterm birth: prevention and management.* Chichester, West Sussex; Hoboken, NJ: Wiley-Blackwell; 2010.
19. Meis PJ, Klebanoff M, Thom E, et al. Prevention of recurrent preterm delivery by 17 alpha-hydroxyprogesterone caproate. *The New England journal of medicine.* 2003;**348**(24):2379–85.
20. Owen J, Hankins G, Iams JD, et al. Multicenter randomized trial of cerclage for preterm birth prevention in high-risk women with shortened midtrimester cervical length. *American journal of obstetrics and gynecology.* 2009;**201**(4):375.e1–8.
21. National Collaborating Centre for Women and Children's Health. *Diabetes in pregnancy management of diabetes and its complications from preconception to the postnatal period.* NICE Guideline No. 3. London: National Institute for Health and Care Excellence (NICE); 2015 Feb 25.
22. ACOG Task Force on Hypertension in Pregnancy. *Hypertension in pregnancy.* Washington, DC: American College of Obstetricians and Gynecologists; 2013: 47–51.
23. ACOG Committee Opinion No. 518: Intimate partner violence. *Obstetrics and gynecology.* 2012;**119**(2 pt 1): 412–17.
24. Workowski KA, Berman S, CDC. Sexually transmitted diseases treatment guidelines, 2010. *MMWR recomm rep.* 2010 Dec 17;**59**(RR-12):1–110.
25. WHO. *Consolidated guidelines on the use of antiretroviral drugs for treating and preventing HIV infection: recommendations for a public health approach.* Geneva: World Health Organization; 2013.
26. ACOG Practice Bulletin No. 86: Viral hepatitis in pregnancy. *Obstetrics and gynecology.* 2007;**110**(4):941–56.
27. ACOG Practice Bulletin No. 131: Screening for cervical cancer. *Obstetrics and gynecology.* 2012; **120**(5):1222–38.
28. ACOG Practice Bulletin No. 140: Management of abnormal cervical cancer screening test results and cervical cancer precursors. *Obstetrics and gynecology.* 2013;**122**(6):1338–67.
29. House TE, Williams BL, Jr., Meares GM, Hester LL, Jr. Pregnancy complicated by urinary tract infections. *Obstetrics and gynecology.* 1969;**34**(5):670–4.
30. Merkatz IR, Nitowsky HM, Macri JN, Johnson WE. An association between low maternal serum alpha-fetoprotein and fetal chromosomal abnormalities. *American journal of obstetrics and gynecology.* 1984;**148**(7):886–94.
31. Wald NJ, Cuckle HS, Densem JW, et al. Maternal serum screening for Down's syndrome in early pregnancy. *BMJ.* 1988;**297**(6653):883–7.
32. Renier MA, Vereecken A, Van Herck E, et al. Second trimester maternal dimeric inhibin-A in the multiple-marker screening test for Down's syndrome. *Human reproduction.* 1998;**13**(3):744–8.
33. Cole LA, Shahabi S, Oz UA, et al. Hyperglycosylated human chorionic gonadotropin (invasive trophoblast antigen) immunoassay: a new basis for gestational Down syndrome screening. *Clinical chemistry.* 1999;**45**(12):2109–19.
34. Wapner RJ. First trimester aneuploidy screening: results of the NICHD multi-center study. *American journal of obstetrics and gynecology.* 2002;**185**(S70).
35. Dunstan FD, Nix AB. Screening for Down's syndrome: the effect of test date on the detection rate. *Annals of clinical biochemistry.* 1998;**35**(Pt 1):57–61.
36. Jenkins TM, Wapner RJ. Integrated screening for Down's syndrome. *The New England journal of medicine.* 1999;**341**(25):1935; author reply 6.
37. Rhoads GG, Jackson LG, Schlesselman SE, et al. The safety and efficacy of chorionic villus sampling for early prenatal diagnosis of cytogenetic abnormalities. *The New England journal of medicine.* 1989;**320**(10): 609–17.
38. Saura R, Gauthier B, Taine L, et al. Operator experience and fetal loss rate in transabdominal CVS. *Prenatal diagnosis.* 1994;**14**(1):70–1.
39. Odibo AO, Gray DL, Dicke JM, et al. Revisiting the fetal loss rate after second-trimester genetic amniocentesis: a single center's 16-year experience. *Obstetrics and gynecology.* 2008;**111**(3):589–95.
40. Bianchi DW, Platt LD, Goldberg JD, et al. Genome-wide fetal aneuploidy detection by maternal plasma DNA sequencing. *Obstetrics and gynecology.* 2012;**119**(5):890–901.
41. ACOG Committee Opinion No. 545: Noninvasive prenatal testing for fetal aneuploidy. *Obstetrics and gynecology.* 2012;**120**(6):1532–4.
42. Crane JP, LeFevre ML, Winborn RC, et al. A randomized trial of prenatal ultrasonographic screening: impact on the detection, management, and outcome of anomalous fetuses. The RADIUS Study Group. *American journal of obstetrics and gynecology.* 1994;**171**(2):392–9.
43. Nyberg DA, Souter VL, El-Bastawissi A, et al. Isolated sonographic markers for detection of fetal Down syndrome in the second trimester of pregnancy. *Journal of ultrasound in medicine: official journal of the*

American Institute of Ultrasound in Medicine. 2001;**20**(10):1053–63.

44. Carpenter MW, Coustan DR. Criteria for screening tests for gestational diabetes. *American journal of obstetrics and gynecology.* 1982;**144**(7):768–73.
45. Coustan DR. Screening and diagnosis of gestational diabetes. *Seminars in perinatology.* 1994;**18**(5):407–13.
46. Iams JD, Goldenberg RL, Meis PJ, et al. The length of the cervix and the risk of spontaneous premature delivery. National Institute of Child Health and Human Development Maternal Fetal Medicine Unit Network. *The New England journal of medicine.* 1996;**334**(9):567–72.
47. Romero R, Nicolaides K, Conde-Agudelo A, et al. Vaginal progesterone in women with an asymptomatic sonographic short cervix in the midtrimester decreases preterm delivery and neonatal morbidity: a systematic review and metaanalysis of individual patient data. *American journal of obstetrics and gynecology.* 2012;**206**(2):124.e1–19.
48. Cahill AG, Odibo AO, Caughey AB, et al. Universal cervical length screening and treatment with vaginal progesterone to prevent preterm birth: a decision and economic analysis. *American journal of obstetrics and gynecology.* 2010;**202**(6):548.e1–8.
49. Colin Y, Cherif-Zahar B, Le Van Kim C, et al. Genetic basis of the RhD-positive and RhD-negative blood group polymorphism as determined by Southern analysis. *Blood.* 1991;**78**(10):2747–52.
50. ACOG Committee Opinion No. 485: Prevention of early-onset group B streptococcal disease in newborns. *Obstetrics and gynecology.* 2011;**117**(4):1019–27.
51. ACOG Practice Bulletin No. 145: Antepartum fetal surveillance. *Obstetrics and gynecology.* 2014;**124**(1): 182–92.
52. ACOG Practice Bulletin No. 107: Induction of labor. *Obstetrics and gynecology.* 2009;**114**(2 Pt 1):386–97.
53. ACOG Committee Opinion No. 561: Nonmedically indicated early-term deliveries. *Obstetrics and gynecology.* 2013;**121**(4):911–15.
54. Towers CV, Freeman RK, Nageotte MP, et al. The case for amniocentesis for fetal lung maturity in late-preterm and early-term gestations. *American journal of obstetrics and gynecology.* 2014;**210**(2):95–6.
55. ACOG Committee Opinion No. 559: Cesarean delivery on maternal request. *Obstetrics and gynecology.* 2013;**121**(4):904–7.
56. ACOG Practice Bulletin No. 146: Management of late-term and postterm pregnancies. *Obstetrics and gynecology.* 2014;**124**(2 Pt 1):390–6.

Chapter 13

Pregnancy termination

Jennifer Lesko and Kari Braaten

Introduction

In developed nations, women spend many of their reproductive years trying to avoid pregnancy. Even with the availability of modern contraception, contraceptive gaps and failures are common; the United States has unintended pregnancy rates as high as 50%.[1, 2] Approximately one in five US pregnancies ends in abortion, and as many a one-third of all women will have an abortion by the time they are 45 years old.[3] Physicians can expect that a substantial number of their patients will seek or have undergone this common procedure. It is imperative that physicians counsel patients appropriately and neutrally regarding their pregnancy options.

This chapter will focus on counseling for patients with undesired pregnancy as well as appropriate management of both medical and surgical abortion in the office.

Unintended pregnancy

Unintended pregnancy is defined as one that is either mistimed or unwanted. Mistimed pregnancies occur when a woman becomes pregnant at a time when she did not desire conception though she would like a pregnancy in the future. Unwanted pregnancies occur when a women does not want to be pregnant currently or at any time in the future.[4] In 2008, 51% of all pregnancies in the United States were considered unintended, and the unintended pregnancy rate among women aged 15–44 was 54/1,000.[4, 5]

Women who continue unintended pregnancies are at increased risk of adverse social, economic, and health outcomes for both the mother and the child. Unintended births are associated with delays in prenatal care, smoking during pregnancy, lack of breastfeeding, poor health for the child, and poor outcomes for the mother and mother-child relationship.[4, 6] Women with unintended pregnancies are disproportionately impoverished, younger, more likely to be single and of underrepresented minority groups, and less likely to have completed high school. Nearly twice as many births resulting from unintended pregnancy are paid for by public insurance programs. The subsequent costs of unintended pregnancy to society are also quite high and include children's medical expenses, pregnancy-related care, and other government benefits for the woman and her children.[7]

Publicly funded family planning clinics have been found to be effective at promoting consistent and effective contraceptive use. Additionally, large studies like the Contraceptive CHOICE study, have demonstrated reductions in rates of unintended pregnancy, repeat abortions and teenage births when highly effective, long-acting, reversible methods are provided to patients at no cost.[1, 8]

Accessibility of abortion services

Internationally, abortion is not widely available; many countries currently have or have had restrictions on abortion accessibility. As a result, unsafe, illegal abortions are responsible for the majority of maternal morbidity and mortality in early pregnancy.[9] However, abortion was made legal in the United States in 1973 with the Supreme Court decision *Roe v Wade*. This protected a women's right to obtain an abortion before viability without government interference, and consequently decreased the rates of severe morbidity and mortality in the United States.

Despite this legal precedent, and the prevalence of the procedure, abortion remains less accessible to women than many other medical procedures. Recently, a barrage of new legal constraints has been passed on a state-by-state level, making it increasingly more difficult for women to obtain abortions.

Office Care of Women, ed. Martin E. Olsen and Botros Rizk. Published by Cambridge University Press.

Distance and providers

In 2011, 89% of US counties had no abortion clinics or abortion providers; 38% of women live in these counties. There has been a notable decline in both the number of abortion clinics and providers, and many US women now have to travel great distances to obtain an abortion.[10, 11] Many providers offer abortion only early in pregnancy; women needing later abortions have far fewer options.[11]

Cost

The cost of an abortion can be prohibitive for many women. In the United States, women who seek abortion are often low income, and many states do not provide government coverage for abortions. The median charges for early abortions of less than 10 weeks gestational age was $480 for surgical abortion and $500 for medication abortion. For women in need of services at greater than 20 weeks gestational age, costs were substantially higher, with a median charge in 2011 and 2012 of $1,350.[10, 12] This does not include indirect costs such as travel, child care, and missed wages.

Legal concerns

Individual state laws increasingly play a role in reducing access to abortion. In 30 US states, more than 205 abortion restrictions were enacted between 2011 and 2013; which is more than the entire previous decade.[13]

Several types of laws aim to restrict women's access to abortion. These include requirements for factually incorrect counseling or ultrasound viewing, parental consent or notification, limits on gestational age, bans on private insurance coverage, limitations on the use of evidence-based medical abortion protocols, and restrictions on what types of providers can administer medical abortion. New laws require abortion providers to comply with regulations like those of ambulatory surgical centers or to have admitting privileges at nearby hospitals. The costs of compliance with these laws are high; providers are frequently forced to renovate or close their clinics, while local hospitals are reluctant to grant privileges.[13] These regulations disproportionately affect the poorest and most socially disadvantaged women.

It is imperative that physicians are aware of the laws surrounding abortion in the jurisdiction in which they practice before embarking on the provision of abortion services in their offices.

Harassment

Many patients are forced to endure harassment when they seek an abortion. More than 80% of clinics experience picketing from anti-abortion protestors, and these intimidating activities serve to increase the stigma surrounding abortion.[12] Providing abortion in an office setting may help decrease harassment and normalize the procedure as part of the full spectrum of obstetric and gynecologic care.

Counseling, patient education, and informed consent

Counseling of a patient seeking abortion must include a discussion of all pregnancy options: continuing the pregnancy and raising the child, continuing the pregnancy and choosing adoption, or undergoing abortion. If a woman is uncertain about her choice, abortion should be delayed until she is certain of her decision.[14–17] When the decision has been made to proceed with abortion, she must then be counseled about the methods of abortion. Since the majority of abortions occur in the first trimester, most women have the option of medical or surgical abortion.

Table 13-1 gives an overview of the comparisons of medical and surgical abortion. Both methods are highly effective in the first trimester. Surgical abortion requires anesthesia and is completed faster, where as medical abortion is more private, patient-driven, takes more time, and results in more overall cramping and blood loss. Despite these differences, when women are counseled appropriately about what to expect, satisfaction rates are very high with both methods.[14–17]

Additional consideration must be paid to government-mandated protocols for abortion counseling including waiting periods, scripted patient information, and ultrasound requirements. These protocols are purported to help women make more informed decisions but many of them have not been found to improve care. They are often medically inaccurate.[18]

It is important to address patient's mental health and to assess their emotional support needs. Patients in a vulnerable emotional state or with a lack of personal support, may benefit from a referral to other health and social service agencies or hotlines.[18]

Finally, contraceptive counseling is a critical component of informed consent. Patients should be informed about their options for preventing a subsequent unintended pregnancy.

Table 13-1 A comparison of medical abortion and surgical abortion

	Medical abortion	Surgical abortion
Success rates	95–95%	98%
Need for additional procedure	2%–5% will need curettage for continued pregnancy, bleeding	2% will need repeat curettage for bleeding, retained products
Gestational age limits	4–10 weeks GA	4 weeks GA to viability*
Typical number of visits	2	1
Bleeding expectations	Heavy for several hours; like a period for 2 weeks	Usually period-like or lighter for 2 weeks
Analgesia	Oral NSAIDs, narcotics	Oral or IV sedation PCB
Infection risks	0.02%	1% but decreased with use of prophylactic antibiotics
Surgical risks	None	Anesthesia risks, cervical injury, uterine perforation
Risks to current pregnancy, if ongoing	Exposure to teratogenic medications	Increased risk of miscarriage
Effects on future pregnancy	None	None
Contraception initiation	Immediate for oral contraceptives. Implants at 1-week follow-up.	Immediate post-abortal initiation of all types.

* Limits are based on ability to follow very early pregnancy with serial serum hCGs afterward to ensure pregnancy has been evacuated. On the other end of the spectrum, many providers do not provide surgical abortions after the first trimester in their gynecologic office.

Medical evaluation

Before a woman undergoes a first trimester abortion, a full medical history should be obtained. Many women with stable, chronic medical conditions such as hypertension, diabetes, or asthma may be safely managed in the office setting.[19] Consultation with the patient's primary care physician or specialist may be necessary before deciding whether women with uncontrolled chronic diseases should be referred to a hospital based setting for a surgical abortion. Such conditions include history of stroke, impaired renal function, hepatic disease with elevated prothrombin time, cardiomyopathy, active lupus flare, pulmonary hypertension, and severe psychiatric illness.[19] This consultative process must be expedited for the medically complex patient, as delaying abortion care may place vulnerable women at risk of complications with increasing gestational age.[20]

Once a patient is deemed eligible to undergo abortion in the office setting, confirmation of pregnancy with a urine pregnancy test or ultrasound is necessary.

Physical exam should confirm normal vital signs and no evidence of an active pelvic infection. Laboratory evaluation includes Rh (D) antigen status, sexually transmitted infection testing for chlamydia per Centers for Disease Control and Prevention (CDC) recommendations, and anemia screening.

Determining gestational age

Clinicians typically date pregnancy from the first day of the last menstrual period (LMP). This method of dating can be inaccurate for women with irregular periods, who were using contraception when they became pregnant, or who are postpartum and breastfeeding. Other patients may not experience pregnancy symptoms. A bimanual exam is useful to estimate uterine size and position, but a fibroid uterus or obesity may confound the ability to accurately date a pregnancy. Increasingly, more abortion providers will confirm gestational age with an ultrasound.[21, 22] Ultrasound can also identify uterine anomalies or ectopic pregnancy prior to attempting a procedure.

Although ectopic pregnancy tends to be less frequent in the abortion population, women with risk factors or symptoms should be evaluated for ectopic pregnancy prior to offering medical or surgical abortion.[15, 23] If ultrasound does not confirm an intrauterine or ectopic pregnancy, but the patient is highly motivated to have an abortion on that day, she may safely undergo uterine aspiration with tissue inspection and human chorionic gonadotropin (hCG) follow-up to rule out ectopic pregnancy or failed abortion.[23, 24] Facilities must be able to track these patients and send out pathology specimens if products of conception are not definitely identified. Additionally, these women must be counseled that they will need follow-up appointments, blood draws, and possible ultrasounds to confirm resolution of the pregnancy.[23]

Medical abortion

Medical abortion medications

Mifepristone is a progesterone antagonist derived from norethindrone that promotes decidual necrosis, cervical softening, increased uterine contractility, and prostaglandin sensitivity. Misoprostol is a prostaglandin E1 analogue that causes uterine contractions and cervical softening.

Candidates for medical abortion

Most women will qualify for medical abortion if they are of the appropriate gestational age. Absolute contraindications include hemoglobin less than 9.5 g/dL, confirmed or suspected ectopic pregnancy, intrauterine device (IUD) in place, current long-term corticosteroid therapy, chronic adrenal failure, known coagulopathy, anticoagulant therapy, and intolerance or allergy to mifepristone or misoprostol. Furthermore, women with severe liver, renal, respiratory, vascular or cardiac disease may not be appropriate candidates. Patients who cannot comply with follow-up, desire a quick resolution of undesired pregnancy, or cannot understand the instructions, may be better served by a surgical procedure.[15]

Regimens

FDA-approved regimen

The only regimen approved by the Food and Drug Administration (FDA) in the United States is 600 mg of mifepristone administered orally, followed by misoprostol 400 mcg administered orally 48 hours later. The efficacy of this regimen is 92% up to 42 days of gestation. This regimen is not routinely recommended or used.

Evidence-based regimens

Other evidence-based regimens are considered superior to the FDA-approved regimen for both efficacy and safety. The most successful regimen consists of mifepristone 200 mg orally, followed by misoprostol 800 mcg, taken buccally, vaginally, or sublingually 24–48 hours later with success rates of 95%–99% up to 63 days gestational age.[15, 25] An alternative option with similar success rates is the use of vaginal misoprostol 800 mcg six hours or less after taking mifepristone.[26] A recent study also demonstrated a success rate of 93% among women 63–70 days gestational age.[27] Figure 13-1 depicts the mifepristone medication and the associated patient agreement.

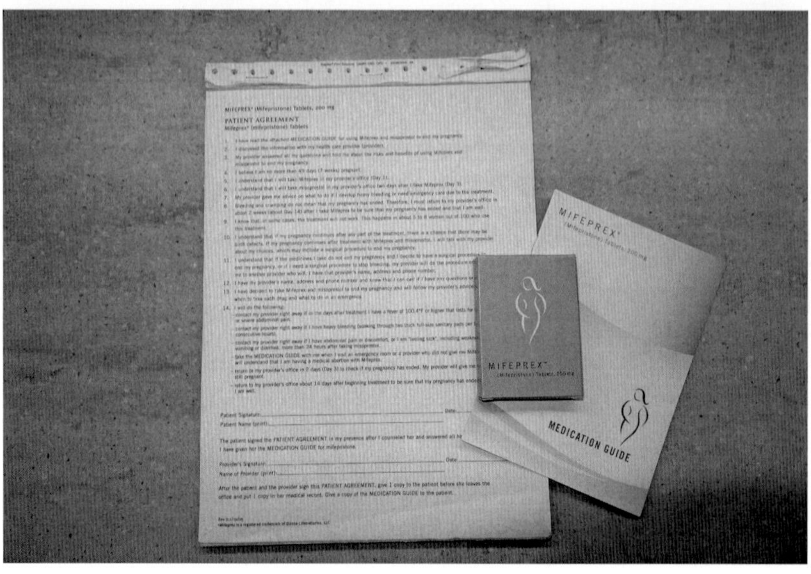

Figure 13-1 Medical abortion medication (mifepristone) and patient agreement (Danco).

Table 13-2 Patient expectations of medication abortion

What to expect after taking the misoprostol pills at home:

1. Cramping and bleeding are normal.
2. Symptoms will start two to four hours after taking misoprostol and will be heaviest when the pregnancy is expelled.
3. It can be normal to have lemon-sized blood clots and to soak up to two pads an hour for two hours.
4. The side effects of misoprostol include nausea, vomiting, dizziness, mild fever, and chills for 24 hours.

When to call about an emergency:

1. Fever of 100.4°F (38°C) or higher for more than 24 hours after taking misoprostol
2. Soaking more than two maxi pads an hour for more than two hours
3. Passing greater than lemon-sized blood clots for two hours or more
4. Bleeding heavily for more than 12 hours in a row
5. Severe vomiting and inability to eat or drink for more than six hours
6. Abdominal pain or cramping that does not improve with oral NSAIDs, narcotics, heating pads, or rest
7. Weakness, nausea, abdominal pain, vomiting, diarrhea more than 24 hours after taking misoprostol

Adverse events

Bleeding and cramping are normal side effects of the medical abortion. Table 13-2 illustrates the expectations that should be discussed with women for medical abortion and recovery.

Adverse effects are typically mediated by dose and route of misoprostol. These include nausea, vomiting, diarrhea, headaches, dizziness, and low-grade fevers. Oral or sublingual administration more commonly results in gastrointestinal side effects as compared to vaginal and buccal routes. Adjunct medications – non-steroidal anti-inflammatory drugs (NSAIDs), narcotics, and anti-emetics – may be helpful in mediating side effects.

Follow-up

Follow-up is required to confirm that the abortion is complete. Ultrasound has traditionally been the gold standard to confirm expulsion of the gestational sac. It is normal to see blood products and decidua on ultrasound, and in the absence of excessive bleeding, these findings do not represent need for uterine evacuation.[15, 28]

Prerequisite follow-up ultrasound may be a barrier to medical abortion for some women.[29] Assessing symptomatology in conjunction with a serum human chorionic gonadotropin (hCG) level is an accurate way of ensuring completion of the procedure while minimizing the number of in-person visits.[28, 29] An 80% decrease in serum hCG values one week after abortion is highly correlated with completed abortion and results in fewer surgical interventions than ultrasound follow-up. Blood draws may also be more accessible for patients than ultrasound.[29, 30]

Complications

Complications from medical abortion are rare and generally fall into the categories of excessive bleeding, infection, retained gestational sac, and ongoing pregnancy.

Excessive bleeding requiring emergent curettage occurs in approximately 0.2% of patients within the first 24 hours. It is imperative that providers offering medical abortion have training in surgical abortion or be able to refer to a physician who does.[15]

Serious infections are extremely rare after medical abortion. The most serious infections that have been associated with medical abortion are caused by the clostridial species.[31] Suspicions of intrauterine or systemic infection after medical abortion should prompt patient admission to the hospital for evaluation, broad-spectrum antibiotics, and supportive management.[15]

Evidence of a persistent gestational sac on ultrasound without evidence of fetal cardiac activity or continued development, may be managed expectantly, as long as the patient does not have continuing symptoms of pregnancy or prolonged excessive bleeding. The sac may pass spontaneously, even two weeks after mifepristone. Other options include repeating a dose of the misoprostol or undergoing surgical evacuation.[15]

The rate of ongoing pregnancy after medical abortion is less than 1%. If an ongoing pregnancy is diagnosed, uterine aspiration is suggested. If the patient strongly wishes to avoid surgical intervention a repeat dose of misoprostol may be attempted, which will successfully expel the pregnancy 36% of the time.[32]

Mifepristone and misoprostol are considered teratogenic, with increased risks of several congenital anomalies. Patients with ongoing pregnancies should be encouraged to undergo additional treatment to complete their abortions.[15]

First trimester surgical abortion

The appropriate office candidate

When performing surgical abortion in an office setting, providers should ensure that technical comfort with the procedure exists. Emergency precautions must be in place. Patients with more complex scenarios may be safer in a surgical center or hospital setting. Such complexities include suspected ectopic pregnancy with undiagnosed adnexal mass, uterine anomaly or significant cavity distorting lesion, uterine infection or sepsis, hemodynamic instability, or anemia with hemoglobin of less than 8 mg/dL.

MVA, EVA, dilators, and cannula

Abortion can be performed in the office with a standard set of tools that include a suction device, cannula, and dilators (Figure 13-2).

Both electric and mechanic suction apparatuses are available. The Mechanical Vacuum Aspirator (MVA) is a 60-mL syringe cylinder that creates up to 60 mmHg of pressure and can accommodate up to a 14 mm cannula for evacuation of the uterus. The MVA is typically quieter than an Electric Vacuum Aspirator (EVA), but may require multiple passes at higher gestational ages. The EVA is an electric suction machine with single-use tubing that can accommodate cannulas used to evacuate any sized uterus. MVAs and EVAs are equally efficacious in completing an abortion in the first trimester with equivalently low rates of complications. Patients may prefer the quiet of the MVA; however, providers prefer the EVA for its greater speed and ease of use at later gestational ages.[33, 34]

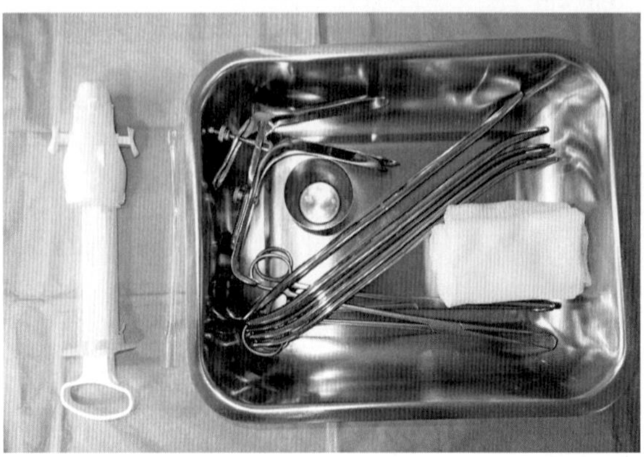

Figure 13-2 Surgical abortion equipment (from left to right: MVA, cannula, speculum, sterile cup for lidocaine, Pratt dilators, sterile gauze, ring forceps, tenaculum).

Rigid or flexible cannulas are available. Providers typically choose the cannula size that is roughly equivalent to gestational age in weeks. There are no differences in cervical injury, infection, blood transfusion, incomplete abortion, or need for repeat aspiration based on cannula types.[34] For dilator choice, the Society of Family Planning advocates for tapered dilators such as Pratt or Denniston. Blunt Hegar dilators may require more force and increase the risk of perforation.[35]

Cervical preparation

There is insufficient evidence to support the use of universal cervical preparation for patients in the first trimester, beyond dilation with mechanical dilators. This is based on very low rates of cervical injuries and clinically apparent uterine perforation in the first trimester, which are 0.1/10,000 to 10/10,000 and 0.1/1,000 to 4.0/1,000, respectively. The risks of these injuries are increased in certain subgroups; therefore, the Society of Family Planning recommends cervical preparation for adolescents, especially if the gestational age is greater than 12 weeks; all women greater than 12–14 weeks gestational age; and any women with initially difficult dilation.[35]

Misoprostol is the standard cervical preparation given prior to first trimester abortion in the office setting. It is inexpensive, it starts working within 2 hours, and it can be administered by a variety of different routes. It is most commonly given vaginally or buccally because these routes result in fewer gastrointestinal side effects while still maximizing cervical preparation. The recommended dose is 400 mcg administered three to four hours prior to the procedure.[35, 36] Although osmotic dilators can been used for cervical ripening prior to procedures, they typically require overnight placement for optimal effect.

The surgical abortion procedure

After consents have been signed, the patient is placed in the dorsal lithotomy position. A bimanual exam is performed to confirm the position and the size of the uterus. A speculum is placed and the cervix identified. The cervix may be cleansed with betadine, chlorhexadine or saline.[37] Then 1 mL or 2 mL of 1% lidocaine is injected at the anterior lip of the cervix and a tenaculum is placed. A paracervical block may be used at this point for analgesia (see "Pain Management"). The cervix is then sequentially dilated with sterile dilators to admit a suction cannula of the appropriate size.

If using an MVA, the plunger is withdrawn and locked to create suction, and the appropriately sized cannula is attached to the syringe with care to keep the tip of the cannula sterile. The cannula is then passed into the uterine cavity, the valves are opened to activate the suction, and the contents of the uterus are aspirated using a twirling or back-and-forth motion. If using an EVA, the cannula is attached to the tubing, the thumb switch is closed to generate suction, and a similar motion is employed to evacuate the uterus.

The uterus is considered empty when involution is palpated, there is a uniformly gritty or sandpaper sensation with passage of the cannula over the endometrium, and there is no evidence of additional tissue passing through the cannula.

After aspiration is complete, the products are inspected by rinsing them with water and then floating them over a backlight to identify tissue. Depending on gestational age, a gestational sac, chorionic villi, blood, decidua, and possibly fetal parts can be seen (Figures 13-3 and 13-4). If the villi are hydropic or there is suspicion of a molar pregnancy, the tissue should be sent for pathologic evaluation. If a pregnancy cannot be confirmed, a repeat aspiration may be performed. The tissue may be sent for pathologic analysis to identify whether an intrauterine pregnancy is present, serial serum hCG levels should be followed, and the patient should receive ectopic precautions.

Once the abortion is deemed complete, all instruments should be removed from the vagina and bleeding should be evaluated. The patient should be monitored to ensure that her vitals are normal and that her bleeding and pain are appropriate. Once the patient is stable to go home, she should be given discharge instructions and emergency contact information.

Complications

Complications of first trimester abortion are extremely rare with a rate of less than 1% for any complication and a hospitalization rate of only 0.3%.[38] Hemorrhage is among the more common complications and may be caused by uterine atony, abnormal placentation, cervical laceration, coagulopathy, or retained products of conception.[39] Uterine perforations occur in 0.1/1,000 to 0.3/1,000 of procedures, and are usually at the fundus,

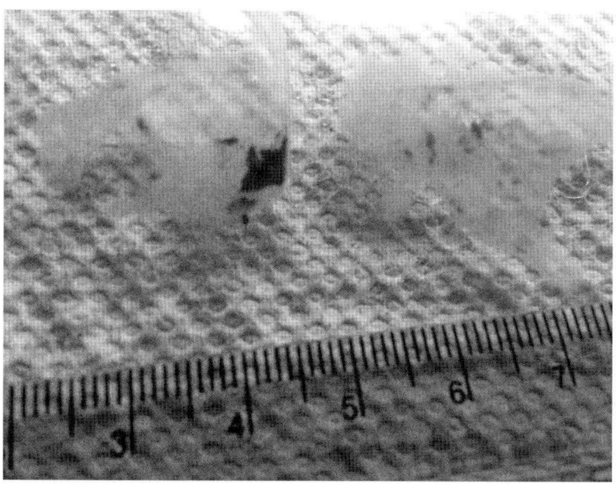

Figure 13-3 Uterine aspirate and products of conception at six weeks gestation.

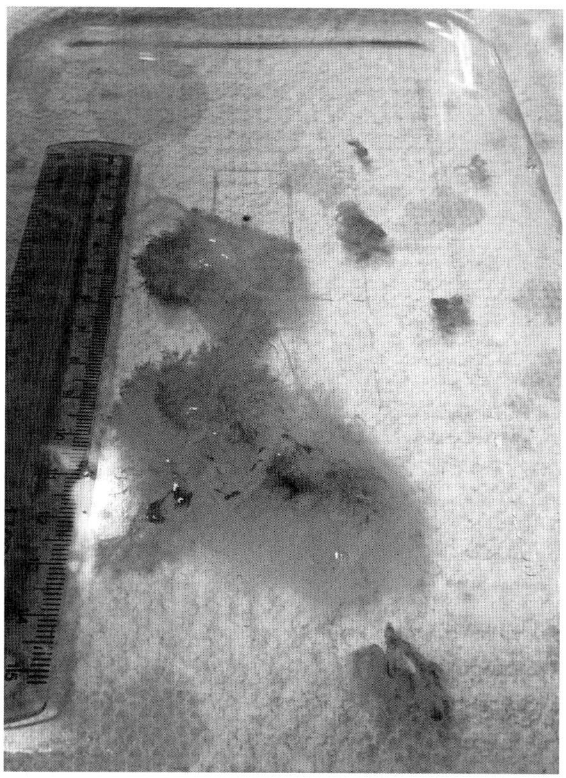

Figure 13-4 Uterine aspirate and products of conception at 10 weeks gestation.

Table 13-3 First trimester surgical abortion complications and management

Surgical complication	Management
Hemorrhage	• Speculum exam for cervical lacerations • Ultrasound to assess for retained products, free fluid in pelvis • Obtain IV access and administer fluids • Uterine massage • Uterotonic medications: methylergonovine maleate 0.2 mg IM (contraindicated in hypertension); misoprostol 400 mcg–800 mcg PR • Intrauterine placement of sterile Foley bulb for tamponade • With continued bleeding or suspicion of disseminated intravascular coagulation, transfer to hospital for further care • Consider reaspiration, uterine artery embolization; hysterectomy if bleeding persistent.
Uterine perforation	• Suspected small perforation – monitor for several hours • If vital signs are within normal limits and there is no evidence of peritoneal signs or worsening pain, discharge home with precautions • If severe perforation suspected, transfer to hospital for laparoscopy or laparotomy
Incomplete abortion or ongoing pregnancy	• Repeat aspiration with ultrasound guidance • Can consider administration of misoprostol to expel remaining products of conception if bleeding minimal
Cervical lacerations	• Monsel's solution or silver nitrate at the site of laceration • If larger laceration, a suture may be necessary
Hematometra	• Reaspiration of the uterus • Administration uterotonic medications to prevent recurrence
Post-abortal infections	• Broad spectrum antibiotic management
Vasovagal episodes	• Place patient in Trendelenburg position • Cool compresses • Smelling salts • Administer atropine if no response to above

resulting from the suction cannula.[35] Incomplete abortion may require reaspiration or administration of misoprostol to expel retained tissue. Other complications include cervical lacerations, hematometra, post-abortal infections, ongoing pregnancy, and vasovagal episodes (Table 13-3).

Pain management

Pain management options are influenced by whether the patient is having a medication abortion or a surgical abortion, the clinical setting of the abortion, and patient preference.

Medical abortion

Pain is the most commonly reported side effect during medical abortion and is expected. It most typically occurs after the administration of misoprostol as the uterus begins contracting to expel the pregnancy. Approximately 75% of patients undergoing medical abortion experience pain severe enough to use a narcotic medication. Factors associated with increased analgesic use include increasing gestation, young age, nulliparity, and white race.[40]

Several regimens of pain medications have been studied for medical abortion. The best evidence for pain relief with medical abortion is for NSAIDs. Ibuprofen appears to be superior to acetominophen as well as placebo.[40, 41] Administration of ibuprofen prophylactically on a scheduled basis does not appear to be more beneficial than when taken as needed.[42] Typical pain regimens for medical abortion rely on NSAIDs as the first line pain medication, with additional narcotics or acetominophen with narcotics as needed. Women are generally instructed to take ibuprofen 600 mg–800 mg with the onset of cramping and every four to eight hours as needed. A narcotic medication is available to take in addition if needed.

Surgical abortion

Pain during surgical abortion occurs with several steps of the procedure: the paracervical block, tenaculum placement, cervical dilation, aspiration and post-procedural cramping. Studies report that 78%–97% of women experience at least moderate pain with the procedure and several studies have found pain to be inversely correlated with satisfaction.[43] Factors that increase perception of pain include pre-procedural depression, fear, anxiety, young age, nulliparity, history of pelvic pain/dysmenorrheal, and uterine retroversion, whereas prior vaginal delivery decreases perception of pain.[43]

Approaches to pain during surgical abortion include oral premedication, local anesthesia (paracervical block), IV sedation and deep sedation or general anesthesia. Pain management is often driven by the type of facility and can safely and adequately be administered at a reasonable cost.

Paracervical block

A paracervical block of local anesthetic has been shown to provide pain relief during abortion.[44] No particular type of local anesthetic has been proven more effective than others; however lidocaine and chloroprocaine have less toxicity than bupivacaine. There is improved pain control with buffered compared to plain lidocaine, and deep injection compared to superficial. A slower injection makes the paracervical block itself less painful. A four-site block does not appear to offer benefit over a two-site block, and there does not appear to be a difference between cervical or vaginal vault injections.[44]

Premedications

Medications that can be taken prior to an abortion procedure have been investigated because of their ease of use and potential for patient self-administration. Types of medications that have been evaluated for potential pain relief include NSAIDs, oral benzodiazepines, oral narcotics, and prostaglandins.

NSAIDs have become a mainstay of pain control for abortion procedures. They are most commonly given prior to the procedure, and then recommended to women to be taken on an as-needed basis after their procedure. The most commonly used NSAIDs are oral ibuprofen and naproxen, and parenteral ketorolac sodium. Whether NSAIDs improve procedural pain is unclear; however, they do decrease post-operative pain as compared to placebo.[45] There is no benefit for parenteral NSAIDs such as ketorolac with patients who can tolerate oral medications.[46] Prophylactic ibuprofen should be given 60–90 minutes prior to the procedure, which is early enough to provide maximal effect.

Oral benzodiazepines, oral narcotics and cervical preparation are commonly used with misoprostol but do not appear to decrease procedural pain; they do in many cases increase side effects.[47] It is therefore generally felt that these medications should not be used for the purpose of reducing pain.

IV sedation and general anesthesia

Many abortion providers offer some form of intravenous sedation. Sedation is a spectrum, and the amount of sedation that an abortion provider is able to offer depends on staffing, medication availability and safety. Minimal sedation is defined by a normal level of responsiveness to verbal stimulation, without any effect on cardiopulmonary function. Moderate sedation, also sometimes termed "conscious sedation," typically involves parenteral medications such as fentanyl and midazolam. Patients retain purposeful response to verbal or tactile stimulation, and no airway intervention is required. Spontaneous ventilation may be affected but remains adequate, and cardiovascular function is usually maintained. Moderate sedation can be administered by an appropriately trained abortion provider, and requires safety features, including nursing staff, supplemental oxygen, and the ability to manage over-sedation or airway difficulties. Deep sedation should not be administered in an office setting without these resources.

In randomized studies, moderate IV sedation with fentanyl and midazolam provides improved pain control over placebo and increases patient satisfaction. Minimal or low-dose sedation does not appear to offer benefit.[40] Women who choose between local anesthesia only and IV sedation report similar levels of satisfaction, suggesting that expectations and self-perception of pain tolerance play an important role in the experience of pain.[48]

Antibiotic management

Upper genital tract infection after first trimester surgical or medical abortion is extremely rare with a rate of less than 1%. Antibiotic prophylaxis has been studied extensively in both the medical and surgical abortion populations.[37]

A number of randomized controlled trials have been conducted to evaluate whether benefit of prophylactic antibiotics in surgical abortion exists. Although the benefit may be more likely in populations at high risk, including those with a history of chlamydia cervicitis or previous pelvic inflammatory disease, a systematic review found a clinically and statistically significant reduction in postabortal infections when prophylactic antibiotics were used in all patients.[49] Thus, the recommendations of the American College of Obstetrics and Gynecology and the Society of Family Planning is to prescribe antibiotic prophylaxis for surgical abortion. A preferred regimen is 100 mg of doxycycline given prior to the procedure and then a dose of 200 mg after the procedure.[37, 50]

The recommendations for medical abortion are less clear. Since medical abortion is not an invasive procedure, the theoretical risk of infection should be less than of surgical abortion. A large multicenter study at several Planned Parenthood abortion clinics found a significant decrease in infection rates and infection-related mortality when two simultaneous interventions were implemented: changing the route of misoprostol from vaginal to buccal and implementing a seven-day course of antibiotics. It has been difficult to determine whether this was a result of antibiotics or decreasing the risk of vaginal contamination with misoprostol.[51, 52] The Society of Family Planning does not routinely recommend antibiotic prophylaxis with medical abortion.[15, 37]

Contraceptive counseling and initiation

Treatment for unintended, undesired pregnancy presents a unique opportunity to counsel patients about preventing future unintended pregnancy. Patients should be counseled regarding their contraceptive options with consideration of their health status, any potential contraindications, and emphasis on the most effective methods. Research from the Contraceptive CHOICE project has demonstrated that women who choose highly effective, long-acting, reversible methods of contraception (LARC) including the levonorgestrel intrauterine device (IUD), the copper IUD, and the etonorgestrel implant are highly satisfied with their method, use it for longer than other methods, and have a reduction in unintended pregnancy rates.[53]

It is safe to initiate most forms of contraception immediately in both surgical and medical abortion patients. Patients may start using combined hormonal birth control on the day of their procedure or the day of mifepristone administration. It is also safe to place an intrauterine device or implant following a surgical abortion as long as there are no contraindications or evidence of infection.[54] Most patients can receive an IUD, implant, or depot medroxyprogesterone at their medical abortion follow-up visit.[15]

Concluding remarks

Unintended pregnancy affects women worldwide. It is a physician's responsibility to counsel women about their options. When a woman opts to proceed with abortion, she should receive factually accurate counseling. When performed according to evidence-based protocols with the use of aseptic techniques and appropriate antibiotics, abortion is an extremely safe procedure with rare complications and few risks to future pregnancies. Following abortion, it is important to establish a contraceptive plan to help the patient prevent future unintended pregnancies.

References

1. Finer LB, Zolna MR. Unintended pregnancy in the United States: incidence and disparities, 2006. *Contraception* 2011 Nov;**84**(5):478–85.
2. Institute of Medicine (US) Committee on Unintended Pregnancy, 1995.
3. Jones RK, Kavanaugh ML. Changes in abortion rates between 2000 and 2008 and lifetime incidence of abortion. *Obstet Gynecol* 2011 Jun;**117**(6):1358–66.
4. Finer LB, Zolna MR. Shifts in intended and unintended pregnancies in the United States, 2001–2008. *Am J Public Health* 2014 Feb;**104**(Suppl 1):S43–8.
5. Pazol K, Creanga AA, Burley KD, et al. Abortion surveillance – United States, 2010. *MMWR Surveill Summ* 2013 Nov 29;**62**(8):1–44.
6. Barber JS, Axinn WG, Thornton A. Unwanted childbearing, health, and mother-child relationships. *J Health Soc Behav* 1999 Sep;**40**(3):231–57.
7. Sonfeld A, Kost K. *Public Costs from Unintended Pregnancies and the Role of Public Insurance Programs in Paying for Pregnancy and Infant Care: Estimates for 2008*. New York: Guttmacher Institute, 2013.
8. Peipert JF, Madden T, Allsworth JE, Secura GM. Preventing unintended pregnancies by providing no-cost contraception. *Obstet Gynecol* 2012 Dec;**120**(6): 1291–7.

9. Sedgh G, Singh S, Shah IH, et al. Induced abortion: incidence and trends worldwide from 1995 to 2008. *Lancet* 2012 Feb 18;**379**(9816):625–32.

10. Jones RK, Zolna MR, Henshaw SK, Finer LB. Abortion in the United States: incidence and access to services, 2005. *Perspect Sex Reprod Health* 2008 Mar;**40**(1):6–16.

11. Jones RK, Jerman J. Abortion incidence and service availability in the United States, 2011. *Perspect Sex Reprod Health* 2014 Mar;**46**(1):3–14.

12. Jerman J, Jones RK. Secondary measures of access to abortion services in the United States, 2011 and 2012: gestational age limits, cost, and harassment. *Womens Health Issues* 2014 Jul–Aug;**24**(4):e419–24.

13. Boonstra HD, Nash E. A Surge of State Abortion Restrictions Puts Providers – and the Women They Serve – in the Crosshairs. *Guttmacher Policy Review* 2014;**17**(1):9–15.

14. Creinin MD. Randomized comparison of efficacy, acceptability and cost of medical versus surgical abortion. *Contraception* 2000 Sep;**62**(3):117–24.

15. ACOG Committee on Practice Bulletins – Gynecology. ACOG Practice Bulletin No. 143: Medical management of first-trimester abortion. *Obstet Gynecol* 2014 Mar;**123**(3):676–92.

16. Rorbye C, Norgaard M, Nilas L. Medical versus surgical abortion: comparing satisfaction and potential confounders in a partly randomized study. *Hum Reprod* 2005 Mar;**20**(3):834–8.

17. Henshaw RC, Naji SA, Russell IT, Templeton AA. Comparison of medical abortion with surgical vacuum aspiration: women's preferences and acceptability of treatment. *BMJ* 1993 Sep 18;**307**(6906):714–17.

18. Gould H, Perrucci A, Barar R, et al. Patient education and emotional support practices in abortion care facilities in the United States. *Womens Health Issues* 2012 Jul–Aug;**22**(4):e359–64.

19. Guiahi M, Davis A, Society of Family Planning. First-trimester abortion in women with medical conditions. *Contraception* 2012 Dec;**86**(6):622–30.

20. Bartlett LA, Berg CJ, Shulman HB, et al. Risk factors for legal induced abortion-related mortality in the United States. *Obstet Gynecol* 2004 Apr;**103**(4): 729–37.

21. Kulier R, Kapp N. Comprehensive analysis of the use of pre-procedure ultrasound for first- and second-trimester abortion. *Contraception* 2011 Jan; **83**(1):30–3.

22. O'Connell K, Jones HE, Simon M, et al. First-trimester surgical abortion practices: a survey of National Abortion Federation members. *Contraception* 2009 May;**79**(5):385–92.

23. Lichtenberg ES, Paul M, Society of Family Planning. Surgical abortion prior to 7 weeks of gestation. *Contraception* 2013 Jul;**88**(1):7–17.

24. Edwards J, Carson SA. New technologies permit safe abortion at less than six weeks' gestation and provide timely detection of ectopic gestation. *Am J Obstet Gynecol* 1997 May;**176**(5):1101–6.

25. von Hertzen H, Huong NT, Piaggio G, et al. Misoprostol dose and route after mifepristone for early medical abortion: a randomised controlled noninferiority trial. *BJOG* 2010 Sep;**117**(10):1186–96.

26. Creinin MD, Fox MC, Teal S, et al. A randomized comparison of misoprostol 6 to 8 hours versus 24 hours after mifepristone for abortion. *Obstet Gynecol* 2004 May;**103**(5 Pt 1):851–9.

27. Winikoff B, Dzuba IG, Chong E, et al. Extending outpatient medical abortion services through 70 days of gestational age. *Obstet Gynecol* 2012 Nov;**120**(5): 1070–6.

28. Grossman D, Grindlay K. Alternatives to ultrasound for follow-up after medication abortion: a systematic review. *Contraception* 2011 Jun;**83**(6):504–10.

29. Clark W, Bracken H, Tanenhaus J, et al. Alternatives to a routine follow-up visit for early medical abortion. *Obstet Gynecol* 2010 Feb;**115**(2 Pt 1):264–72.

30. Dayananda I, Maurer R, Fortin J, Goldberg AB. Medical abortion follow-up with serum human chorionic gonadotropin compared with ultrasonography: a randomized controlled trial. *Obstet Gynecol* 2013 Mar;**121**(3):607–13.

31. Cohen AL, Bhatnagar J, Reagan S, et al. Toxic shock associated with *Clostridium sordellii* and *Clostridium perfringens* after medical and spontaneous abortion. *Obstet Gynecol* 2007 Nov;**110**(5):1027–33.

32. Reeves MF, Kudva A, Creinin MD. Medical abortion outcomes after a second dose of misoprostol for persistent gestational sac. *Contraception* 2008 Oct; **78**(4):332–5.

33. Bird ST, Harvey SM, Beckman LJ, et al. Similarities in women's perceptions and acceptability of manual vacuum aspiration and electric vacuum aspiration for first trimester abortion. *Contraception* 2003 Mar;**67**(3): 207–12.

34. Kulier R, Fekih A, Hofmeyr GJ, Campana A. Surgical methods for first trimester termination of pregnancy. *Cochrane Database Syst Rev* 2001;**4**:CD002900.

35. Allen RH, Goldberg AB, Board of Society of Family Planning. Cervical dilation before first-trimester surgical abortion. *Contraception* 2007 Aug;**76**(2): 139–56.

36. Kapp N, Lohr PA, Ngo TD, Hayes JL. Cervical preparation for first trimester surgical abortion. *Cochrane Database Syst Rev* 2010 Feb 17;**2**:CD007207.

37. Achilles SL, Reeves MF, Society of Family Planning. Prevention of infection after induced abortion: release date October 2010: SFP guideline 20102. *Contraception* 2011 Apr;**83**(4):295–309.

38. Weitz TA, Taylor D, Desai S, et al. Safety of aspiration abortion performed by nurse practitioners, certified nurse midwives, and physician assistants under a California legal waiver. *Am J Public Health* 2013 Mar;**103**(3):454–61.

39. Kerns J, Steinauer J. Management of postabortion hemorrhage: release date November 2012 SFP Guideline #20131. *Contraception* 2013 Mar;**87**(3):331–42.

40. Jackson E, Kapp N. Pain control in first-trimester and second-trimester medical termination of pregnancy: a systematic review. *Contraception* 2011 Feb;**83**(2): 116–26.

41. Avraham S, Gat I, Duvdevani NR, et al. Pre-emptive effect of ibuprofen versus placebo on pain relief and success rates of medical abortion: a double-blind, randomized, controlled study. *Fertil Steril* 2012 Mar;**97**(3):612–15.

42. Raymond EG, Weaver MA, Louie KS, et al. Prophylactic compared with therapeutic ibuprofen analgesia in first-trimester medical abortion: a randomized controlled trial. *Obstet Gynecol* 2013 Sep;**122**(3):558–64.

43. Renner RM, Jensen JT, Nichols MD, Edelman AB. Pain control in first-trimester surgical abortion: a systematic review of randomized controlled trials. *Contraception* 2010 May;**81**(5):372–88.

44. Renner RM, Nichols MD, Jensen JT, et al. Paracervical block for pain control in first-trimester surgical abortion: a randomized controlled trial. *Obstet Gynecol* 2012 May;**119**(5):1030–7.

45. Suprapto K, Reed S. Naproxen sodium for pain relief in first-trimester abortion. *Am J Obstet Gynecol* 1984 Dec 15;**150**(8):1000–1.

46. Braaten KP, Hurwitz S, Fortin J, Goldberg AB. Intramuscular ketorolac versus oral ibuprofen for pain relief in first-trimester surgical abortion: a randomized clinical trial. *Contraception* 2014 Feb;**89**(2):116–21.

47. Micks EA, Edelman AB, Renner RM, et al. Hydrocodone-acetaminophen for pain control in first-trimester surgical abortion: a randomized controlled trial. *Obstet Gynecol* 2012 Nov;**120**(5): 1060–9.

48. Allen RH, Kumar D, Fitzmaurice G, et al. Pain management of first-trimester surgical abortion: effects of selection of local anesthesia with and without lorazepam or intravenous sedation. *Contraception* 2006 Nov;**74**(5):407–13.

49. Low N, Mueller M, Van Vliet HA, Kapp N. Perioperative antibiotics to prevent infection after first-trimester abortion. *Cochrane Database Syst Rev* 2012 Mar 14;**3**:CD005217.

50. ACOG Committee on Practice Bulletins – Gynecology. ACOG Practice Bulletin No. 104: antibiotic prophylaxis for gynecologic procedures. *Obstet Gynecol* 2009 May;**113**(5):1180–9.

51. Fjerstad M, Trussell J, Sivin I, et al. Rates of serious infection after changes in regimens for medical abortion. *N Engl J Med* 2009 Jul 9;**361**(2): 145–51.

52. Trussell J, Nucatola D, Fjerstad M, Lichtenberg ES. Reduction in infection-related mortality since modifications in the regimen of medical abortion. *Contraception* 2014 Mar;**89**(3):193–6.

53. Winner B, Peipert JF, Zhao Q, et al. Effectiveness of long-acting reversible contraception. *N Engl J Med* 2012 May 24;**366**(21):1998–2007.

54. Okusanya BO, Oduwole O, Effa EE. Immediate postabortal insertion of intrauterine devices. *Cochrane Database Syst Rev* 2014 Jul 28;**7**:CD001777.

Chapter 14

Office care of the pediatric-adolescent gynecologic patient

Nancy Sokkary and Jessica Francis

Introduction

Pediatric and adolescent gynecology (PAG) is a vast and quickly growing field within obstetrics and gynecology. The goal of PAG is to bridge the gap between the world of pediatrics and adult medicine in the area of obstetrics and gynecology. Some gynecologic issues are difficult to address in the general pediatric setting; however, most children and adolescents do not have an established gynecologist. PAG serves as a home for those patients who may find it difficult or intimidating to seek care.

The subspecialty was born from the notion that young patients with gynecologic problems would best be served by providers who had expertise in both fields and work with interdisciplinary teams.[1] More than 30 years ago the first edition of a text devoted to PAG was published. Now there are ten fellowship programs, multiple annual conferences, and a journal entirely dedicated to PAG. As the field has grown, so too has quality research. We now have evidence-based workups and treatment algorithms specific to this patient population that can hopefully be used by general gynecology providers.[2]

Scope of the specialty

Pediatric and adolescent gynecology includes a wide array of gynecologic issues. This chapter will review the global approach to a pediatric/adolescent patient in the gynecology clinic. It will also outline the clinical steps specific for evaluating and treating adolescents with heavy menstrual bleeding, vulvovaginitis, and abnormal pubertal development.

Menorrhagia

Abnormal uterine bleeding is the most common reason for adolescents to visit the gynecologist.[3] Up to 40% of adolescents report heavy menstrual bleeding (HMB), defined as more than eight days of bleeding, more than 80 mL of blood loss, or more than eight pads per day. This can have a large impact on medical health but also mental well-being. For some adolescents, heavy bleeding results in missed school, decreases in physical activity, and low energy. Perhaps most importantly, it may be a sign of an underlying bleeding disorder. It has been reported that anywhere from 10% to 48% of adolescents with HMB have an underlying bleeding disorder, and HMB is the single most common presenting symptoms in women with bleeding disorders.[3]

Vulvovaginitis

Vulvovaginitis is one of the most common gynecologic complaints among prepubertal females, although the true incidence is unknown.[4, 5] The pediatric population is at increased risk of developing vulvar and vaginal infections and irritation for several reasons. From shortly after birth until puberty, the vagina is in an atrophic state with little estrogen exposure, low glycogen, and a neutral pH of 6.5. In addition, these girls have not yet developed the protective barriers such as hair and labial fat pads. Finally, this age group is at high risk of infection due to poor hygiene and proximity of the rectum to the vulva and vaginal introitus.[6]

Delayed puberty

Delayed puberty is thought to affect about 3% of young women.[7] It is defined as absence or incomplete development of secondary sex characteristics by the age at which 95% of children in that cultural group have already initiated these changes. We do know that young black females are likely to enter puberty earlier than Hispanic girls, who are in turn likely to enter puberty earlier than Caucasian girls. The most likely diagnosis is that of constitutional delay. Other possible etiologies of delayed puberty include chronic disease, autoimmune disorders, nutritional deficiencies, tumors

Office Care of Women, ed. Martin E. Olsen and Botros Rizk. Published by Cambridge University Press.

(central nervous system, gonadal, or adrenal), and primary ovarian insufficiency (POI). In one large case series, 50 diagnoses were identified that led to pubertal delay.[8]

Precocious puberty

Precocious puberty can be a very difficult diagnosis, as the cause can range from a variant of normal development to high-risk pathologic causes including malignancy. Different professional groups consider precocious puberty as the onset of secondary sexual development before the age of six to eight years in girls. The threshold for evaluation can be very difficult to establish, however, and has been debated over the years due to differences between girls of varying ethnicities. That being said, the younger a patient presents with secondary sex characteristics, the more assertive the clinician should be in evaluating the patient. The main concern regarding evaluation for precocious puberty is that pathology may be missed if we are too rigid with an age cut-off for evaluation.[9] Clinicians should use their best judgment and operate on a case-by-case basis.

Precocious puberty can be classified as gonadotropin-dependent (GDPP) or gonadotropin-independent (GIPP) based on the pathologic process resulting in the pubertal changes. GDPP is often referred to as central precocious puberty, as it implies that the source of stimulation is the hypothalamus. GIPP is referred to as peripheral precocious puberty, as the source of stimulation is often from an ovarian or other peripheral mass.

Other common presenting complaints seen in PAG clinics include oligomenorrhea, primary amenorrhea, and contraception. Polycystic ovarian syndrome effects between 11% and 26% of adolescents.[10] Although müllerian anomalies and disorders of sexual differentiation are considered rare, ongoing research in PAG is contributing greatly to understanding diagnosis and therapy.[11] PAG is also invested in preventing teen pregnancy with use of long-acting reversible contraceptive methods and providing contraception to adolescents with complex medical comorbidities. Although these areas are an integral part of PAG, they are covered in other chapters or are beyond the scope of this text and will not be reviewed here.

Approach to the pediatric/adolescent patient

Sensitivity, comfort, and a nonpatronizing attitude are of the utmost importance. When addressing gynecologic topics with a young population, it is paramount to appear comfortable and at ease with topics that can be awkward for children and adolescents to discuss such as vaginal discharge or pain, details of their menstrual cycle, and sexual history. There are several techniques that can be used to facilitate a comfortable visit. Explain the appointment and physical exam that will be done in advance.[1] Using models or parents to demonstrate appropriate parts of the history and exam can be helpful. Give the patient control by allowing her to decide when to do the exam and who will be in the room for it. Allowing the patient to participate will give her a sense of control. The patient, for example, may help with collection of swabs or measurements if needed.

Confidentiality is a unique and complicated aspect for PAG patients. It is important that the provider, patient, and guardian understand the importance, benefits, and limits of confidentiality in this setting. The Guttmacher Institute has published "An overview of Minors' Consent Law" that is easily accessible online. This document outlines the laws regarding consent by a minor for contraceptive services, sexually transmitted infection services, prenatal care, adoption, and abortion. In most states the consent laws apply to patients over the age of 12.[12] Like many confidentiality clauses, this can be broken if the patient is deemed to be a risk to herself or others. Clinics that have a high volume of PAG patients may choose to have their confidentiality rules posted; others have a sheet that patients and guardians can review. Regardless of what is done on a systems level, it is important that the provider inform anyone accompanying the minor that part of the history will be done in private. It should also be explained to the patient what information, if any, will be relayed to the parent or guardian. Although confidentiality is paramount, the patient should be encouraged to confide in her guardian when appropriate.[13]

Certain resources can be very helpful in the clinical setting. Models, as previously mentioned, are helpful to demonstrate development and anatomy. Pictures are truly valuable for young patients. Use of a flip chart of normal anatomy or images from the internet will increase patient comprehension of simple and complex gynecologic issues. The internet cannot be underestimated. Several websites, Facebook pages, and online support groups exist for patients with genetic disorders such as Turner's syndrome, müllerian agenesis, and Von Willebrand disease. Bedsider.org is

Table 14-1 Menstrual history

- Age of menarche
- Interval between periods
- Number of days of bleeding
- Number of pads/tampons used per day
- Presents of soiling
- Presents of clotting

Table 14-2 Vulvovaginitis history

- Type of discomfort: itch, burn, sting, sore
- Location of discomfort
- Timing (night/day)
- Erythema
- Discharge: color and odor

a fantastic resource for sexually active teens, their parents, and providers.

History

The history should be collected in a manner that will put the child or adolescent at ease. Sensitive questions may come up during the history, and these must be handled in a respectful and professional manner.[6] Often the parent will have to give part or the entire history. However, if the patient is old enough to speak, it is important to include her in the history by making eye contact with the patient and asking her questions directly; the guardian may have to assist. Additionally, the patient should always be given the opportunity to talk to the provider in private.

Heavy menstrual bleeding

Patients presenting with HMB should always be asked about their menstrual cycle in detail (see Table 14-1). When collecting or tracking this history, it can be useful to use a calendar. Many teenagers have smartphones with applications that can also help to track the menstrual cycle. Review of systems should include questions regarding easy bruising, frequent nosebleeds, prolonged healing of small wounds, bleeding complications with larger wounds/surgeries, and unexplained blood in the stool.[14] A personal or family history of anemia requiring a blood transfusion is also suggestive of a bleeding disorder. It is imperative to know about any previous medical history or medications that may contribute to heavy bleeding such as aspirin or anticoagulants. If anovulation is being considered on the differential, then androgenizing symptoms should be asked about to rule out PCOS such as acne, hirsutism, and alopecia.

Vulvovaginitis

Collecting a history from a prepubertal patient about vulvovaginitis takes great patience and collaboration with the parent or guardian. It's often helpful to start with a review of systems that are seemingly unrelated to the vaginal area, such as history of allergies, eczema, or dermatitis, type of soap and detergent used at home, physical activities that could exacerbate the symptoms (horseback riding and swimming), recent infections, and medications.[4] Questions specific to the vulvovaginal symptoms are reviewed in Table 14-2. It is also important to discuss bowel habits, assess hygiene, and rule out foreign body. Finally, sexual assault/abuse should be addressed with the guardian and the patient in private, if the patient is old enough to communicate. Abuse should be considered in patients with changes in behavior such as nightmares, new onset enuresis, or unexplained abdominal pain.[6]

Delayed puberty

An extensive history will provide the physician with valuable information to help differentiate between constitutional delay and pathologic delay of puberty. First and foremost, a detailed history of timing and order of development of secondary sex characteristics should be obtained. This includes growth velocity plotted over time. Next, personal medical history should be discussed, including chronic disease, neurologic symptoms, ability to smell, weight changes, disordered eating, sexual activity, emotional stress, acne, and hirsutism. The discussion also includes surgical history as well as any history of chemotherapy or radiation therapy. This personal medical history can be obtained in conjunction with a review of systems in order to cover all pertinent points. Next, a neonatal history should be performed. This should include information regarding maternal medication use during pregnancy, any pregnancy complications, and history of other pregnancy outcomes. Family history is also very important, as constitutional delay can be familial.[15] Additionally, parental height is important in determining height potential in the child undergoing evaluation.

Precocious puberty

The history-taking portion of the workup is critical, as it can help the clinician determine whether GIPP or GDPP is more likely. It is important to obtain information regarding the sequence and timing of pubertal development. If the sequence and timing mirrors that of normal puberty, but at a younger age, this is suggestive of GDPP. Alternatively, if the pubertal progression deviates from the normal sequence and timing, then a peripheral source of gonadal hormones (GIPP) is more likely to be the issue.[16]

Accurate information regarding how quickly puberty is progressing is also very important. This is a reflection of how long the patient has been exposed to sex hormones. Aspects of family and medical history that should be addressed are similar to those described for the evaluation of delayed puberty. In addition, possible exposure to exogenous hormones should be investigated.

Physical exam of the pediatric/adolescent patient

The exam should begin with a full explanation of what will be done. It is important to have a chaperone in the room with the provider in addition to anyone that will make the patient feel more comfortable, usually a parent or guardian. If the adolescent prefers that no one else be in the room, this request should be respected. The exam should always start with the least invasive portions such as neck or back. A gynecologic exam can be embarrassing and uncomfortable for patients. For younger pediatric patients it can helpful to have them sit with their guardian in a frog leg position, the patient resting on the lap of the guardian with feet together and knees bent and spread laterally. An exam of the outside genitalia should be done first without touching the patient at all. When it is necessary to examine the hymen, urethra, or vaginal introitis, the labia majora can be lightly grasped and pulled distally instead of laterally.

Heavy menstrual bleeding

For HMB the exam is fairly focused. Height, weight, and blood pressure are important because they may help guide the treatment options (discussed later in the chapter). Palpation of the thyroid should be done, and a close exam of skin should be done to look for excessive bruising or poor wound healing. This is also an opportunity to evaluate Tanner staging and do a genital exam in patients that are sexually active; however, neither of these things are necessary for HMB evaluation. Again, if PCOS is considered in the differential, signs of androgen access such as hirsutism, acne, and alopecia should be noted.

Vulvovaginitis

An exam should start with a general evaluation of the skin looking for any evidence of dermatitis. The anogenital region needs to be examined more thoroughly. The patient should be placed in either frog-leg or knees-to-chest position described earlier. First examine the mons, labia majora, clitoral hood, and inguinal region evaluating for discoloration, edema, and general hygiene. The rectum and perineum should also be well visualized, focusing on hygiene and presence of abnormal lesions such as ulcers or fissures. With gentle traction the urethra, clitoris, labia minora, and vaginal introitus can be examined. Effort should be made to assure the hymen is intact and there are no distal vaginal lacerations. It is usually not necessary to do an invasive speculum exam in this patient population. If there is suspicion for a foreign body or a lesion originating from the proximal vagina, an exam under anesthesia with vaginoscopy should be considered.

Delayed puberty

Critical components of the examination for delayed puberty include height and weight, neurologic assessment, assessment of skin and skeletal structure for any congenital anomalies, and Tanner staging to assess sexual maturity (see Figure 14-1). The axilla, breasts, and genitals should be examined last. The genitals should be evaluated for vaginal patency as well as estrogen effect. Usually an external genital exam will suffice.

Precocious puberty

In addition to the standard thorough examination, there are a few key components to focus on when evaluating for precocious puberty. Height velocity should be determined, as this can offer insight into whether the source of hormone exposure is peripheral versus central. The skin should be thoroughly inspected for café-au-lait spots, which are seen in McCune-Albright syndrome. Additionally, all noted secondary sex characteristics should be classified as

Breast Development

1. Elevation of the papilla only. Prepubertal
2. Elevation of breast and papilla as a small mound (breast budding)
3. Enlargement of breast and areola with no separation of contours
4. Further enlargement with projection of areola and papilla to form secondary mound above the level of the breast
5. Projection of the papilla only with recession of the areola to the general contour of the breast.

Pubic Hair Development

1. No pubic hair. Prepubertal
2. Sparse growth of long, straight, slightly pigmented hair along the labia
3. Course, dark, curlier hair extending to the mons
4. Adult hair spreading over the mons but not to the medial surface of the thighs
5. Adult hair spreading to the medial thighs; distributed in an inverse triangle

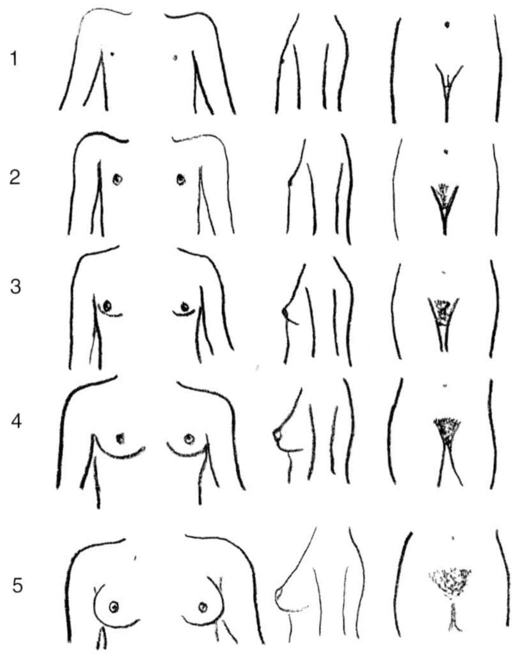

Figure 14-1 Tanner staging in females.

virilizing or feminizing, as this can help narrow down possible sources of sex hormones.[17] Pubertal staging should be performed on every individual, regardless of timing of puberty (see Figure 14-1).

Laboratory analysis

Many issues in PAG do not require any laboratory assessment, for example labial adhesions and dysmenorrhea. Laboratory analysis is guided by the presenting symptom, with the exception of a urine pregnancy test that can be done routinely in any postpubertal female.

Heavy menstrual bleeding

There are a very specific set of labs that should be done for adolescents presenting with HMB since menarche: complete blood count, thyroid-stimulating hormone, INR, PT, PTT, and a Von Willebrand panel which includes Factor 8, Ristocetin cofactor activity, and Von Willebrand factor antigen. If blood products are necessary, it is imperative to draw these labs before transfusion is started. The American College of Obstetricians and Gynecologists (ACOG) supports testing adolescents with HMB since menarche for Von Willebrand disease. This is because of the prevalence as well as positive impact of early diagnosis.[18] HMB in adolescents can be due to bleedings disorders other than Von Willebrand disease such as platelet dysfunction and factor deficiencies. If there is a high index of suspicion referral to a hematologist should be made for additional testing.[14]

Vulvovaginitis

Prepubescent patients that present with nonspecific vulvovaginal symptoms and have an exam that is consistent with poor hygiene do not need any labs. Counseling on proper hygiene is usually sufficient.[5] If the symptoms are severe or persistent, it is useful to do a bacterial swab. There is limited data on how to best attain a sample in this population. A small saline moistened swab can be inserted directly into the vagina if the patient tolerates it. Alternatively, sterile water can be introduced via a feeding tube or small catheter, with valsalva the water will come out and the sample can be taken from there. The sample can be sent for culture, gram stain, or used to perform a wet mount. If abuse is suspected, *N. gonorrhea* and *Chlamydia trachamotis* must be considered. Cultures can be sent and the cervical probe for nucleic acid amplification tests can be used vaginally. In cases of suspected abuse a specialist in assault should be involved as there are often specific protocols for how cultures and tests need to be collected and performed. Pediatric patients may have vulvovaginal infections from a wider variety of organisms than adult patients; organisms such a *Beta Streptococcus* and *Shigella* are known pathogens for pediatric vulvovaginitis. It is frequently necessary to notify the laboratory that testing for respiratory and enteric pathogens is also required in addition to the usual vaginal pathogens.

Delayed puberty

Several laboratory tests may aid in the evaluation of delayed puberty. Some, all, or none of these may be necessary based on the history and physical exam findings. Labs that could provide additional information include a CBC, BUN, creatinine, glucose, electrolytes, and liver function tests. Labs more specifically related to delayed puberty are follicle-stimulating hormone (FSH), luteinizing hormone (LH), estradiol, prolactin, thyroid-stimulating hormone (TSH) and free T4. An x-ray of the hand and wrist for bone age can also provide very valuable information and often dictates the next step in the workup. If diagnosis is made a chromosome analysis and florescent in situ hybridization (FISH) for sex androgen determining region Y (SRY) should be performed, at which point a pediatric endocrinologist or gynecologist should be involved.

Since delayed puberty can be attributed to a variety of causes, imaging of the pelvis may be important to rule out any anatomic abnormalities of the vagina, cervix, or uterus. If these structures are intact, then uterine size and ovarian volume should be evaluated. These values provide information regarding whether or not these structures have undergone estrogen stimulation.

Precocious puberty

When precocious puberty is suspected, based on history and examination findings, the initial laboratory workup is similar to that listed earlier including FSH, LH, estradiol, TSH, and prolactin. Androgens (testosterone, androstenedione, DHEAS, and 17 OHP) should be measured if the patient has isosexual development.

If LH levels are markedly elevated at baseline, then GDPP can be diagnosed without additional testing. If not, a gonadotropin-releasing hormone (GnRH) stimulation test will clarify a diagnosis. When needed, a GnRH stimulation test can distinguish patients with GDPP, GIPP, and normal pubertal variants. Levels of LH are measured at baseline and then after GnRH administration.[19]

Based on the results of the stimulation test, additional laboratory or radiologic evaluation may be indicated. If a diagnosis of GDPP is made, imaging of the brain will be necessary to rule out a central nervous system (CNS) lesion. Serum testosterone and estradiol levels will be helpful to establish the degree of pubertal advancement and can also be followed if therapy is initiated.

Abdominal and pelvic ultrasound should be obtained to identify any ovarian mass and if there is evidence of post-pubertal uterine and ovarian development.[9] A radiographic bone age should be determined, as this will help to guide therapy.

Treatment

Heavy menstrual bleeding

In the outpatient clinical setting there are multiple very effective options to control bleeding. Hormonal therapy has long been used and proven effective time and time again.[20] For the patient that is actively bleeding and has been bleeding excessively an oral contraceptive pill (OCP) taper is a good place to start. Most tapers are based on anecdotal experience or reports from experts. One commonly used taper is any 35 mcg combination OCP three times a day for a week, twice a day for a week, then one pill daily. The addition of an anti-emetic is often helpful if dosing more than one pill a day. Contraceptive rings and patches can be used with similar efficacy to oral pills for maintenance. For patients who have undesired side effects from combination contraception or a contraindication to estrogen, several progesterone only options exist. The most commonly used progesterone methods for adolescents with HMB are depo medroxyprogesterone acetate and levonorgestrel intrauterine devices. In patients with severe bleeding disorders, 104 mg of depo medroxyprogesterone acetate can be given subcutaneously to avoid risk of hematoma; side effects are similar to that of intramuscular administration.[21] The levonorgestrel intrauterine device has proven to be very effective in controlling HMB in the adolescents, particularly those that have failed other medical management.[22]

Antifibrinolytics have recently become more commonly used for patients with heavy bleeding. Aminocaproic acid and tranexamic acid are the two that are available in the United States, both in IV and PO form. They are typically taken multiple times a day for three to seven days during active bleeding. It can be used in conjunction with or independent of hormonal methods.[23]

Vulvovaginitis

The treatment for vulvovaginitis is entirely dependent on the etiology. Nonspecific vulvovaginitis can be addressed with hygiene counseling such as using scent free, dye free soaps and detergents, wearing white cotton underwear, voiding with legs wide open, and wiping from front to back. In the initial period sitz baths followed by a barrier cream or low dose steroid such as A+D ointment, or hydrocortisone ointment can be recommended to keep the area clean and dry. Hand washing and loose-fitting clothing should also be encouraged.[4, 6]

In the case of a positive culture, antibiotics should only be used if the cultured organism is not normal flora of the vagina. The most common pathogenic agents to cause vulvovaginitis are *S. pyogenes*, *H. influenza*, and *E. vermicularis*; these should be treated with PO penicillin, amoxicillin, and mebendazole, respectively.[4] *Candida albicans* and *C. glabrata* are also causative agents of infectious vulvovaginitis. The first-line treatment is a topical antifungal for *C. albicans*, whereas *C. glabrata* often necessitates a long course of 1% boric acid cream. Rarely, abnormal vulvar or vaginal discharge and itching can be due to condylomata acuminate or genital herpes. Genitals warts can be treated with either liquid nitrogen or carbon-dioxide laser therapy; however, if they are asymptomatic they can be followed up for 60 days as they may spontaneously resolve.[4] Genital herpes is treated with acyclovir or an equivalent. Although neither genital warts nor herpes is diagnostic of sexual abuse, possible abuse should certainly be investigated in a pediatric patient presenting with either finding.

Labial adhesions and lichen sclerosis are not infections, but the hypoestrogenic state of prepubescent females puts them at risk for both conditions. Labial adhesions may, however, increase the risk of vulvovaginal infections that may manifest as irritation, discharge, or itching. The first-line treatment for labial adhesions is estrogen cream, however recent studies have shown that betamethasone cream is equally effective.[24] The labial adhesions should *not* be separated forcefully in the office. Manual separation is required only if urinary outflow is disrupted and when rarely needed should be performed in a setting with anesthesia.

Lichen sclerosis often presents as itching in the vulvar area; the exam is usually consistent with hypopigmented vulvar skin and loss of architecture. This condition has been diagnosed in the prepubertal population more frequently than previously. Treatment is a topical high dose steroid such as clobetasol twice daily.[25]

Finally if trauma or foreign body is suspected as a cause of a vulvovaginal complaint, surgical intervention may be required. An exam under anesthesia with a vaginoscopy can be both diagnostic and therapeutic. If a foreign body is identified it can be removed and the vagina well cleaned. Vaginoscopy is performed in the operating room with use of a small diameter cystoscope. The pressure from the distending medium (usually sterile water) and clasping the labia together will allow the vaginal mucosa to distend for a survey of the cavity.[6]

Delayed puberty

If the evaluation is negative for a disease process, patients with delayed puberty may not require any treatment. It is known that the most common etiology of delayed puberty is constitutional, so it is expected that these patients will enter puberty and achieve full sexual maturation as well as predicted height without any intervention. However, when treatment is required, it is aimed at the cause of the problem, if known. For many patients with chronic disease, optimization of that condition can often lead to initiation of puberty. For patients with estrogen deficiency, regardless of the root cause, estrogen replacement, with eventual cyclic progesterone, will be necessary to achieve breast growth, uterine growth (and eventually menses), adult height, and bone protection. Calcium and vitamin D supplementation is imperative.[26]

In patients with significantly compromised height, growth hormone may also be indicated. These patients should be managed in conjunction with an endocrinologist to ensure they are receiving an appropriate dose of growth hormone as well as to monitor any side effects.

Precocious puberty

The treatment of GIPP depends on the underlying cause. It is important to identify a cause and treat it promptly, as GIPP can lead to GDPP if left untreated. There are not, however, sufficient data to support treatment of precocious puberty for the sole purpose of minimizing the potential psychosocial side effects of early menses and pubertal development.[19]

When GDPP is diagnosed, there may be a CNS lesion that can be treated. When this is not the case, the primary treatment is a GnRH agonist. The goal of this therapy is not to stop progression of secondary sex characteristics, but rather to optimize the patients' adult height potential. Considerations for treatment include age, rate of maturation, and height potential. Several formulations of GnRH agonists exist, and options can be tailored to individual patient needs.

Screening

A PAG clinic presents the opportunity to screen for multiple medical and psychosocial comorbidities. If patients are old enough to talk they should be screened for abuse and assault. All adolescents are screened in private regarding sexual intercourse, drugs, and alcohol use. This serves as an opportunity to intervene early with proper testing and contraception. The menstrual cycle is now considered a portion of the vital signs; it is a good screening tool for disorders discussed earlier such as bleeding disorders and abnormal pubertal development.

Prevention

Interactions with pediatric and adolescent patients in gynecology clinics can serve as preventative visits. From a public health stand point, screening for, counseling, and treating sexually transmitted infections in the adolescent population is of the utmost importance. The United States of America has the highest teen birth rate among developed nations. Since 2010 there has been a national Teen Pregnancy Prevention Initiative aimed at decreasing teen pregnancy. Educating adolescents in gynecology clinic about effective contraception is an important part of this initiative. Gynecologists and other adolescent care providers who provide contraception to adolescents should be comfortable recommending and placing long-acting reversible contraception (IUD's and implants are discussed in Chapter 2) in this age group.[27]

The early diagnosis of the conditions described previously is important to prevent severe complications. For example, bleeding disorders that are found around the time of menarche can prevent complications with surgical and obstetric interventions in the future.[14] Additionally, proper diagnosis and treatment can prevent or decrease missed school and work. Early recognition of abnormal pubertal development can increase efficacy of treatment options and prevent long-term sequelae such as short stature.

Concluding remarks

Pediatric and adolescent gynecology is a vast and expanding field. Because children and adolescents have a number of gynecologic complaints, gynecologists and all women's health providers should be comfortable providing children and adolescents care. Some common problems dealt with in the population are relatively simple to address when armed with the proper information. Excellent PAG care serves as an opportunity to establish a relationship with patients who are often neglected and at high risk.

References

1. Lara-Torre E. The physical exam in the pediatric and adolescent patient. In: Sanfilippo JS, editor. *Clinical Pediatric and Adolescent Gynecology*. New York: Informa Healthcare; 2009, pp. 140–51.
2. Hillard PJ. What's clinically relevant and new in pediatric and adolescent gynecology? *Current opinion in obstetrics & gynecology*. 2012 Oct;**24**(5):273–4. PubMed PMID: 22954762.
3. Frishman GN. Evaluation and treatment of menorrhagia in an adolescent population. *Journal of minimally invasive gynecology*. 2008 Nov–Dec;**15**(6): 682–8. PubMed PMID: 18971130.
4. Dei M, Di Maggio F, Di Paolo G, Bruni V. Vulvovaginitis in childhood: best practice & research. *Clinical obstetrics & gynaecology*. 2010 Apr;**24**(2):129–37. PubMed PMID: 19884044.
5. Yilmaz AE, Celik N, Soylu G, et al. Comparison of clinical and microbiological features of vulvovaginitis in prepubertal and pubertal girls. *Journal of the Formosan Medical Association = Taiwan yi zhi*. 2012 Jul;**111**(7): 392–6. PubMed PMID: 22817817.
6. Emans SJ. Vulvovaginal problems in the prepubertal child. In: Emans SJ, Laufer MR, Goldstein DP, editors. *Pediatric and Adolescent Gynecology*. Fifth ed.

Philadelphia: Lippincott Williams & Wilkins; 2005, pp. 83–119.

7. Rosenfield RL. Clinical review 6: diagnosis and management of delayed puberty. *Journal of clinical endocrinology and metabolism*. 1990 Mar;**70**(3):559–62. PubMed PMID: 2407749. Epub 1990/03/01. eng.
8. Sedlmeyer IL, Palmert MR. Delayed puberty: analysis of a large case series from an academic center. *Journal of clinical endocrinology and metabolism*. 2002 Apr;**87** (4):1613–20. PubMed PMID: 11932291. Epub 2002/04/05. eng.
9. Emans SJ. Precocious puberty. In: Emans SJ, Laufer MR, Goldstein DP, editors. *Pediatric and Adolescent Gynecology*. Fifth ed. Philadelphia, PA: Lippincott Williams & Wilkin; 2005, pp. 156–80.
10. Connor EL. Adolescent polycystic ovary syndrome. *Adolescent medicine: state of the art reviews*. 2012 Apr;**23**(1):164–77, xii. PubMed PMID: 22764561.
11. Grimbizis GF, Campo R, on behalf of the Scientific Committee of the Congenital Uterine Malformations common Eshre/Esge working group: Stephan Gordts SBMGVTTCLCDA. Clinical approach for the classification of congenital uterine malformations. *Gynecological surgery*. 2012 May;**9**(2):119–29. PubMed PMID: 22611348. Pubmed Central PMCID: 3338910.
12. Institute G. *An Overview of Minors' Consent Law*. New York: State Policies in Brief; 2013.
13. Sowinska-Przepiera E, Jarzabek-Bielecka G, Andrysiak-Mamos E, et al. [Legal aspects in pediatric and adolescent gynecology]. *Ginekologia polska*. 2013 Feb;**84**(2):131–6. PubMed PMID: 23668060.
14. Ahuja SP, Hertweck SP. Overview of bleeding disorders in adolescent females with menorrhagia. *Journal of pediatric and adolescent gynecology*. 2010 Dec;**23**(6 Suppl):S15–21. PubMed PMID: 20934893.
15. Sedlmeyer IL, Hirschhorn JN, Palmert MR. Pedigree analysis of constitutional delay of growth and maturation: determination of familial aggregation and inheritance patterns. *Journal of clinical endocrinology and metabolism*. 2002 Dec;**87**(12):5581–6. PubMed PMID: 12466356. Epub 2002/12/06. eng.
16. Hill NC, Oppenheimer LW, Morton KE. The aetiology of vaginal bleeding in children. A 20-year review. *British journal of obstetrics and gynaecology*. 1989 Apr;**96**(4):467–70. PubMed PMID: 2751960.
17. Tavassoli FA, Norris HJ. Sertoli tumors of the ovary. A clinicopathologic study of 28 cases with ultrastructural observations. *Cancer*. 1980 Nov 15;**46** (10):2281–97. PubMed PMID: 7427869.
18. Committee on Practice B-G. Practice bulletin no. 128: diagnosis of abnormal uterine bleeding in reproductive-aged women. *Obstetrics and gynecology*. 2012 Jul;**120**(1):197–206. PubMed PMID: 22914421.
19. Carel JC, Eugster EA, Rogol A, et al. Consensus statement on the use of gonadotropin-releasing hormone analogs in children. *Pediatrics*. 2009 Apr;**123**(4):e752–62. PubMed PMID: 19332438.
20. Wilkinson JP, Kadir RA. Management of abnormal uterine bleeding in adolescents. *Journal of pediatric and adolescent gynecology*. 2010 Dec;**23**(6 Suppl):S22–30. PubMed PMID: 20869283.
21. Guilbert ER, Kaunitz AM. Depo-Provera and skeletal health: reviewing the evidence; developing and disseminating a consensus. *Contraception*. 2009 Mar;**79**(3):165–6. PubMed PMID: 19185667.
22. Chi C, Pollard D, Tuddenham EG, Kadir RA. Menorrhagia in adolescents with inherited bleeding disorders. *Journal of pediatric and adolescent gynecology*. 2010 Aug;**23**(4):215–22. PubMed PMID: 20471874.
23. Lukes AS, Moore KA, Muse KN, et al. Tranexamic acid treatment for heavy menstrual bleeding: a randomized controlled trial. *Obstetrics and gynecology*. 2010 Oct;**116**(4):865–75. PubMed PMID: 20859150.
24. Myers JB, Sorensen CM, Wisner BP, et al. Betamethasone cream for the treatment of pre-pubertal labial adhesions. *Journal of pediatric and adolescent gynecology*. 2006 Dec;**19**(6):407–11. PubMed PMID: 17174831.
25. Powell J, Wojnarowska F. Childhood vulvar lichen sclerosus: an increasingly common problem. *Journal of the American Academy of Dermatology*. 2001 May;**44**(5):803–6. PubMed PMID: 11312428.
26. Emans SJ. Delayed puberty. In: Emans SJ, Laufer MR, Goldstein DP, editors. *Pediatric and Adolescent Gynecology*. Fifth ed. Philadelphia: Lippincott; 2005, pp. 181–213.
27. Committee on Adolescent Health Care Long-Acting Reversible Contraception Working Group TACoO, Gynecologists. Committee opinion no. 539: adolescents and long-acting reversible contraception: implants and intrauterine devices. *Obstetrics and gynecology*. 2012 Oct;**120**(4):983–8.

Chapter 15

Amenorrhea

Melanie Altizer and Patrice M. Weiss

Introduction

Amenorrhea is the absence of menstruation. It can be the result of transient, intermittent, or permanent conditions. Further classification divides amenorrhea into two distinct subsets, primary and secondary amenorrhea. Primary amenorrhea is used to describe the absence of menses by age fifteen in the presence of secondary sexual characteristics. It can also be used to describe those patients who exhibit the absence of both menses and secondary sexual characteristics by age 12–13.[1] Secondary amenorrhea refers to the cessation of menses for more than three cycles or six months in women who have undergone menarche. The goal of treatment in primary amenorrhea is restoration of normal growth and development. In secondary amenorrhea, the goal may be focused on restoring fertility.

Approximately 3%–4% of reproductive aged women, not including those who are pregnant or breastfeeding, are diagnosed with amenorrhea. Of the cases of primary amenorrhea, 40% are the result of endocrine factors and the remaining 60% are attributed to abnormalities of development.[2] The most common cause of secondary amenorrhea is pregnancy.

For the purpose of diagnosing and treating amenorrhea, attempting to distinguish between the historical definition of primary and secondary amenorrhea may be misleading. Practically, the workup of amenorrhea should be approached by level of menstrual cycle control. The basic levels of control are the hypothalamic-pituitary axis, ovary, uterus, and vagina. Workup of the patient with primary amenorrhea includes all the causes linked to secondary amenorrhea; diagnoses lined mainly with primary amenorrhea are listed in Table 15-1.

Table 15-1 Conditions associated exclusively with primary amenorrhea

Gonadal dysgenesis
Swyer syndrome
46, XY gonadal dysgenesis
46, XX gonadal dysgenesis.
Turner's syndrome
Müllerian agenesis
Imperforate hymen
Transverse vaginal septum
Cervical atresisa
Androgen insensitivity syndrome

Normal menstrual cycle

In order to completely understand amenorrhea along with its causes and treatments, knowledge of the normal menstrual cycle is essential. There are many levels of control of the menstrual cycle and a problem at any level can lead to amenorrhea. The cascade of regulation of menstrual function begins with environmental stimuli that act on the central nervous system (CNS). In turn, the hypothalamus secretes gonadotropin-releasing hormone (GnRH) in a pulsatile manner. The GnRH released by the hypothalamus then exerts an effect on the anterior pituitary to cause release of follicle-stimulating hormone (FSH) and luteinizing hormone (LH). FSH and LH exert end organ effect on ovarian follicular development and regulation of estrogen and progesterone production. The uterine lining changes in response to ovarian estrogen and progesterone production. This ultimately results in menses.

Causes of amenorrhea

Hypothalamic

Dysfunction of the hypothalamus is a common cause of secondary amenorrhea but can also cause primary amenorrhea. Menstrual abnormalities resulting from hypothalamic causes can be mild leading to luteal phase dysfunction, moderate resulting in

Office Care of Women, ed. Martin E. Olsen and Botros Rizk. Published by Cambridge University Press.

disorders of follicle development and anovulation or severe resulting in hypothalamic amenorrhea. Hypothalamic amenorrhea is commonly associated with excessive physical activity, nutritional disturbances, or emotional and mental stressors.

Other causes of hypothalamic dysfunction leading to abnormalities of the menstrual cycle include eating disorders such as anorexia and bulimia, excessive exercise, congenital GnRH deficiency (Kallmann's syndrome), and rarely, mutations in the GnRH receptor.

Hypothalmic amenorrhea is a diagnosis made by the exclusion of other causes of hypogonadotrophic-hypogonadaism (diminished function of gonads due to suboptimal secretion of the gonadotropins FSH and LH). Hypothalamic amenorrhea is characterized by low to normal serum FSH levels in the setting of low estrogen levels. These findings occur in the absence of any pituitary causes. Most women with hypothalamic amenorrhea have abnormal patterns of GnRH secretion that cause abnormalities in pituitary gonadotropin release and subsequent menstrual disturbances.[2]

Treatment of amenorrhea associated with hypothalamic dysfunction is often multifactorial and dependent upon the cause. Those who suffer from an eating disorder frequently require intense multidisciplinary treatment with a dietician, physician, and mental health-care provider in order to address issues with nutrition, electrolyte abnormalities, osteoporosis, and intensive cognitive behavioral therapy.[3] Oral contraceptives are seldom useful in the treatment of patients with amenorrhea resulting from an eating disorder. Physiologic hormone supplementation or oral contraceptives are an option for those with exercise-induced amenorrhea and can play a role in preserving bone health and the prevention of osteoporosis. Ovulation induction may ultimately be required to help these patients achieve pregnancy.[4] All patients with hypothalamic amenorrhea should be on calcium supplementation for bone health. Finally, patients with congenital GnRH deficiency can be treated with exogenous gonadotropins.

Pituitary

Many conditions of the anterior pituitary can result in amenorrhea. Tumors are the most common pituitary cause and of these, benign pituitary adenomas account for approximately 90% of all pituitary tumors. There are multiple different types of benign pituitary adenomas, each named for their cell type. The most common of these is prolactinoma. Among the other less common types of adenomas are thyrotroph, somatotroph, corticotroph, and gonadotroph. Malignant tumors of the pituitary are rare. Other non-hormone-secreting tumors that can affect the anterior pituitary and subsequently lead to amenorrhea include meningiomas, craniopharyngiomas, gliomas, chordomas, and metastatic tumors. In addition to neoplasms, other systemic and localized entities can cause pituitary dysfunction. These include, tuberculosis, sarcoidosis, cyts, and fatty deposits. These can all lead to compressive damage of the pituitary. Finally, infiltration of the pituitary by lymphocytes, (hemochromatosis), radiation, surgical damage, or infarction (Sheehan's syndrome) can compromise pituitary function.[2]

Diagnosis of pituitary abnormalities is typically made with a combination of lab work and imaging studies such as MRI. For the purpose of this chapter, the discussion of diagnosis and treatment will focus primarily on prolactinoma. Patients with prolactin-secreting adenoma can present with a variety of complaints including headache, amenorrhea, visual changes, and galactorrhea.[5] Functional adenomas cause elevated prolactin levels. Patients with significantly elevated prolactin levels, greater than 100 ng/mL, should undergo an MRI to assess for macro or microadenoma.[6] It should be noted that modest elevations in prolactin levels also occur as the result of stress, nipple stimulation, sex, and sleep. MRI should also be obtained in patients who are amenorrheic with normal prolactin levels if they have headaches, visual disturbances, or any other CNS symptoms suggestive of mass lesion.

Prolactin causes amenorrhea by suppressing GnRH secretion. Negative feedback from hypothalamic dopamine controls prolactin release. Therefore, first line medical treatment of amenorrhea caused by prolactin-secreting adenoma is often by administration of a dopamine agonist.[8] The two most commonly used are bromocriptine and cabergoline. Nonfunctional adenomas can result in amenorrhea by mass effect and compression on the pituitary stalk. In these patients, transphenoidal resection is the treatment of choice. Resection is also used in functional adenomas that failure conservative medical therapy. Radiation therapy can be used in cases that are refractory to medical and surgical therapy.

Ovarian disorders

Among the most common causes of amenorrhea are disorders of the ovary. They are responsible for many cases of both primary and secondary amenorrhea. Ovarian dysfunction can have many causes including polycystic ovary syndrome (PCOS), obesity, thyroid disease, chronic anovulation, and prolactin-driven processes. In addition, disorders that result in ovarian failure also cause amenorrhea and will be the primary focus of the discussion of ovarian disorders presented in this chapter.

Ovarian failure results when scant or no follicles are present that can produce estradiol in response to pituitary stimulation with gonadotropins. The occurrence of amenorrhea will be determined by the time in one's life when ovarian follicles are depleted. This can occur at any point in an individual's life, from embryonic development to menopause.

Gonadal dysgenesis

Gonadal dysgenesis is one of the most common causes of primary amenorrhea, accounting for approximately 30%–40% of cases.[2] It is characterized by incomplete or defective gonad formation. The cause can either arise from problems with the structure or number of chromosomes. The most common cause of gonadal dysgenesis is Turner's syndrome.

Turner's syndrome

Turner's syndrome is usually the result of a 45, XO karyotype.[7] Other causes may include structural problems with the X chromosome. Turner's syndrome may also be expressed through varying degrees when only some of the body's cells are affected. This is known as mosaicism.[8] The typical Turner's syndrome phenotype is that of short stature, webbed neck, absence of sexual development, low set ears, widely spaced nipples, short fourth metacarpels, posterior hairline, and increased carrying angle at the elbow. In addition to their specific phenotypical appearance, patients with Turner's syndrome present clinically with primary amenorrhea and absent secondary sex characteristics. They also exhibit poor growth during childhood. Once the diagnosis of Turner's syndrome is made, the patient should be routinely monitored for the development of cardiac conditions, thyroid abnormalities, renal abnormalities, and other disorders including celiac disease and diabetes.[2]

Other forms of gonadal dysgenesis exist and include Swyer syndrome 46, XY and 46, XX gonadal dysgenesis.

Premature ovarian failure

Premature ovarian failure usually refers to amenorrhea that occurs before the age of 40. It has many causes and the patients exhibit a variety of phenotypes. These patients usually experience a hypergonadotrophic-hypogonadal state. Typically, premature ovarian failure occurs after onset of menarche but it can also occur before menarche as well. Patients with ovarian failure may have episodes of intermittent ovarian function.[9] Ovarian failure can have multiple causes including chromosomal abnormalities, fragile X mutations, radiation therapy, chemotherapy, autoimmune disorders, and galactosemia. Premature ovarian failure results from accelerated follicular atresia or disorders in follicular development. In most patients, a single cause is never identified.[10]

The diagnosis of premature ovarian failure can be made by demonstration of a low estradiol level in the setting of consistently elevated FSH levels.

Treatment of ovarian failure should include appropriate psychological and emotional support in addition to management of any associated autoimmune disease, hormone therapy, and fertility issues. Patients affected by premature ovarian failure are at significant risk for depression and often describe feeling a sense of loss. Counseling and support groups should be offered.[11, 12] Hormone replacement with estrogen and progestin or oral contraceptive pills (OCPs) is important to promote bone health and prevent vasomotor symptoms in addition to vaginal atrophy and should continue until approximately age 50, when most women begin to experience a decline in ovarian function.[10, 13] Calcium and vitamin supplementation are also important for bone health.[14] Those patients interested in fertility can explore the option of in vitro fertilization (IVF) with donor oocytes.

Uterine and genital outflow tract disorders

Disorders of the genital outflow track are the result of failure of vertical fusion or failure of müllerian duct development during embryonic development. They most often present during the time of puberty with primary amenorrhea. There is a group of outflow tract disorders where the patients usually present with secondary amenorrhea as the result of damage to the cervix or endometrium with subsequent scar tissue formation from trauma or infection. These patients usually have developmentally normal genital tract structures.

Imperforate hymen

Imperforate hymen is a congenital condition that causes obstruction of the vaginal opening. It occurs when there is failure of the hymen to perforate during development in utero. This happens when the sinovaginal bulbs fail to canalize along with the rest of the vagina.[2] Patients usually present during adolescence with complaints of primary amenorrhea and cyclic pelvic and abdominal pain sometimes with accompanying urinary complaints secondary to accumulation of obstructed menstrual flow. On physical exam, these patients exhibit normal secondary sexual development. The vagina may be distended, and there is no obvious vaginal opening. Instead, a blue, bulging perineal membrane, caused by hematocolpos, is usually noted.

Treatment consists of surgical resection of the hymen to relieve the obstruction and allow for the menstrual fluid to drain. This should be done as soon as possible after diagnosis to decrease the chance of infertility related to reproductive tract scar tissue formation from inflammation caused by accumulated menstrual fluid. Surgical treatment is accomplished by making a cruciate incision in the hymen and subsequent excision of the central portion of tissue. Topical estrogen cream is often applied for a brief period of time to promote adequate healing of the vaginal tissue.

Imperforate hymen most often occurs as a sporadic event but can rarely be found in multiple members of the same family.[2]

Transverse vaginal septum and cervical atresia

Transverse vaginal septum is caused by failure of the vaginal plate, formed by fusion of the sinovaginal bulbs, to canalize during embryonic development.[2] Patients with a transverse vaginal septum present much like those with an imperforate hymen. They most often have complaints of cyclic pelvic and abdominal pain by build-up of obstructed menstrual flow. Like those with an imperforate hymen, patients with a transverse vaginal septum exhibit normal secondary sex characteristics. Unlike those with imperforate hymen, these patients have a normal vaginal orifice along with a shortened vagina and absence of a visible cervix on physical exam. Physical exam is also remarkable for a palpable hematocolpos proximal to the level of the vaginal obstruction. Having the patient perform a valsalva maneuver can help differentiate between cases of imperforate hymen and transverse vaginal septum. An imperforate hymen will bulge during valsalva maneuver whereas a transverse vaginal septum will not.[2, 15]

Pelvic ultrasound is useful in determining the level and extent of obstruction of the collected menstrual fluid. An MRI, on the other hand, can give more detail of the patient's anatomy, which can be beneficial for purposes of surgical planning. As with imperforate hymen, prompt surgical correction should be undertaken to prevent infertility related to obstruction of menstrual fluid outflow. The surgical approach involves excising the septum and then joining the upper and lower margins of the vagina. This sometimes requires a tissue graft if the septum excised was extremely thick.

Cervical atresia has less obvious management options and controversy exists regarding the best treatment approach. Some experts favor hysterectomy whereas others favor a more conservative approach in an attempt to preserve fertility.[16] These patients are also at significant risk of developing endometriosis and adhesions.

Müllerian agenesis

Müllerian agenesis, also known as Mayer-Rokitansky-Kuster-Hauser syndrome, is a common cause of primary amenorrhea. It occurs with almost as much frequency as gonadal dysgenesis. The cause is most often unknown. Müllerian agenesis usually occurs sporadically but has also been associated with chromosomal abnormalities.[2]

The usual presentation is during puberty with primary amenorrhea. These patients have normal breast and pubic hair development, and there is no visible vagina on physical exam. Rudimentary uterine structures may be present to varying degrees with normal or atrophic fallopian tubes. A small percentage of these patients may have functional endometrial tissue and can suffer from painful hematometra.

Skeletal and urologic anomalies may also be present in cases of müllerian agenesis. Coexisting urologic anomalies can range from unilateral renal agenesis and horseshoe kidney to a duplication of the collecting system. Skeletal anomalies include hemivertebrae, scoliosis, and limited range of motion. The ovaries arise from different embryologic structures and are usually normal in patients diagnosed with müllerian agenesis. They can, however, also be hypoplastic.[2]

Diagnosis is primarily made by history and physical examination. Pelvic ultrasound can help determine the structure of any existing reproductive organs. MRI can provide for definitive information if needed.[17]

The goal of treatment is creating a functional vagina either with progressive dilation or surgical procedures such as the McIndoe or Vecchietti. These patients can have normal sexual function. In addition, they can have genetic offspring through IVF technologies.[18, 19]

Androgen insensitivity syndrome

Androgen insensitivity syndrome (AIS), commonly referred to as testicular feminization, is the third most common cause of primary amenorrhea. Patients with AIS have a normal 46, XY karyotype. Their testes produce both testosterone and anti-müllerian hormone. AIS is caused by a genetic abnormality in the androgen receptor gene that results in end organ resistance to the effects of androgen activity.[20] This resistance prevents the process of normal masculinization of both internal and external genital structures. These patients are born with normal external female genitalia due to absence of androgen action but have absent internal female genitalia due to the action of anti-müllerian hormone. As a consequence, the vagina is a short, blind pouch.

AIS patients have a normal physical exam at birth and typically exhibit normal growth and development in childhood. At puberty, they gain breast development secondary to the peripheral conversion of androgens to estrogen that acts on the breast tissue to stimulate development.[21] Given the lack of ovarian progesterone, the areolae and nipples are often small and pale and the breasts lack significant glandular development. Physical exam is also remarkable for absent pubic and axillary hair as a result of lack of androgen effects on peripheral end organs. The testicles may be partially descended and found in the inguinal cavity, or be completely contained within the abdomen.

Primary amenorrhea is the usual presenting complaint for patients with AIS. As previously discussed, they have breast development but absent pubic and axillary hair. They will also have an absent cervix and a small, blind ending vaginal canal. Serum testosterone levels will be in the normal male range and the high female range.

Treatment of patients with AIS has two major areas of focus.[2] The first is creation of a functioning vagina and the second is removal of gonadal tissue to prevent development of a neoplastic process. As with müllerian agenesis, creation of a functional vagina can either be accomplished through progressive dilation or surgical creation of a neo-vagina. Once puberty is complete, the gonads are surgically removed because there is a 2%–5% risk of developing testicular cancer after age 25.[22]

Cervical stenosis

Cervical stenosis can cause partial or complete obstruction of the cervical opening and most often results from operative procedures on the cervix to treat dysplasia. Patients usually present with complaints of progressively worsening dysmenorrhea and continued spotting after their period resulting from obstructed menstrual flow.[23] Diagnosis can be made clinically by attempted passage of a uterine sound or cervical Os finder™.[2] The treatment is surgical dilation of the stenotic cervical canal and subsequent drainage of any existing hematometra. For added protection against uterine perforation, some providers perform the dilation under ultrasound guidance.

Asherman syndrome

Asherman syndrome is a condition that results from the formation of intrauterine adhesions that can cause partial or total obstruction of the uterine cavity. This usually occurs following trauma to the uterus or infection.[24] Any condition that causes inflammation in the uterus, such as endometriosis, retained products of conception, or septic abortion, places a patient at risk for the development of Asherman syndrome.[10] It can also occur following cesarean section, hysteroscopy/dilation and curettage (D&C), and myomectomy.[25] It is a rare complication of uterine artery embolization.

Patient presentation usually includes dysmenorrhea, difficulty becoming pregnant, or recurrent miscarriage in the setting of recent history of uterine instrumentation or inflammation. Rarely, patients may present with complete amenorrhea.[25]

Diagnosis first begins with a suspicion based on patient history. Ultrasound can reveal any retained fluid within the uterus. Sonohysterogram or hysterosalpingogram can delineate the extent of the obstruction as well as the location. Hysteroscopy can establish a definitive diagnosis.

Treatment is accomplished through resection of uterine adhesions via operative hysteroscopy.

A balloon is often subsequently inserted into the uterus for a period of time to prevent immediate postoperative occlusion of the endometrial cavity. Some providers also utilize estrogen supplementation for three to four weeks post resection to promote healing of the endometrium.[26] Recurrence rates are high and many patients require retreatment.[27] The ultimate goal of treatment is to relieve any discomfort from the obstructed flow of menstrual fluid and restoration of fertility.

Evaluation

As with any other medical condition, the evaluation of a patient with amenorrhea must start with a detailed history and physical examination to determine specifically if the patient has primary or secondary amenorrhea. This forms the basis and foundation for the rest of the workup, diagnosis, and treatment. A systematic approach that separates the reproductive system into levels of control provides a useful foundation on which to begin. The function of each level must me assessed and a cause for any dysfunction identified and proper treatment initiated.

History

It is often helpful to begin with a detailed gynecologic history to include timing of onset of puberty and menarche. It's also important to determine the presence or absence of premenstrual symptoms as well as cyclic pelvic and abdominal pain. Cyclic pelvic pain in the setting of primary amenorrhea is suggestive of outflow tract obstruction such as that which occurs secondary to imperforate hymen or transverse vaginal septum. In patients presenting with cyclic pelvic pain and secondary amenorrhea, the possibility of Asherman syndrome or cervical stenosis should be considered in the setting of recent uterine instrumentation, trauma, or infection. Patients affected by PCOS often describe irregular and infrequent menstruation since the onset of menarche. In addition, they may complain of acne and hirsuitism secondary to androgen excess. Patients suffering from hypothalamic causes of amenorrhea often describe situations of extreme stress, both mental and physical or extreme exercise or state of malnutrition. Premature ovarian failure usually follows a course of gradual intermenstrual lengthening and progressively decreasing amounts of menstrual flow. It is also not uncommon for patients to complain of menopausal symptoms such as hot flashes and vaginal dryness. This process ultimately leads to amenorrhea. A history of any chronic illness is important as amenorrhea often results from a number of long standing medical conditions. Visual changes, seizures, and headaches may indicate a CNS lesion impacting hypothalamic or pituitary function. Congenital adrenal hyperplasia may present with worsening hirsuitism or extreme virilization. Elevated prolactin levels, resulting from prolactinoma, can cause galactorrhea and nipple discharge. In addition to personal medical history, family history is also important when seeing a patient for amenorrhea. Key elements of family history include cases of delayed puberty, infertility, and premature ovarian failure.

Physical

The physical exam should begin with measurement of the patient's height, weight, and body mass index. Palpation of the thyroid gland and assessment of Tanner staging are essential components of the physical exam.[28] Short statue is a characteristic of patients with gonadal dysgenesis. Low body weight can be associated with disorders involving the hypothalamus.[20] Breast development is an indicator of endogenous estrogen production and exposure as well as its effects on end organ tissue.[28] Milky discharge, or galactorrhea is suggestive of hyperprolactinemia. Patients with PCOS may be obese and suffer from acne or other skin changes such as acanthosis nigricans. Dry, coarse skin suggests hypothyroidism whereas soft moist skin suggests hyperthyroidism. Signs of virilization can be found in patients with congenital adrenal hyperplasia. Examination of the external and internal genital tract can reveal outflow tract obstructions or absent and malformed organs. Patients with ovarian failure may show evidence of atrophic vaginal tissue from diminished estrogen exposure. The presence of pubic hair development is an indicator of the effects of endogenous androgen exposure. Finally, a patent vaginal opening and normal cervix would rule out disorders such as transverse vaginal septum and imperforate hymen as well as AIS and müllerian agenesis.

Laboratory testing

The first step in laboratory evaluation of amenorrhea is a pregnancy test. Pregnancy is the most common cause of secondary amenorrhea. In the presence of a negative pregnancy test, the following initial lab tests should be obtained: thyroid-stimulating hormone (TSH), prolactin, FSH, and LH. If a patient has signs of androgen excess such as hirsuitism, dehydroepiandrosterone sulfate (DHEAS), testosterone, androstenedione, and 17-OH progesterone should be obtained. These tests can help differentiate the source of androgen excess between the adrenal gland and ovary. In the setting of chronic disease, CBC, liver enzymes, BUN, and creatinine should be obtained along with a urinalysis.

In certain instances, a karyotype may be necessary, especially in cases of suspected Turner's syndrome.

Imaging

Pelvic ultrasound can be used to confirm the presence or absence of the uterus and to evaluate the structure of the ovaries. A saline sonohysterogram or hysterosalpingogram may be useful in cases of suspected Asherman syndrome. MRI is often obtained to evaluate for potential pituitary or hypothalamic lesions.[29]

Concluding remarks

Amenorrhea is a common gynecological complaint and can pose a significant diagnostic and therapeutic challenge to the clinician. There can be many causes, some of which are multifactorial. For descriptive purposes, amenorrhea is often described in terms of primary or secondary amenorrhea. Primary amenorrhea refers to absence of menses by age 15 in the presence of normal development of secondary sexual characteristics or the absence of both menses and secondary sexual characteristics by age 12–13. Secondary amenorrhea is typically defined as the cessation of menses for more than three cycles or six months in women who have undergone menarche. The initial patient workup can seem overwhelming and confusing unless a logical, stepwise approach is consistently followed with each patient. The hallmark of determining an appropriate diagnosis and treatment plan begins with a proper patient history and physical exam. Next, the appropriate diagnostic lab work and imaging studies must be employed. Finally, once an etiology is determined, treatment can begin. Treatment of amenorrhea is driven by both the cause of the amenorrhea and the desires of the patient. Treatment should be directed at correcting any underlying pathology including surgical correction of any outflow tract obstruction and the restoration of normal ovarian function to promote proper bone and reproductive health.

Lastly, in addition to treating the physical consequences of amenorrhea, the clinician must also be aware of the psychological consequences and be prepared to address them. Amenorrhea and the resulting potential impaired fertility can take a devastating toll on both the patient and her family. As a result, anyone caring for a patient with amenorrhea must not only assess and treat the physical sequelae but must also address any mental and emotional concerns as well.

References

1. Practice Committee of the American Society for Reproductive Medicine. Current evaluation of amenorrhea. *Fertility and Sterility* 2006; **86**: 148.
2. Fritz MA, Speroff L. *Clinical Endocrinology and Infertility*, 8th ed. Philadelphia: Lippincott Williams & Wilkins, 2010: 435–94.
3. Kreipe RE, Yussman SM. The role of the primary care practitioner in the treatment of eating disorders. *Adolesc Med* Feb 2003; **14**(1): 133–47.
4. Martin KA, Hall JE, Adams JM, Crowley WF Jr. Comparison of exogenous gonadotropins and pulsatile gonadotropin-releasing hormone for induction of ovulation in hypogonadotropic amenorrhea. *J Clin Endocrinol Metab* 1993; **77**: 125.
5. Melmed S, Casanueva FF, Hoffman AR, et al. Diagnosis and treatment of hyperprolactinemia: an Endocrine Society clinical practice guideline. *J Clin Endocrinol Metab* 2011; **96**: 273.
6. Casanueva FF, Molitch ME, Schlechte JA, et al. Guidelines of the Pituitary Society for the diagnosis and management of prolactinomas. *Clin Endocrinol (Oxf)* 2006; **65**: 265.
7. Saenger P. Turner's syndrome. *N Engl J Med* 1996; **335**: 1749.
8. Zhong Q, Layman LC. Genetic considerations in the patient with Turner syndrome – 45, X with or without mosaicism. *Fertil Steril* 2012; **98**: 775.
9. Nelson LM, Anasti TN, Kimzey LM, et al. Development of luteinized graafian follicles in patients with karyotypically normal spontaneous premature ovarian failure. *J Clin Endocrinol Metab* 1994; **79**: 1470.
10. Nelson LM. Clinical Practice: primary ovarian insufficiency. *N Engl J Med* 2009; **360**: 606.
11. Groff AA, Covington SN, Halversor LR, et al. Assessing the emotional needs of women with spontaneous premature ovarian failure. *Fertil Steril* 2005; **83**: 1734–41.

12. Greil AL. Infertility and psychological distress: a critical review of the literature. *Soc Sci Med* 1997; **145**: 1679–704.

13. Crofton PM, Evans N, Bath LE, et al. Physiological versus standard sex steroid replacement in young women with premature ovarian failure; effects on bone mass acquisition and turnover. *Clin Endocrinol (Oxf)* 2010; **73**: 707.

14. North American Menopause Society. *The role of calcium in peri- and postmenopausal women: 2006 position statement of the North American Menopause Society*. 2006; **13**: 862–77.

15. Rock JA, Azziz R. Genital anomalies in childhood. *Clinical Obstet Gynecol* 1987; **30**: 682.

16. Fujimoto VY, Miller JH, Klein NA, Soules MR. Congential cervical atresia: report of seven cases and review of the literature. *Am J Obstet Gynecol* 1997; **177**(6): 1419–25.

17. Mazouni C, Girard G, Deter R, et al. Diagnosis of mullerian anomalies in adults; evaluation of practice. *Fertil Steril* 2008; **89**: 219.

18. ACOG Committee on Adolescent Health Care. ACOG Committee Opinion No. 274, July 2002: Nonsurgical diagnosis and management of vaginal agenesis. *Obstet Gynecol* 2002; **100**: 213.

19. Edmonds DK. Congenital malformations of the genital tract and their management. *Best Pract Res Clin Obstet Gynecol* 2003; **17**: 19.

20. Gustafson ML, Donahoe PK. Male sex determination: current concepts of male sexual differentiation. *Annu Rev Med* 1994; **45**: 505.

21. Katz VL, Lentz GM, Lobo RA, Gorshenson DM. *Comprehensive Gynecology*, 5th ed. St. Louis: Mosby; 2007: 933–61.

22. Verp MS, Simpson JL. Abnormal sexual differentiation and neoplasia. *Cancer Genet Cytogenet* 1987; **25**: 191.

23. Baldauf JJ, Dreyfus M, Ritter J, et al. Risk of cervical stenosis after large loop excision or laser conization. *Obstet Gynecol* 1996; **88**: 933.

24. Deans R, Abbott J. Review of intrauterine adhesions. *J Minim Invasive Gynecol* 2010; **17**: 555.

25. March CM. Asherman's syndrome. *Semin Reprod Med* 2011; **29**: 83.

26. March CM. Management of Asherman's syndrome. *Reprod Biomed Online* 2011; **23**: 63.

27. AAGL Advancing Minimally Invasive Gynecology Worldwide. AAGL practice report: practice guidelines for management of intrauterine synechiae. *J Minim Invasive Gynecol* 2010; **17**: 1.

28. Klein DA, Poth MA. Amenorrhea: an approach to diagnosis and management. *America Family Physician* 2013; **87**(11): 781–8.

29. Master-Hunter T, Heiman D. Amenorrhea: evaluation and treatment. *American Family Physician* 2006; **73**(8): 1374–82.

Chapter 16

Abnormal uterine bleeding

Jeanette Lager, James Gregg, and Laurie Swain

Introduction

Abnormal uterine bleeding (AUB) accounts for one-third of ambulatory gynecology visits in premenopausal women and more than 70% of visits for perimenopausal and postmenopausal women.[1] Given the prevalence of patients seen with this complaint, this chapter will review the epidemiology, nomenclature, diagnosis, and management of this common disorder.

Terminology

Normal menses occurs every 21–35 days with regularity of ±2 days and lasts 5–7 days. Less than 80 mL of blood is lost during a normal cycle. Although menses is usually regular during the reproductive years, variations in menstrual timing are common near the time of menarche and perimenopause. During the first five to seven years after menarche, the cycle length is typically longer and then shortens in length until the cycles become regular. Perimenopause is the time period from the onset of cycle irregularity until one year after the last menses. During this time the cycles initially may increase in frequency and then decrease in frequency until menses stop altogether. Menopause, the cessation of menses, is defined as 12 months of amenorrhea.[2]

Until recently, abnormal uterine bleeding was classified by descriptors of frequency and volume of vaginal bleeding. *Menorrhagia* was defined as heavy, regular menses. *Oligomenorrhea* was defined as menstrual cycles greater than 35 days to 3 months in duration. *Polymenorrhea* was defined as cycles occurring at intervals less than 21 days. *Metrorrhagia* was the term used to describe irregular cycles, and *menometrorrhagia* was defined as heavy, irregular cycles. The term *dysfunctional uterine bleeding* (DUB) defined abnormal uterine bleeding where no clear etiology could be identified.[3]

Woolcock and his colleagues noted confusion among providers with regards to abnormal uterine bleeding terminology. Additionally, the overlapping terms and variable definitions limited study comparison and planning of multicenter trials.[4] Although previous terminology described characteristics of AUB, the terms did not incorporate etiology, which often determines the treatment options. Thus, a new classification for AUB was first proposed in 2005 by the International Federation of Gynecology and Obstetrics (FIGO) which was supported by American College of Obstetricians and Gynecologists (ACOG) in July 2012 in the practice bulletin on the diagnosis of AUB in reproductive-aged women.[3, 5] This section summarizes this recently adopted nomenclature.

Abnormal uterine bleeding (AUB) is defined as bleeding from the uterine corpus that is abnormal in regularity, volume, and/or timing in a nonpregnant woman.[5] Acute AUB is an episode of heavy bleeding that, in the opinion of the provider, requires immediate intervention. Chronic AUB is defined as the presence of AUB for the majority of the previous six months. It is possible to have an acute exacerbation of AUB that requires medical or surgical intervention with a known underlying cause of chronic AUB. Based on this new classification, descriptions of bleeding flow or pattern, such as AUB followed by heavy menstrual bleeding (HMB) and intermenstrual bleeding (IMB), should be used in place of menorrhagia, metrorrhagia, and menometrorrhagia. For example, a woman with menstrual cycles that are heavy or prolonged would be classified as having AUB/HMB. HMB is excessive blood loss which is considered blood loss >80 mL, but should be based clinically on a patient's perception of their menses. IMB is uterine bleeding that occurs between clearly defined cycles and may occur at the same time in each cycle or in an irregular pattern. As an example, mid-cycle spotting that occurs as a result of an endometrial polyp would be considered AUB/IMB.

Office Care of Women, ed. Martin E. Olsen and Botros Rizk. Published by Cambridge University Press.

Further classification is based on structural and nonstructural causes, known by the acronym PALM-COEIN. PALM describes the structural abnormalities, and COEIN represents the nonstructural etiologies (see Table 16-1).

Structural terminology: PALM

As shown in Table 16-1, PALM stands for structural etiologies of AUB, which include polyp (AUB-P), adenomyosis (AUB-A), leiomyoma (AUB-L), and malignancy or hyperplasia (AUB-M).

Endometrial polyps are hyperplastic growths of endometrial glands, blood vessels and stroma that project into the endometrium.[6] They are often asymptomatic, but women may present with AUB/HMB, postcoital spotting, and prolonged menses. The specific mechanism that causes bleeding is unclear but some theories include mechanical distention of the endometrium and stromal congestion within the polyp leading to venous stasis and apical necrosis. Risk factors include increasing age, hypertension, obesity, and tamoxifen use.[7, 8]

Table 16-1 PALM-COEIN classification system

PALM	COEIN
Polyp	**C**oagulopathy
Adenomyosis	**O**vulatory
Leiomyomas	**E**ndometrial
Hyperplasia and other **m**alignancies	**I**atrogenic
	Not yet classified

Source: Adapted from the FIGO Working Group on Menstrual disorders. [5]

Adenomyosis is a condition where endometrial glands invade the myometrium. This leads to symptoms of dysmenorrhea and HMB. In the past, there were no radiographic findings described to identify adenomyosis. Rather, the diagnosis was found after hysterectomy on pathological specimen and as an incidental finding at the time of autopsy. Since radiological findings have been described on transvaginal ultrasound and magnetic resonance imaging (MRI), there are limited data on risk factors. The following characteristics have been associated with adenomyosis: multiparity, endometriosis, leiomyomas, previous uterine surgery, and increasing age.[9]

Leiomyomas are smooth muscle tumors of the myometrium which may be submucosal, intramural, subserosal or a combination of these categories. The PALM-COIEN terminology further subclassifies leiomyomas, based on location and number (see Table 16-2). Patients with submucosal myomas can

Table 16-2 FIGO subclassification of myomas [5]

Type	Number	Location
Submucosal	0	Pedunculated intracavitary
	1	<50% intramural
	2	≥50% intramural
Other	3	Contacts endometrium, 100% intramural
	4	Intramural
	5	Subserosal ≥50% intramural
	6	Subserosal < 50% intramural
	7	Subserosal pedunculated
	8	Other (specify – e.g., cervical, broad ligament, parasitic)
Hybrid leiomyomas		Classification that refers to the relationship to the endometrium and the serosa. The classification lists the first number as the relationship to the endometrium, followed by a hyphen, and then the number that represents the relationship to the serosa.

Table 16-3 Risk factors for endometrial cancer [4]

Increasing age
Weight >90 kg (200 lbs.)
Anovulatory cycles (e.g., PCOS)
Early menarche
Late menopause
Nulliparity
Infertility
Diabetes mellitus
Tamoxifen use
Family history of endometrial or colon cancer

present with heavy menstrual bleeding, infertility, or recurrent pregnancy loss.[10] Leiomyomas may also be associated with a normal bleeding pattern but can present with bulk symptoms, such as pelvic pressure, polyuria, and constipation. African-American ethnicity, early menarche, multiparity, and family history of myomas are all risk factors for myomas. Myomas are less frequent among smokers.[11]

Endometrial hyperplasia is the result of abnormal proliferation of the endometrium, which can progress to carcinoma.[12] Conditions associated with unopposed estrogen increase the risk of endometrial cancer. Table 16-3 lists the risk factors for endometrial hyperplasia and cancer. Symptoms of endometrial hyperplasia may include postmenopausal bleeding, AUB or intermenstrual spotting. Endometrial hyperplasia is classified based on histology as simple or complex hyperplasia, with or without atypia. The classification correlates with the risk of progression to cancer. The likelihood of progression of endometrial hyperplasia to endometrial cancer was demonstrated in a retrospective review of 170 women who had at least a one-year delay between diagnosis and hysterectomy (Table 16-3):[13]

- simple hyperplasia without atypia – 1 (1%) of 93 patients
- complex hyperplasia without atypia – 1 (3%) of 29 patients
- simple hyperplasia with atypia – 1 (8%) of 13 patients
- complex hyperplasia with atypia – 10 (29%) of 35 patients

The differences in each of the subgroups were not statistically significant but suggested a trend. The regression rate of hyperplasia in simple hyperplasia, complex hyperplasia and atypical hyperplasia were 80%, 79%, and 58%, respectively. Once a hyperplastic or malignant condition is diagnosed, it is then classified by the appropriate FIGO or World Health Organization (WHO) classification.

Nonstructural terminology: COEIN

The acronym COEIN refers to the nonstructural etiologies: coagulopathy (AUB-C), ovulatory (AUB-O), endometrial (AOB-E), iatrogenic (AOB-I), and entities that have not yet been classified (AUB-N) (see Table 16-1).

Coagulopathic abnormalities should be considered in women with a lifelong history of HMB or symptoms concerning for prolonged bleeding. Approximately 13% of women presenting with a complaint of AUB/HMB are diagnosed with Von Willebrand disease, based on a systematic review of nine studies with a total of 988 women with AUB/HMB.[14] Initial screening is appropriate for women who present with:[15]

HMB since menarche

or

One of more of the following:

1. postpartum hemorrhage
2. surgery-related bleeding
3. bleeding associated with dental work

or

Two or more of the following:

1. bruising one to two times per month
2. epistaxis one to two times per month
3. frequent gum bleeding
4. family history of bleeding disorder

Of note, AUB-C classification also includes AUB related to treatment with warfarin, heparin, or low molecular weight heparin.

Regular menstrual cycles are evidence of a functional hypothalamic-pituitary-ovarian (PTO) axis and thus ovulatory cycles. When a patient's cycle becomes irregular, this may suggest that the etiology of the abnormal bleeding is related to anovulation. Anovulatory women may present with little or no menses at all, or heavy, irregular bleeding. Ovulatory

Table 16-4 Medications that can cause AUB

Anticoagulants	Hormonal	Psychiatric	Other
Coumadin	Corticosteroids	Lithium	Rifampin
Heparin	Hormonal contraceptives	Tricyclic antidepressants	Phenytoin
Aspirin	Tamoxifen	Selective serotonin reuptake inhibitors	Ginseng
	Hormone replacement therapy	Antipsychotic medications	Ginkgo biloba

dysfunction can be caused by endocrinopathies, adrenal lesions, or central nervous system (CNS) lesions that may disrupt the PTO axis.

Endometrial causes of AUB are the result of an imbalance of locally active substances such as prostaglandin F2 alpha and prostaglandin E2, or infection. Patients present with cyclic menstrual bleeding without another definable cause of AUB that is identified. Regulation of menstrual bleeding is dependent on the appropriate and coordinated release of pituitary and ovarian hormones, which in turn affect the local balance of prostaglandins, tissue plasminogen activator, and prostacyclins. Disruption of this can lead to intermenstrual spotting or prolonged menses, and is also considered an endometrial etiology (AUB-E).[6, 16, 17]

Iatrogenic causes of AUB include medications and medical devices that may be used to address AUB or have known side effects of AUB. Gonadal steroid medications may cause bleeding between scheduled cycles, which is termed "break-through bleeding." Other medication, such as tricyclic antidepressants can affect dopamine metabolism and may interfere with ovulatory function. Table 16-4 lists medications that can contribute to iatrogenic causes of AUB, such as hormonal medications, anticoagulants, psychiatric medications, herbal supplements, antibiotics, and tobacco use.

Anticoagulants affect normal hemostasis and can result in AUB/HMB. Although this can be considered an iatrogenic cause, note that this is classified as AUB-C (coagulopathy). This is because the effect on hemostasis is similar in management to inherited disorders of hemostasis.

AUB-N (*not yet classified*) includes etiologies that may not fit in the other categories. Chronic endometritis and arterio-venous malformation are examples of AUB-N. This provides a category for emerging etiologies that may not fit in the other categories.

Evaluation

History and physical exam

The pattern of AUB guides further testing and treatment. Reviewing the current bleeding pattern, including frequency, duration, and volume serves to direct evaluation and identify the likely causes of AUB. The review of systems should be focused on symptoms of anemia, thyroid disease, hyperandrogenism, and hypothalamic dysfunction. The sexual history and contraceptive history will assess the possibility of pregnancy or infectious causes and identify medications that may contribute to AUB. A detailed menstrual history may reveal lifelong HMB, suggestive of a coagulopathy or irregular bleeding suggests ovulatory dysfunction due to endocrinopathy or may raise concern for hyperplasia or carcinoma. The medical history can identify chronic diseases that cause AUB, and a careful review of both prescription and nonprescription medications should be performed to identify medications that can contribute to AUB (see Table16-4).

The physical examination includes vital signs to evaluate for signs of anemia. The patient should be evaluated for signs of hyperandrogenism and polycystic ovarian syndrome including increased BMI, hirsuitism, and acanthosis nigricans. An abdominal and pelvic exam is imperative for all women who present with AUB. Blood in the vault, active bleeding from the cervical Os, clot size, and quantity should be noted. The pelvic exam can exclude nonuterine causes of bleeding, such as vaginal trauma or cervical lesions. The bimanual exam assesses uterine size, contour, and tenderness. A large, irregularly shaped uterus would suggest the possibility of myomas. Adenomyosis may reveal a diffusely tender, enlarged, globular uterus on exam. Additional tests, such as a Pap smear, cervical

Table 16-5 Causes, symptoms, and additional diagnostic tests for AUB

Causes	Symptoms	Diagnostic test to consider:
Coagulopathy	HMB, family history of coagulopathy or personal history of easy bruising or epistaxis	Von Willebrand factor, ristocetin cofactor, PT/PTT, platelet count (CBC)
Thyroid disease	Heat or cold intolerance, menstrual irregularities, dry skin	Thyroid-stimulating hormone
Polycystic ovarian syndrome	Weight gain, hirsuitism, acne	Dehydroepiandrosterone sulfate, free testosterone
Hypothalamic dysfunction	Stress, eating disorders, extreme weight loss	Follicle-stimulating hormone/luteinizing hormone
Prolactinemia/ prolactinoma	Amenorrhea, nipple discharge	Prolactin
Congenital adrenal hyperplasia	Acne, hirsuitism	Morning 17-OHP in the early follicular phase
Androgen producing tumors	Hirsuitism	Dehydroepiandrosterone sulfate, testosterone, cortisol

cultures, and endometrial biopsy can be performed as appropriate.

Laboratory evaluation

Initial labs for AUB may include:

- complete blood count (CBC) for patients with HMB or chronic bleeding
- urine or serum pregnancy test, if there is any possibility of pregnancy

Irregular cycles may be due to physiologic causes of anovulation such as adolescence, perimenopause, pregnancy, and lactation. If the review of symptoms suggests other tests should be included as clinically indicated. Table 16-5 lists diagnostic tests based on specific symptoms.

If the patient has risk factors for a coagulopathy as described in the section for AUB-C, Von Willebrand factor, ristocetin cofactor, and hematology consultation should be considered.

Uterine assessment

Uterine assessment should be performed when a structural cause of AUB is suspected. Uterine abnormalities may be evaluated with radiologic imaging or hysteroscopy. Radiographic studies include transvaginal ultrasound (TVUS), sonohysterography, and magnetic resonance imaging (MRI). Computed tomography (CT) has less utility in benign gynecology because soft tissue delineation is limited. For this reason, pathological findings on CT are followed up with additional testing. TVUS is first line for evaluation because it is less time consuming for the patient, relatively low cost and less invasive than other modalities. However, the utility of TVUS is limited when evaluating intracavitary abnormalities, such as endometrial polyps and submucosal myomas, which are frequently implicated as structural causes of AUB. The sensitivity and specificity of TVUS for the evaluation of intracavitary uterine abnormalities are 56% and 73%, respectively, whereas the sensitivity and specificity for sonohysterography are 81.3% and 100%, and are 87.5% and 100% for hysteroscopy, respectively.[18] Thus if the ultrasound is nondiagnostic, sonohysterography or hysteroscopy should be considered. Figures 16-1 and 16-2 show examples of transvaginal ultrasound and sonohysterography for endometrial polyps.

Sonohysterography is performed by placing a small balloon catheter intracervically through which saline is injected at the time of TVUS. This is well

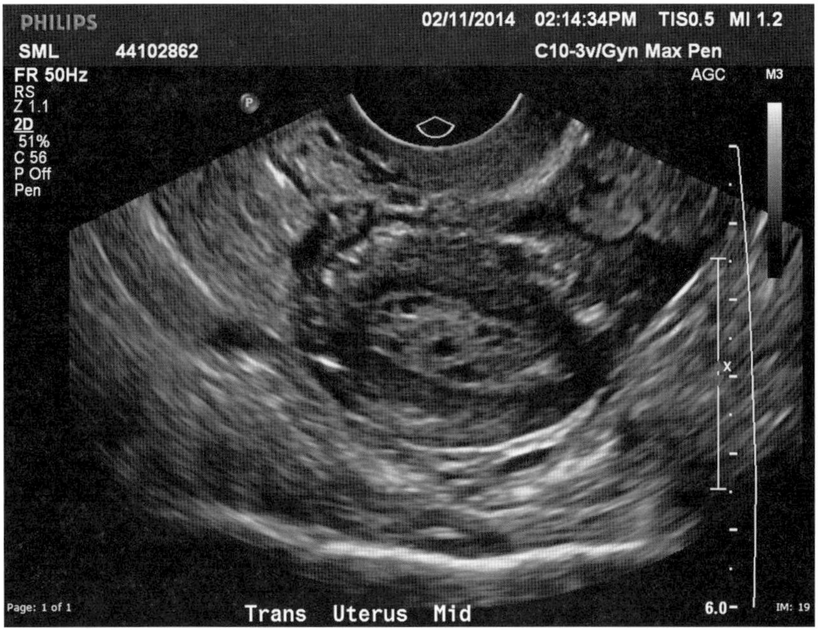

Figure 16-1 Transvaginal ultrasound showing endometrial polyp. Grayscale image shows a thickened endometrial stripe, which can be a nonspecific finding. Hysterosonogram or MRI is recommended to classify lesion.

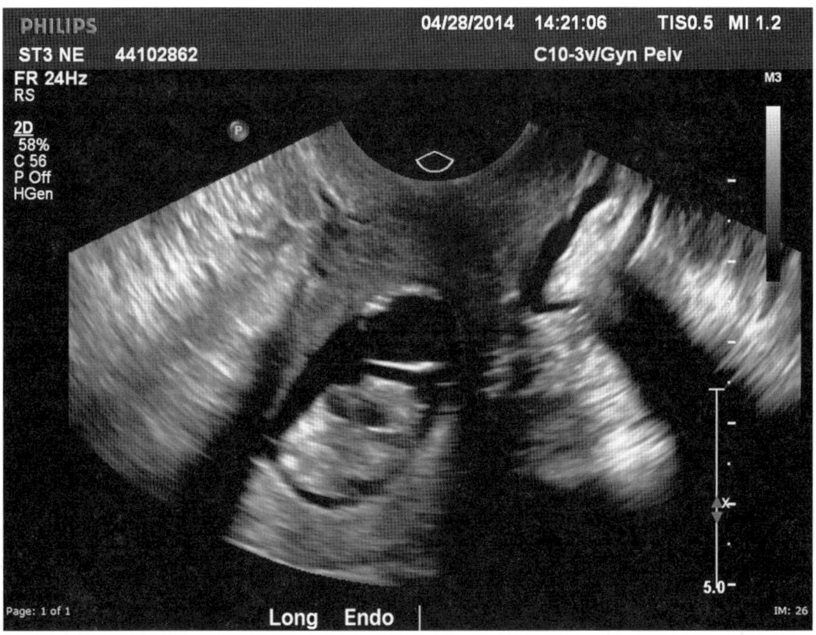

Figure 16-2 Hysterosonogram image after balloon deployed and saline infused into endometrial cavity. An endometrial polyp is seen with a stalk, and fluid is noted around the majority of the polyp.

tolerated by patients and provides immediate information regarding location, size, and depth of intracavitary myomas as well as endometrial polyps. An additional advantage of SIS is the ability to classify the type of submucosal myoma based on the degree of intramural involvement. This information is pivotal for surgical planning and counseling.

Hysteroscopy provides direct visualization of the endometrial cavity and can be performed in the office or operating room. Directed biopsies can be

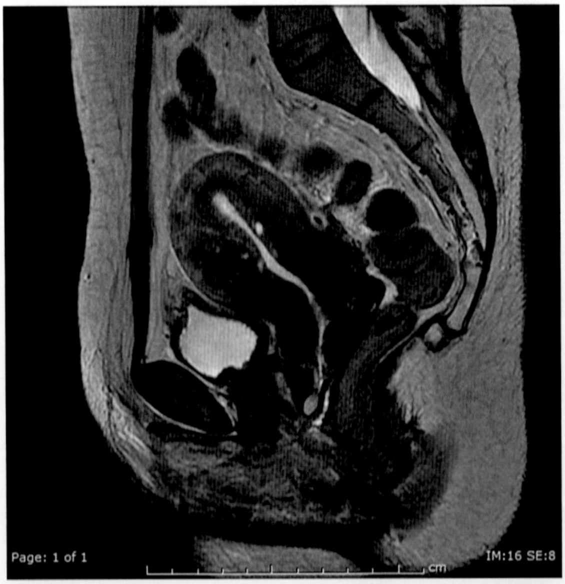

Figure 16-3 MRI sagittal T2-weighted fast spin echo shows diffuse widening of the low signal intensity junctional zone consistent with adenomyosis. High signal intensity linear striations and punctate foci of high signal present.

performed if indicated, and hysteroscopy has the advantage of being both a diagnostic and therapeutic modality depending on the instruments available.

MRI is relatively noninvasive, provides excellent tissue delineation, and provides multiplanar images. MRI can provide detailed information regarding size, location and number of uterine masses. MRI can also identify junctional thickening, which is suggestive of adenomyosis. Figures 16-3 shows an example of adenomyosis on t-2 weighted MRI image.

Histologic assessment

Histologic assessment of the endometrium is easy to perform in the office and may provide information about the presence of premalignant and malignant conditions of the endometrium (AUB-M). Endometrial specimens may be obtained using an endometrial pipelle, dilation and curettage (D&C), or hysteroscopically directed biopsies. Endometrial biopsy can be performed in the office and is excellent for detecting hyperplasia with atypia and endometrial cancer with a sensitivity and specificity of 82.3% and 98% for hyperplasia with atypia and 91% and 98% in detecting endometrial cancer, respectively.[19] However, endometrial sampling using a pipelle is a blind evaluation of the endometrium, has been shown to sample an average of 4% of the endometrium, and may miss a focal endometrial lesion.[20] For this reason, hysteroscopy with direct biopsies may be more appropriate for investigation of focal endometrial lesions. In clinical situations where a larger sample of tissue is needed, the endometrial biopsy is nondiagnostic, or an endometrial biopsy is unable to be performed in the office, dilation and curettage with or without hysteroscopy can be performed.

Endometrial sampling should be performed in women who have an increased risk for endometrial hyperplasia or cancer (Table 16-3). In women older than 45 years, endometrial sampling is recommended by ACOG for any AUB. In women older than 19 years and younger than 45 years, endometrial sampling should be considered in women with a history of chronic anovulatory cycles or persistent AUB unrelieved by medical therapy. In adolescents younger than 19 years, endometrial sampling is rarely necessary for evaluation given the limited cases of hyperplasia or malignancy in this population.[21]

Management

Medical management

Several factors should be considered in the management of AUB. Clinical diagnosis determines the appropriate treatment options. Additionally, one should clarify the patients' perspective on severity of symptoms, desire for future fertility or contraception, and preferences for treatment. These factors allow for shared decision to clarify options, review patient values, and potentially increase compliance of treatment.[22]

Figure 16-5 summarizes the evaluation to direct treatment. In cases where the treatment is related to ovulatory dysfunction, medical management is first line therapy. Medical management is also useful for structural etiologies as a long-term treatment or to temporarily manage symptoms. Medical treatment is useful as a bridge to menopause in a perimenopausal patient, and in the preoperative period to optimize comorbid conditions, such as anemia and diabetes.

Medical treatments are hormonal or nonhormonal. A patient may have risk factors or comorbidities where certain treatments are contraindicated and should not be used to treat AUB. For example, contraindications to combined oral contraceptives include previous thromboembolic event or stroke, history of an estrogen dependent tumor, active liver disease,

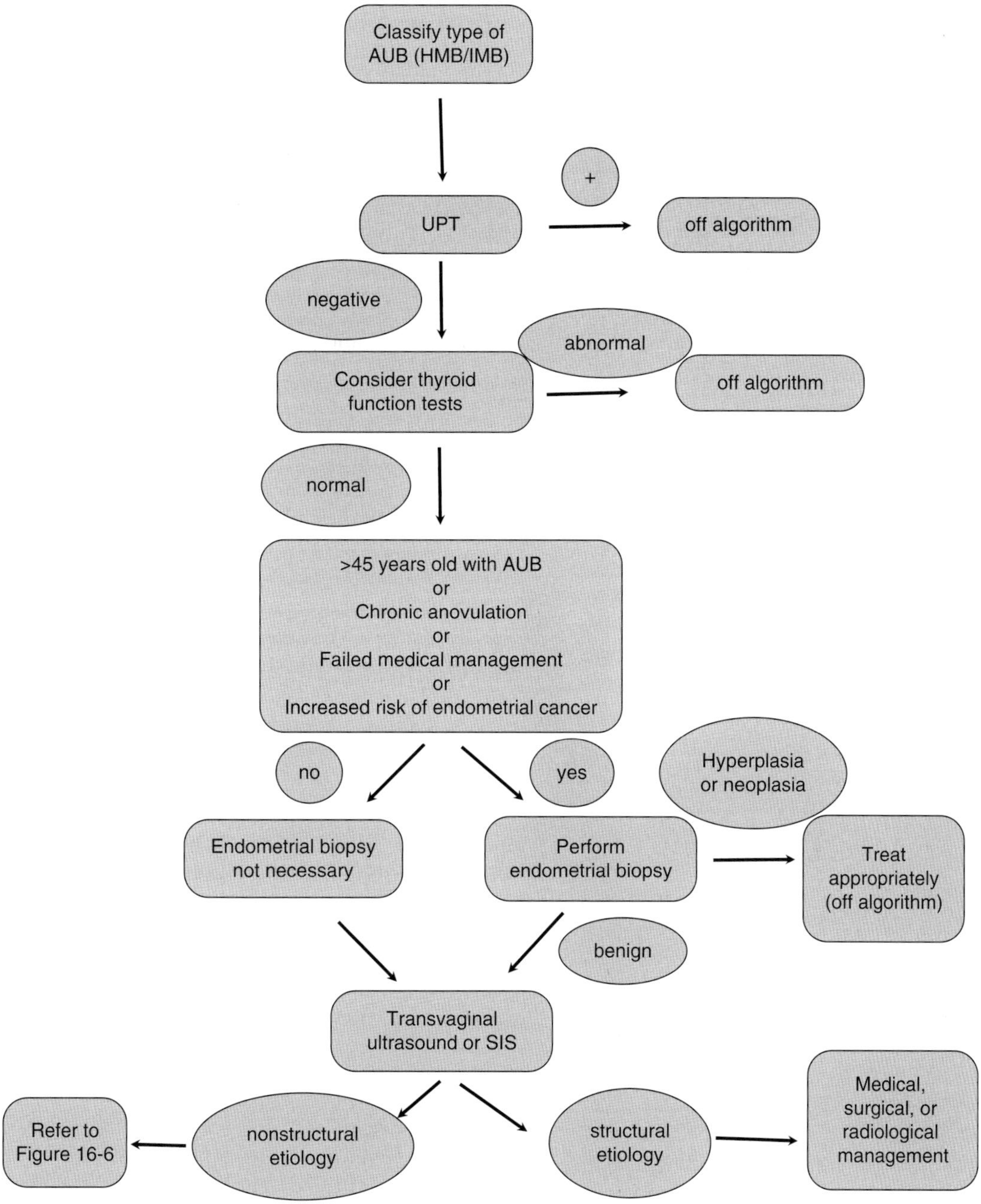

Figure 16-4 Algorithm to evaluate nonpregnant women for AUB.

pregnancy, hypertriglyceridemia, migraine with aura, tobacco use of more than 15 cigarettes per day, and age greater than 35 years. The Centers for Disease Control and Prevention (CDC) released medical eligibility criteria for contraceptive use, which can be found at www.cdc.gov/mmwr/preview/mmwrhtml/rr5904a1.htm?s_cid=rr5904a1_e. This site is an excellent resource for patients that have comorbidities or contraindications that preclude a particular treatment regimen.

Medical management of AUB consists of hormonal therapies and non-hormonal therapies. Medical management options are described in Figure 16-6 and the specific medications are listed in Table 16-6.

Table 16-6 Medications for AUB

Medication	Dosage	Additional information
Estrogen-progestin contraceptives	Estrogen 20 mcg–35 mcg ethinyl estradiol Progestin: norethindrone or norethindrone acetate (>1 mg) or levenogestrel (≥150 mcg)	Regimen may either be cyclic or continuous
Levonorgestrel IUD	Levonorgestrel 20 mcg/24 hours	May be used for 5 years
Progestin	Medroxyprogesterone acetate 20 mg–40 mg daily Megestrol acetate 40 mg–80 mg daily Norethindrone acetate 5 mg–10 mg	Regimen may be continuous or taken 14 days of the month; however, it is not effective to reduce blood flow when taken in the luteal phase in ovulatory women
Nonsteroidal anti-inflammatory drugs	Mefenamic acid 500 mg three times daily Naproxen 500 mg, repeat dose in 3–5 hours, then 250 mg–500 mg twice daily Ibuprofen 600 mg daily	Regimen is taken during menses only
Antifibrinolytic	Tranexamic acid 1,300 mg three times daily	Regimen is taken for a maximum of 5 days, during menses

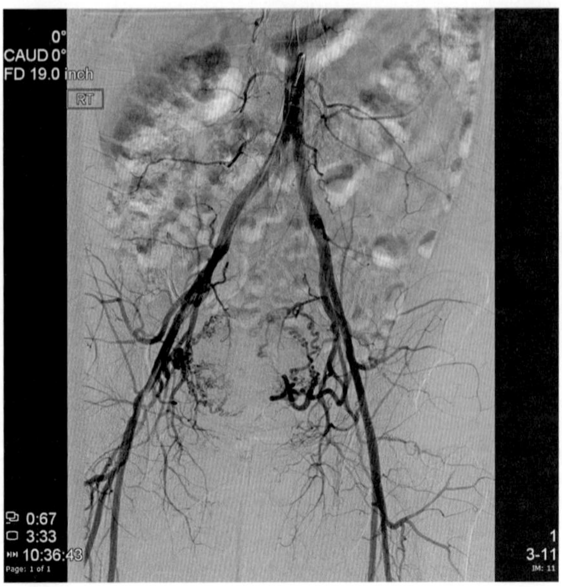

Figure 16-5 UAE flush pelvic aortogram.

Estrogen-progestin oral contraceptive pills (OCPs) have been shown to regulate bleeding patterns and reduce blood flow compared to placebo (47% vs. 9%) and may be taken cyclically or continuously.[23] When OCPs were compared to levenorgestrel IUD, the IUD resulted in less blood loss (87% vs. 35%).[24] The levonorgestrel IUD has been demonstrated to decrease menstrual blood loss by 74%–97% after one year of use in patients with AUB/HMB and has been shown to increase hemoglobin levels.[25, 26] The levonorgestrel IUD is well tolerated with adherence rates of 79.5%.[26] The most common reason for discontinuing use was irregular bleeding, which is most common for women in the first three months. After six months, most women report no bleeding to very light bleeding.[27] Oral progestin is effective for AUB but is less effective than OCPs or the levenogestrel IUD. The progestin only pill is useful for patients that have a contraindication for combination OCPs. [For a detailed list of contraindications associated with contraceptive methods, refer to www.cdc.gov/reproductivehealth/unintendedpregnancy/usmec.htm for the US Medical Eligibility Criteria (US MEC).]

Nonsteroidal anti-inflammatory drugs (NSAIDs) reduce menstrual blood volume by reducing prostaglandin synthesis in the endometrium. This leads to vasoconstriction and decreased blood flow. NSAIDs have been shown to reduce HMB compared to placebo, but are not as effective as the hormonal methods. In a systematic review of seven studies, there was

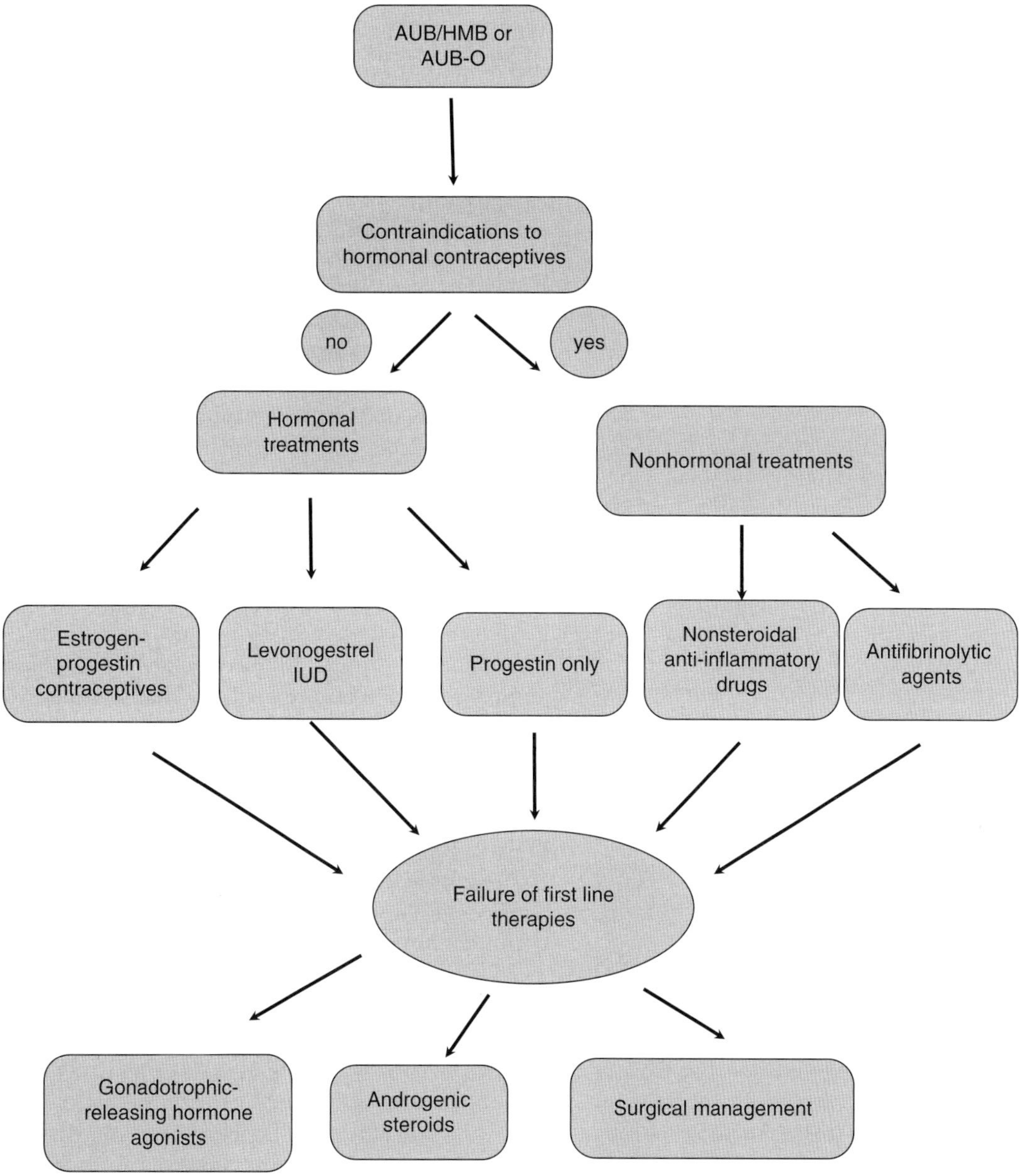

Figure 16-6 Algorithm for medical management of AUB.

no evidence of a difference between different NSAIDs in a reduction of HMB.[27]

Transexamic acid, an antifibrinolytic agent, was approved by the Food and Drug Association (FDA) in 2009 for the treatment of menorrhagia. Antifibrinolytics inhibit plasminogen activators that normally cause fibrinolysis and are more abundant in women with HMB. Antifibrinolytics have been shown to reduce blood loss and improve limitation of physical activities, work inside and outside of the home, and perceived blood loss when compared to placebo.[28] There is a concern for thrombosis associated with transexamic acid and it is contraindicated in patients with a history of thrombosis or with concurrent use of a combination hormonal contraception.

Surgical management

Some causes of AUB are amenable to medical therapy, whereas some are best managed surgically. Furthermore, some women are unsatisfied with or do not desire long-term medical management of their AUB. Several surgical options exist and are discussed here.

Endometrial ablation

Endometrial ablation is a procedure used to reduce uterine bleeding by destroying the endometrial lining. Historically, resectoscopic ablation was performed using a hysteroscope and roller ball or wire loop. Now global ablative techniques are more common and use bipolar radiofrequency, hot liquid-filled balloon, cryotherapy, circulating heated water or microwave energy. Endometrial ablation is contraindicated in women who desire future fertility, have known or suspected endometrial hyperplasia or cancer (AUB-M), have a pelvic infection, or have had previous transmyometrial uterine surgery. Endometrial ablation has been shown to reduce menstrual blood flow, and may cause amenorrhea. Patient satisfaction is high, approximately 90% in one year.[30] However, there is a risk of subsequent surgery in cases where AUB or dysmenorrhea persists. The rate of additional surgical treatment for AUB at two to five years postoperatively is 21%–25%, depending on the technique.[30] Success may be lower in women with adenomyosis (AUB-A) (RR or OR1.7).[31]

Myomectomy

Surgical options for patients who are diagnosed with AUB-L include myomectomy, myolysis, or hysterectomy. Myomectomy may be performed hysteroscopically, laparoscopically, robotic-assisted, or through a laparotomy incision (open myomectomy). A hysteroscopic approach is appropriate for type 0 (intracavitary) or type 1 (where greater than 50% of the myoma is intracavitary), but is less effective in completely removing a type 2 (less than 50% of the myoma is submucosal). Both laparoscopic and open myomectomy can access subserosal, intramural, and submucosal fibroids. Laparoscopic myomectomies are associated with less anemia, a shorter hospital stay and quicker recovery, and longer operative duration as compared to open procedures.[32] Regardless of the surgical approach for myomectomy, the risk of myoma recurrence is 20% after laparoscopic myomectomy and 18 percent of open myomectomies.[32] Recurrent myomas are more likely in women who have multiple myomas than single myomas at the time of surgery. One retrospective study reviewed myoma recurrence in 145 women after open myomectomy. The risk of recurrent myomas after five years was 74% in patients with multiple myomas and 11% in those with single myomas. The rate of reoperation after multiple and solitary myomectomy were 62% and 9%, respectively.[33] The potential need for cesarean after myomectomy due to the risk of uterine rupture is an important consideration.

Myolysis

A relatively new technique is laparoscopic ultrasound-guided radiofrequency volumetric thermal ablation for symptomatic fibroids. A prospective, single arm study of 31 women showed improved symptom severity scores of 59.7%, 71.7%, and 82.0% at 3, 6, and 12 months, respectively.[34] Thirty-six month data from a prospective trial of 135 women was published in 2013 which showed improved symptom severity scores. In this study, there was an 11% reintervention rate, which included 2 myomectomies, 11 hysterectomies, and 1 uterine artery embolization. This study was limited by the lack of a comparison group; however, there are currently studies underway which will compare a laparoscopic ultrasound-guided radiofrequency volumetric thermal ablation to other treatments for fibroids.[35]

Hysterectomy

Hysterectomy is the most common gynecologic surgical procedure and is the definitive treatment for AUB. After hysterectomy, 96% of patients have reported that surgery had somewhat or completely resolved the gynecological problem.[36] Hysterectomy can be performed with or without the removal of ovaries. The benefits of concomitant removal of ovaries include reduced need for subsequent surgery (estimated 3%–8% of women undergoing hysterectomy),[37] reduction of breast cancer in premenopausal women, and reduction of ovarian cancer in all ages. The decision to perform bilateral oophorectomy is based on age, pathologic findings, and risk factors and patient preference. The surgical approach depends on uterine size, uterine dimensions, past medical and surgical history, and the experience and expertise of the surgeon. If possible, a vaginal approach is preferable, followed by laparoscopic or robotic assisted hysterectomy, then total abdominal hysterectomy.[38, 39, 40]

Large uteri can be removed laparoscopically utilizing morcellation techniques. This has been performed vaginally and abdominally in a closed and open system. In April 2014, the FDA released a safety communication that discourages the use of power morcellation in women with uterine fibroids due to the risk of inadvertent spread of undiagnosed cancer.[41] In December 2013, the Society of Gynecologic Oncologists released a statement.[42] Soon after the FDA communication, the American College of Obstetricians and Gynecologists and the Association of Gynecologic Laparoscopists have also released statements addressing morcellation of uterine fibroids due to the risk of inadvertent spread of cancer.[43, 44] The risk of uterine sarcoma has been estimated as less than 1 in 1,000 [42] and as high as 1 in 350 women [41] As a result of this concern, there are a number of hospitals that are not performing open power morcellation because of this risk. Open morcellation should not be performed if there is a concern for malignancy and patients should be counseled regarding the potential risks associated with this procedure. The minimally invasive techniques associated with morcellation result in shorter recovery and less blood loss than an open procedure. At this time, there is an active discussion on morcellation techniques and strategies to reduce this risk.

Radiological procedures

Several radiological treatments including uterine artery embolization (UAE) magnetic resonance guided-focused ultrasound (MRg-FUS), and energy based leiomyoma ablation have been used to treat AUB. As UAE is well researched and the most commonly performed radiological procedure, the most extensive discussion will be on UAE.

Uterine artery embolization

Uterine artery embolization is an endovascular procedure performed to produce hemorrhagic infarction of symptomatic uterine fibroids while maintaining endometrial and myometrial perfusion. The primary symptom for which women seek treatment for fibroids is menorrhagia.[45] Symptomatic fibroids usually result in heavy menstrual cycles with an increase in the length of the cycle and the number of days of heavy bleeding. Additional symptoms include pain and pressure associated with the mass effect of large uterine fibroids.

Magnetic resonance (MR) imaging should be used to evaluate patients before and after UFE. The assessment should include fibroid location, number, and size and the presence or absence of enhancement. Contrast enhanced MR also allows for the evaluation of the pelvic vasculature with assessment of the origins of the uterine arteries. MRI is used to identify patients that might be at a higher risk of a complication, such as fibroid expulsion, and have an effect on outcome, such as adenomyosis.[45] Pre-procedural MRI has been shown to affect case management, as evidenced by increased diagnostic confidence and allowing for an immediate change in treatment plan.[46] MR imaging is the most accurate imaging modality for detection of mimics of fibroids including adenomyosis, solid adnexal masses, focal myometrial contractions, and occasionally uterine leiomyosarcomas.[47]

Certain anatomic fibroid subtypes may affect management decisions. Intracavitary fibroids are more likely to be expelled after embolization and may present with lower abdominal pain and cramping and possible infection. These patients may require further gynecologic intervention. Pedunculated subserosal fibroids with a narrow stalk have been suggested to be a contraindication to embolization due to the risk of detachment, but the risk has been studied and no instances of detachment were noted. Cervical fibroids may be resistant to complete hemorrhagic infarction due to alternative blood supply to the cervix.[45]

Absolute contraindications include current pregnancy, known or suspected gynecologic malignancy, and current uterine or adnexal infection. Relative contraindications include contrast material allergy, coagulopathy, and renal failure.

Uterine artery embolization is accomplished via a catheter-based approach in which the common femoral artery is accessed and then the ipsilateral and contralateral uterine arteries are selected, usually with a microcatheter, and then embolized with particles.

The internal iliac artery terminates into anterior and posterior divisions. The branches of the anterior division include the inferior gluteal, obturator, internal pudendal, vesical, middle hemorrhoidal, uterine, and vaginal arteries. The branches of the posterior division include the superior gluteal, iliolumbar, and lateral sacral arteries. Due to the anterior and posterior orientation of the divisions, the selection of the anterior division is facilitated with a contralateral anterior oblique projection.

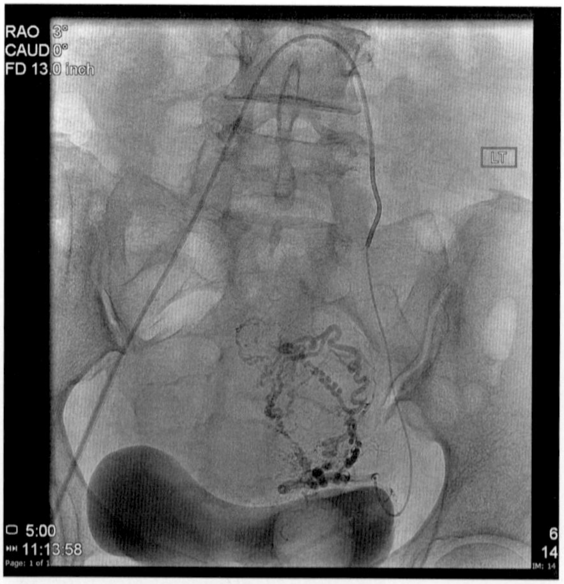

Figure 16-7 UAE of selected uterine artery.

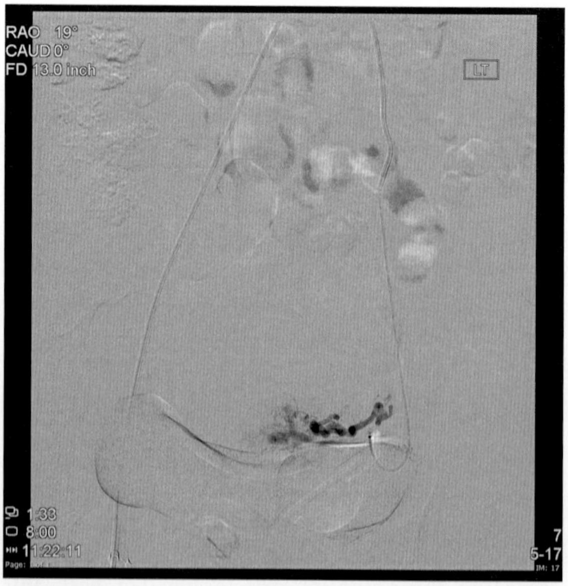

Figure 16-8 UAE post embolization.

The uterine artery is the first or the second branch of the anterior division of the internal iliac artery in 51% of cases.[47] In 6% of cases, the uterine artery is the first branch of the internal iliac artery above the level of the inferior gluteal and superior gluteal arteries; and in 15%–40% of the general population, the internal iliac artery terminates in a trifurcation with the uterine artery origin positioned between the anterior and posterior divisions.[47] In the latter two cases, the selection of the uterine artery is facilitated by an ipsilateral anterior oblique projection.

The presence of uterine fibroids usually results in the hypertrophy and distortion of the uterine arteries, which supply both the normal myometrium and the fibroids. The uterine artery has a characteristic U shape with a descending portion extending along the lateral pelvic wall, a transverse portion extending medially into the lower pelvis across the distal ureter at the level of the cervix, and an ascending portion extending superiorly along the lateral margin of the uterus. The uterine artery will typically have a corkscrew type appearance beginning in the ascending portion that will perfuse numerous collaterals to hyper-enhancing fibroids. The vesical and vaginal arteries usually originate from the transverse portion of the uterine artery. Safety of the procedure necessitates selection of the uterine artery into the ascending portion of the vessel to prohibit misadministration of embolic material into the vesical and vaginal arteries. Selection of the uterine artery into the distal corkscrew portion of the vessel assures a safe working position for embolization. A flush pelvic aortogram may be necessary if the characteristic uterine artery is not visualized, as the supply to the fibroids may originate from the ovarian arteries (see Figure 16-6).

Complete occlusion of the uterine arteries with stasis of contrast material is the usual angiographic endpoint when embolization is performed with nonspherical polyvinyl alcohol particles (see Figure 16-7).[47] Embolization is stopped when a standing column of contrast material is observed or when reflux of contrast is noted within the proximal ascending portion of the uterine artery (see Figure 16-8). With the administration of microspheres, the target of the embolization is the perifibroid arterial plexus, and embolization of the main uterine artery may be spared, with the angiographic endpoint becoming "near stasis" of the uterine artery with a "pruned-tree" appearance.[47]

Major complications include fibroid passage, infectious disease (endometritis, pelvic inflammatory disease, tubo-ovarian abscess, pyomyoma), deep venous thrombosis, pulmonary embolism, ovarian dysfunction, fibroid regrowth, and uterine necrosis. Fibroids in contact with the endometrial surface, including submucosal fibroids or intramural fibroids with a submucosal component, pose an increased risk for fibroid passage.[48] In many cases, the fibroid is expelled spontaneously. Hysteroscopic resection is reserved for cases in which the patient is symptomatic or the fibroid is only partially infarcted, and is still firmly attached to the uterine wall.[48] Women over 45 years of age are at increased risk for ovarian dysfunction after uterine artery embolization because they have a higher prevalence of uterine-ovarian arterial anastomoses (43% of cases) compared with women under 45 years of age (<5%).[48] UAE is a radiological procedure that uses a transcutaneous femoral artery approach to identify the vascularity to leiomyomas and embolize the arterial supply using particulate embolic material, usually polyvinyl alcohol particles of triacryl gelatin microspheres. This is often performed using a unilateral approach but may be performed bilaterally depending on the location and vascularity of the myomas.[45] Pre-procedure evaluation includes magnetic resonance imaging to document the vascularity, number, location and size of myomas, adenomyosis, or other uterine conditions. UAE has been shown to improve AUB/HMB, pelvic pressure, and pelvic pain. Two multicenter randomized trials, EMbolization versus hysterecoMY (EMMY) and Randomized Trial of Embolization versus Surgical Treatment for Fibroids (REST) compared UAE to hysterectomy (EMMY) or hysterectomy and myomectomy (REST). Both trials showed similar symptom relief, quality of life and patient satisfaction in the surgical and UAE treatment arms.[46, 47] Absolute contraindications for UAE include pregnancy, known or suspected gynecologic malignancy, current uterine or adnexal infection. Relative contraindications include allergy to contrast material, renal failure and known coagulopathy.[45]

Magnetic resonance imaging-guided focused ultrasound surgery

Magnetic resonance imaging-guided focused ultrasound surgery (MRg-FUS) is procedure that utilizes MRI for localization of the leiomyomas and real-time feedback for the use of high-intensity ultrasound waves that converge at a precise target point within the fibroid causing protein denaturation, irreversible cell damage and coagulative necrosis. MRg-FUS was FDA approved for the treatment of uterine leiomyomas in 2004, and several short-term studies that show volume reduction of myomas, but further research is needed to evaluate long-term results.[49]

There are other radiological modalities that are currently being evaluated for the treatment of AUB. These technologies can have a tremendous impact on treatment options for AUB and may expand the options for treatment.

Concluding remarks

Abnormal uterine bleeding is a common reason women present to their provider. This chapter discusses the current FIGO classification system (PALM-COIEN). Evaluation of AUB should include a detailed history, review of systems, and physical exam. Imaging and endometrial assessment are often useful in determining diagnosis and treatment. Once the etiology is determined, the appropriate medication or surgical therapy may be performed. Minimally invasive therapies and radiological treatments continue to be developed and will add to the spectrum of modalities available for the treatment of AUB.

References

1. Fraser IS, Langham S, Uhl-Hochgraeber K. Health-related quality of life and economic burden of abnormal uterine bleeding. *Expert Rev Obstet Gynecol* 2009; **4** (2):179–189.
2. Speroff L, Glass RH, Kase NG. *Clinical gynecology and infertility*. 6th ed. Baltimore, MD: Lippincott Williams & Wilkins; 1999.
3. American College of Obstetricians and Gynecologists. ACOG Practice Bulletin No. 128: Diagnosis of abnormal uterine bleeding in reproductive-aged women. *Obstet Gynecol* 2012; **128**(4): 1–11.
4. Woolcock JG, Critchley HO, Munro MG, et al. Review of the confusion in current and historical terminology and definitions for disturbances of menstrual bleeding. *Fertility and sterility* 2008; **90**(6): 2269–2280.
5. Munro MG, Critchley HO, Broder MS, et al. FIGO Working Group on Menstrual Disorders. FIGO classification system (PALM-COEIN) for causes of abnormal uterine bleeding in nongravid women of reproductive age. *Int J Gynaecol Obstet* 2011; **113**(1): 3–13.
6. Smith SK, Abel MH, Kelly RW, et al. Prostaglandin synthesis in the endometrium of women with ovular dysfunctional uterine bleeding. *Br J Obstet Gynaecol* 1981; **88**(4): 434–442.
7. Cohen I. Endometrial pathologies associated with postmenopausal tamoxifen treatment. *Gynecol Oncol* 2004; **94**: 256–266.
8. Dreisler, E, Sorenson SS, Lose G. Endometrial polyps and associated factors in Danish women aged 36–74 years. *American Journal of Obstetrics and Gynecology* 2009; **200**(2): 147.e1–e6.

9. Thomas JS, Clark JF. Adenomyosis: a retrospective view. *Journal of the National Medical Association* 1989; **81**(9): 969.
10. American Association of Gynecologic Laparoscopists (AAGL): Advancing Minimally Invasive Gynecology Worldwide. AAGL practice report: practice guidelines for the diagnosis and management of submucous leiomyomas. *Journal of Minimally Invasive Gynecology* 2012; **19**(2): 152.
11. Day Baird D, Dunson DB, Hill MC, et al. High cumulative incidence of uterine leiomyoma in black and white women: ultrasound evidence. *American Journal of Obstetrics and Gynecology* 2003; **188**(1): 100–107.
12. Marsden DE, Hacker NF. The classification, diagnosis and management of endometrial hyperplasia. *Reviews in Gynaecological Practice* 2003; **3**(2): 89–97.
13. Kurman RJ, Kaminski PF, Norris HJ. The behavior of endometrial hyperplasia: a long-term study of "untreated" hyperplasia in 170 patients. *Obstetrical & Gynecological Survey* 1986; **41**(1): 58–61.
14. Shankar M, Lee CA, Sabin CA, Economides DL, et al. Von Willebrand disease in women with menorrhagia: a systematic review. *BJOG: An International Journal of Obstetrics & Gynaecology* 2004; **111**(7): 734–740.
15. Kouides PA, Conard J, Peyvandi F, et al. Hemostasis and menstruation: appropriate investigation for underlying disorders of hemostasis in women with excessive menstrual bleeding. *Fertil Steril* 2005; **84**(5): 1345–1351.
16. Gleeson NC. Cyclic changes in endometrial tissue plasminogen activator and plasminogen activator inhibitor type 1 in women with normal menstruation and essential menorrhagia. *Am J Obstet Gynecol* 1994; **171**(1): 178–183.
17. Smith SK, Abel MH, Kelly RW, et al. A role for prostacyclin (PGi2) in excessive menstrual bleeding. *Lancet* 1981; **1**(8219): 522–524.
18. Kelekci S, Kaya E, Alan M, et al. Comparison of tranvaginal sonography, saline infused sonography, and office hysteroscopy in reproductive-aged women with or without abnormal uterine bleeding. *Fertil Steril* 2005; **84**: 682–686.
19. Dijkhuizen FP, Mol BW, Brolmann HA, et al. The accuracy of endometrial sampling in the diagnosis of patients with endometrial carcinoma and hyperplasia: a meta-analysis. *Cancer* 2000; **89**(8): 1765–1772.
20. Rodriguez GC, Yaqub N, King ME. A comparison of the pipelle device and the Vabra aspirator as measured by endometrial denudation in hysterectomy specimens: the pipelle devices samples significantly less of the endometrial surface than the Vabra aspirator. *Am J Obstet Gynecol* 1993; **168**: 55–59.
21. American College of Obstetricians and Gynecologists. ACOG Practice Bulletin No. 136: Management of abnormal uterine bleeding associated with ovulatory dysfunction. *Obstet Gynecol* 2013; **136**: 1–10.
22. Politi MC, Han PK, Col NF. Communicating the uncertainty of harms and benefits of medical interventions. *Med Decis Making* 2007; **27**: 681.
23. Stewart A, Cummins C, Gold L, et al. The effectiveness of the levonorgestrel-releasing intrauterine system in menorrhagia: a systematic review. *BJOG*. 2001 Jan; **108** (1): 74–86. Review. PubMed PMID: 11213008.
24. Lowe RF, Prata N. Hemoglobin and serum ferritin levels in women using copper releasing or levonogestrel-releasing intrauterine devices: a systemic review. *Contraception* 2013; 486.
25. Monteiro I, Bahamondes L, Diaz J, et al. Therapeutic use of levonorgestrel-releasing intrauterine system in women with menorrhagia: a pilot study(1). *Contraception* 2002; **65**: 325–328.
26. Lethaby AE, Cooke I, Rees M. Progesterone or progestogen-releasing intrauterine systems for heavy menstrual bleeding. *Cochrane Database Syst Rev* 2005; **19**: CD002126.
27. Stewart A, Cummins C, Gold L, et al. The effectiveness of the levonorgestrel-releasing intrauterine system in menorrhagia: a systematic review. *BJOG: An International Journal of Obstetrics & Gynaecology* 2001; **108**: 74–86. doi: 10.1111/j.1471-0528.2001.00020.x
28. Lethaby A, Farquhar C, Cooke I. Antifibrinolytics for heavy menstrual bleeding. *Cochrane Database Syst Rev* 2000; **2**: CD000249.
29. Lukes AS, Moore KA, Muse KN, et al. Tranexamic acid treatment for heavy menstrual bleeding: a randomized controlled trial. *Obstet Gynecol* 2010; **116**: 865–875(I).
30. Lethaby A, Hickey M, Garry R, Penninx J. Endometrial resection / ablation techniques for heavy menstrual bleeding. *Cochrane Database Syst Rev* 2009; **4**: CD001501.
31. El-Nashar SA, Hopkins MR, Creedon DJ, et al. Prediction of treatment outcomes after global endometrial ablation. *Obstet Gynecol* 2009; **113**: 97.
32. Jin C, Hu Y, Chen XC, et al. Laparoscopic versus open myomectomy–a meta-analysis of randomized controlled trials. *Eur J Obstet Gynecol Reprod Biol* 2009; **145**: 14.
33. Hanafi M. Predictors of leiomyoma recurrence after myomectomy. *Obstet Gynecol* 2005; **105**(4): 877–881.
34. Garza Leal JG, Hernandez Leon I, Castillo Saenz L, et al. Laparoscopic ultrasound-guided radiofrequency volumetric thermal ablation of symptomatic uterine leiomyomas: feasibility study using the Halt 2000 Ablation System. *J Minim Invasive Gynecol* 2011; **18**: 364–371.

35. Berman JM, Guido RS, Leal JG, et al. Three-year outcome from the Halt trial: a prospective analysis of radiofrequency volumetric thermal ablation of myomas. *The J Minim Invasive Gynecol* 2014 Sep–Oct; **21**(5): 767–774. doi: 10.1016/j.jmig.2014.02.015. Epub 2014 Mar 5.
36. Kjerulff KH, Rhodes JC, Langenberg PW, et al. Patient satisfaction with results of hysterectomy. *Am J Obstet Gynecol* 2000; **183**: 1440.
37. Plockinger BJ, Kolbl H. Development of ovarian pathology after hysterectomy without oophorectomy. *J Am Coll Surg* 1994; **178**: 581–585.
38. Nieboer TE, Johnson N, Lethaby A, et al. Surgical approach to hysterectomy for benign gynaecological disease. *Cochrane Database of Syst Rev* 2009 Jul 8; **3**: CD003677. doi: 10.1002/14651858.CD003677.pub4.
39. ACOG. Committee Opinion No. 444: Choosing the route of hysterectomy for benign disease. *Obstet Gynecol* 2009; **114**(5): 1156–1158.
40. AAGL Advancing Minimally Invasive Gynecology Worldwide. AAGL position statement: route of hysterectomy to treat benign uterine disease. *J Minim Invasive Gynecol* 2011; **18**(1): 1–3.
41. US Food and Drug Administration. Laparoscopic Uterine Power Morcellation in Hysterectomy and Myomectomy: FDA Safety Communication. www.fda.gov/MedicalDevices/Safety/AlertsandNotices/ucm393576.htm. (Accessed April 28, 2014.)
42. Society of Gynecologic Oncology. Position statement on morcellation. www.sgo.org/newsroom/position-statements-2/morcellation. (Accessed April 28, 2014.)
43. Association of Gynecologic Laparoscopists. Member update on laparoscopic uterine power morcellation in hysterectomy and myomectomy. www.aagl.org/aaglnews/aagl-member-update-fda-issues-safety-communication-on-laparoscopic-uterine-power-morcellation-in-hysterectomy-and-myomectomy. (Accessed April 28, 2014.)
44. American College of Obstetricians and Gynecologists. ACOG Statement: FDA Issues Safety Communication on Laparoscopic Uterine Power Morcellation in Hysterectomy and Myomectomy. www.acog.org/About_ACOG/Announcements/FDA_Issues_Safety_Communication_on_Laparoscopic_Uterine_Power_Morcellation. (Accessed April 28, 2014.)
45. Bulman JC, Ascher AM, Spies JB. Current concepts in uterine fibroid embolization. *Radiographics* 2012; **32** (6): 1735–1750.
46. Omary RA, Vasireddy S, Chrisman HB, et al. The effect of pelvic MR imaging on the diagnosis and treatment of women with presumed symptomatic uterine fibroids. *J Vasc Interv Radiol* 2002; **13**(11): 1149–1153.
47. Deshmukh SP, Gonsalves CF, Guglielmo FF, Mitchell DG. Role of MR imaging of uterine leiomyomas before and after embolization. *Radiographics* 2012; **32**: E251–E281.
48. Kitamura Y, Ascher SM, Cooper C, et al. Imaging manifestations of complications associated with uterine artery embolization. *Radiographics* 2005; **25**: S119–S132.
49. Funaki K, Fukunishi H, Funaki T, Kawakami C. Mid-term outcome of magnetic resonance-guided focused ultrasound surgery for uterine myomas: from six to twelve months after volume reduction. *J Minim Invasive Gynecol* 2007; **14**(5): 616–621.

Chapter 17

Office care of sexually transmitted infections

Joanna Hooper and Lawrence Leeman

Introduction

Sexually transmitted infections (STI) can result in infertility, ectopic pregnancy, cervical cancer, and neonatal transmission. The bacterial STIs usually respond to antibiotic treatment; however, infection with human papillomavirus (HPV) or herpes simplex virus (HSV) may be life long. Psychological distress after the diagnosis of an STI is common due to concerns regarding the source of the infection, potential clinical sequelae, and the effect on sexuality and relationships.

Chlamydia and gonorrhea

Cervicitis caused by chlamydia and gonorrhea is typically asymptomatic. About 6%–14% of women report symptoms with chlamydia cervicitis, and approximately 30% of women are symptomatic with gonorrhea cervicitis.[1, 2] Nonspecific symptoms include abnormal discharge, inter-menstrual or post-coital bleeding which may be mistaken for bacterial vaginosis, or dysfunctional uterine bleeding. The less common condition of chlamydia urethritis should be considered in women with sterile pyuria, particularly younger women at increased risk of chlamydial infection.

Unfortunately, women often present with later stage manifestations of gonococcal or chlamydial infection including pelvic inflammatory disease (PID) and ectopic pregnancy. PID increases the risk of tubal pregnancy, from 15% with the first occurrence, to 75% after three episodes of PID, and the number of episodes is associated with increased risk of tubal infertility.[3, 4]

Epidemiology

Young age is the primary nonmodifiable risk factor for chlamydia and gonorrheal infection, with prevalence highest for women age 25 and younger. Young age is a risk factor both because of age-related changes in sexual behavior, and the possibility of acquired immunity from repeat infections.[5] Chlamydia is the most common reportable bacterial infection in the United States with 467.7 cases per 100,000 people in 2012.[6] Other risk factors for acquiring *C. trachomatis* include previous infection, a history of having had another sexually transmitted infection, a new sex partner within the last three months, and inconsistent use of condoms.[7] The reported incidence is approximately twice as high in women; this may be due to increased screening of women.[8]

Gonorrhea is the second most common reportable bacterial STI with a rate of 108.7 cases per 100,000 women in 2012. Rates of gonorrhea infection among African-American women are about 15 times higher than for Caucasian women in the United States.[8]

Pathophysiology

C. trachomatis is a gram-negative obligate intracellular bacterium, which has an affinity for columnar epithelium that lines mucous membranes. Chlamydia most commonly initially infects the cervix and occasionally the urethra. It can later ascend the genital tract and cause pelvic inflammatory disease. Cervical infection with *C. trachomatis* is typically asymptomatic. *C. trachomatis* can also infect pharyngeal and rectal cells; these infections are also typically asymptomatic and can therefore be spread to partners through oral or anal sex. *C. trachomatis* can infect the conjunctiva of newborns during vaginal delivery leading to conjunctival scarring and blindness if untreated.

Neisseria gonorrhea is a gram-negative diplococci that needs to be intracellular for multiplication. Most commonly it infects the columnar epithelium of the cervix, then ascends the genital tract potentially causing pelvic inflammatory disease. Gonococcal cervicitis is typically asymptomatic, but symptoms can be nonspecific including dyspareunia, lower abdominal and pelvic pain, or a purulent vaginal discharge. Gonococcal

Office Care of Women, ed. Martin E. Olsen and Botros Rizk. Published by Cambridge University Press.

urethritis, with dysuria and purulent urethral discharge, is less common.

Screening recommendations

The Centers for Disease Control and Prevention (CDC) recommends that all sexually active patients 25 years of age and younger be screened annually regardless of symptoms or other risk factors. Women older than 25 years of age who are deemed to be high risk based on risk factors just described should also be screened.[9] Women who have sex only with women are still at risk of contracting chlamydia and therefore should be tested using the same criteria as heterosexual women. The CDC and the US Preventive Task Forces (USPTF) recommend that pregnant women be screened with each pregnancy.

Nucleic acid amplification tests (NAAT) are the recommended method for chlamydia and gonorrheal testing due to higher sensitivity and specificity than other tests; a single swab tests for both.[10] Endocervical collection of the specimen is common, however alternatives that do not require a speculum examination may increase acceptability to patients and compliance with screening. Vaginal NAAT swabs or first catch urine specimens can be collected by patients.

Providers may consider testing women at risk of oral or rectal infection by swabbing the pharynx or rectum as approximately 10% of chlamydia and 31% of gonorrhea cases would be missed in women without extra-genital testing.[11] However, the number of women needed to screen to detect 1 case is 70, and specific guidelines have not been made with regard to routine extra-genital screening.[12]

A follow-up test for both gonorrhea and chlamydia is recommended three months after treatment.[13] NAAT results may still be positive despite adequate treatment if collected within three weeks of treatment as nucleic acids from the infection could still be present. Antibiotic resistant gonorrhea is increasing, and women with treatment failure or recurrent infection should have an endocervical culture with antibiotic sensitivities sent. Antibiotic resistance for chlamydia is rare, and a persistent positive result is typically from reinfection from the same partner.[10]

Treatment

The CDC recommends treatment for chlamydia with either a single 1 g of oral azithromycin, or 100 mg of doxycycline (for nonpregnant women only) by mouth twice daily for one week. The ease of the single dose improves adherence, which may be further increased by observed administration.[14] Treatment failures after doxycycline or azithromycin are usually due to reinfection; 15%–30% of women treated for chlamydia become reinfected.[13] Partner treatment is essential to minimize risk of reinfection.

Two agents are required to treat *N. gonorrhea* because of resistance to several antibiotics (fluoroquinolones, penicillins, sulfonamides, and tetracycline). The current recommended first-line treatment is ceftriaxone 250 mg IM and 1 gram of PO azithromycin or doxycycline 100 mg PO BID for seven days. Given the ease of one dose versus seven days of treatment, azithromycin is preferred over the doxycycline. The combination of the antibiotics provides synergy to treat gonorrhea regardless of co-infection status with *C. trachomatis*.[15]

An alternate regimen, although less favored due to antibiotic resistance, includes cefixime 400 mg PO once plus either one dose of 1 g of azithromycin or the weeklong course of doxycycline. Another alternative is monotherapy with 2 g of oral azithromycin, which is the only option for patients who have an allergy to cephalosporins. CDC no longer recommends cefixime as a first-line choice due to lower serum levels than ceftriaxone and growing resistance. If cefixime or monotherapy with azithromycin is used, the recommendation is to collect a culture at site of infection in one week as a trial of cure test.[14] For treatment failure, the patient should receive 250 mg of IM ceftriaxone and 2 g of oral azithromycin, an endocervical culture with antibiotic sensitivities should be collected, and consultation with an infectious disease or family planning specialist is recommended.[14] A clinical trial by the CDC and the National Institute of Health in 2013 showed that regimens using oral azithromycin in combination with injectable gentamicin, or oral azithromycin with oral gemifloxacin were effective in treating gonorrhea with cure rates of 100% and 99.5%, respectively. The regimens were poorly tolerated, are not considered first line choices, but offer clinicians an alternative therapy option.[16]

Pelvic inflammatory disease

Epidemiology

Pelvic inflammatory disease (PID) encompasses infections of the upper female genital tract that including salpingitis, endometritis, tubo-ovarian abscess and/or pelvic peritonitis. The downstream sequelae of PID include ectopic pregnancy and tubal infertility. *Neisseria gonorrhea* and *Chlamydia trachomatis* are the "classic" organisms responsible for PID and are present in about 65%–75% of cases of PID; however, PID infections are commonly polymicrobial. Anaerobic vaginal bacteria, gardnerella vaginalis, enteric gram-negative rods, mycoplasma hominus, and ureaplasma urealyticum have all been implicated as causal organisms. The PEACH Trial demonstrated that women with PID associated with chlamydia or mycoplasma had symptoms for a week longer prior to seeking medical evaluation than women with *N. gonorrhea* associated PID. This suggests that gonorrheal PID has a more acute and severe presentation.[17]

Prevention

Two approaches to prevent the sequelae of PID are to screen and treat chlamydia and gonorrhea at the stage of asymptomatic cervicitis and to treat sexually active women with mild symptoms when these are suspicious for PID. The British POPI study demonstrated that 9.5% of 74 women with untreated asymptomatic chlamydia cervicitis developed PID within 12 months.[18] Although most women with tubal infertility do not have a known history of PID, a World Health Organization (WHO) study demonstrated serological evidence of prior chlamydia or gonorrhea infection in 93% of women with bilateral tubal infertility compared to 40% of fertile controls subjects.[19]

Clinical presentation and diagnosis

The presentation of PID may include pelvic or abdominal pain, fever, leukocytosis, elevated ESR or c-reactive protein, mucopurulent cervical or vaginal discharge, and white blood cells (WBCs) on wet mount; however even when several of these findings are present, specificity and sensitivity remain low. A classic study of Swedish women showed that even when using the most specific findings (fever >38.3°C/100.9°F, elevated ESR, and adnexal tenderness), PID confirmed by laparoscopic salpingitis was only present in 65% of the women studied.[20] Additionally, if all three findings were required for diagnosis, sensitivity was low, and failed to detect 35% of cases of laparoscopic-confirmed salpingitis.

Many cases of PID have mild nonspecific symptoms resulting in delayed diagnosis. Laparoscopic diagnosis of Salpingitis may be considered definitive, but the test is expensive and its invasive nature limits its use to women with mild symptoms. Increased rates of tubal infertility and ectopic pregnancy have led to concerns about under treatment; therefore, in 2002 the CDC expanded recommendations for empiric treatment. All sexually active young women or other women at risk for STDs should receive antibiotic treatment if they have pelvic or abdominal pain not explained by another etiology along with the presence of cervical motion, uterine or adnexal tenderness.[14]

Treatment

Most women with suspected PID can be treated in the outpatient setting with outcomes equivalent to inpatient parenteral antibiotic treatment. Exceptions may include women with severe symptomatic illness including those with high fever, tubo-ovarian abscess, pregnancy, inability to tolerate oral medications, or peritoneal signs in whom another form of acute abdomen cannot be ruled out. Failure to respond to oral antibiotics within three days is another indication for inpatient treatment with parenteral antibiotics. The three recommended outpatient regimens include 14 days of doxycycline 100 mg PO BID along with any one of the following: one dose of ceftriaxone 250 mg IM, cefoxitin 2 g IM with probenicid 1 g oral, or other third-generation parenteral cephalosporin.[15] Metronidazole 500 mg orally twice a day (BID) for 14 days may be used as part of the initial treatment, although this is optional based on 2010 CDC recommendations. Oral quinolones and oral cefixime are no longer recommended as first-line treatment for outpatient PID treatment due to resistant *Neisseria gonorrhea*.[21] All women with PID should be reevaluated in three days. Women with tubo-ovarian abscess need a minimum of 24 hours of inpatient parenteral antibiotics. CDC recommended parenteral regimens include IV cefotetan or cefoxitin with IV or oral doxycycline, or intravenous clindamycin and gentamicin.[15] Women with an intrauterine device (IUD) in place should not have routine removal; removal has not shown improved outcomes. If no improvement occurs after 72 hours of treatment, removal should be considered.[22] Male partners within 60 days of diagnosis should be treated, and if there have been no partners within the last 60 days, then the last partner should be treated.

Herpes simplex virus

Herpes simplex viruses are double-stranded DNA viruses. During the initial infection, virions travel up the nerve roots to the ganglia where they can remain latent. Reactivation of latent viral infection can occur traveling back down the nerve to cause cutaneous symptoms typically including painful blisters or ulcers. Women may be totally asymptomatic from their HSV infection.[23] HSV-2 is transmitted though sexual contact as well as perinatal transmission. Genital HSV-1 can be transmitted through oral contact as well as vaginal or anal intercourse.[23]

Epidemiology

About two-thirds of the US population are seropositive for HSV-1. Most acquired the oro-labial form nonsexually during childhood. Adults who acquire HSV-1 are much more likely to acquire the virus through sexual activity. HSV-2 is less common; approximately 17% of the adult US population is sero-positive for HSV-2.[24, 25] HSV has a short incubation period of 2–12 days; patients typically can accurately identify the person who infected them.[26] People who share information about infection with their partners are less likely to infect their partners, likely due to protective measures.[27]

Natural history

Previous infection with HSV-1 does not decrease the rate of HSV-2 acquisition; however, patient's previously infected with HSV-1 who acquire HSV-2 are less likely to be symptomatic.[28] Women who have HSV-2 are more likely to experience recurrences than those with genital HSV-1, and the recurrences tend to be more severe. The duration of the primary infection appears to be positively correlated with increased number of recurrences. 90% of symptomatic persons with genital HSV-2 infection will have a recurrence compared to 57% of patients with primary genital HSV-1.[29, 30] A woman previously infected with the oro-labial form of HSV-1 appears to be protected against genital HSV-1.[31] Additionally, people who are already infected with HSV-2 are unlikely to subsequently acquire HSV-1.[32]

Viral shedding occurs more frequently with HSV-2 than HSV-1. Within the first year of acquisition of the infection, viral shedding occurs on 30% of days and does not seem to be correlated with the presence of a lesion, and often precedes symptoms.[33]

Screening and diagnosis

The USPSTF recommends against routine serological screening for herpes in asymptomatic persons, and IgM testing is not a reliable indicator of recent infection.[34] Serological testing may be useful for women with recurrent genital symptoms or atypical symptoms who had a negative NAAT, or patients who have been told they have HSV based on clinical symptoms, but who do not have a laboratory diagnosis. One can also consider testing HIV+ persons who present for STD testing.[15]

Prevention and treatment of genital HSV

There is no cure for HSV infection. Antiviral therapy can reduce symptoms, morbidity, and duration of viral shedding, but it has no impact on eradicating the disease or on latent HSV. Treatment during a primary or secondary outbreak does not decrease recurrence.[35]

Consistent condom use can reduce the spread to an unaffected partner. Perfect condom use (100% of the time) results in 30% lower risk of spreading HSV to the unaffected partner.[36] Consistent condom use along with suppressive therapy with antiviral medication can reduce transmission rates by 55%.[37]

Primary HSV can be particularly painful and prolonged (19 days vs. 10 days duration on average for a recurrence), so it should be treated with antivirals. Acyclovir, famciclovir, and valacyclovir are all extremely well tolerated with a very low risk of toxicity and appear to have similar efficacy (see Table 17-1).[38, 39]

Perinatal transplacental transmission to the fetus with subsequent neonatal infection occurs in 30%–50% of neonates when vaginal delivery occurs with active genital lesions of a primary infection compared to only 3% in women having a vaginal delivery with active lesions due to a recurrent infection.[40] Pregnant women with a primary infection during pregnancy should be treated with antivirals to decreased duration and severity of symptoms as well as decrease viral shedding.

Confirmation with viral or serological testing should be considered in patients with only a clinical diagnosis. Pregnant women with a history of recurrent active genital herpes should be offered suppressive treatment with antivirals starting at 36 weeks and through the remainder of the pregnancy.[41] Additionally, if active genital lesions are present at the time of delivery, cesarean delivery should be

Table 17-1 Dosing for antivirals for herpes simplex virus [15, 72]

	Primary infection treatment	Chronic suppressive therapy for recurrent disease	Episodic treatment for recurrent disease	Suppressive therapy in pregnancy (starting @36 w)
Acyclovir	400 mg TID *or* 200 mg 5 × /day for 7–10 days	400 mg BID	800 mg BID *or* 200 mg 5 × /day	400 mg TID
Famciclovir	250 mg TID for 7 days	250 mg BID	125 mg BID	Limited data in pregnancy
Valacyclovir	1g BID for 10 days	1 g daily (or 500 mg daily for pts <9 episodes/yr)	500 mg BID × 3 days	500 mg BID

performed; however, lesions on the sacrum or thigh may be covered to facilitate safe vaginal delivery.[41] The routine screening of women for serological evidence of genital herpes infection is not recommended.

Patients with primary HSV infections may have severe dysuria secondary to ulcerations near the urethra, or difficulty urinating because of sacral nerve root involvement. In such cases adjunctive pain medications or catheterization may be needed.

Patients with complicated HSV [meningitis or central nervous system (CNS) involvement, disseminated HSV, pneumonitis, or hepatitis] require parenteral administration of antivirals.

Syphilis

Reported primary and secondary syphilis in 2013 was nearly 10 times more common in men than women. This increased rate of infection appears to be primarily among men who have sex with men; nearly 75% of cases are within this cohort.[42]

The highest risk women are those aged 20–24 (3.9/100,000 in 2012).[42] Despite the low incident rates, syphilis is considered a major public health risk among women due to the serious morbidities of congenital and tertiary syphilis. A high coinfection rate with HIV exists as the genital sores make it easier to transmit HIV.[43] Socioeconomic disparities also are associated with higher rates of syphilis.[43] Syphilis reporting is important, as insuring partners of index cases receive testing and treatment.[44]

Pathophysiology

The causative organism for syphilis is the spirochete *Treponemal pallidum*.[45] Syphilis has three stages: primary, secondary, and tertiary. Transmission occurs during the primary stage from direct contact with a syphilitic sore through vaginal, anal, or oral sex. Transplacental infection can occur. People are infectious in the primary and secondary stages but may be completely asymptomatic during these stages.

Primary syphilis is characterized by a chancre that typically appears on the genitals approximately three weeks after sexual contact with a syphilis infected individual. The chancre may be on the vaginal wall or cervix; it is a raised erythematous appearing lesion that is often painless and lasts for three to six weeks. Dark-field microscopy or immunofluorescent stains of exudate from the chancre would show many spirochetes.

Approximately 75% of patients with untreated primary syphilis will develop secondary syphilis. The secondary stage of the disease is characterized by spread of the spirochetes to mucocutaneous tissues and skin. Clinically it can present as condyloma lata, palmar rash, diffuse rash (Figure 17-1), or lymphadenopathy. Condyloma lata are raised silvery gray plaques that appear typically in moist areas such as the axilla, inner thighs, and anogenital area. Patients can develop additional superficial spirochete-containing lesions in mucous membranes. Patients typically then go on to develop a latent phase that can last several years during which time milder versions of the superficial lesions can periodically recur.

Tertiary syphilis occurs in one-third of untreated patients and most frequently manifests as cardiovascular syphilis, which causes syphilitic aortitis that can lead to aortic aneurysm and aortic valve insufficiency. Less frequently, tertiary syphilis manifests as neurosyphilis. Neurosyphilis presents as tabes dorsalis, meningovascular disease, and general paresis. Late benign syphilis, or gummatous syphilis, is characterized by gummas

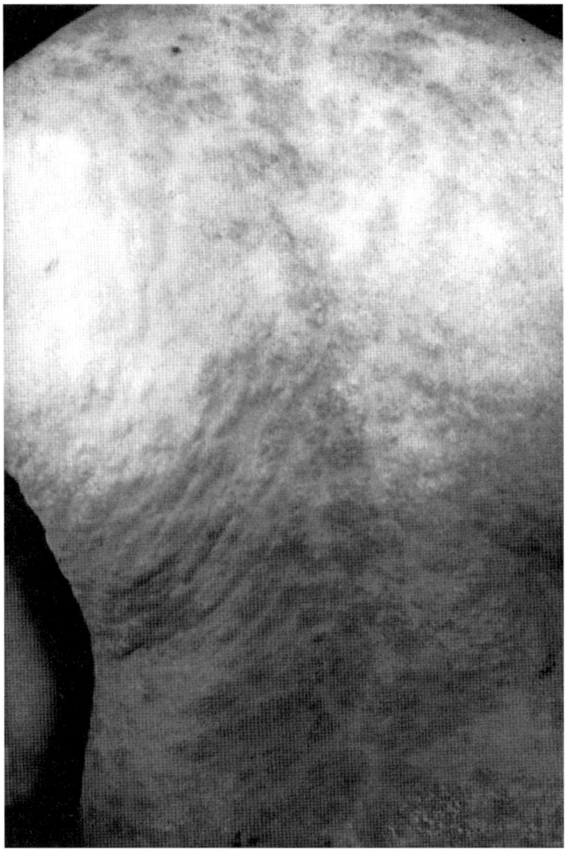

Figure 17-1 This patient presented with a secondary syphilitic rash covering his back representing the systemic spread of the *Treponema pallidum* bacteria. (Courtesy of CDC/Dr. Gavin Hart.)

that can form on the bone, skin, liver, or mucous membranes, particularly of the oropharynx. Tertiary syphilis has become rare since the advent of penicillin.

Screening and testing

Syphilis screening of women should include every pregnant woman at the first prenatal visit, commercial sex workers, persons in correctional facilities, persons infected with HIV, persons who exchange sex for drugs, and patients with genital ulcers consistent with chancres. Routine screening in asymptomatic low-risk individuals is not recommended.[46]

Traditionally, testing for *T. pallidum* was conducted by initially performing the nonspecific, quantitative, rapid plasma reagin test (RPR). RPR has good sensitivity, however, due to poor specificity a confirmatory treponemal test, is indicated, most

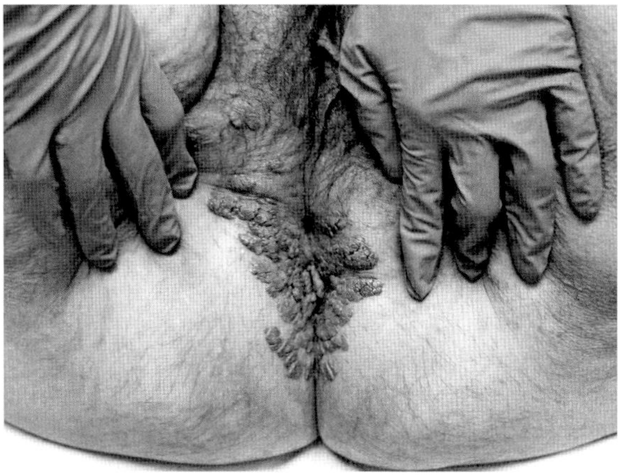

Figure 17-2 Also known as "condyloma lata," this photograph depicts the appearance of what was determined to be secondary syphilitic lesions on a patient's perineum. Condyloma lata lesions are smooth, moist, and flat, whereas condylomata acuminatum lesions, though similar, are cauliflower-like, dry, and bulky, respectively. (Photo courtesy of CDC/Joyce Ayers.)

commonly the Fluorescent Treponemal Antibody absorption test (FTA-ABS).

Recently more sensitive and specific *T. pallidum* immunoassays have been developed that are being used as the initial screening test, with the RPR for confirmation.[47] One issue is that *T. pallidum* IgG will persistently be positive in people who have a history of successfully treated infection. The RPR can help distinguish patients with active infection from patients with treated infection, as quantitative titer should fall after treatment. The documentation of the history of treatment as well as prior and current RPR titers is part of the evaluation of a positive treponemal test.

Condyloma lata lesions (Figure 17-2) are smooth, moist, and flat, while condylomata acuminatum lesions, though similar, are cauliflower-like, dry, and often bulky.[48]

Treatment

Penicillin is the antibiotic of choice and has been proven clinically over many decades of experience to be effective. For early primary and secondary infection, the CDC recommends the use of Benzathine penicillin G (Bicillin L-A) due to its long half-life which effectively treats the slowly multiplying spirochete This should not be confused with Bicillin C-R, which has a significantly shorter half-life and has been shown to not be effective. Benzathine penicillin G should be given in one dose of 2.4 million units IM.[49]

For latent syphilis, intramuscular Benzathine penicillin G 2.4 million units should be given weekly for three weeks. There is no evidence of penicillin resistance; however, macrolide resistance has begun to emerge. Therefore penicillin remains the treatment of choice for pregnant penicillin-allergic patients, who should undergo penicillin desensitization.[49]

One possible complication of treatment is the Jarisch-Herxheimer reaction, which includes fever, myalgias, malaise, and typically occurs within the first 24 hours of treatment for early syphilis. It can be managed with antipyretics and should not prevent treatment.

For penicillin-allergic patients with early syphilis who are not pregnant, alternative treatment options include doxycycline 100 mg by mouth twice a day for 14 days or 2 g of oral azithromycin in one dose in patients with medication compliance problems. The doxycycline is preferred as resistance is emerging to azithromycin.

For latent syphilis in the penicillin-allergic patient, a longer course of antibiotics is required; patients should receive doxycycline 100 mg by mouth twice daily for 28 days.[50]

Genital ulcers

Herpes simplex virus and syphilis are the most common causes of genital ulcers; however, the differential diagnosis is broad and includes infectious and noninfectious etiologies. Noninfectious causes include sexual trauma, Behcet syndrome, psoriasis, cancer, fixed drug eruptions, and Wegener's graulomatosis.[15, 51] Chancroid (*Haemophilus ducreyi*), granuloma inguinale, and lymphogranuloma venereum are three uncommon STIs that should be considered in evaluation of ulcers that are not clinically consistent and confirmed to be herpetic or syphilitic in origin. Due to the occurrence of ulcers with multiple organisms, all women with genial ulcers should be tested for HSV with PCR test and syphilis with serological testing.

Chancroid presents as a genital or perianal lesion. It is quite uncommon with only 28 cases reported by US state health departments in 2009, although underreporting is suspected.[51] The ulcers are commonly quite painful and are accompanied by unilateral suppurative adenopathy. It is common for chancroid ulcers to be co-infected with HSV. The ulcers should be cultured specifically for *H. ducreyi*; however, laboratory diagnosis is difficult and a commercial PCR is not available. Only about 80% of women with lesions have a successful culture based diagnosis. A probable diagnosis of chancroid can be made if a painful ulcer accompanied by clinical presentation and adenopathy consistent with chancroid are present in a patient after syphilis and HSV have been ruled out. The treatment can be a single intramuscular injection of ceftriaxone (250 mg) or a 1-g oral dose of azithromycin.[15] Alternatives include ciprofloxacin 500 mg oral twice daily for three days or erythromycin 500 mg orally three times a day for seven days. In general, symptoms should start to improve within three days with ulcer resolution in seven days, although larger ulcers may take two weeks or longer to completely resolve. A trial of cure is not needed; however, sexual partners from the 10-day period prior to the occurrence of the genital ulcer should be seen and treated. The infected patient should be rechecked for HIV and syphilis three months after treatment if initial tests were negative.

Granuloma inguinale is very rare in the United States; however, it is endemic in many tropical areas and should be suspected in individuals presenting with a slowly growing germinal or perineal ulcer after travel to these areas. The ulcers are painless, have a beefy red appearance, commonly bleed, and are without accompanying adenopathy. The causative organism is the intracellular gram-negative bacterium *Klebsiella granulomatis*, which is hard to identify. Microscopic examination of biopsy specimen or crushed tissue for Donovan bodies is required. The treatment of choice is azithromycin one gram weekly or 50 mg daily for at least three weeks and until all ulcers have resolved.[15] Doxycycline, ciprofloxacin, erythromycin, and trimethoprim-sulfamethoxazole are alternatives. Sexual contacts within the 60-day period prior to the development of symptoms should be offered treatment.[15]

Lymphogranuloma venereum (LGV) commonly presents in women as tender, unusual unilateral inguinal or femoral adenopathy. Although an ulcer may initially be present, it may no longer be visible at the time of diagnosis. The organism is *Chlamydia trachomatis serovars* L1, L2, and L3 and these may be identified by culture of genital swabs or aspirated suppurative lymph nodes. LGV can be an invasive systemic illness with proctocolitis progressing to fistulas, strictures, and chronic colitis that can be mistaken for inflammatory bowel disease. Treatment is doxycycline by mouth twice daily for 21 days and presumptive treatment after examination should be given to contacts within sixty days of the development of symptoms.[15]

Genital warts

Human papillomavirus (HPV) infection can cause genital warts or cervical dysplasia. More than 140 different HPV viruses exist; about 40 of these have been shown to be sexually transmissible through vaginal, anal, or oral contact. HPV is the most common STI. Thirteen genotypes can cause cervical cancer with HPV 16 and 18 being the highest risk infections. The CDC estimates that 360,000 individuals acquire genital warts each year.[31] About 90% of cases of genital warts are due to HPV genotypes 6 and 11.[52]

The quadrivalent vaccine offers protection against HPV 6, 11, 16, and 18. The bivalent vaccine only covers 16 and 18 and does not have a meaningful effect on the incidence of genital warts. The CDC recommends vaccination for all girls and women from age 11 or 12 through age 26. Vaccination is recommended for all males aged 12–21 or through age 26 for men who have sex with men. For both vaccines, three injections are recommended with the second one to two months after the first dose and the third six months after the first dose.

Vaccination of males with the quadrivalent vaccine is beneficial in decreasing their risk for genital condyloma and anal intraepithelial neoplasia; their female sexual partners risk of cervical cancer and genital condyloma will also be reduced.[53, 54]

Diagnosis

Genital warts (*Condyloma accuminata*) may have a classic verrucous or cauliflower appearance or they may be flat, papular, or keratotic. Or they may resolve prior to detection. Size can range from 1–2 mm up to several centimeters (Figure 17-3).

A singe wart or multiple lesions may be present. The warts can be found on the vulvar, perineal, perianal, vaginal, or cervical areas. Asymptomatic women may experience burning, itching, or pain with intercourse.

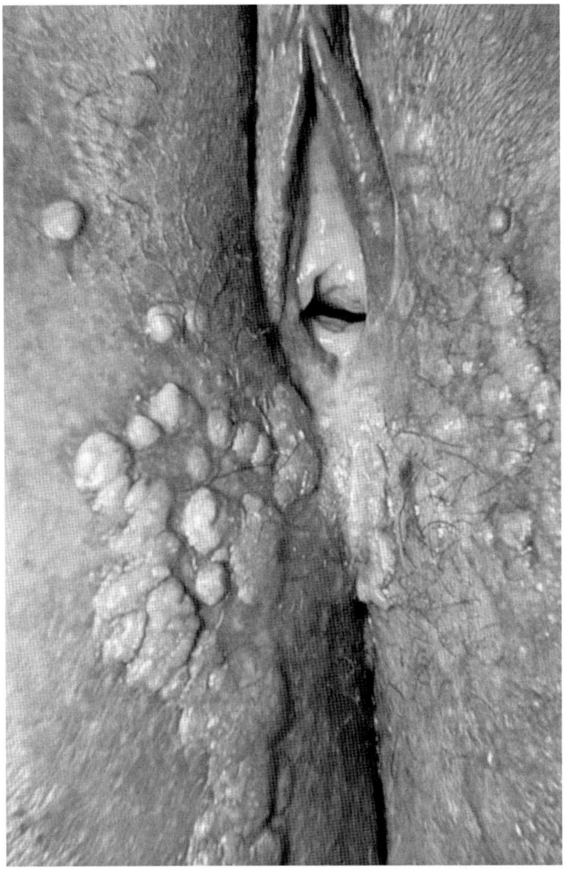

Figure 17-3 Perianal genital warts. (Courtesy of Dr. Alan Waxman of the University of New Mexico.)

Transmission and psychosocial issues

Genital warts are easily transmitted through skin-to-skin contact. The incubation period is most commonly from three weeks to three months. It may be difficult to determine the timing of exposure or specific partner associated with the infection.

Patient psychological stress can be substantial. [55, 56] The presence of genital condyloma can adversely affect self-image, relationships, and sexual activity and cause anxiety and depression. The uncertainty regarding the time to resolution, success of various treatments, concern for HPV-related cancers, and concern of transmission to current or future sexual partners, physical discomfort, and treatment-related limitations on sexual activity are common patient concerns.

Risk of cancer

The genotypes (6 and 11) that commonly cause external genital condyloma are not high risk for cervical cancer induction. Women should have age and history appropriate high-risk HPV screening with Pap testing since they may be infected with multiple HPV genotypes. Women who are 26 years old or younger should be offered HPV vaccination. Modifiable risk factors for cervical cancer include smoking cessation, condom use and limiting the number of sexual partners.

Treatment

Treatment modalities include self-administered home treatments, provider administered outpatient options, and treatments that are usually performed in an operating room setting. It is common for multiple modalities to be sequentially required to successfully eradicate the warts. Spontaneous resolution will occur within 6–12 months in 30%–40% of cases.[57] There is no evidence that treatment will decrease the likelihood of transmission or result in the elimination of the presence of the HPV virus from the genital tract. Even after successful treatment the recurrence rate remains high (13%–65%) indicating that the virus is still present.[52]

Patient applied treatment

Many patients prefer patient-applied treatments that can be administered at home. These include Imiquimod (3.75% or 5%), Podophyllotoxin 0.5%, and Sinecatechins 15%. None of these patient-applied formulations are approved for use in pregnancy.

Imiquimod is as an immune response modifier. The original 5% formulation is applied three times per week at night and washed off in 6–10 hours for up to 16 weeks. The 3.75% Imiquimod cream was approved by the FDA in 2010. It is used daily for two weeks with same requirement to wash off in 6–10 hours. The two-week treatment may be repeated after a two-week rest up to a maximum of eight weeks of treatment. It is available as a dose metered pump.

Podophyllotoxin 5% is an antimitotic drug that induces tissue necrosis. It is applied twice daily for three days. After a four-day "rest period" the treatment is repeated for another three days; a maximum of four cycles can be administered. The solution is applied with a cotton swab and the gel is applied with the fingers. Mild to moderate pain may occur. The newest patient applied treatment is Sinetcatechin 15%, a green tea extract. It is applied three times per day for a maximum of 16 weeks. Side effects include burning, redness, pain, and a vesicular rash.

Physician-administered treatment

Trichloracetic acid (TCA) or bichloracetic acid in 80% solution may be applied weekly or every other week. It must be washed off after six hours and may cause pain and local inflammation. It is safe in pregnancy and may be applied to vagina, anal canal, or perianal area as well as to the vulva or perineum. Cryotherapy is another provider treatment that can be used in a spray form, by cotton applicator, or with a metal cryoprobe. It may be used in pregnancy; however, vaginal application in pregnancy is not appropriate. Carbon dioxide laser may be useful when widespread disease has been resistant to other treatment. Laser requires use of anesthesia or analgesia.

Choice of treatment

For first-time lesions in a single location, TCA or cryotherapy are first-line choices. For first-time warts in multiple locations, the Planned Parenthood Federation of America (PPFA) recommends Imiquimod. Additionally, Imiquimod is recommended for recurrent warts, or failure of TCA or cryotherapy to clear warts in three treatment sessions.[58]

Pregnancy and HPV infection

Genital warts can increase rapidly in size and number during pregnancy. HPV can rarely be transmitted to the infant during birth and cause lower respiratory papillomatosis. The CDC recommends cesarean delivery only if the condylomas enlarge such that the vaginal outlet is obstructed or at risk of excessive bleeding.[15] Due to the potential for rapid proliferation, treatment may be considered early in pregnancy.

Patient applied treatments with imiquimod, sinecatechins, or podofilox are all contraindicated in pregnancy, as is office treatment with podophyllin.[52] Cryotherapy, surgical excision, electrosurgery, CO_2 laser, and chemical treatment with trichloracetic acid all are acceptable treatment options in pregnancy.

Trichomonas

Epidemiology

T. vaginalis is not a reportable disease; best estimates, however, indicate that it is one of the most common nonviral infections. A large study of reproductive aged women in the United States showed overall infection rates of 1.3%. African-American women were found to have higher rates of infection. Trichomonas is more common in women who douche. Infection rates were also associated with increasing age and increased number of sexual partners.[59]

Trichomonas is of public health significance since infection seems to be positively associated with higher rates of HIV acquisition and it's association with preterm delivery.

Pathophysiology

Trichomonas vaginalis is an oval-shaped-flagellated protozoan that typically infects the squamous epithelium of the vagina, but it can also infect the urethra, periurethral glands, and rarely the bladder. It is not found in the oropharynx or rectum. Sexual transmission occurs in penetrative sex between men and women, but transmission between women who have sex with women also occurs. Bacterial vaginosis may coexist. The classic presentation is a foul-smelling frothy discharge, but up to 50% of infected women can be asymptomatic.[60] No natural immune response against *Trichamonas* is mounted; therefore, reinfection between partners is common.

Testing and screening

Testing is performed in women with abnormal vaginal discharge, and screening should be considered in women with risk factors including multiple sex partners, IV drug use, women who exchange sex for drugs, and women who have a history of STI.

Testing can be performed by wet mount if the slide is viewed immediately after collection (see Figure 17-4). Wet mount has a sensitivity of only 60%–70%,[61] whereas newer DNA testing has sensitivities ranging from 69.5% to 96.8%.[62] Cultures can also be used, but the culture has to be immediately processed by the laboratory, or the sensitivity drops very significantly. Cultures are therefore less practical than wet prep or newer NAAT testing.

Treatment

T. vaginalis can be treated by single dose therapy with 2 g of metronidazole by mouth. Alternatively, it can be treated with a seven-day course of metronidazole 500 mg by mouth twice daily. The single dose option can cause more gastrointestinal distress. The partner needs to be treated as well, and both should abstain from sex for one week. Of note, tinidazole has a half-life of 13 hours compared to 6–7 hours for metronidazole, so after tinidazole consumption, a patient should avoid alcohol for at least 72 hours; the alcohol avoidance is less for metronidazole. Some resistance to metronidazole is emerging and tinidazole may be considered in cases of treatment failure. When single-dose treatment with metronidazole has not been curative then a seven-day course should be considered. Vaginal metronidazole preparations are not recommended by the CDC for trichomoniasis. Most treatment "failures" are a result of reinfection.

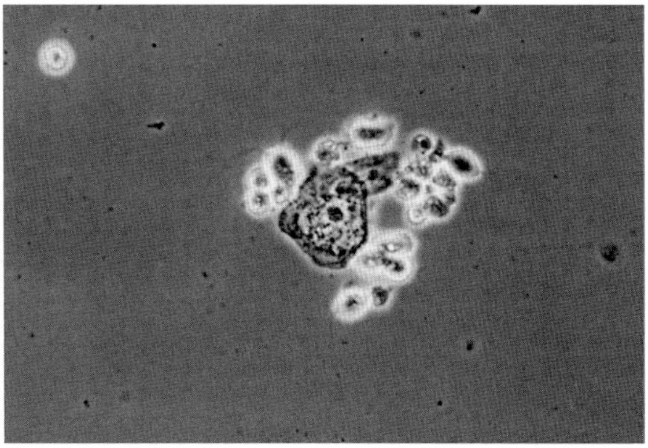

Figure 17-4 This phase contrast wet mount micrograph of a vaginal discharge revealed the presence of *Trichomonas vaginalis* protozoa. (Photo courtesy of the CDC, 1986.)

In pregnancy, symptomatic women can be treated with metronidazole and may tolerate the seven-day course better than the 2-g one-time dose because of the nausea related to pregnancy. Metronidazole is safe to use even in the first trimester of pregnancy and can be used for symptomatic women.[63] In asymptomatic pregnant women, however, treatment has actually been shown to increase rates of preterm delivery (possibly due to disrupted vaginal flora),[64] so treatment may be deferred until 37 weeks in these women.[15]

HIV

Epidemiology

Based on estimates by the WHO and the UNAIDS, at the end of 2013 an estimated 39 million people worldwide were living with HIV. In 2013, there were over 1.5 million AIDS-related deaths. It is estimated that over 70% of new infections occur in sub-Saharan Africa and is spread predominately through heterosexual sex.[65] In the United States the majority of cases are male-to-male sexual transmission, but a quarter of cases occur during heterosexual sex.[66]

Risk factors for HIV acquisition include vaginal or anal intercourse without a condom particularly with new or multiple partners, men who have sex with men, and needle sharing for IV drug use. Sexually transmitted infections that can disrupt the mucosal layer such as syphilis, gonorrhea, chlamydia, trichomonas, or bacterial vaginosis also increases chances of HIV acquisition.[66]

Pathophysiology

Human immunodeficiency virus is a retrovirus that attacks immune and dendritic cells, leaving the body vulnerable to opportunistic infections and cancers.

Transmission typically occurs through transfer of semen or blood through vaginal or anal sex but can also occur with oral sex, needle sticks, breast milk, transplacentally, or during birth.[66]

Screening and prevention

The USPSTF recommends screening all individuals aged 15–65 and those older and younger if risk factors are present, with increased screening intervals for those who are high risk. Pregnant women should also be screened at the beginning of each pregnancy.[67]

There is no cure for HIV/AIDS that will eliminate the virus; however, antiretroviral treatment (ART) can reduce viral loads, improve longevity, and decrease transmission. Transmission can be prevented by condom use, decreasing number of sexual partners, and voluntary male circumcision in high prevalence areas (reduction of up to 60%).[66] Pregnant women who are HIV positive should be treated during prenatal care and labor with ART to prevent vertical transmission.[68] In high prevalence areas, breastfeeding accompanied by antiretroviral treatment may be recommended by each individual country as the benefits of breastfeeding on other forms of infant mortality outweigh the diminished risk of HIV transmission to the infant.[69]

Concluding remarks

Sexually transmitted infections have high morbidity; prevention is optimal. Use of condoms and modification of high-risk sexual activity are the primary preventive methods, and women's health-care providers traditionally have emphasized these recommendations. A review of behavioral sexual reduction counseling by the US Preventive Services Task Force has demonstrated that high-intensity (>2 hours) counseling on sexual risk reduction decreased STI incidence in adolescents (*or* 0.38; 95% CI 0.24 to 0.60) and adults (*or* 0.70; 95% CI 0.56 to 0.87).[70] The USPTF recommended in 2014 that intensive behavioral counseling should be provided for adults at increased risk for STI and all adolescents that are sexually active.[71] All providers should routinely obtain a sexual history. Health-care providers, in collaboration with public health workers, should develop and find creative routes to provide this education.

References

1. Detels, R., et al., The incidence and correlates of symptomatic and asymptomatic *Chlamydia trachomatis* and *Neisseria gonorrhoeae* infections in selected populations in five countries. *Sex Transm Dis*, 2011. **38** (6): pp. 503–9.
2. McCormack, W.M., et al., Clinical spectrum of gonococcal infection in women. *Lancet*, 1977. **1**(8023): pp. 1182–5.
3. Rana, P., et al., Ectopic pregnancy: a review. *Arch Gynecol Obstet*, 2013. **288**(4): pp. 747–57.
4. Westrom, L., et al., Pelvic inflammatory disease and fertility. A cohort study of 1,844 women with laparoscopically verified disease and 657 control women with normal laparoscopic results. *Sex Transm Dis*, 1992. **19**(4): p. 185–92.
5. Brunham, R.C., Immunity to *Chlamydia trachomatis*. *J Infect Dis*, 2013. **207**(12): pp. 1796–7.
6. Centers for Disease Control and Prevention, *Sexually Transmitted Disease Surveillance, 2012*. December 2013, Department of Health and Human Services. Available at: www.cdc.gov/std/stats12/surv2012.pdf. Accessed Dec. 15, 2015.
7. Datta, S.D., et al., Gonorrhea and chlamydia in the United States among persons 14 to 39 years of age, 1999 to 2002. *Ann Intern Med*, 2007. **147**(2): pp. 89–96. Available at: www.cdc.gov/std/stats12/surv2012.pdf. Accessed Dec. 8, 2015.
8. Centers for Disease Control and Prevention, 2012 Sexually Transmitted Diseases Surveillance. 2012 [cited 2014]. Available at: www.cdc.gov/std/stats12/tables/21.htm. Accessed Oct. 18, 2014.
9. Geisler, W.M., Diagnosis and management of uncomplicated *Chlamydia trachomatis* infections in adolescents and adults: summary of evidence reviewed for the 2010 Centers for Disease Control and Prevention Sexually Transmitted Diseases Treatment Guidelines. *Clin Infect Dis*, 2011. **53**(Suppl 3): pp. S92–8.

10. Centers for Disease Control and Prevention, Recommendations for the laboratory-based detection of *Chlamydia trachomatis* and *Neisseria gonorrhoeae*. *MMWR*, 2014. **63**(Rr-2): pp. 1–24.
11. Peters, R.P., et al., Screening of oropharynx and anorectum increases prevalence of *Chlamydia trachomatis* and *Neisseria gonorrhoeae* infection in female STD clinic visitors. *Sex Transm Dis*, 2011. **38**(9): pp. 783–7.
12. Trebach, J.D.1, et al., *Neisseria gonorrhoeae* and *Chlamydia trachomatis* among women reporting extragenital exposures. *Sex Transm Dis*, 2015 May. **42**(5): pp. 233–9.
13. Gaydos, C.A., et al., *Chlamydia trachomatis* reinfection rates among female adolescents seeking rescreening in school-based health centers. *Sex Transm Dis*, 2008. **35**(3): pp. 233–7.
14. Centers for Disease Control and Prevention, Update to CDC's sexually transmitted diseases treatment guidelines, 2010: oral cephalosporins no longer a recommended treatment for gonococcal infections. *MMWR*, 2012. **61**(31): pp. 590–4.
15. Workowski, K.A. and S. Berman, Sexually transmitted diseases treatment guidelines, 2010. *MMWR Recomm Rep*, 2010. **59**(Rr-12): pp. 1–110.
16. National Institutes of Health, Efficacy of Combination Therapies for Gonorrhea Treatment. [Clinical Trial]. Available at: www.clinicaltrials.gov/ct2/show/NCT00926796?term=gemifloxacin&cond=gonorrhea&rank=1. Accessed Dec. 8, 2015.
17. Taylor, B.D., et al., Microbial correlates of delayed care for pelvic inflammatory disease. *Sex Transm Dis*, 2011. **38**(5): pp. 434–8.
18. Oakeshott, P., et al., Randomised controlled trial of screening for *Chlamydia trachomatis* to prevent pelvic inflammatory disease: the POPI (prevention of pelvic infection) trial. *BMJ*, 2010. **340**: p. c1642.
19. Tubal infertility: serologic relationship to past chlamydial and gonococcal infection. World Health Organization Task Force on the Prevention and Management of Infertility. *Sex Transm Dis*, 1995. **22**(2): pp. 71–7.
20. Jacobson, L. and L. Westrom, Objectivized diagnosis of acute pelvic inflammatory disease. Diagnostic and prognostic value of routine laparoscopy. *Am J Obstet Gynecol*, 1969. **105**(7): pp. 1088–98.
21. Mitchell, C. and M. Prabhu, Pelvic inflammatory disease: current concepts in pathogenesis, diagnosis and treatment. *Infect Dis Clin North Am*, 2013. **27**(4): pp. 793–809.
22. Tepper, N.K., et al., Retention of intrauterine devices in women who acquire pelvic inflammatory disease: a systematic review. *Contraception*, 2013. **87**(5): pp. 655–60.
23. Schulte, J.M., et al., HSV-1 and HSV-2 seroprevalence in the United States among asymptomatic women unaware of any herpes simplex virus infection (Herpevac Trial for Women). *South Med J*, 2014. **107**(2): pp. 79–84.
24. Schillinger, J.A., et al., National seroprevalence and trends in herpes simplex virus type 1 in the United States, 1976–1994. *Sex Transm Dis*, 2004. **31**(12): pp. 753–60.
25. Bernstein, D.I., et al., Epidemiology, clinical presentation, and antibody response to primary infection with herpes simplex virus type 1 and type 2 in young women. *Clin Infect Dis*, 2013. **56**(3): pp. 344–51.
26. Blank, H. and H.G. Haines, Experimental human reinfection with herpes simplex virus. *J Invest Dermatol*, 1973. **61**(4): pp. 223–5.
27. Wald, A., et al., Knowledge of partners' genital herpes protects against herpes simplex virus type 2 acquisition. *J Infect Dis*, 2006. **194**(1): pp. 42–52.
28. Langenberg, A.G., et al., A prospective study of new infections with herpes simplex virus type 1 and type 2. Chiron HSV Vaccine Study Group. *N Engl J Med*, 1999. **341**(19): pp. 1432–8.
29. Benedetti, J., L. Corey, and R. Ashley, Recurrence rates in genital herpes after symptomatic first-episode infection. *Ann Intern Med*, 1994. **121**(11): p. 847–54.
30. Engelberg, R., et al., Natural history of genital herpes simplex virus type 1 infection. *Sex Transm Dis*, 2003. **30**(2): pp. 174–7.
31. Reeves, W.C., et al., Risk of recurrence after first episodes of genital herpes. Relation to HSV type and antibody response. *N Engl J Med*, 1981. **305**(6): pp. 315–19.
32. Corey, L., et al., Genital herpes simplex virus infections: clinical manifestations, course, and complications. *Ann Intern Med*, 1983. **98**(6): pp. 958–72.
33. Gupta, R., et al., Valacyclovir and acyclovir for suppression of shedding of herpes simplex virus in the genital tract. *J Infect Dis*, 2004. **190**(8): pp. 1374–81.
34. Wald, A. and R. Ashley-Morrow, Serological testing for herpes simplex virus (HSV)-1 and HSV-2 infection. *Clin Infect Dis*, 2002. **35**(Suppl 2): pp. S173–82.
35. Mertz, G.J., et al., Double-blind placebo-controlled trial of oral acyclovir in first-episode genital herpes simplex virus infection. *JAMA*, 1984. **252**(9): pp. 1147–51.
36. Martin, E.T., et al., A pooled analysis of the effect of condoms in preventing HSV-2 acquisition. *Arch Intern Med*, 2009. **169**(13): pp. 1233–40.
37. Corey, L., et al., Once-daily valacyclovir to reduce the risk of transmission of genital herpes. *N Engl J Med*, 2004. **350**(1): pp. 11–20.

38. Perry, C.M. and D. Faulds, Valaciclovir: a review of its antiviral activity, pharmacokinetic properties and therapeutic efficacy in herpesvirus infections. *Drugs*, 1996. **52**(5): pp. 754–72.

39. Perry, C.M. and A.J. Wagstaff, Famciclovir: a review of its pharmacological properties and therapeutic efficacy in herpesvirus infections. *Drugs*, 1995. **50**(2): pp. 396–415.

40. Brown, Z.A., et al., Genital herpes complicating pregnancy. *Obstet Gynecol*, 2005. **106**(4): pp. 845–56.

41. ACOG Practice Bulletin. Clinical management guidelines for obstetrician-gynecologists. No. 82 June 2007. Management of herpes in pregnancy. *Obstet Gynecol*, 2007. **109**(6): pp. 1489–98.

42. Summary of notifiable diseases – United States, 2010. *MMWR*, 2012. **59**(53): pp. 1–111.

43. Kaplan, J.E., et al., Guidelines for prevention and treatment of opportunistic infections in HIV-infected adults and adolescents: recommendations from CDC, the National Institutes of Health, and the HIV Medicine Association of the Infectious Diseases Society of America. *MMWR Recomm Rep*, 2009. **58**(Rr-4): pp. 1–207; quiz CE1–4.

44. Patton, M.E., et al., Primary and secondary syphilis – United States, 2005–2013. *MMWR Morb Mortal Wkly Rep*, 2014. **63**(18): pp. 402–6.

45. Centers for Disease Control and Prevention and J., Ayers, *Treponemal pallidum* spirochete (image number 2392) accessed from CDC Public Health Image Library. Available at: http://phil.cdc.gov/phil/details.asp?pid=2392. 1969. Accessed Dec. 13, 2015.

46. Calonge, N., Screening for syphilis infection: recommendation statement. *Ann Fam Med*, 2004. **2**(4): pp. 362–5.

47. Syphilis testing algorithms using treponemal tests for initial screening – four laboratories, New York City, 2005–2006. *MMWR*, 2008. **57**(32): pp. 872–5.

48. Centers for Disease Control and Prevention and J., Ayers, Vulvar condyloma lata (image number 11256) accessed from CDC Public Health Image Library. Available at: http://phil.cdc.gov/phil/details.asp?pid=11256. 1969. Accessed Dec. 13, 2015.

49. Centers for Disease Control and Prevention, Diseases Characterized by Genital, Anal, or Perianal Ulcers. 2010 [cited 2014]. Available from: www.cdc.gov/std/treatment/2010/genital-ulcers.htm-syphilis. Accessed Aug. 15, 2014.

50. Centers for Disease Control and Prevention, Management of Persons Who Have a History of Penicillin Allergy. Sexually Transmitted Diseases Treatment Guidelines 2010 [cited 2014]. Available at: www.cdc.gov/std/treatment/2010/penicillin-allergy.htm. Accessed Aug. 15, 2014.

51. Roett, M.A., M.T. Mayor, and K.A. Uduhiri, Diagnosis and management of genital ulcers. *Am Fam Physician*, 2012. **85**(3): pp. 254–62.

52. Nelson, E.L. and C.K. Stockdale, Vulvar and vaginal HPV disease. *Obstet Gynecol Clin North Am*, 2013. **40**(2): pp. 359–76.

53. Campos-Outcalt, D., HPV vaccine is now routinely indicated for males. *J Fam Pract*, 2012. **61**(1): p. 38–40.

54. Korostil, I.A., et al., Near elimination of genital warts in Australia predicted with extension of human papillomavirus vaccination to males. *Sex Transm Dis*, 2013. **40**(11): pp. 833–5.

55. Mortensen, G.L. and H.K. Larsen, The quality of life of patients with genital warts: a qualitative study. *BMC Public Health*, 2010. **10**: p. 113.

56. Hammarlund, K. and M. Nystrom, The lived experience of genital warts: the Swedish example. *Health Care Women Int*, 2004. **25**(5): pp. 489–502.

57. Wiley, D.J., et al., External genital warts: diagnosis, treatment, and prevention. *Clin Infect Dis*, 2002. **35** (Suppl 2): pp. S210–24.

58. Vender, R., et al., Therapeutic options for external genital warts. *J Cutan Med Surg*, 2013. **17**(Suppl 2): pp. S61–7.

59. Sutton, M., et al., The prevalence of *Trichomonas vaginalis* infection among reproductive-age women in the United States, 2001–2004. *Clin Infect Dis*, 2007. **45**(10): pp. 1319–26.

60. Van Der Pol, B., et al., Prevalence, incidence, natural history, and response to treatment of *Trichomonas vaginalis* infection among adolescent women. *J Infect Dis*, 2005. **192**(12): pp. 2039–44.

61. Krieger, J.N., et al., Diagnosis of trichomoniasis. Comparison of conventional wet-mount examination with cytologic studies, cultures, and monoclonal antibody staining of direct specimens. *JAMA*, 1988. **259**(8): pp. 1223–7.

62. Van Der Pol, B., C.S. Kraft, and J.A. Williams, Use of an adaptation of a commercially available PCR assay aimed at diagnosis of chlamydia and gonorrhea to detect *Trichomonas vaginalis* in urogenital specimens. *J Clin Microbiol*, 2006. **44**(2): pp. 366–73.

63. Caro-Paton, T., et al., Is metronidazole teratogenic? A meta-analysis. *Br J Clin Pharmacol*, 1997. **44**(2): pp. 179–82.

64. Klebanoff, M.A., et al., Failure of metronidazole to prevent preterm delivery among pregnant women with asymptomatic *Trichomonas vaginalis* infection. *N Engl J Med*, 2001. **345**(7): pp. 487–93.

65. World Health Organization, HIV/AIDS Fact Sheet No. 360. 2014 [cited 2014]. Available at: www.who.int/mediacentre/factsheets/fs360/en. Accessed Dec. 11, 2014.

66. Centers for Disease Control and Prevention, HIV Risk, Prevention, and Testing Behaviors – National HIV Behavioral Surveillance System: Men Who Have Sex With Men, 20 U.S. Cities, 2011. HIV Surveillance Special Report 8. 2014. Published September [cited 2014]. Available at: www.cdc.gov/hiv/library/reports/surveillance/-special. Accessed Dec. 11, 2014.
67. US Preventive Services Task Force, Final Recommendation Statement: Human Immunodeficiency Virus (HIV) Infection: Screening. December 2014. 2013 April [cited 2014]. Available at: www.uspreventiveservicestaskforce.org/Page/Document/RecommendationStatementFinal/human-immunodeficiency-virus-hiv-infection-screening. Accessed Dec. 13, 2014.
68. Health Human Services, Recommendations for Use of Antiretroviral Drugs in Pregnant HIV-1-Infected Women for Maternal Health and Interventions to Reduce Perinatal HIV Transmission in the United States. 2014 [cited 2014]. Available at: http://aidsinfo.nih.gov/contentfiles/lvguidelines/perinatalgl.pdf. Accessed Dec. 14, 2014.
69. World Health Organization, Guidelines on HIV and Infant Feeding 2010: Principles and Recommendations for Infant Feeding in the Context of HIV and a Summary of Evidence [cited 2014]. Available at: http://whqlibdoc.who.int/publications/2010/9789241599535_eng.pdf?ua=1. Accessed Dec. 13, 2014.
70. O'Connor, E.A., et al., Behavioral sexual risk-reduction counseling in primary care to prevent sexually transmitted infections: an updated systematic evidence review for the US Preventive Services Task Force. *Ann Intern Med*, 2014.
71. LeFevre, M.L., Behavioral counseling interventions to prevent sexually transmitted infections: US Preventive Services Task Force recommendation statement. *Ann Intern Med*, 2014.
72. Garland, S.M. and M. Steben, Genital herpes. *Best Pract Res Clin Obstet Gynaecol*, 2014 Oct. **28**(7): pp. 1098–110.

Chapter 18

Office management of pelvic pain and dyspareunia

Charles Cox

Introduction

Pelvic pain is pain in the lower abdomen and pelvis. Acute pelvic pain (APP) can present as an acute emergency and may be life threatening or it may last up to three months. Chronic pelvic pain (CPP) lasts longer than three months.

Chronic pelvic pain can be cyclical if it is related to the menstrual cycle or non-cyclical. Pelvic pain associated with sexual intercourse is called dyspareunia and often coexists with pelvic pain.

Pelvic pain can be the symptom of a specific pathology of the reproductive, gastrointestinal, urological, neurological, or musculoskeletal system. APP is usually associated with an identifiable cause. The etiology of chronic pelvic pain can be multifactorial. CPP with no identifiable underlying pathology is defined as chronic pelvic pain syndrome.

Pathologies from different systems that cause pelvic pain may present with similar characteristics due the proximity of pelvic organs and the common innervation. Therefore a thorough history and clinical examination is essential to establish an accurate diagnosis or narrow the differential diagnosis.

Acute pelvic pain, chronic pelvic pain, and dyspareunia share common etiologies Their management approach is different, however, and they will be presented separately in this chapter.

Acute pelvic pain

Scope of the problem

Abdominal pain accounts for 5% of total visits to emergency departments; women with pelvic pain represent 12% of this population.[1] The majority are reproductive age. The differential diagnosis of APP is listed in Table 18-1. The severity of the different causes of APP ranges from life-threatening conditions to conditions that can be managed with simple pain relief.

The presentation of even life-threatening conditions can be vague, nonspecific, or involve only symptoms from a system different to the one from which the pathology arises. Women with ectopic pregnancy, for example, may present with gastrointestinal symptoms.[2] A careful clinical assessment aided by laboratory tests and imaging can help to identify women who need surgery or medical treatment and reassure the ones with normal findings. In 80% of women with pelvic pain and a normal pelvic ultrasound the pain improves or resolves without any complication.[3]

Pelvic pain accounts for 25% of referrals for pelvic ultrasound.[3] The cost of surgery performed in the United States for pelvic pain (acute and chronic) is more than $2 billion annually.[4]

Approach to acute pelvic pain

The clinician must urgently assess and resuscitate the acutely ill patient.

Life threatening conditions such as ectopic pregnancy, hemorrhagic corpus luteum, appendicitis, and sepsis must be considered. A pregnancy test and an early ultrasound examination can be essential. It is important to evaluate for conditions that may threaten long-term fertility and the development of chronic pelvic pain such as pelvic sepsis, endometriosis, and accidents to ovarian cysts. The pain should be addressed early. Administration of analgesia does not affect diagnosis and should not be delayed.

If a diagnosis cannot be established, further imaging in the form of CT or MRI can be considered.

Laparoscopy is the gold standard for assessing acute pelvic pain and conditions such as ectopic pregnancy, accidents to ovarian cysts, and appendicitis can be treated with minimally invasive techniques.

Office Care of Women, ed. Martin E. Olsen and Botros Rizk. Published by Cambridge University Press.

Table 18-1 Differential diagnosis of acute pelvic pain

Pregnancy-related complications
1. Miscarriage
2. Ectopic pregnancy
3. Hemorrhagic corpus luteum
Gynecological causes
1. Dysmenorrhea
2. Uterine fibroids (degeneration, extrusion, torsion)
3. Endometriosis
4. Ovarian accidents (rupture, hemorrhage, torsion)
5. Midcycle ovulation pain
6. Ovarian tumors
7. Ovarian hyperstimulation syndrome
8. Pelvic inflammatory disease (endometritis, salpingitis, tubo-ovarian abscess)
9. Hematometra
10. Pelvic adhesions
Gastrointestinal
1. Appendicitis
2. Gastroenteritis
3. Diverticulitis
4. Constipation
5. Irritable bowel syndrome
6. Inflammatory bowel disease
7. Bowel obstruction
Genitourinary
1. Urinary tract infection
2. Painful bladder syndrome
3. Stones
4. Urinary retention
Musculoskeletal
1. Muscle injury
2. Joint inflammation
3. Herniated disc
4. Hernia (incarceration and strangulation)
Other
1. Aortic aneurysm
2. Sickle cell crisis

History

The history should establish the chronology and the characteristics of the pain. The onset, duration, location, intensity, nature, type, radiation, associated symptoms, and alleviating and aggravating factors should be noted. Symptoms related to the urinary, gastrointestinal, musculoskeletal and nervous system should be assessed.

Table 18-2 5 Ps approach for sexual history

- Past history of sexually transmitted disease
- Partners: gender, number in past 12 months, partner involved in sexual relationship with other partners
- Practices: sexual (vaginal, anal, oral), needle or sex toys sharing
- Prevention: use of condoms
- Pregnancy prevention: method of contraception

Table 18-3 Risk factors for PID

1. Sexually active and under 25
2. Multiple partners
3. Partner with additional partners plus the patient
4. History of PID
5. History of untreated STD
6. Use of intrauterine device
7. Douching

The gynecological history should include questions about dysmenorrhea, dyspareunia, abnormal uterine bleeding, and vaginal discharge. History should uncover any recent gynecological procedures that involved instrumentation of the cervix or uterus as these can increase the risk of pelvic inflammatory disease. Previous medical and surgical history and current medications should also be noted. The patient's sexual history will help to stratify the risks for PID.[5] (See Tables 18-2 and 18-3.)

Clinical examination

Examination should include assessment of the patient's general condition and vital signs. Although fever is suggestive of an infectious cause of pelvic pain, it is absent in 60% of patients with PID and in more than 30% of patients with appendicitis. Remember that young women tolerate blood loss well and even with significant bleeding into the abdomen, peritoneal irritation may be a late sign. The absence of signs of peritonitis does not rule out either hemoperitoneum or PID.

The abdomen should be examined for surgical scars, distention, tenderness, signs of peritonitis, and palpable masses. Right upper quadrant tenderness associated with pelvic pain may be indicative of Fitz-Hugh-Curtis syndrome.

A speculum examination of the vagina and cervix may demonstrate discharge, bleeding, or erythema.

A bimanual examination will assess the position and mobility of the uterus as well as the presence of masses or tenderness in the adnexa. Pain on moving the cervix is strongly suggestive of pelvic pathology. Cervical excitation is said to occur in a quarter of women with appendicitis.[6]

The sensitivity of pelvic examination for detecting an adnexal mass is low.[7] Body habitus and tenderness also hinder the palpation of pelvic masses.

Investigations

A urine pregnancy test and urinalysis should be done quickly. A complete blood count and C-reactive protein may be helpful if an infectious cause is suspected. A normal white cell count does not exclude the possibility of PID or appendicitis.

Swabs to detect chlamydia and gonorrhea should be obtained.

Positive results support the diagnosis of PID whereas negative results do not exclude it.

The absence of pus cells in separately obtained endocervical or vaginal swabs has a good negative predictive value for PID.

Imaging

Transvaginal (TVS) and transabdominal (TAS) ultrasound examination of the pelvis can be helpful in establishing a diagnosis. TVS and TAS can identify conditions requiring emergency care such as ruptured ectopic pregnancy, hemorrhagic ovarian cyst, or ovarian torsion. Imaging can assist in the diagnosis of ovarian cysts, tumors, uterine fibroids, and complications of PID such as pyosalpinx, tubo-ovarian abscess. Appendicitis can be diagnosed by ultrasound examination. A normal examination makes the diagnosis less likely.

Computed tomography (CT) can detect acute appendicitis, other bowel pathologies such as inflammatory bowel disease, diverticulitis, infectious colitis, as well as ureteral calculi.

Invasive diagnosis

Diagnostic laparoscopy should be considered in symptomatic women with pregnancy of unknown location in which serum hCG is above the discriminatory zone of 1,000 IU/L–2,000 IU/L and the TVS has failed to demonstrate an intrauterine or ectopic pregnancy. In nonpregnant women diagnostic laparoscopy can be considered if the pain is unresolved after a period of 24–48 hours of observation.

The most common laparoscopic findings in women with nonspecific low abdominal pain were appendicitis, PID, and ovarian cysts. Diagnosis may not be established in 20% of women.[8]

Laparoscopy in women of reproductive age with nonspecific low abdominal pain is associated with an increased rate of specific diagnosis and a shorter hospital stay compared to a wait and see approach.[9]

Treatment of acute pelvic pain

The aim of the treatment is to provide pain relief and address the pathologic process that accounts for the symptoms.

Medical treatment

Analgesia is the mainstay treatment for acute pelvic pain related to dysmenorrhea and endometriosis. Ovulation suppression can be considered to reduce the recurrence of pain due to these conditions.

Fibroid degeneration and ovarian hyperstimulation syndrome are also managed with analgesia.

Nonsteroidal anti-inflammatory drugs (NSAIDs) should be avoided in ovarian hyperstimulation syndrome.

Active observation for 24–72 hours with analgesia can result in resolution of symptoms in 50%–70% of women with nonspecific low abdominal pain and no established diagnosis without an increase in morbidity.[8, 10]

Clinicians should maintain a low threshold for the diagnosis and treatment of PID. Empiric treatment should be given in sexually active women if they present with low abdominal/pelvic pain, if no other cause for the symptoms can be identified and they exhibit cervical, uterine or adnexal tenderness on the clinical examination.[5] A broad spectrum antibiotic treatment is required to cover aerobic and anaerobic bacteria along with chlamydia and gonorrhea. Early initiation of treatment can prevent long-term sequelae.

Treatment for PID is outlined in Chapter 16 and in the CDC guidelines.

Surgical treatment

Surgical treatment should be considered as a matter of urgency in unstable women with ruptured ectopic pregnancy, hemorrhagic ovarian cysts, and sepsis secondary to appendicitis, or ruptured tubo-ovarian abscess.

Preservation of viable ovarian tissue in symptomatic women with suspected ovarian torsion is more likely to happen if detorsion of the ovary takes place within 48 hours from the onset of the symptoms. In these cases detorsion of the ovary, even if it appears dark purple or black, has been associated with good clinical outcome with little short- or long-term morbidity.[12]

Diagnostic laparoscopy for acute low abdominal pain results in higher rates of specific diagnoses than a wait and see approach.[9] In the conservative approach, however, up to 50% of women may not need surgery without any negative clinical effects.[8]

Prevention

Prevention of acute pelvic pain can be achieved mainly through prevention of sexually transmitted diseases. This can result in prevention of acute pelvic inflammatory disease and ectopic pregnancy.

Sexually active women can reduce the risk of getting STDs by using a barrier method of contraception, having annual screening for chlamydia if they are under 25 or having a screening after a new sexual relationship.

In order to prevent reinfection, sexual partners should be offered screening and treatment in cases of PID. Sexual intercourse should be avoided until the treatment course is completed. Repeat testing for STIs two to four weeks after the treatment should be considered if the symptoms persist.

Chronic pelvic pain

Scope of the problem

Chronic pelvic pain is persistent intermittent or constant pain perceived in structures related to the pelvis. It can be a symptom of a specific pelvic organ pathology or a syndrome in the absence of an underlying pathology. Prevalence for reproductive age women is between 14.7%–25%.[13, 14]

Pelvic pathology, history of abuse, and psychological morbidity are predisposing factors for CPP.[15]

Chronic pelvic pain has a negative impact on women's activity at home, at work, and on their relationships.[16] A US-based study showed that 3.9% of women with CPP missed at least a day of work per month due to their symptoms.[16] Similarly 18% of employed women in the UK were off work for at least one day each year.[17] Many well-defined conditions can account for CPP (Table 18-4).

Table 18-4 Causes of chronic pelvic pain

Causes
Gynecological
Endometriosis
Adenomyosis
Pelvic adhesions
Fibroids
Pelvic congestion syndrome
Ovarian cysts, tumors
Ovarian remnant syndrome
Residual ovary syndrome
Gastrointestinal
Irritable bowel syndrome
Inflammatory bowel disease
Constipation
Diverticular disease
Colorectal malignancy
Urological
Painful bladder syndrome/interstitial cystitis
Chronic urinary tract infection
Urolithiasis
Bladder malignancy
Musculoskeletal
Myofascial pain
Degenerative disk disease
Pelvic floor myalgia and spasms
Nerve entrapment syndromes

Approach to chronic pelvic pain

It should be remembered that patients with chronic pelvic pain may have discomfort arising from more than one system. Patients will often have a history of consultations with other specialties, and a variety of investigations may have already been performed. Specific questioning may be necessary. Psychological morbidity and physical or sexual abuse are associated with chronic pelvic pain.

The practitioner must assess the degree to which the pain is interfering in the patient's professional, sexual, and social life. Exploration of her thoughts about the pain, factors related to the onset of pain, and what strategies improve the pain should be undertaken.

The patient can be reassured that her condition is common and that after investigations it is likely that long-term fertility is not affected. She should be made aware that laparoscopy, despite being the gold standard for the investigation of pelvic pain, is often negative; although it may show minor degrees of endometriosis or adhesions, these are unlikely to be the cause of pain. These minor findings may be fastened onto with a resulting increase in unnecessary treatment and invasive procedures. The woman deserves to know that laparoscopy is a frequent and profitable gynecological procedure but is not without its risks and complications.

History

Details about the duration, characteristics, and chronology of pain should be obtained. A pain diary for two to three menstrual cycles is helpful to identify aggravating and alleviating factors. Events or situations that women associate with the onset of pain and describe them as traumatic can be suggestive of underlying psychological trauma must be addressed. Women should be asked about red flag symptoms that may need urgent investigations and referral to a specialist (Table 18-5). Full body pain maps prompt women to report the location of the pain and rate the intensity of the pain on a scale from 0 to 10 on every area they experience pain. Symptoms that indicate some of the common pathologies of CPP should be elicited (Table 18-6).

Women should be asked about their mood, sleep, and appetite. The two-question Patient Health Questionnaire-2 can be used as a screening tool for depression (Table 18-7). A score of 3 or more requires further evaluation of the woman for depressive disorder.[18] Women with history of child or adult abuse are more likely to have and report CPP.[19, 20] In a safe, private setting with no one known to the woman present, the patient should be asked whether she has been threatened or hurt currently, in the past, or whether she has been forced to do something sexually that she did not desire.[21]

The impact of CPP on the ability to perform daily activities should be explored and documented. Women should be asked how the pain has affected their role in their family, their relationship, their performance at work, and their social life. Previous medical, surgical history and prior investigations and treatment should be noted. It is useful to establish the results of previous investigations and the effect of previous treatments.

Women should be invited to express their concerns about their pain and any possible explanations about causation that they may have heard. It is essential to establish the patient's expectations at the initial consultation. Such information will help the clinician to tailor the interventions accordingly, clarify any misconceptions and shape their expectations. Questionnaires such as the one designed by the International Pelvic Pain Society (www.pelvicpain.org/pdf/FRM_Pain_Questionnaire.pdf) can facilitate

Table 18-5 Red flag symptoms

- Unexplained weight loss
- Bleeding per rectum
- Irregular perimenopausal vaginal bleeding
- Postmenopausal or postcoital bleeding
- Hematuria

Table 18-6 Symptoms of common conditions of CPP

Endometriosis	Dysmenorrhea, dyspareunia, infertility
Painful bladder syndrome	Urinary frequency, urgency; pain before, during, or after voiding
Irritable bowel syndrome	Onset of pain associated with change in frequency or appearance of stools; pain improves with defecation.
Musculoskeletal problems	Pain varies with movements and posture

Table 18-7 The Patient Health Questionnaire-2

Over the past 2 weeks how often have you been bothered by any of the following problems?	Not at all	Several days	More than half the days	Nearly every day
Little interest or pleasure in doing things	0	1	2	3
Feeling down, depressed, or hopeless	0	1	2	3

a thorough pre-visit history and prompt to screen common causal conditions of chronic pelvic pain.

Clinical examination

Clinical examination of the abdomen may demonstrate the site of tenderness. Scars should be noted, and clinicians should check for scar hypersensitivity. The abdomen should be examined for highly localized trigger points. Light localized pressure on these points may elicit local tenderness or vigorous pain occasionally paired with a muscle twitch.

A cotton swab can be used to identify areas of tenderness on the vulva and the introitus.

A single-digit vaginal examination is advisable in women with CPP. The pelvic floor muscles should be palpated at rest and during contraction. The tone and areas of tenderness should be noted.

Specific palpation of the urethra, bladder base and vaginal walls should follow and the utero-sacral ligaments, posterior vaginal fornix and recto-vaginal septum should be examined for nodularity and localized tenderness.

The examination of the uterus should include an evaluation of the shape, size, and mobility. Areas of tenderness should be noted and motion tenderness elicited by gentle movement of the cervix should be checked (cervical excitation).

The adnexal areas should be examined for tenderness or palpable masses.

On speculum examination the vaginal walls, fornices, and cervix should be examined. Signs of infection, endometriotic implants, and cervical lesions can be identified. The pelvic support of the bladder, urethra, vagina, uterus, and rectum should be documented.

As chronic pelvic pain can be musculoskeletal in origin, an assessment of posture, back and pelvic joints should be included in the clinical examination. Women should be examined for scoliosis, pelvic asymmetry, and tenderness over sacroiliac joints and the symphysis pubis.

A normal clinical examination does not preclude the possibility of an anatomic condition responsible for CPP. Up to 50% of women with normal clinical examination have abnormal laparoscopic findings.[22]

Investigations

The basic laboratory examination in CPP should include a complete blood count, C-reactive protein, urinalysis and urine culture. All sexually active women should also be offered screening for sexual transmitted diseases. CA-125 should be considered postmenopausal women with pelvic pain or new onset irritable bowel syndrome (IBS) symptoms.[23]

Pelvic ultrasound is a useful test to evaluate pelvic masses and diagnose adenomyosis. If the transvaginal pelvic ultrasound is normal and there is no evidence of localized pelvic tenderness or reduced ovarian mobility during the examination, then the likelihood of identifying relevant pathology at laparoscopy is 20%.[24]

MRI of pelvis can be of value in the diagnosis of deep infiltrating endometriosis, adenomyosis, fibroids, and their complications. MRI venography may help in the diagnosis of pelvic congestion syndrome in women with relevant clinical symptoms.[25]

Invasive diagnosis

Laparoscopy can be helpful in establishing a diagnosis of CPP if the history is suggestive of endometriosis or pelvic adhesions, if there are abnormal findings in the clinical examination and in adolescents who did not respond to conservative treatment.

Laparoscopy is the investigation of choice for the diagnosis of endometriosis. It has a positive predictive value of 93.3% and a negative predictive value of 41.9%.[26] Endometriosis has been found in 29%–45% of women who had laparoscopy for CPP.[27]

Pelvic adhesions are found in up to 38%–55% of women with CPP.[28] Adhesions are more likely to account for pain if they are dense, they distort the pelvic anatomy, and their location correlates with the area of pain and tenderness.

An increased pelvic pathology compared with adults has been found in symptomatic adolescents. Hence a laparoscopy can be helpful in young women who do not respond to conservative treatment.

Similarly 90% of women with abnormal findings in clinical examination were found to have abnormal laparoscopic findings.[27]

Approach to treatment

The approach to treatment is determined by the working differential diagnosis, symptoms severity, fertility aspirations, previous treatments, and personal wishes and concerns (Table 18-8). Clinicians and patients may initially choose a conservative approach to treat the most common or the most likely diagnoses

Table 18-8 Management options of irritable bowel syndrome

- General advice about diet
- Gluten free or low-FODMAP (fermentable oligosaccharides, disaccharides, monosaccharides, and polyols) diets.
- Adjust fiber intake. Consider soluble fibers and psyllium. Avoid insoluble fiber (bran).
- Consider laxatives (avoid lactulose) or antimotility agent to achieve soft, well-formed stools depending on symptoms.
- Peppermint oil
- Antispasmodic agents when required
- If the preceding are not helpful, then low-dose tricyclic antidepressants can provide symptom and pain relief.
- If TCAs are ineffective, then selective serotonin reuptake inhibitors can be considered.
- If symptoms persist after 12 months, then referral for psychological interventions such as cognitive behavioral therapy or hypnotherapy is advisable.
- Linaclotide, lubiprostone can be used in constipation-predominant IBS.

Table 18-10 Causes of superficial dyspareunia

- Skin diseases (dermatitis, dermatoses)
- Vulvodynia
- Congenital vaginal anomalies
- Pelvic floor spasm
- Vaginal dryness hypoestrogenism
- Vulvovaginitis
- Desquamative inflammatory vaginitis
- Iatrogenic (radiation, post surgery, obstetric lacerations)

according to the clinical assessment; this leaves invasive diagnosis and surgical treatment for the nonrespondents. Women with fertility concerns may opt for an early invasive diagnosis and surgical treatment as conservative methods involving contraception may not be suitable for them.

Various comorbidities are prevalent in women with CPP; the treatment of CPP should aim to minimize pain from each of the pelvic organs involved (Tables 18-9 and 18-10). Long-term medical care may be required as a single intervention frequently does not achieve a major therapeutic improvement or a complete cure.

Table 18-9 Treatment options for women with painful bladder symptoms

- Education about the syndrome and its management
- Behavioral modifications: fluid management, diet, bladder training, pelvic floor muscle relaxation
- Stress management practices for stress-induced flare-ups
- General body exercise and physiotherapy to address myofascial trigger points
- Oral analgesia
- Oral medications: amitriptyline, hydroxyzine, pentosan polysulfate; combination of the last two results in better response
- Intravesical treatment: lidocaine, heparin, dimethyl sulphoxide, hyaluronic acid
- Cystoscopy with low pressure hydrodistention
- Cystoscopic treatment of Hunner's lesions with laser or electrocautery
- Intravesical botulinum toxin

Treatment of chronic pelvic pain

Analgesia

Simple analgesics (paracetamol, NSAIDs) can be considered in the initial management. If they fail to improve the pain or the functional status over a short period of time, they should be stopped. NSAIDs are effective in the treatment of dysmenorrhea.[29]

Opioids can be used for chronic pain in nonmalignant conditions. There are no controlled studies on the use of opioids in CPP. Given the lack of their effectiveness in CPP and their side effects the decision for the use of opioids in CPP should be made on individual basis by clinicians experienced in their use.

Hormonal-based treatment

Ovarian suppression by continuous use of the combined oral contraceptive pill or use of a vaginal contraceptive ring or transdermal patch can result in improvement of pain in endometriosis, adenomyosis, and pelvic congestion syndrome as well as in noncyclic CPP.[29, 30] Moreover cyclical variation of pain due to IBS or PBS may also respond.

Progestagens and a levonorgestrel-releasing intrauterine system have a similar effect on endometriosis- and adenomyosis-associated pain.

Progestogen (medroxyprogesterone acetate) at a dose of 30 mg a day for six months was associated with a reduction of pain in pelvic congestion syndrome.[30] Women should be informed of the possible weight gain during this treatment.

GnRH agonists are also effective in the treatment of endometriosis and better than progestogen for pain associated with pelvic congestion syndrome.[31] Hormonal add-back therapy is recommended to prevent bone loss and hypoestrogenic symptoms. The use of GnRH agonists is licensed for six months and the combination with HRT is safe and effective for up to two years.[32] There is evidence to suggest that the combination is safe for up to 10 years.[33] See Chapter 25 for further discussion of endometriosis.

Medical treatment of neuropathic pain

Medications that modulate neuropathic pain can be used for the treatment of CPP. Evidence for benefit in CPP is limited, but they have been effective in the management of other painful syndromes including IBS, painful bladder syndrome.

A reduction in pain can be achieved by amitriptyline and/or gabapentin. The combination of both is most effective and gabapentin alone was more effective than amitriptyline alone.[34]

Pregabalin and duloxetine are used for the management of neuropathic pain in non-specialist settings. There is lack of evidence for their effectiveness in CPP. Tramadol can also be considered for the short-term management (less than four weeks) of neuropathic pain. All neuropathic medications have side effects that limit their use. Therefore it is advisable to start with a low dose and increase it slowly.

Physiotherapy

Physiotherapy as part of a multidisciplinary approach has been found to be beneficial.[35] It is likely to be beneficial if myofascial trigger points have been found during the examination.

Neuromodulation

Spinal cord stimulation is a treatment option for adults with pain of neuropathic origin. It is effective in the management of painful bladder syndrome.[36] Its role in the management of chronic pelvic pain is yet to be established.

Psychological therapy

Psychological intervention in general can improve pain experience and motor function in women with CPP.[37] The combination of MPA and psychological therapy resulted in nearly three quarters of women reporting >50% pain relief from pelvic congestion syndrome.[38]

Surgery

Pain reduction or improvement in the quality of life has been reported even after diagnostic laparoscopies.[39] This could happen due to the impact of having a laparoscopy on women's beliefs about their health.[40] In endometriosis, reduction of pelvic pain can be achieved by ablation or excision of peritoneal endometriosis, cystectomy of ovarian endometriomas, and removal of deep endometriosis. Some women with CPP may benefit from adhesiolysis if more conservative measures have failed to address CPP.

Hysterectomy may result in pain reduction if the pain is associated with adenomyosis, endometriosis, or symptomatic fibroids. The absence of these pathologies is a risk factor for persistent pain following the procedure.[41] A therapeutic trial with GnRH agonists prior to hysterectomy is advisable.

The effectiveness of presacral neuroctomy has not been demonstrated. Laparoscopic uterosacral nerve ablation is also ineffective in the management of CPP.[42]

Prevention

Primary prevention of CPP is a challenge due the unclear and multifactorial origin of the disease.

Secondary prevention can be achieved by screening sexually active women for sexually transmitted diseases and treating them accordingly. Periodic screening for physical and/or sexual abuse is recommended for all women. Talking, managing and avoiding these violent experiences can prevent the long-term effects such as CPP.

The primary aim of tertiary prevention should be the development of a good therapeutic relationship with the woman. An empathetic approach to the problem of CPP can be therapeutic in itself. Both physical and psychological aspects of care should be addressed early in the consultation process. Women should also be encouraged to take an active role in managing their symptoms.

Table 18-11 Pertinent points in history

History	Clinical significance
Obstetric Perineal injuries in childbirth	10%–14% superficial dyspareunia 12 months postpartum [47]
Medical Diabetes Sjögren's syndrome	Vaginal dryness, candidiasis Vaginal dryness
Surgical Anterior or posterior vaginal wall repair Prolapse surgery using mesh	De novo dyspareunia 15–30% [48] 15% [49]
Medications Antidepressants, antipsychotics GnRH agonists	Decreased arousal, decreased lubrication Vaginal dryness
Contraception Low-dose estrogen combined contraceptive pill Depot medroxyprogesterone acetate	Decreased lubrication Decreased lubrication
Allergy to latex	Irritation from the use of condoms

Dyspareunia

Dyspareunia is genital pain experienced just before, during or after intercourse. It is one of the most frequently reported comorbidities in women with CPP with rates ranging from 15% to 88%.[43]

Dyspareunia affects 8%–21% of women.[13] It is considered primary when the symptoms occur from the onset of sexual activity and secondary when it occurs after a period of pain free intercourse.

The term "de novo dyspareunia" is used to describe new onset sexual pain following vaginal surgery.

Dyspareunia can be further divided into superficial (introital) and deep depending on the location of the pain. The causes of dyspareunia differ for each subtype. Deep dyspareunia can result from any condition that is responsible for acute or chronic pelvic pain.

The causes of superficial dyspareunia are outlined in Table 18-11.

Approach to the patient

Women can be reluctant to discuss sexual pain; clinicians should include questions about sexual activity and pain in routine assessment. Patients should be encouraged to voice their concerns, their views about the cause of the pain and their expectations from the consultation. Involvement of the partner in the consultation should be encouraged but remains the decision of the patient.

Some women may not be able to tolerate a vaginal examination. In this case the following options may be appropriate

- Defer the examination for another visit
- Offer referral to another colleague or specialist nurse for the examination
- Use premedication
- Use small-size speculums
- Conduct the clinical assessment under anesthesia

A women should be reassured that she is in control of the examination and can ask it to be stopped at any time. Clinicians need to ascertain whether the tenderness elicited during the examination reproduces the pain that the woman describes.

History

The location of the pain helps to differentiate between superficial and deep dyspareunia and may point to structures responsible for the pain. Onset and chronology of pain should be explored. Patients should be asked if the problem is lifelong or acquired. In cases of primary dyspareunia, congenital abnormalities of the vagina must be excluded. When it is acquired, the situation that triggered the symptoms needs to be explored.

Pain before intercourse suggests a phobic attitude with tension of the pelvic floor muscles.

Pain at entry is associated with causes of superficial dyspareunia. Pain after intercourse could be due to mucosal irritation, pelvic congestion syndrome, or pelvic floor dysfunction. Women should be asked if the pain is constant, intermittent, or provoked. Situations or positions during intercourse that trigger the pain should be noted.

The characteristics of sexual pain vary depending on the cause. The pain in superficial dyspareunia is described as burning, splitting, tearing, sore, or a dull ache. Deep dyspareunia may be described as shooting, cramping pain, dull ache or "something is being bumped."

The relationship of dyspareunia to the menstrual cycle is important as cyclic pain can be suggestive of endometriosis or adenomyosis. The pain intensity and the impact of pain on the course of sexual activity should be noted.

Clinicians should enquire about the other aspects of sexual function. As a response to sexual arousal, the vaginal lubrication increases, the upper end of the vagina lengthens and the uterus elevates into the pelvis.[44] Lack of arousal not only affects lubrication but it may allow sensitive areas to come into contact with the penis. Failure to achieve orgasm can result in pelvic venous congestion and dull ache following intercourse.

A sexual history will provide useful information about current and past sexual practices. Dyspareunia can result from a wide range of pathologies and it is important to enquire about other associated symptoms and take a thorough gynecological, medical, and surgical history. Pertinent points are summarized in Table 18-12.

Examination

Clinical examination of dyspareunia is similar to the previously discussed examination for chronic pelvic pain with some additional steps. The external genitalia should be examined for signs of dermatitis-erythema, scaling, fissuring and vulvar skin conditions such as lichen sclerosus, or lichen planus. A moistened cotton-tipped applicator can be used to elicit tenderness in the vulva and vaginal vestibule. According to Friedrich, vulvar vestibulitis syndrome (VVS) is defined as (1) severe pain with vestibular touch or attempted vaginal entry, (2) tenderness to cotton swab pressure localized to the vulvar vestibule, and (3) physical findings confined to various degrees of vestibular erythema.[45] It is advisable to start touching from the vulva toward the introitus and record the findings on a diagram. Similar testing can be performed during the speculum examination to elicit abnormal sensitivity from the cervix or the vault in posthysterectomy women.

Investigations

Urinalysis, measurement of vaginal pH, and microscopy can guide the initial management in cases of dyspareunia in the presence of abnormal vaginal discharge. Vaginal and cervical swabs for culture can be considered if clinically indicated. Vulval biopsies can confirm diagnosis in vulval dermatoses and rule out malignancy in suspicious appearing lesions. In cases of deep dyspareunia, a pelvic ultrasound is recommended.

Treatment

A multidisciplinary approach may be necessary. If the dyspareunia is secondary to a specific pelvic pathology then a referral to the appropriate specialty is recommended. Referrals to other health-care professionals such as physiotherapists, pain specialists, and psychosexual specialists may be necessary to manage the different aspects of dyspareunia

Superficial dyspareunia

A discussion with the couple about the physiologic body changes during sexual response can facilitate a better understanding of dyspareunia and can engage both partners in the treatment plan.

Written information in the form of patient information leaflets is well received by women. Abstinence from penetrative sexual activity may be indicated until the sexual pain is addressed.

Women should be advised about vulvar hygiene and elimination of potential vulvar skin irritants. Vulvar skin disease such as dermatitis or dermatoses (lichen planus, lichen sclerosus) can be treated with local steroid creams. The potency of the prescribed steroids and length of treatment depends on the severity of the disease and the response to treatment. The chronicity of these conditions may required a maintenance dose in the form of a twice a week application may be necessary.

In vaginal atrophy and dyspareunia due to hypoestrogenism, lubricants can provide temporary relief but it can be followed by vaginal irritation. Moisturizers provide a transient benefit and may be the treatment of choice when estrogen therapy is ineffective or contraindicated. Systemic hormone replacement therapy can achieve symptom relief in 75% of women. Local estrogen treatment is the treatment of choice. Creams may have an advantage over the vaginal ring and tablets due to the added lubrication they offer. Up to 90% of women will experience improvement in their symptoms within four to six weeks. Low-dose local vaginal estrogen treatment can be considered for as long as the symptoms persist.[46] Ospemifene, a novel selective estrogen receptor modulator is an effective and safe treatment for dyspareunia associated with postmenopausal vulvar and vaginal atrophy.[47]

Recurrent candidiasis can be treated with topical or oral azoles. Weekly doses and longer courses of treatment may be necessary.

Local anesthetic agents can be considered in women with vulvodynia or vestibulitis. They should be used with caution as sensitization to these agents can worsen the symptoms. Local steroid creams are sometimes applied to the vestibule two or three times a week. Medications for neuropathic pain as described in the CPP section can also been used for unprovoked vulvodynia/vestibulitis. Local excision of the painful vestibule can improve symptoms especially if it is combined with postoperative psychosexual therapy in refractory cases but does carry the risks associated with operative procedures.

Botulinum toxin injected into levator muscles has been used successfully in the treatment of refractory vaginismus.[48]

After sexual education has occurred and once good pelvic floor relaxation has been obtained, desensitization exercises can be used to help women achieve penetration. The patient uses by her finger or different sizes vaginal dilators. Cognitive behavioral therapy can be helpful if there is marked anxiety, fear, or erroneous thoughts that interfere with sexual function.

Deep dyspareunia

The use of combined hormonal contraceptive or vaginal contraceptive ring or transdermal contraceptive patch can reduce dyspareunia associated with endometriosis and adenomyosis. If GnRH agonists are used the add-back therapy is advisable to avoid the effects of hypoestrogenism. Surgical excision of deep infiltrating endometriosis improves dyspareunia and quality of sex life significantly.

If pelvic congestion is suspected, ovarian suppression by 30 mg of MPA for six months or GnRH agonists can improve pelvic pain. Embolization of the ovarian veins can achieve improvement in pain ranging from 58% to 83%.[49] Hysterectomy with bilateral oophorectomy can also reduce pain.[50]

Concluding remarks

Pelvic pain and dyspareunia are common symptoms that warrant careful investigation and early diagnosis to reduce the risk of the conditions becoming long-term and crippling conditions threatening fertility and general health. The differential diagnosis is broad and the management challenges to the provider are more significant than some other diagnoses. Successful treatment of these conditions is very important to the patients and very satisfying to the health-care team.

References

1. Powers RD, Guertler AT. Abdominal pain in the ED: stability and change over 20 years. *Am J Emerg Med* 1995;**13**:301–3.
2. Centre for Maternal and Child Enquiries (CMACE). Saving Mothers' Lives: reviewing maternal deaths to make motherhood safer: 2006–08. The Eighth Report on Confidential Enquiries into Maternal Deaths in the United Kingdom. *BJOG* 2011;**118**(Suppl. 1):17.
3. Harris RD, Holtzman SR, Poppe AM. Clinical outcome in female patients with pelvic pain and normal pelvic US findings. *Radiology* 2000;**216**:440–443.
4. Reiter RC, Gambone JC. Nongynecologic somatic pathology in women with chronic pelvic pain and negative laparoscopy. *J Reprod Med* 1991;**36**:253–259.
5. Workowski KA, Berman S; Sexually transmitted diseases treatment guidelines 2010. Centers for Disease Control and Prevention (CDC). *MMWR Recomm Rep* 2010 Dec 17;**59**(RR-12):1–110. Erratum in: *MMWR Recomm Rep* 2011 Jan 14;60(1):18.
6. Bongard F, Landers DV, Lewis F. Differential diagnosis of appendicitis and pelvic inflammatory disease: a prospective analysis. *American Journal of Surgery* 1985;**150**(1):90–6.
7. Padilla LA, Radosevich DM, Milad MP. Accuracy of the pelvic examination in detecting adnexal masses. *Obstet Gynecol* 2000;**96**(4):593–8.
8. Morino M, Pellegrino L, Castagna E, et al. Acute nonspecific abdominal pain: a randomized, controlled trial comparing early laparoscopy versus clinical observation. *Ann Surg* 2006;**244**:881–8.
9. Gaitán HG, Reveiz L, Farquhar C. Laparoscopy for the management of acute lower abdominal pain in women of childbearing age. *Cochrane Database Syst Rev* 2011;**1**: CD007683. doi:10.1002/14651858.CD007683.pub2.
10. Decadt B, Sussman L, Lewis MO, et al. Randomized clinical trial of early laparoscopy in the management of acute non-specific abdominal pain. *Br J Surg* 1999;**86**: 1383–6.
11. DeWitt J, Reining A, Allsworth JE, Peipert JF. "Tuboovarian Abscesses: Is Size Associated with Duration of Hospitalization & Complications?" *Obstetrics and Gynecology International* 2010; 2010, Article ID 847041, 5 pages. doi:10.1155/2010/847041.
12. Cohen SB, Wattiez A, Seidman DS, et al. Laparoscopy versus laparotomy for detorsion and sparing of twisted ischaemic adnexa. *JSLS* 2003;**7**:295–9.
13. Latthe P, Latthe M, Say L, et al. WHO systematic review of prevalence of chronic pelvic pain: a neglected reproductive health morbidity. *BMC Public Health* 2006;**6**:177.
14. Ahangari A. Prevalence of chronic pelvic pain among women: an updated review. *Pain Physician* 2014;**17**:E 141–7.
15. Latthe P, Mignini L, Gray R, et al. Factors predisposing women to chronic pelvic pain: systematic review. *BMJ* 2006 Apr 1;**332**(7544):749–55.

16. Mathias SD, Kupperman M, Liberman RF, et al. Chronic pelvic pain: prevalence, health-related quality of life, and economic correlates. *Obstet Gynecol* 1996;**87**:321–7.
17. Zondervan KT, Yudkin PL, Vessey MP, et al. The community prevalence of chronic pelvic pain in women and associated illness behaviour. *Br J Gen Pract* 2001;**51**:541–7.
18. Kroenke K, Spitzer RL, Williams JB. The patient health questionnaire-2: validity of a two-items depression screener. *Medical Care* 2003;**41**:1284–94.
19. Jamieson DJ, Steege JF. The association of sexual abuse with pelvic pain complaints in a primary care population. *Am J Obstet Gynecol* 1997;**177**: 1408–12.
20. Raphael KG, Widom CS, Lange G. Childhood victimization and pain in adulthood: a prospective investigation. *Pain* 2001;**92**:283–93.
21. Gottlieb AS. Domestic violence: a clinical guide for women's health care providers. *Obstetrician & Gynaecologist* 2012;**14**:197–202.
22. Howard FM. The role of laparoscopy in the evaluation of chronic pelvic pain: pitfalls with a negative laparoscopy. *J Am Assoc Gynecol Laparosc* 1996;**4**:85–94.
23. National Institute for Health and Clinical Excellence. Ovarian Cancer. The recognition and initial management of ovarian cancer. *NICE clinical guideline 122*. London: NICE; 2011 [http://guidance.nice.org.uk /CG122/NICEGuidance/pdf/English].
24. Okaro E, Condous G, Khalid A, et al. The use of ultrasound-based "soft marker" for the predictions of pelvic pathology in women with chronic pelvic pain – can we reduce the need of laparoscopy. *BJOG* 2006;**113** (3):251–6.
25. Meneses LQ, Uribe S, Tejos C, et al. Using magnetic resonance phase-contrast velocity mapping for diagnosing pelvic congestion syndrome. *Phlebology* 2011;**26**:157–61.
26. Albee RB Jr, Sinervo K, Fisher DT. Laparoscopic excision of lesions suggestive of endometriosis or otherwise atypical in appearance: relationship between visual findings and final histologic diagnosis. *J Minim invasive Gynaecol* 2008;**15**:32–7.
27. Marana R, Paielli FV, Muzii L, et al. [The role of laparoscopy in the evaluation of chronic pelvic pain.] *Minerva Ginecol* 1993;**45**:281–6.
28. Kresch AJ, Seifer DB, Sachs LB, Barrese I. Laparoscopy in 100 women with chronic pelvic pain. *Obstet Gynecol* 1984;**64**:672–4.
29. Dunselman GA, Vermeulen N, Becker C, et al. ESHRE guideline: management of women with endometriosis. *Hum Reprod* 2014 Mar;**29**(3):400–12. doi:10.1093/ humrep/det457.
30. Soysal ME, Vicdan K, Soysal S, Ozer S. A controlled trial of goserelin and medroxyprogesterone acetate in the treatment of pelvic congestion. *Human Reproduction* 2001;**16**(5):931–9.
31. Brown J, Pan A, Hart RJ. Gonadotrophin-releasing hormone analogues for pain associated with endometriosis. *Cochrane Database Syst Rev* 2010;**12**: CD008475. doi:10.1002/14651858.CD008475.pub2.
32. Farmer JE, Prentice A, Breeze A, et al. Gonadotrophin-releasing hormone analogues for endometriosis: bone mineral density. *Cochrane Database Syst Rev* 2003;**4**: CD001297. doi:10.1002/14651858.CD001297.
33. Bedaiwy MA, Casper RF. Treatment with leuprolide acetate and hormonal add-back for up to 10 years in stage IV endometriosis patients with chronic pelvic pain. *Fertil Steril* 2006;**86**:220–2.
34. Sator-Katzenschlager SM, Scharbert G, Kress HG, et al. Chronic pelvic pain treated with gabapentin and amitriptilyne. *Wiener Medizinische Wochenschrift* 2005;**117**(21–22):761–8.
35. Peters AA, van Dorst E, Jellis B, et al. A randomized clinical trial to compare two different approaches in women with chronic pelvic pain. *Obstet Gynecol* 1991;**77**:740–4.
36. Srivastava D. Efficacy of sacral neuromodulation in treating chronic pain related to painful bladder syndrome/interstitial cystitis in adults. *J Anaesthesiol Clin Pharmacol* 2012;**28**:428–35.
37. Haugstad GK, Haugstad TS, Kirste UM, et al. Mensendieck somatocognitive therapy as treatment approach to chronic pelvic pain: results of a randomized controlled intervention study. *Am J Obstet Gynecol* 2006 May;**194**(5):1303–10.
38. Farquhar CM, Rogers V, Franks S, et al. A randomized controlled trial of medroxyprogesterone acetate and psychotherapy for the treatment of pelvic congestion. *Br J Obstet Gynaecol* 1989 Oct;**96**(10):1153–62.
39. Swank DJ, Swank-Bordewijk SC, Hop WC, et al. Laparoscopic adhesiolysis in patients with chronic abdominal pain: a blinded randomised controlled multi-centre trial. *Lancet* 2003;**361**(9365):1247–51.
40. Elcombe S, Gath D, Day A. The psychological effects of laparoscopy on women with chronic pelvic pain. *Psychol Med* 1997;**27**:1041–50.
41. Hillis SD, Marchbank PA, Peterson HB. The effectiveness of hysterectomy for chronic pelvic pain. *Obstetrics and Gynecology* 1995;**86**(6):941–5.
42. Daniels JP, Middleton L, Xiong T, et al. Individual patient data meta-analysis of randomised evidence to assess the effectiveness of laparoscopic uterosacral nerve ablation in chronic pelvic pain. *Hum Reprod Update*. 2010 Nov–Dec;**16**(6):568–76.
43. Andrews J, Yunker A, Reynolds WS, et al. *Noncyclic Chronic Pelvic Pain Therapies for Women: Comparative*

Effectiveness [Internet]. Rockville (MD): Agency for Healthcare Research and Quality (US); 2012 Jan. (Comparative Effectiveness Reviews, No. 41.) Available from: http://www.ncbi.nlm.nih.gov/books/NBK84586. Assessed July 2014.

44. Schultz WW, van Andel P, Sabelis I, Mooyaart E. Magnetic resonance imaging of male and female genitals during coitus and female sexual arousal. *BMJ* 1999 Dec 18–25;**319**(7225):1596–600.

45. Friedrich EG. Vulvar vestibulitis syndrome. *J Reprod Med* 1987 Feb; **32**(2):110–14.

46. Sturdee DW, Panay N; International Menopause Society Writing Group. Recommendations for the management of postmenopausal vaginal atrophy. *Climacteric* 2010 Dec;**13**(6):509–22.

47. Cui Y, Zong HT, Yan HL, et al. Treating dyspareunia associated with postmenopausal vulvar and vaginal atrophy: a systematic review and meta-analysis. *J Sex Med* 2014;**11**:487–97.

48. Ferreira JR, Souza RP. Botulinum toxin for vaginismus treatment. *Pharmacology* 2012;**89**(5–6): 256–9.

49. Smith PC. The outcome of treatment for pelvic congestion syndrome. *Phlebology* 2012 Mar;**27** (Suppl 1):74–7.

50. Beard RW, Kennedy RG, Gangar KF, et al. Bilateral oophorectomy and hysterectomy in the treatment of intractable pelvic pain associated with pelvic congestion. *Br J Obstet Gynaecol* 1991;**98**:988–92.

Chapter 19

Office management of pelvic masses

Elaine Stickrath

Introduction

A diagnosis of pelvic mass is anxiety provoking for both the patient and provider alike. Pelvic masses are common. It is estimated that up to 80% of women have a pelvic mass of some kind, with the most common being uterine myoma.[1] Given that 40%–70% of women in the United States have fibroids and another 5%–10% of women will undergo surgery for an ovarian mass, this is a problem that all providers will encounter.[2, 3] Providers should feel comfortable evaluating and managing pelvic masses and must know when to refer these patients.

A high index of suspicion for a pelvic mass needs to be present at the time of the initial patient evaluation in order to make the diagnosis. Many patients are asymptomatic; others present with vague symptoms. The incidence of adnexal masses in the asymptomatic population is about 0.17%–5.9%.[4] In those with an adnexal mass, the physical exam is only about 51% sensitive, even in the setting of masses that are more than 5 cm.[5] Physical exam is often also limited by other factors, including patient discomfort and a high body mass index.

Clinician goals when seeing patients with pelvic masses are to determine the organ of origin, to consider the likelihood of a malignancy, and to decide what or if treatment is necessary. This requires a combination of history, exam findings, imaging, and lab analysis. This combined approach for patients with a pelvic mass will be reviewed in detail to guide practitioners in their management and referral process.

Initial evaluation of a pelvic mass

The initial evaluation begins with a thorough history, review of systems, and physical exam. When obtaining the history, it is important to elicit any current symptoms. Many women with a pelvic mass will describe pain, pelvic pressure, menstrual changes, urinary frequency, changes in bowel habits, and possibly changes in eating habits such as early satiety. In addition to eliciting symptoms, it is also important for the physician to complete a thorough medical and surgical history as these can influence management if a pelvic mass is diagnosed. After completing the history, a review of systems is critical. Many women with a pelvic mass have nonspecific symptoms and may not be attribute these symptoms to a single disease process. Table 19-1 highlights findings on review of systems that should trigger a provider to be suspicious of a possible pelvic mass.

Next, a thorough physical exam should be performed including vital signs, evaluation of the head, neck, breasts, heart, and lungs. During the abdominal exam, the provider should focus on any distention, abnormality of bowel sounds, palpable fluid wave indicating ascites, and any palpable masses. If rebound or guarding is present, this indicates a more acute process that may require prompt surgical intervention.

The comprehensive pelvic exam should consist of inspection of the external genitalia, speculum exam, bimanual exam, and recto-vaginal exam. A speculum exam is useful as it can show a cervical mass or

Table 19-1 Review of systems findings consistent with a pelvic mass

- Pelvic pain
- Pelvic pressure
- Frequent urination
- Changes in bowel habits
- Early satiety
- Abdominal distention
- Abnormal bleeding
- Dyspareunia
- Cyclic pain
- Dysmenorrhea

Office Care of Women, ed. Martin E. Olsen and Botros Rizk. Published by Cambridge University Press.

Table 19-2 Pelvic mass physical exam findings concerning for malignancy

- Fixed
- Irregular
- Nodularity in the recto-vaginal septum
- Solid
- Bilateral

Table 19-3 Differential diagnosis of a pelvic mass

Gynecologic
• Myoma
• Ectopic pregnancy
• Functional cyst
• Benign ovarian neoplasm
• Tubo-ovarian abscess
• Hydrosalpinx
• Endometrioma
• Ovarian malignancy
Nongynecologic
• Diverticular abscess
• Appendiceal abscess
• GI malignancy
• Bladder enlargement
• Bladder diverticulum
• Metastatic disease

a deviated cervix. A cervix that is significantly deviated may indicate a displaced uterus from a proximal mass, or an enlarged uterus due to myomas. Next, in the bimanual exam, the size, mobility, and shape of the uterus should be evaluated. Myomas are the most common pelvic mass; this diagnosis should be high on the differential. Once the uterus is assessed, the adnexa should be palpated. The size, mobility, contour, and consistency of the mass should be described. The opposite adnexa should be assessed for bilaterality. A recto-vaginal exam is useful for palpating a retroverted uterus, or any mass in the posterior cul de sac. Nodularity of the recto-vaginal septum can be detected, or a mass arising from the rectum can be diagnosed. Table 19-2 lists physical exam findings that are concerning for a malignancy.

Because pelvic masses are quite common, and often asymptomatic, many women are diagnosed at the time of imaging for another indication. These women should have the same evaluation as described above.

Once a pelvic mass has been diagnosed, whether incidentally or during the physical exam, it is important to gather further information to aid in making a diagnosis. First, the clinician should start with a broad differential diagnosis. Pelvic masses can arise from the reproductive tract, but it is also important to consider masses of GI or GU origin. Table 19-3 includes a differential diagnosis for a pelvic mass. An important consideration is to determine benign conditions from malignant pathologies.

Imaging

Imaging studies are indicated for any patient with exam findings consistent with a pelvic mass. Patients whose complaints correspond with a high clinical suspicion for pelvic mass based on history and review of systems may also be candidates for imaging. The limitations of the pelvic exam have already been discussed; therefore, this exam cannot be relied upon with certainty. Some situations do exist when imaging has not proven to be beneficial. If the diagnosis of uterine myomas can be made clinically, an ultrasound may not be needed. Cantuaria, et al. showed that there is a strong correlation in the setting of uterine fibroids between the bimanual exam, ultrasound findings and the uterine weight at the time of hysterectomy.[6] This study concluded that imaging did not add any benefit but did add increased cost to the care of the patient. Conversely, an argument can be made that treatment options other than surgery may be considered based on the size or location of fibroids or additional pathology may be encountered which could change management decisions. The author therefore suggests imaging of patients with known or suspected pelvic mass.

Transvaginal ultrasound (TVUS) is the imaging modality of choice for visualizing pelvic anatomy.[7] Transvaginal ultrasound is very effective. The pooled sensitivity and specificity for greyscale transvaginal ultrasound in the diagnosis of an adnexal mass is 0.82%–0.91% and 0.68%–0.81%, respectively.[8] When morphologic findings are combined with Doppler studies, the pooled sensitivity and specificity improve to 0.89% and 0.91%.[8] Effectiveness combined with widespread availability, relatively low cost, lack of radiation exposure and general tolerability makes TVUS the best modality for evaluating the pelvis.

Computed tomography (CT) scans are used quite commonly and often incidentally lead to the diagnosis of a pelvic mass. Many patients, in fact, present to their providers with unexpected findings from a CT scan. Typically these patients will need a TVUS to further define the mass as the specificity of CT scan is inferior to

TVUS. The pooled sensitivity is 0.90% and specificity is 0.75%.[8] CT scan thus is good at detecting a mass but is not as good as ultrasound at characterizing or diagnosing the etiology of the mass. In addition, CT scans incur the disadvantage of radiation exposure. CT scans can be helpful in evaluation of a malignant pelvic mass, as CT is superior at detecting metastatic disease, ascites, and lymph node enlargement.

Magnetic resonance imaging (MRI) is another imaging modality that does not involve radiation exposure. It does, however, incur a much greater cost than ultrasound. MRI has not been shown to be superior to ultrasound for the diagnosis of pelvic mass. The pooled sensitivity and specificity are 0.91% and 0.88%, respectively.[8] As with CT, MRI is good at diagnosing a mass, but it not as good as TVUS at characterizing the mass.

Positron emission tomography (PET) scans have also been studied for the diagnosis of pelvic masses. This modality shows a pooled sensitivity of 0.67% and specificity of 0.79%.[8] Given that PET scans are not superior in the detection of a pelvic mass and are significantly more expensive than a TVUS, they are not routinely recommended.

Management of pelvic masses

This chapter will focus on masses of gynecologic origin. Examples of non gynecologic pelvic masses are those arising from the urinary tract or bowel (see Table 19-1). When a nongynecologic mass is diagnosed, an appropriate referral can be made. A diagnosis based on imaging can at times be confusing, in situations, it is best to involve other experts for management assistance.

Emergent management of pelvic mass

Ectopic pregnancy

The first step in management of a gynecologic mass is to determine the acuity of the clinical condition. Certain gynecologic masses present as surgical emergencies, one of which is an ectopic pregnancy. A full discussion of the management of ectopic pregnancies is included in Chapter 11. A urine pregnancy test should always be ordered in the initial evaluation of a pelvic mass in a premenopausal woman. If positive, the adnexal mass should be considered an ectopic pregnancy until proven otherwise. Ectopic pregnancies are most commonly noted on ultrasound as hypoechoic round structures near to, but separate from, the ovary. Ideally, a gestational sac or even crown rump length can be seen, but when diagnosed early, ectopic pregnancies may simply appear as a vascular hyperechoic mass (Figure 19-1). In the office setting, patients may present with an early pregnancy and associated cramping or bleeding. Those patients should be referred for

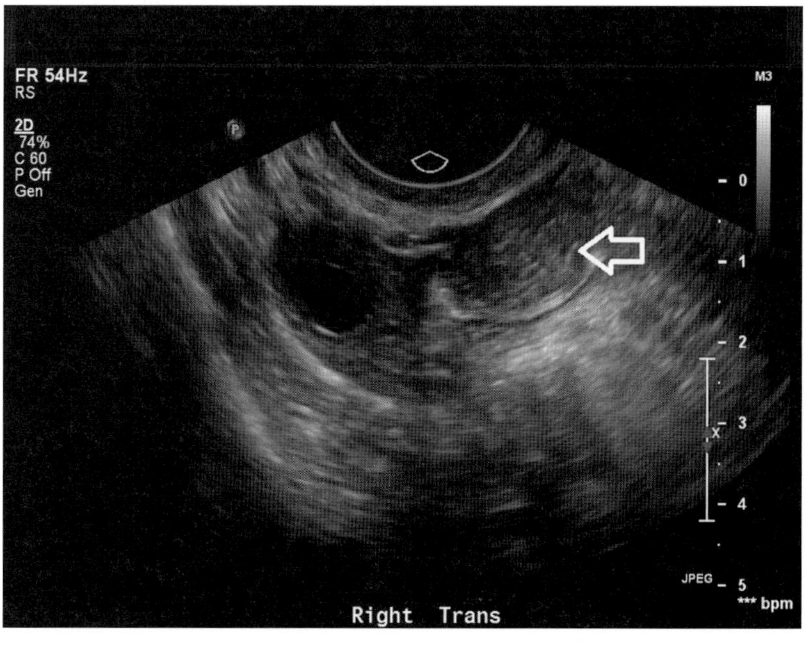

Figure 19-1 An ectopic pregnancy is seen as a hyperechoic mass immediately adjacent to, but separate from, the ovary. The ectopic is labeled with the arrow and is to the right of the normal appearing ovary (corpus luteum present).

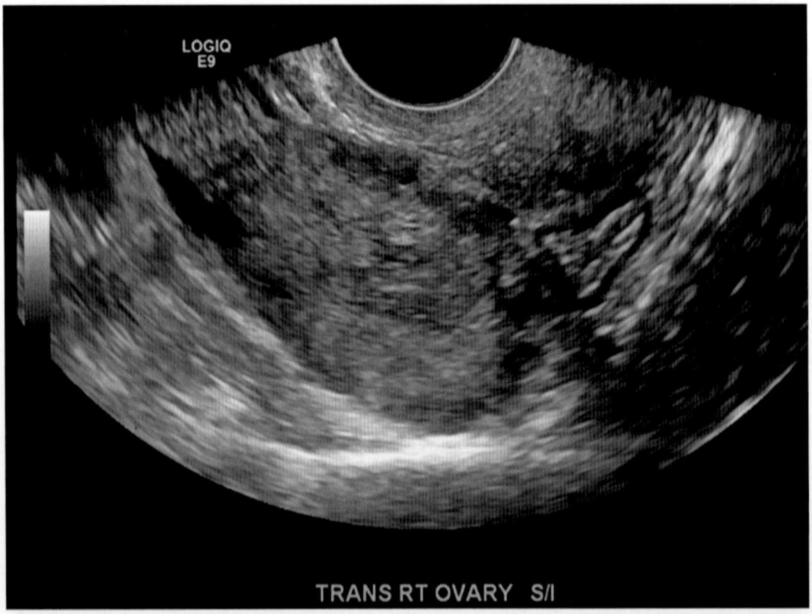

Figure 19-2 A torsed adnexa without an obvious ovarian mass. The ovary is abnormal in its size, shape, and edematous appearance. It is uniformly hyperechoic and does not have crisp borders typically seen with a normal ovary.

an urgent ultrasound to determine the pregnancy location in order to make the diagnosis of an ectopic pregnancy as early as possible.

Adnexal torsion

Another gynecologic pelvic mass presenting as an emergency is adnexal torsion. Patients experiencing torsion usually have acute onset of pain, often with nausea and vomiting. They may have signs of peritoneal irritation such as rebound or guarding. The overall prevalence is about 2.7%.[9] Torsion occurs more commonly on the right.[9] Adnexal pathology is present in about 50%–80% of torsed adnexa.[9] In the setting of torsion, the ovary tends to have a rounder, more edematous appearance with increased volume (Figure 19-2). The use of Doppler flow imaging alone to make the diagnosis of adnexal torsion is unreliable and clinical judgment should always be used over Doppler studies. Doppler flow studies are very sensitive; when flow is absent, this is essentially diagnostic. However, when flow is present, there is a high false negative rate. In studies of surgically confirmed ovarian torsion, up to 60% had blood flow present on Doppler studies.[10, 11]

Once the diagnosis is made, prompt intervention is needed to save the ovary and prevent future sequelae including necrosis, febrile illness and potential sepsis. Laparoscopic surgery is recommended with untwisting of the adnexa. The decision to remove any associated pathology after detorsing the adnexa can be a difficult one. Most associated cysts are physiologic and do not require removal. When a pathologic cyst is present, such as with a mature teratoma, it is beneficial to the patient to have the lesion removed to prevent recurrence. Surgery on ischemic and edematous adnexa can, however, result in bleeding. The bleeding risk must be weighed against the risk of recurrence and the risk of a second operative procedure if removal is delayed as some authors suggest.[11] Once the adnexa is detorsed, the return of ovarian function is quite good even if the intraoperative appearance is worrisome. In a review of five studies looking at subsequent ovarian function as measured by follicular development, subsequent appearance on ultrasound, as well as function during ovarian stimulation, 88%–100% of detorsed ovaries regained normal function.[11]

Tubo-ovarian abscess

A tubo-ovarian abscess (TOA) may be diagnosed in an acutely ill patient. TOAs are typically found in patients presenting with acute pelvic inflammatory disease (PID). Physical exam findings include fever, cervicitis, cervical motion tenderness, and abdominal pain. The patient may have a palpable mass in the adnexa. Imaging of the adnexa may show a pyosalpinx; this is a dilated tubular structure filled with complex fluid. Typically, pyosalpinx is seen by transvaginal ultrasound with an estimated sensitivity ranging from 83% to 93%.[12, 13] Pelvic inflammatory disease complicated by tubo-ovarian abscess requires inpatient admission and intravenous antibiotic therapy. If the patient does not improve, surgical drainage may be necessary. It is important to recognize this type of pelvic mass because the diagnosis of TOA excludes the possibility of outpatient management and necessitates inpatient parenteral treatment for PID.

Nonemergent management of pelvic mass

Uterine myomas

The most common pelvic masses are uterine myomas. The etiology, diagnosis, and management of uterine leiomyomata will be discussed in detail in Chapter 20. It is important to consider uterine myoma in the differential diagnosis of a uterine mass, but they should also be considered when a mass is located adjacent to the uterus, or even in the adnexa as pedunculated myomas are often confused with complex ovarian masses.

Nonovarian adnexal masses

Several other adnexal masses do not arise from the ovary such as paratubal cysts, hydrosalpinx, or tubo-ovarian abscess. Paratubal cysts are simple, thin walled cystic structures in the adnexa that appear to be separate from the ovary. On exam, they are nearly impossible to differentiate from an ovarian cyst, but on ultrasound imaging, they move separately from the ovary. They are typically stable over time or slow growing and are less likely to regress than a simple ovarian cyst. Hydrosalpinx is a dilated tube, typically seen as filled with simple fluid on ultrasound. These are difficult to palpate on physical exam, and are typically asymptomatic. Hydrosalpinx can arise from prior pelvic infection with tubal damage, such as a prior tubo-ovarian abscess, prior ectopic pregnancy or from prior tubal surgery. Uterine myomas can also be present at the uterine cornual region or in the broad ligament and can be interpreted as adnexal masses. Physical exam is helpful in these patients as the mass will be solid, smooth, and firm, and it will move in conjunction with the uterus.

Ovarian masses

Ovarian masses can be seen at the time of imaging for a suspected mass palpated during an exam, or are often found incidentally when the pelvis is imaged for another reason. The differential diagnosis for ovarian masses is broad and cannot be covered comprehensively in this chapter, but the most common ovarian masses will be reviewed. When evaluating an ovarian mass, it is important to first classify the mass as physiologic or pathologic.

Physiologic ovarian cysts

Examples of physiologic or functional cysts include dominant follicles, corpus lutea, or hemorrhagic corpus lutea. These are the most commonly seen cysts during an ultrasound. Although normal, they are typically commented on by the interpreting physician, and the information is subsequently relayed to the patient. This can cause anxiety for the patient as these common cysts are often interpreted as being abnormal. Physiologic cysts, however, simply illustrate that the ovary is working properly, producing dominant follicles and ovulating. In this situation, reassurance can be given to the patient. The vast majority of simple cysts of the ovary resolve without intervention. Modesitt, et al. followed nearly 3,000 unilocular ovarian cysts in postmenopausal women. In those with simple cysts less than 10 cm, none developed ovarian cancer and nearly all resolved spontaneously.[14] It is suggested that simple cysts less than 5 cm do not even need repeat imaging. If the diagnosis of a physiologic cyst is less clear, or if the cyst is complex due to hemorrhage within the cyst (Figure 19-3), repeat imaging with expectant management should be the treatment of choice rather than any other intervention. Ovulation suppression should be considered if these cysts are bothersome to the patient. The recommended interval of reimaging is somewhat controversial, but most suggest around 8–12 weeks allowing time for the functional cyst to resolve completely.

Pathologic ovarian masses – benign

A wide variety of benign masses of the ovary exist. The most common are mature cystic teratomas, endometriomas, fibromas, and cystadenomas. Each of these has a different appearance on ultrasound, findings on exam, and management.

Mature cystic teratomas, also called dermoids, are the most common benign ovarian mass seen in the premenopausal patient. They are filled with tissue from every germ cell line, giving them classic findings of internal fat, hair, and even teeth (Figure 19-6).

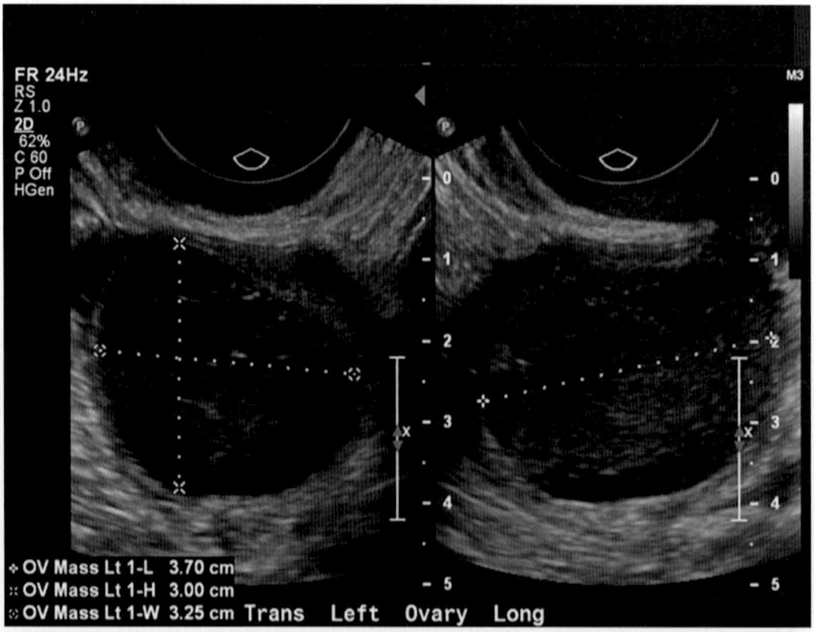

Figure 19-3 Hemorrhagic cyst.

On exam, they are usually mobile, smooth walled, and can range in size from a few centimeters to more than 10 cm. They are bilateral about 15% of the time; bilaterality should be taken into consideration when performing a physical exam and reviewing imaging studies. Because they are filled with dense tissue, mature teratomas have a higher risk of torsion than some other masses and should be removed.

Endometriomas are often diagnosed as part of the workup for clinically significant endometriosis. In patients with dysmenorrhea, a physical exam with a fixed, painful pelvic mass is suspicious for an endometrioma. These are commonly palpated in the posterior cul de sac, and are sometimes best examined with a recto-vaginal exam. On ultrasound imaging, they are filled with homogenous low-level echoes without vascularity (Figure 19-4). The homogenous material seen on ultrasound is old blood, which is seen surgically as a "chocolate cyst." The differential diagnosis of this type of mass should include a hemorrhagic cyst as these can sometimes have a similar appearance. Reimaging of this type of cyst is recommended, and if persistent, the diagnosis of endometrioma can presumptively be made. No intervention is needed if a patient is asymptomatic. However, if the woman is symptomatic, surgery may be necessary to remove the endometrioma with fulguration of any other implant areas for pain relief.

Ovarian fibromas are the most common benign solid tumor of the ovary. They are typically small and very slow growing. They are firm on pelvic exam, but are still mobile and smooth. On ultrasound the finding of a homogenous, solid, avascular mass that is relatively stable over time is most consistent with a fibroma. They do not require removal if they are asymptomatic and stable, but surgical removal of any pathologic ovarian mass is a reasonable option after weighing the risks and benefits. A rare disorder called Meigs' syndrome occurs with fibromas in conjunction with ascites and pleural effusions. Removal of the mass results in resolution of the fluid collections. This only occurs in 2% of fibromas and should not be a driving factor to remove the mass, but should be considered in a female patient presenting with unexplained ascites and pleural effusion.[2]

A more common type of benign, but pathologic, ovarian mass is the cystademoma. Cystadenomas are further divided into serous or mucinous type. Serous cystadenomas are palpated as soft, smooth, and mobile masses on pelvic exam. They are seen on ultrasound imaging as thin walled, mostly hypoechoic cysts with some uniform complexity to the internal fluid, thereby differentiating them from simple cysts (Figure 19-5). These cysts are persistent on ultrasound; this differentiates them from physiologic cysts. Mucinous cystadenomas are similar in that they are thin walled and cystic on ultrasound, but

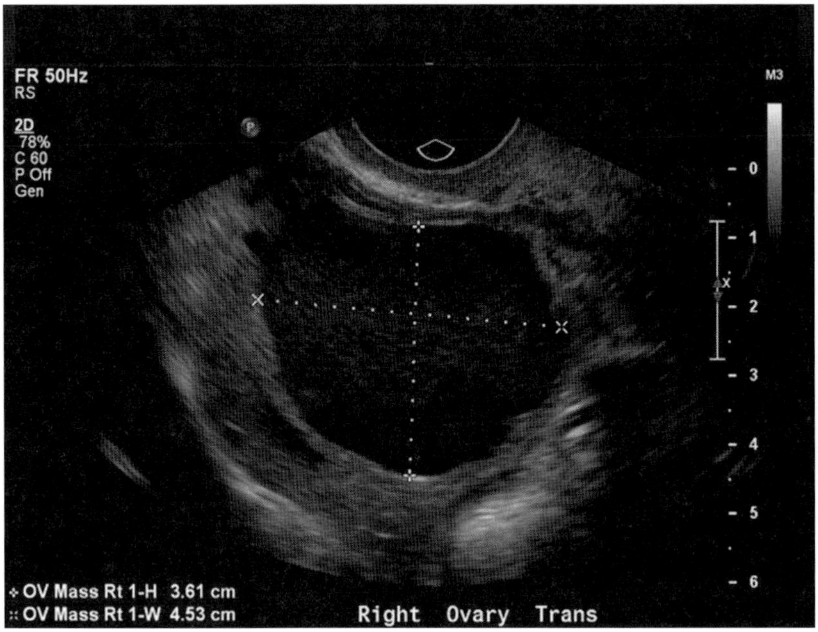

Figure 19-4 Endometrioma.

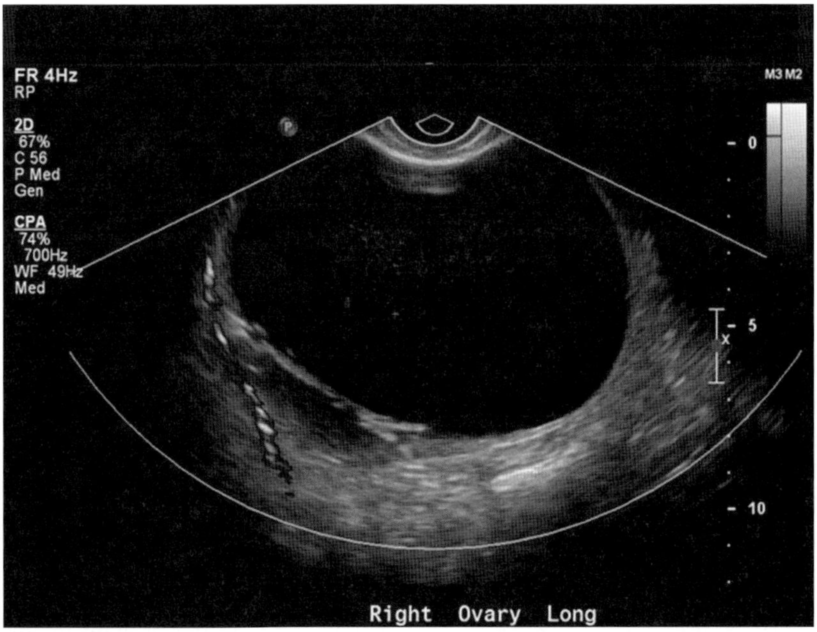

Figure 19-5 Serous cystadenoma.

they are filled with a more hyperechoic fluid making them more complex in appearance. These two types of cystadenomas can also be differentiated based upon size. Mucinous cystadenomas can be extremely large, not uncommonly up to 20 cm in size, whereas other benign ovarian cysts rarely grow to that size.

Pathologic ovarian masses – malignant

The differentiation between benign and malignant ovarian masses is difficult and can be very anxiety provoking for providers. The diagnosis of a late-stage ovarian malignancy is rarely missed, but the diagnosis of an early malignancy is difficult to make.

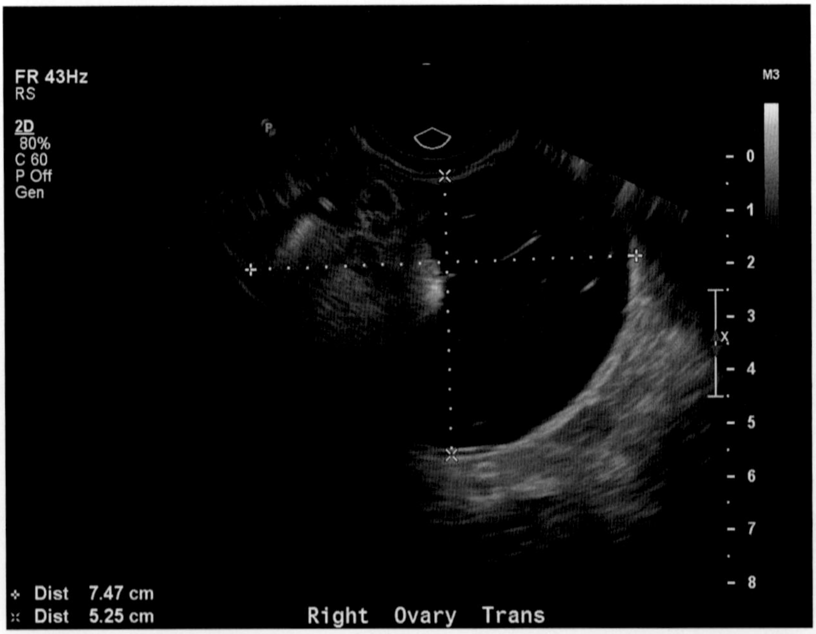

Figure 19-6 Mature cystic teratoma.

There is no screening test that can reliably diagnose an ovarian cancer before the patient is symptomatic. Even the use of advanced imaging techniques may fail to differentiate between benign and malignant processes. The combination of a thorough history, exam, review of imaging and laboratory analysis gives health-care providers the ability to discern when a patient should have an ovarian mass removed by a gynecology specialist and when the patient needs to be referred to a gynecologic oncology subspecialist for further care.

A history and review of systems should focus on any weight change, feelings of early satiety, abdominal bloating, and abdominal pain. Patients at highest risk of ovarian cancer are postmenopausal women, patients with late menopause, or those with a history of infertility. Protective factors include prior hysterectomy or tubal ligation, use of oral contraceptive pills, and nuliparity.[15] Family history is also a major factor and should be elicited in detail. Women with a strong family history of breast or ovarian cancer may qualify for genetic testing. Patients with BRCA1 have a 39%–46% chance of developing ovarian cancer, and those with BRCA2 mutations have a 12%–20% risk of ovarian cancer in their lifetime.[16] Women who should be offered BRCA testing are outlined in Table 19-4.

On physical exam, palpation of an advanced pelvic cancer reveals a fixed, firm, nodular mass. This may be palpated abdominally, during a bimanual exam, or during a rectal exam. When the recto-vaginal septum demonstrates nodularity, this usually indicates a more advanced stage. If the malignancy arises from the uterus or cervix, a fungating mass may be seen or palpated vaginally. Bilaterality should be assessed. An abdominal fluid wave can be present in patients with ascites. The ascites is caused by lymph node involvement of the malignancy.

As previously discussed, if an adnexal mass is palpated on exam, TVUS is the imaging method of choice. Masses that raise concern for malignancy are complex on ultrasound. These complex findings can be in the form of multiple septations, a mixture of cystic and solid components, or nodularity at the periphery. Fluid in the posterior cul de sac can potentially represent ascitic fluid. The vascularity seen in malignant masses also helps to differentiate them from benign masses. When using Doppler flow to evaluate a mass, it is normal to have flow at the periphery of a benign mass as this is flow to the normal ovarian cortex. However, if there are solid components or nodularity at the periphery with vascular flow, that should raise concern for a malignant lesion. These findings on imaging, in combination with the patient's history, can help guide the provider in determining the likelihood of a malignancy.

If a malignant mass is suspected, laboratory analysis of tumor markers can be helpful. There are rare

Table 19-4 Patients recommended to have genetic testing

Genetic testing is **recommended** (20%–25% chance of having a genetic predisposition to breast and ovarian cancer):
• Personal history of both breast and ovarian cancer • Ovarian cancer and a first- or-second degree relative with ovarian cancer or premenopausal breast cancer • Ovarian cancer and Ashkenazi Jewish descent • Breast cancer before age 50 and a first- or second-degree relative with ovarian cancer or a male relative with breast cancer • Ashkenazi Jewish with breast cancer at age 40 or younger • Those with a first- or second-degree relative with known BRCA mutation
Genetic testing should be **offered** (5%–10% risk of having a genetic predisposition to breast or ovarian cancer):
• Breast cancer diagnosed before the age of 40 • High-grade serous cancer of the ovary, peritoneum, or fallopian tube diagnosed at any age • Bilateral breast cancer • Ashkenazi Jewish descent and breast cancer diagnosed before the age of 50 • Breast cancer and two first- or second-degree relatives with breast cancer • Unaffected patient with a first- or second-degree relative who meets any of the preceding criteria.

forms of ovarian cancer, typically present in younger women, that require evaluation of AFP, inhibin, quantitative hCG and LDH. Table 19-6 gives information on each lab and associated mass. The most commonly ordered lab test to evaluate potential ovarian cancer is a CA125 level. This test is more useful in post-menopausal women because of its low specificity in the premenopausal female. The CA125 can be falsely elevated by fibroids, endometriosis, inflammatory bowel disease, or other inflammatory conditions of the pelvis. However, in the setting of a suspicious mass, this lab test should be obtained no matter the patient's age; interpretation must be with caution. CA125 is certainly recommended in a postmenopausal woman with a complex ovarian mass. Ova1 is a newer test that combines CA125 level, transferrin, prealbumin, apolipoprotein AI and beta 2 microglobulin. These values are interpreted with special software and a score on a scale of 1 to 10 is assigned. If the patient is premenopausal, a score of less than 5 is considered low risk and 5 or greater is high risk. If the patient is postmenopausal, the cut-off lowers to 4.4. The idea behind this test is that if the score is in the low-risk range, a general gynecology specialist can feel more confident performing the surgery; if a patient has a high-risk score, the patient should be referred to a gynecologic oncology subspecialist for the surgery. The initial trial with Ova1 reported sensitivity of 92.5% and specificity of 42.8% along with a positive predictive value of 42.3% and a negative predictive value of 92.7%.[17] This test should only be used when an adnexal mass is present and should not be used as a screening test. It seems that, based on this initial data, if the patient tests into the high-risk group a fairly large number of them will turn out to have a benign lesion; only very few will have a malignancy when scoring in the low-risk category.

Numerous scoring methods and other attempts at standardizing the evaluation of masses have been attempted to assist in the differentiation between benign and malignant processes, but none have proven successful. Recommendations for referral to cancer subspecialists exist from the Society of Gynecologic Oncology and from the American Congress of Obstetrics and Gynecology; see Table 19-5. These recommendations may be helpful in deciding when to refer a patient to a subspecialist preoperatively, but they have not been shown to be particularly effective at diagnosing an early stage cancer. Many of the criteria for referral are indicative of late stage disease. One study looking at the performance of these guidelines found them to be 79.2% sensitive and 69.8% specific in premenopausal patients and 93.2% sensitive and 59.9% specific in postmenopausal women.[18]

Concluding remarks

Pelvic masses can arise from the uterus, fallopian tubes, ovaries, or other nongynecologic organs such as the bowel or bladder. The evaluation should begin with a thorough history, review of systems, and

Table 19-5 Guidelines for referral to a gynecologic oncologist

Premenopausal

- CA125 level greater than 200 u/mL
- Ascites
- Evidence of distant metastasis (by exam or imaging)
- First-degree relative with breast or ovarian cancer

Postmenopausal

- Elevated CA125 level
- Ascites
- Nodular or fixed pelvic mass
- Evidence of distant metastasis (by exam or imaging)
- First degree relative with breast or ovarian cancer

Source: Im, SS et al., Validation of referral guidelines for women with pelvic masses. *Obstetrics and Gynecology* 2005; 105: 35–41.

Table 19-6 Laboratory workup of germ cell and sex cord-stromal tumors of the ovary

Serum marker	Associated ovarian tumor
Inhibin	Granulosa cell tumor
LDH	Dysgerminoma
β-hCG	Embryonal cell tumor
AFP	Sertoli-leydig tumor
AFP and LDH	Endodermal sinus tumor

physical exam. Next, imaging, usually with transvaginal ultrasound, should be obtained to aid in the diagnosis. Laboratory workup can then be tailored to the findings. Once all of these components are assembled, the appropriate management and referral, if needed, can be done. The comprehensive evaluation outlined in this chapter leads to the best care of this challenging diagnosis.

References

1. Baird, DD. High cumulative incidence of uterine leiomyoma in black and white women; ultrasound evidence. *Am J Obstet Gynecol* 2003; **188**(1): 100–7.
2. Marshall, LM. Variation in the incidence of uterine leiomyoma among premenopausal women by age and race. *Obstet Gynecol* 1997; **90**(6): 967–73.
3. American Congress of Obstetricians and Gynecologists. Committee on Gynecology Practice. ACOG Practice Bulletin No. 83. Management of adnexal masses. *Obstet Gynecol* 2007 July; **110**: 201–14.
4. Lentz, GM. *Comprehensive Gynecology*, 6th edition. Philadelphia: Elsevier Mosby, 2012.
5. Padilla, LA. Limitations of the pelvic examination for evaluation of the female pelvic organs. *Int J Gynecol Obstet* 2005 January; **88**(1): 84–8.
6. Cantuaria, GH. Comparison of binmanual examination with ultrasound examination before hysterectomy for uterine leiomyoma. *Obstet Gynecol* 1998; **92**(1): 109–12.
7. Agency for Healthcare Research and Quality. Management of adnexal mass. Evidence Based Report/Technology Assessment No. 130. AHRQ 2006. Available at: www.ahrq.gov/downloads/pub/evidence/pdf/adnexal/adnexal.pdf. Accessed July 2014.
8. Chiou S. Adnexal torsion: new clinical and imaging observations by sonography, computed tomography, and magnetic resonance imaging. *American Institute of Ultrasound Medicine* 2007; **26**(10): 1289–1301.
9. Bider D. Clinical, surgical and pathologic findings of adnexal torsion in pregnant and nonpregnant women. *Surg Gynecol Obstet* 1991; **173**(5): 363–6.
10. Pena J. Usefulness of Doppler sonography in the diagnosis of ovarian torsion. *Fertility and Sterility* 2000; **73**(5): 1047–50.
11. Oelsner G. Adnexal torsion. *Clinical Obstetrics and Gynecology* 2006; **49**(3); 459–63.
12. Lande, MC. Adnexa and cul-de-sac abnormalities: transvaginal sonography. *Radiology* 1988; **166**(2): 325–32.
13. Lee, DC. Sensitivity of ultrasound for the diagnosis of tubo-ovarian abscess: a case report and literature review. *Journal of Emergency Medicine* 2011; **40**(2): 170–5.
14. Modesitt, SC. Risk of malignancy in unilocular ovarian cystic tumors less than 10 centimeters in diameter. *Obstet Gynecol* 2003; **102**(3): 594–9.
15. Booth, M. Risk factors for ovarian cancer: a case-control study. *Br J Cancer* 1989; **60**(4): 592–98.
16. American Congress of Obstetricians and Gynecologists. ACOG Practice Bulletin No. 103. Hereditary breast and ovarian cancer syndrome. *Obstet Gynecol* 2009 April; **113**(4): 957–66.
17. Ueland, FR. Effectiveness of a multivariate index assay in the preoperative assessment of ovarian tumors. *Obstet Gynecol* 2011; **117**(6): 1289–97.
18. Dearking, AC. How relevant are ACOG and SGO guidelines for referral of adnexal mass? *Obstet Gynecol* 2007; **110**(4): 841–8.

Chapter 20

Office management of incontinence

Ayman M. Elnaqa and Khaled Afifi

Background and prevalence

Urinary incontinence (UI) is the complaint of any involuntary leakage of urine. The prevalence of urinary incontinence varies widely due to differences in definition. Many of those affected will not admit to having continence difficulties. It is estimated that UI affects 30%–60% of middle-aged and older women in the community, and up to 80% of female nursing home residents. Despite this high prevalence, UI is both underreported and undertreated.[1–4] UI may seriously influence the physical, psychological, and social well-being of affected individuals. The impact on the families and carers of women with UI may be profound, and there are considerable resource implications for health services.

Risk factors

Risk factors for UI can be classified as predisposing, obstetric and gynecologic, and promoting factors. Predisposing factors include race (Caucasian women are more susceptible), genetics, congenital defects, and neurologic abnormalities. Obstetric and gynecologic factors include pregnancy/childbirth/parity, pelvic surgery and radiotherapy, and pelvic organ prolapse. Promoting factors include increased age, comorbidities such as diabetes and vascular disease, changes in mobility, obesity, conditions associated with increased abdominal pressure, cognitive impairment, urinary tract infection, and medications such as oral estrogen substitutes, diuretics, and anticholinergic agents.[5]

Types of incontinence

Stress incontinence is the involuntary leakage of urine with effort or exertion, sneezing, coughing, or laughing. These activities result in increased intra-abdominal pressure. This overcomes the sphincter closure mechanism in the absence of a bladder contraction. It is often caused by weakened pelvic muscles. Stress incontinence is the most common type of urinary incontinence in younger women.

Urge incontinence is the involuntary leakage of urine accompanied by or immediately preceded by a strong desire to pass urine. It is generally caused by an oversensitive bladder. Urge incontinence is more common in elderly women. In younger women, urge incontinence may be due to interstitial cystitis. It is termed detrusal overactivity (DO) if there is no identifiable condition and detrusor hyperreflexia if it is a result of a known neurologic lesion.[6] Most patients who present with these symptoms have an idiopathic inability to suppress detrusor contractions.

Although the term "overactive bladder" (OAB) is often used interchangeably with "urge incontinence," it has a slightly different meaning. Overactive bladder is not actually a diagnosis, but refers to a constellation of symptoms associated with urge incontinence. These include urgency, frequency, and nocturia (which may or may not include incontinence).

Mixed incontinence is the combination of stress and urge incontinence. Mixed incontinence is the most common type of urinary incontinence for women overall. The aim of the physician is to identify which type of incontinence is more distressing for the patient and treat it first.

Overflow incontinence is the dribbling and/or continuous leakage associated with incomplete bladder emptying, often caused by impaired detrusor contractility or, more rarely, by bladder outlet obstruction. Outlet obstruction can be seen in women with severe pelvic organ prolapse or prior anti-incontinence surgery. Weak detrusor contraction can be due to diabetic neuropathy, multiple sclerosis, low spinal cord injury, radical pelvic surgery, or secondary to medications such as psychotropic medications.

Functional incontinence occurs in otherwise continent individuals who are unable to get to the toilet in

Office Care of Women, ed. Martin E. Olsen and Botros Rizk. Published by Cambridge University Press.

time. This can be due to cognitive, psychological, or physical impairments. Many functionally impaired women can also have other forms of urinary incontinence; therefore, this is a diagnosis of exclusion.

Total incontinence is a rare form of urinary incontinence due to an anatomic bypass of the normal continence mechanism. Examples of this include urinary fistula, ectopic ureters, and urethral diverticulae.

Transient incontinence due to acute and reversible causes is called transient incontinence. It is more common in elderly. Although transient UI is more likely in persons with lower urinary tract abnormalities, correction of the precipitating factor remains effective in the majority of cases.

Table 20-1 summarizes causes of transient incontinence that can be easier recalled using the mnemonic "DIAPPERS."[7]

Table 20-1 Causes of transient urinary incontinence

Delirium
Infection (Urinary Tract)
Atrophic urethritis or vaginitis
Pharmacology (i.e., diuretics, anticholinergics)
Psychological disorders (especially depression)
Endocrine disorders (i.e., diabetes)
Restricted mobility (i.e., post-operative)
Stool Impaction

Evaluation of patients with urinary incontinence

Most cases of urinary incontinence can be diagnosed based on patient history, symptom assessment, physical examination, and urinalysis. Initiation of noninvasive treatment does not require an extensive workup.

History

A thorough history is the basis of evaluation. It allows the clinician to make a diagnosis, assess the severity and duration of the incontinence and its effect on the quality of life. Detailed medical, obstetric, and surgical history can identify contributing factors and delineate comorbidities which can influence management. Medical conditions such as diabetes, neurological conditions, cognitive impairment, and cardiac and lung disease should be noted.[8] Table 20-2 shows medications that can potentially affect the bladder function.

Estrogen status should be identified together with the intake of hormonal replacement therapy. Previous abdominal and vaginal surgery as well as pelvic radiation should be identified.

Social history includes exercise, smoking, and the amount and type of food/fluid intake as well as environmental issues such as social, cultural, and physical environment. One should also inquire about consumption of bladder irritants (caffeinated products,

Table 20-2 Potential medication effects on continence

Anticholinergic agents	Reduce detrusal contractions, cognitive impairment, constipation	Retention of urine
Cholinesterase inhibitors	Increase detrusal contractions	Urge
Calcium channel blockers	Reduce detrusal contractions, constipation	Retention of urine
ACE inhibitors	induced cough	Stress
Diuretics	Increase urine volume	Urge, Retention of urine
Antipsychotics	Reduce detrusal contractions, constipation, confusion	Retention of urine, Functional
Benzodiazepines	Sedation	Functional
SSRIs	Increase detrusal contractions, sedation	Urge, Functional
Opioids	Reduce detrusal contractions, constipation, confusion	Retention of urine, Functional
Tricyclic antidepressants	Reduce detrusal contractions, sedation	Retention of urine, Functional
Selective alpha blockers	Relax bladder outlet	Stress
Hormone replacement therapy	Ineffective urethral closure	Urge, Stress

Table 20-3 Causes of transient urinary incontinence

0 = no visible or palpable contraction
1 = a very weak contraction, often barely perceived as a flick
2 = a weak but clearly perceived contraction
3 = well perceived, but is not maintained when moderate finger pressure is applied
4 = a contraction with good force, but not maintained when intense finger pressure is applied
5 = maximum strength with strong resistance to oppositional pressure.

alcohol, acidic foods, and drinks). Excessive fluid intake (more than six to eight 8-oz glasses of fluid per day) should be noted.

Lower urinary tract symptoms

Lower urinary tract symptoms can be divided into three groups: storage, voiding, and post-micturition symptoms.

Storage symptoms

Storage symptoms include leakage with exertion such as coughing, sneezing, laughing, bending or lifting. Physicians should enquire about the duration of incontinence, the amount of leakage perceived, and the daily pad usage.

Overactive bladder symptoms include daytime frequency and nocturia, urgency, and urge incontinence. Bladder sensation should be categorized as normal, increased, reduced, or absent.[8]

Voiding symptoms

Hesitancy, straining to void, terminal dribbling in addition to the speed of flow should be noted. Urine stream can be described as normal, slow stream, splitting, or spraying of the urine or intermittent stream. Associated symptoms such as dysuria, pain, or hematuria should be noted.

Post-micturition symptoms

Post-micturition symptoms include feeling of incomplete emptying after passing urine, with or without post-micturition dribble. In addition, one should also inquire about consumption of bladder irritants (caffeinated products, alcohol, acidic foods and drinks). Excessive fluid intake (more than six to eight 8-oz glasses of fluid per day) should be noted.

Sexual history

Dyspareunia, vaginal dryness, and incontinence should be noted. It is helpful to define urine leakage as during penetration, during intercourse, or at orgasm if present.

Symptoms associated with pelvic organ prolapse

Symptoms that suggest prolapse include feeling of a lump, statements such as "something coming down," sensation of vaginal pressure or fullness, heaviness, dragging sensation, low backache, or the need to digitally replace the prolapse in order to defecate or micturate.

Bowel symptoms

Information regarding associated fecal incontinence, frequency of bowel movements, length of time to evacuate, and whether the patient must splint her vagina or perineum during defecation should be obtained. Associated genital and lower urinary tract pain could indicate an underlying pathology.

Functional incontinence assessment

Many patients are incontinent due to poor adaptation to the environment rather than a genuine bladder or bowel problem. The assessment of environmental factors such as clothing and underwear, room floors, and access to toilets (including light switches) are useful when assessing a patient with incontinence, particularly in elderly patients. Referral to occupational therapy for detailed assessment should be considered.

Family and caregivers may be encouraged to discuss history, goals of care, and treatment for individuals with dementia only if the individual is incapable of accurate reporting or weighing treatment decisions.

Examination

General examination should assess the overall patient health and functional status. Evaluate extremities for edema, which can increase nocturia, especially in frail elderly patients

The body mass index (BMI) of the patient should be checked. The prevalence of both UUI and SUI increases proportionately with rising body mass index;[9] weight loss (>5%) in obese women improves UI.[10]

Abdominal examination

An enlarged palpable bladder or any pelvic or abdominal mass can cause pressure symptoms on the bladder. The presence of any scar from previous surgery should be noted. The kidney should be examined for size and tenderness. A back examination for any scars indicating previous surgery or trauma should be carried out.

Vaginal examination

A thorough vaginal examination should be performed. It is best performed in dorsal lithotomy position. The use of Sim's speculum can facilitate the visualization of the vaginal wall. Having the patient stand with one foot on a step stool is helpful if one suspects vaginal prolapse. The vulva and perineum should be inspected for the presence of atrophy or skin excoriation. Atrophic vagina could be associated with increased urinary tract infection and increased urethral and bladder sensitivity. Excessive descent of the urethra-bladder neck area with Valsalva maneuver can be associated with stress incontinence. Any existing prolapse should be noted. Bimanual examination is then performed to assess the size of the uterus and the presence of any pelvic mass.

The National Institute of Clinical Excellence (NICE) does not recommend the routine use of Q-tip, Bonney, Marshall, and Fluid-Bridge tests in the assessment of women with UI.[11]

Cough stress test

The aim of the test is to objectively demonstrate urinary incontinence. The patient is instructed to attend with a reasonably full bladder, and then instructed to cough or to do the Valsalva maneuver. Leakage of urine during the test indicates a positive test result. If no urine leak is observed, the test can be repeated in standing position. A large cystocoele should be reduced prior to the test to avoid a falsely negative test. Incontinence that occurs with cough is thought to be secondary to stress incontinence, but if it occurs a few seconds after a cough, it may be secondary to an uninhibited detrusor contraction.[12] The test is reliable, especially in women with a diagnosis of pure genuine stress incontinence.[13]

Pelvic floor muscle function

Pelvic muscle tone can be assessed by placing an examining finger 5 cm inside the vaginal introitus in the 5 o'clock and 7 o'clock positions. Muscle tone can be qualitatively defined by the tone at rest and the strength of a voluntary or reflex contraction as strong, weak, or absent or by a validated grading system (e.g., Oxford 1–5) (Figure 20-1).[14]

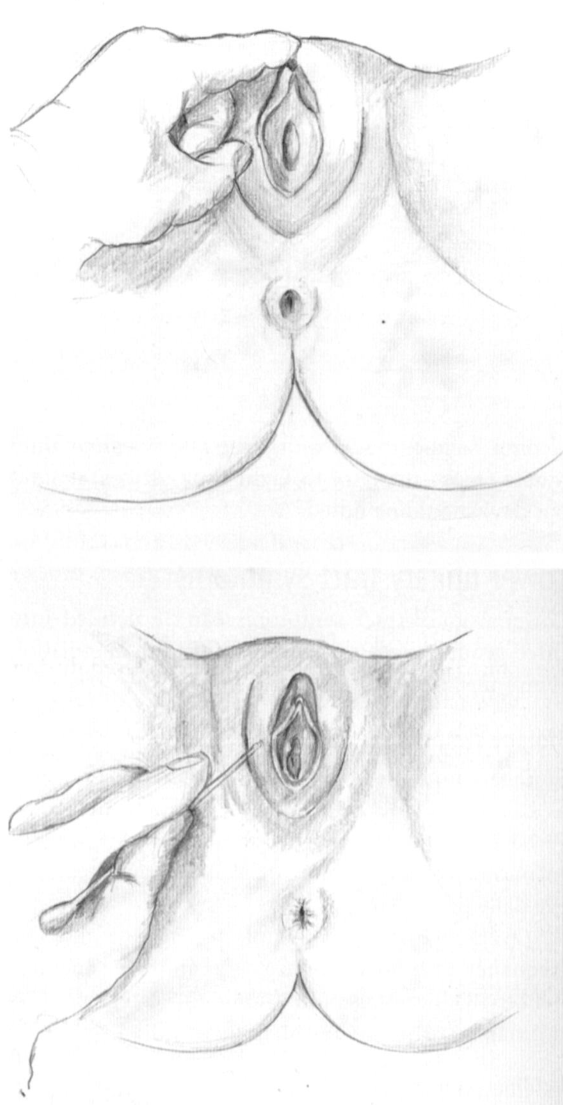

Figure 20-1 (*Upper*) Clitoral and (*lower*) Bulbocavernosus reflexes. Gentle tapping the clitoris or light stroke to the labia majora produce a reflex contraction of the external anal sphincter muscle.

Rectal examination

Health-care providers should check for fecal impaction, masses, presence of piles, or rectal mucosal prolapsed. The rest of the rectal examination is actually a detailed neurologic examination because the same sacral roots (S2–S4) innervate the external urethral sphincter and the anal sphincter. This will be dealt with later with the neurological examination.

Neurological assessment

A brief neurological examination should be part of any assessment for urinary incontinence. The patient's history should rule out any history of spinal cord trauma, tumor, multiple sclerosis, central lumbar disc prolapse, pelvic surgery, or irradiation.

Mental state cognitive function should be assessed, especially in elderly ladies. If concern is raised regarding memory deficits, confusion, or depression, referral for formal testing is essential.

Mobility is assessed by observing the patient while walking into the examining room and getting on and off the examining table. The patient's gait, balance, and the needs of assistance should be noticed.

If a neurological condition is suspected, a detailed neurological assessment is needed.

The ability of the patient to voluntarily contract the external anal sphincter should be assessed during a rectal examination.

Pudendal nerve (supply pelvic floor muscles and striated urinary sphincter and anal sphincter) and pelvic nerves (innervate the detrusor smooth muscle of the bladder and internal urinary sphincter) arise from the sacral segments (S2–S4).

The following reflexes could be of value in assessing patients with suspected neurological condition: ankle reflex (S1–S2), planter reflex (S2–S3), anal reflex (wink) (S2–S4), and bulbocavernousus reflex (S2–S4).The anal reflex and bulbocavernosus reflex are absent in 20% of normal people; hence, the absence of these reflexes are not necessarily pathologic.

Bladder diary

A bladder diary is a 24-hour record of the type and amount of fluid consumed, the number and volume of voids and leaks per hour, and what the patient was doing at the time of each leak. It serves as a diagnostic tool as well as a record of each patient's baseline condition. Events associated with incontinent episodes can help guide the diagnosis (e.g., leaking while unlocking the front door suggests an overactive bladder). The document can also uncover problematic types of intake such as excessive caffeine consumption or drinking after dinnertime, which can lead to increased nocturia. The bladder diary also serves as a good reference to judge the success of treatment. NICE has recommended encouraging women to complete a diary for a minimum of three days covering variations in their usual activities, such as both working and leisure days.

Quality-of-life questionnaire

Several studies have shown that clinicians tend to underestimate the degree of interference perceived by patients due to urinary incontinence.[15] Therefore an objective assessment of the impact of UI on quality of life is an essential part of evaluating patients. It includes assessment of the physical, functional, social, and emotional well-being of an individual. The International Continence Society (ICS) has recommended the use of a quality-of-life questionnaire (QoL) to evaluate the impact of urinary incontinence on patient life and to audit the effectiveness of treatment. There are several QoLs available, many of which are validated for different languages. The following incontinence-specific QoLs have been validated and recommended when therapies are being evaluated: ICIQ, BFLUTS, I-QoL, SUIQQ, UISS, SEAPI-QMM, ISI, and KHQ.[11]

Investigation

Laboratory tests

Urinalysis

Urinalysis should be performed in all cases at the initial assessment to exclude underlying pathology.[16] A clean catch urinalysis should be obtained. NICE has recommended that the urine dipstick needs to include the followings: blood, glucose, protein, leukocytes and nitrites in the urine (Figure 20-2).[11] Urine specific gravity should be checked, especially in patients who are suspected to have polydipsia, nocturia, or renal concentration abnormalities.

Post-void residual

The measurement of post-void residual (PVR) urine volume should be part of the initial assessment. The most accurate method of determining PVR urine volumes is catheterization, which is associated with increased risk of urinary infection and discomfort for the patient. Bladder ultrasound scanning has been introduced as an alternative noninvasive method. PVR of less than 100 mL is normal and more than 200 mL may be associated with obstruction or reduced bladder contractility. In older patents, PVR of 25% of total bladder volume is considered normal.[16]

Pad test

The pad test provides objective information about the severity of incontinence. To standardize the test, the ICS introduced the one-hour pad-weighing test, which measures the urine loss and weight gain of a perineal pad during a standard provocation exercise. Weight gain of more than 2 g per hour is considered as positive.[8] NICE has recommends not to use pad tests in the routine assessment of women with UI.[11]

Special tests

Special tests such as cystourethroscopy or urodynamics may be of assistance in diagnosis. These tests should be applied in a select fashion and be used to address specific diagnostic questions.

Urodynamic study

Urodynamics (UDA) is a general term used for all tests of bladder and urethral function. It is used to obtain information about urine storage and emptying. It is widely used as an addition to clinical diagnosis, to confirm diagnosis, and to provide prognostic information or when clinical diagnosis is difficult because of unclear history.

Several studies did not recommend the routine use of urodynamics before surgery for women who are likely to have genuine stress incontinence. The use of UDA did not improve outcome, and clinical evaluation alone was not found to be inferior to UDA.[17, 18]

NICE recommends not performing multichannel cystometry, ambulatory urodynamics, or videourodynamics before starting conservative management or for women where pure stress incontinence is diagnosed based on detailed history and examination. UDA can be performed in women who have symptoms of OAB leading to a clinical suspicion of detrusor overactivity, symptoms suggestive of voiding dysfunction, anterior compartment prolapse, or had previous surgery for stress incontinence. Ambulatory urodynamics or videourodynamics can be considered after conventional urodynamics if the diagnosis is unclear.[11]

Treatment

Before planning for treatment, it is important to discuss whether the patient wants to receive treatment, the extent of treatment that is acceptable to the patient, patient goals and expectations of treatment, available patient care, and systems for support.

The aim of treatment is to reduce urinary incontinence and improve quality of life. A personalized and tailored multicomponent, stepped approach that is focused on symptoms the patient considers most bothersome is the key to successful outcome.[19]

Regardless of the approaches used, it is up to the individual patient to determine whether she considers her incontinence to be successfully managed. Different women will have different perceptions of what is bothersome and what is tolerable.

Conservative management

Conservative treatment does not involve surgery. These include lifestyle interventions; physical, behavioral, drug and, complementary therapies; and non-therapeutic interventions (such as products that collect or contain leakage). Physical and behavioral therapies and/or lifestyle interventions are also considered preventive measures.

The ICS defines "conservative treatment" as therapies that are usually low cost and managed principally by the person with UI with instruction/supervision from a health-care professional. They differ from other forms of incontinence management, in that they have a low risk of adverse effects and do not prejudice other subsequent treatments.[8]

Nonpharmacologic options

Lifestyle modifications

There is a lack of high-quality prospective controlled trials evaluating the effects of modifying lifestyle factors in women with UI or OAB. However, there is some evidence to suggest that weight loss for moderately and morbidly obese women will reduce UI episodes. Dietary change such as avoiding foods and drinks that can adversely affect normal bladder function (caffeinated products, alcohol, and acidic or spicy products) may be of value. Small clinical trials do suggest that decreasing caffeine intake improves continence, and carbonated drinks increase the risk of OAB.

Although no conclusive association between smoking and urinary incontinence has been found, there are some studies that have shown smoking to be a possible risk factor for UI.[20] Certainly the cough that smoking can cause can be an aggravating factor in stress incontinence. Smoking cessation for patients with stress UI or stress-predominant mixed UI should be offered.

Patients often reduce their fluid intake in an effort to control UI symptoms. To avoid the risk of urinary tract infections, constipation, and dehydration, patients generally should not lower their intake below six to eight 8-oz glasses of fluid each day. Because excessively small or large urine output can contribute to urinary incontinence, reduction of fluid intake in patients who are drinking excessive amounts should be encouraged to adjust their fluid intake to produce a 24-hour urinary output of between 1,000 mL and 2,000 mL.[21]

Patients should avoid constipation as chronic straining may be a risk factor for urinary incontinence and genital organ prolapse.

Drugs that influence bladder function need to be reviewed; anticholinergics and beta blockers can cause overflow incontinence.

Urinary incontinence can be caused or exacerbated in patients with impaired mobility; reduction of physical barriers to toileting and mobility (e.g., selecting clothing that is easier to manage, mobility aids, and living area rearrangement) is important.

These same interventions are also effective for prevention of incontinence.

Physical therapy

Physical therapy should be offered as first-line therapy for the management of urgency, stress, and mixed urinary incontinence. Physical therapy has been found to be more effective and to provide more sustained improvement in symptoms than pharmacologic therapy.[21, 22]

Pelvic floor muscle exercises -- Pelvic floor muscle exercises (PFME) should be offered as first-line conservative therapy for women with stress, urgency, or mixed urinary incontinence.

PFME are based on the principle of strength training and involve squeezing and releasing the pelvic floor muscles. These contractions increase the strength and tone of the pelvic floor. This increases the force of urethral closure, which in turn prevents stress incontinence during an abrupt increase in intra-abdominal pressure. An assessment of pelvic floor muscle function should be undertaken prior to instigation of any pelvic floor muscle intervention.[21] Digital vaginal assessment is suitable for measuring pelvic floor muscle strength and endurance.

PFME are effective in the treatment of stress and mixed urinary incontinence, but there is insufficient evidence to assess their efficacy in the treatment of urge incontinence. Expert opinion suggests that pelvic floor muscle exercises may have a role in treatment of urge incontinence in combination with bladder training.[21]

A wide range of pelvic floor muscle training (PFMT) regimens are reported in the literature. Programs need to be tailored for the individual patient. The basic recommended regimen involves three sets of 8–12 slow-velocity contractions sustained for 6–8 seconds each, performed 3–4 times a week and continued for at least 20 weeks.[19] NICE recommends that pelvic floor muscle training programs comprise at least eight contractions performed three times per day.[11] Besides occasional cases of pain or discomfort, no other adverse effects were noted. In studies of up to one year, higher intensity PFMT regimens confer greater subjective cure or improvement than lower intensity regimens. Perineometry or pelvic floor electromyography should not be used as biofeedback as a routine part of PFMT.[11]

Biofeedback -- Most data regarding biofeedback relate its use in conjunction with PFME, rather than as an isolated intervention. Biofeedback was found to be no more effective than pelvic floor muscle exercises alone in alleviating symptoms of urinary incontinence.[21]

Evidence does not indicate additional benefit from biofeedback with PFME in comparison with PFMT alone in treating UI. Biofeedback with PFME is more costly than PFME alone and therefore is not cost-effective given a lack of additional benefit.[11]

Vaginal cones -- Two high-quality systematic reviews found that the use of weighted vaginal cones is effective in reducing symptoms of stress incontinence.[21] No evidence was found to suggest that use of vaginal cones is more effective than PFME alone. Compared with PFMT, cones are associated with more adherence problems. Vaginal cones are not suitable for all women and are inappropriate for use in some circumstances, such as when there is a moderate to severe prolapse, too narrow or too capacious a vagina causing difficulty with insertion or misplacement of the cone, untreated atrophic vaginitis, vaginal infection, or during menstruation or pregnancy.[11]

Electrical stimulation -- The current literature on the effectiveness of using electrical stimulation in treating urinary incontinence is inconclusive. This is largely due to the wide range of electrical stimulation parameters used in studies. There is a lack of consistency in the electrical stimulation protocols employed in available studies. There is limited evidence for the benefit of electrical stimulation versus sham electrical stimulation in the treatment of urgency UI. There is no evidence of additional benefit for electrical stimulation in combination with PFME compared with PFME alone. The most recent recommendation from NICE [11] does not recommend the routine use of electrical stimulation in the treatment of women with OAB. Electrical stimulation and/or biofeedback should be considered in women who cannot actively contract pelvic floor muscles in order to aid motivation and adherence to therapy.

Magnetic therapy -- Magnetic therapy aims to stimulate the pelvic floor muscles and/or sacral roots by placing them within an electromagnetic field. There are limited data on the use of magnetic therapy for UI, and its role in the treatment of women with UI is unclear.[11]

Behavioral therapies

Behavioral therapy involves an individual learning new patterns of response or reestablishing previously learned behavior to fit in with what is considered usual. Women with OAB (wet or dry) usually void more frequently than usual due to urgency. Women with stress UI also often void more frequently in the belief that they will preempt an involuntary urine loss associated with any increase in intra-abdominal pressure.

Various toileting programs have been used. Bladder training (also described as bladder retraining, bladder drill, bladder reeducation or bladder discipline) actively involves the individual attempting to increase the interval between the desire to void and the actual void. This may occur by mandatory schedules in which the individual may not use the toilet between set times for voiding, or a self-scheduled regimen where the patient gradually increases her inter-voiding times, and may use the toilet between times if the urgency becomes unbearable.[11]

Bladder training -- Bladder training is an appropriate first-line treatment for urgency urinary incontinence, and it is also effective for stress and mixed urinary incontinence. The goal is to have a schedule for voiding once every 2–4 hours. A woman who feels an urge to urinate outside the schedule should try to hold it for more and more minutes each time until she can keep the schedule. Timed voiding is done only when the patient is awake. Bladder training lasting for a minimum of six weeks should be offered as first-line treatment to women with urgency or mixed UI.

A multicomponent behavioral program that includes bladder training and PFME may confer a greater short-term benefit to women with stress, urgency, or mixed UI, but in the long term, combination and monotherapies are equally effective. If women do not achieve satisfactory benefit from bladder training programs, the combination of an OAB drug with bladder training should be considered if frequency is a troublesome symptom.[11]

Prompted voiding and timed voiding -- Prompted voiding and timed voiding are toileting programs used in people who are not capable of independent toileting, such as the cognitively impaired. Prompted voiding teaches people to initiate their own toileting through requests for help and positive reinforcement from carers. It has been used in institutionalized patients with cognitive and mobility problems. They are asked regularly if they wish to void and only assisted to the toilet when there is a positive response.[11]

Timed voiding (scheduled, routine, or regular toileting) is a passive toileting assistance program that is initiated and maintained by a caregiver (e.g., for patients who cannot participate in independent toileting). Toileting is fixed by time or event, on a regular schedule or on a schedule to match the patient's voiding pattern. The aim is to avoid incontinence episodes rather than restore bladder function.[11]

Prompted voiding and timed voiding strategies lead to reduced leakage episodes in cognitively impaired patients.

Neurostimulation

Neurostimulation is the alteration of neural pathways by the application of a stimulus (electrical or chemical) to a targeted site of the body. The exact mechanism of neurostimulation is unclear.

Neurostimulation of the sacral nerve roots may be achieved by direct conduction of electrical impulses from a lead implanted into the sacrum (percutaneous sacral neurostimulation [P-SNS]) by transcutaneous neurostimulation (T-SNS) delivered by surface electrodes applied directly over the sacrum in the region of the sacral nerve roots.

An alternative route for stimulation is through the retrograde stimulation of impulses through the posterior tibial nerve. Posterior tibial nerve stimulation may be delivered by surface electrodes (transcutaneous posterior nerve stimulation [T-PTNS]) or using a fine needle inserted close to the actual nerve (percutaneous posterior tibial nerve stimulation [P-PTNS]).

In an office setting, only T-SNS, P-PTNS, or T-PTNS are suitable in clinical practice. The current recommendations from NICE don't support the use of T-SNS or T-PTNS in treatment of OAB, although some women have found some satisfactory relief from symptoms using T-PTNS.[11]

NICE concluded that P-PTNS should not be offered routinely for treatment of OAB unless there has been a multidisciplinary team (MDT) review, and conservative management including OAB drug treatment has not worked adequately, and the woman does not want botulinum toxin A or percutaneous sacral nerve stimulation.[11]

Alternative conservative management options

Alternative conservative management of UI includes the use of products that collect or contain leakage (e.g., absorbent products, urinals and toileting aids, catheters) and products used to prevent leakage (e.g., devices that support the bladder neck, intra- or extra-urethral devices).

Absorbent products, urinals, and toileting aids -- Pads and pants are ineffective in the treatment of UI, and there is no evidence to support the use of hand-held urinals and toileting aids in the treatment of UI. In women who do not wish to pursue active interventions for UI, absorbent products, urinals, and toileting aids are an alternative management option. The use of these products should be considered for women awaiting definitive treatment.

Pads and protective garments may be the only method of managing UI after treatment of contributing comorbidities in frail older women with no or minimal mobility, advanced dementia, and/or nocturnal UI.[21] To prevent skin breakdown with the use of pads and protective garments, skin-barrier creams, such as Vaseline, may be useful.

Catheters -- Bladder catheterization (intermittent or indwelling urethral or suprapubic) should be considered for women whose persistent urinary retention causes incontinence, symptomatic infections, or renal dysfunction, and who cannot otherwise be corrected. Health-care professionals should be aware that the use of indwelling catheters in urgency UI may not result in continence. Intermittent catheterization is associated with reduced risk of UTI compared with indwelling catheterization. Suprapubic catheterization is preferable to indwelling urethral catheterization owing to reduced risk of urethral and other complications such as symptomatic UTI and "bypassing."

Clean intermittent urethral catheterization is offered to women with urinary retention who can be taught to self-catheterize or who have a carer who can perform the technique

Indications for the use of long-term indwelling urethral catheters for women with UI include chronic urinary retention in women who are unable to manage intermittent self-catheterization, skin wounds, pressure ulcers, or irritations that are being contaminated by urine, distress or disruption caused by bed and clothing changes and when a woman expresses a preference for this management.

Products to prevent leakage -- Several devices exist that temporarily prevent urinary incontinence episodes. They are classified as (a) intravaginal devices (e.g., continence guard, also known as the ConveenContiguard), (b) meatal devices (e.g., FemAssist), and (c) intraurethral devices or urethral plug (e.g., the ViVa Plug, also called Alive).

Some women find these products beneficial for occasional use in certain circumstances as a preventive strategy. There is limited evidence of efficacy in their management of UI. Adverse effects, in particular UTI, are very common. NICE does not recommend the use intravaginal and intraurethral devices for the routine management of UI in women.[11] Women should not consider such devices other than for occasional use when necessary to prevent leakage, such as during physical exercise.

Complementary therapies

Women who do not find conventional treatments acceptable often explore the use of complementary therapies for UI and as adjuncts to conventional treatments.

Poor-quality evidence shows that acupuncture may reduce nocturia and both stress and urgency incontinence in the short term (up to four weeks), but it is unclear whether any particular acupuncture treatment is more effective than others.

There is limited evidence that hypnotherapy for women with UI secondary to detrusor overactivity offers some benefit over the short term (up to six months). About half of women relapsed over a two-year period. There is a lack of evidence on herbal medicines for UI or OAB.[11]

Pharmacologic options

Estrogens

The evidence for the efficacy of estrogens in treating stress incontinence in women is conflicting. A meta-analysis showed that, when taken alone for a short period (three to six months), estrogens had a higher cure and improvement rate compared with placebo. The likelihood of cure or improvement with estrogen therapy was approximately a quarter higher for urge incontinence than stress incontinence. There is no evidence to support the routine use of intravaginal estrogens for the treatment of UI.[11]

Adrenoreceptor agonists

Drugs with an alpha 1A-adrenoreceptor agonist effect, such as ephedrine, pseudoephedrine, phenylpropanolamine, and methoxamine, have been used to treat stress incontinence. These drugs are not selective for urethral alpha adrenoreceptors, and the potential for side effects has limited their use.

Combined noradrenaline and serotonin reuptake inhibitors

Duloxetine is a serotonin and noradrenaline reuptake inhibitor that acts chiefly in the sacral spinal cord. It is thought that the resultant increase in pudendal nerve activity increases urethral sphincter contraction and closure pressure. It is licensed for use in moderate to severe stress UI.

Duloxetine use in the short term was shown to be associated with a reduction in leakage episodes, an increased voiding interval, and improved quality of life in women with stress UI or mixed UI where stress-related leakage is the predominant symptom. Adverse effects, particularly nausea, and discontinuation rates are very common (more than 10%). There is a lack of long-term safety data. The combination of duloxetine and PFME is more effective than no treatment. However, current NICE guidelines do not recommend the use of duloxetine as a first-line treatment or the routine offering as a second-line treatment for women with stress UI. It may be offered as second-line therapy if women prefer pharmacological to surgical treatment or are not suitable for surgical treatment. Women should be adequately counseled about adverse effects, and duloxetine should be used only as part of an overall management strategy in addition to pelvic floor muscle exercises. A four-week trial of duloxetine is recommended for women with moderate to severe stress incontinence. Follow-up occurs again after 12 weeks of therapy to assess progress and determine whether it is appropriate to continue treatment.[11]

Antidepressants

Several tricyclic antidepressants have been reported to have beneficial effects in urge incontinence but only imipramine has been widely used in this context. There are no good quality randomized controlled trials (RCTs) to support its use in detrusor overactivity, and its cardiotoxic side effects limit its use. Imipramine has been used clinically to treat stress incontinence, but no RCTs are available to support its use.[21]

Antimuscarinics

Several antimuscarinics such as darifenacin, fesoterodine, oxybutynin (immediate release), oxybutynin (extended release), oxybutynin (transdermal), oxybutynin (topical gel), propiverine, propiverine (extended release), solifenacin, tolterodine (immediate release), tolterodine (extended release), trospium, and trospium (extended release) are effective in reducing detrusor overactivity and hence urgency and urge incontinence. The drugs depress both voluntary and involuntary detrusor contractions by blocking muscarinic receptors on the bladder smooth muscle. There is a lack of evidence for a difference in effectiveness between OAB drugs. Few women achieve adequate long-term outcomes to continue treatment beyond one year. OAB drug treatment should be considered for women who have not achieved success with conservative management alone. It can also be considered as an adjunct to conservative management.[11]

Oxybutynin immediate release (IR) preparation has the highest incidence of side effects. Darifenacin has been shown to have less central nervous system or cardiac antimuscarinic related adverse effects.

Sustained release (SR) preparations have been shown to be associated with a lower incidence and severity of side effects than SR preparations.[21]

A therapeutic trial of antimuscarinics can be offered before establishing the cause of the OAB symptoms as detrusor overactivity.

Beta-3-adrenoreceptor agonist

Mirabegron (Betmiga) is a beta-3-adrenoreceptor agonist. It activates beta-3-adrenoreceptors causing the bladder to relax, which helps it to fill and also to store urine. It has a marketing authorization in the UK for the symptomatic treatment of urgency, increased micturition frequency, and/or urgency incontinence as may occur in patients with OAB. NICE has recommended mirabegron as an option for treating the symptoms of overactive bladder only for people in whom antimuscarinic drugs are contraindicated or clinically ineffective, or have unacceptable side effects.[23]

Flavoxate

The mechanism of action of flavoxate is not well understood, but it has an inhibitory action on the smooth muscle of the bladder and no antimuscarinic properties. Studies of the efficacy of flavoxate have shown mixed results but there is no evidence to support it use in UI or OAB.[21]

Concluding remarks

Most women with stress, urge, or mixed urinary incontinence are suitable for initial assessment and conservative management in an office setting. Urodynamic assessment is not necessary prior to conservative treatment as it does not improve or predict outcome of conservative treatments. An important proportion of women with voiding dysfunction have underlying conditions such as neuropathy, diabetes, medication side effects, or a pelvic mass which should be addressed prior to initiating a therapeutic plan for incontinence.

References

1. Goode PS, Burgio KL, Richter HE, Markland AD. Incontinence in older women. *JAMA*. 2010 Jun 2;**303**(21):2172–81.
2. Herderschee R, Hay-Smith EJ, Herbison GP, et al. Feedback or biofeedback to augment pelvic floor muscle training for urinary incontinence in women. *Cochrane Database Syst Rev*. 2011;(7):CD009252.
3. Markland AD, Vaughan CP, Johnson TM, 2nd, et al. Incontinence. *Med Clin North Am*. 2011 May;**95**(3): 539–54, x–xi.
4. Keyock KL, Newman DK. Understanding stress urinary incontinence. *Nurse Pract*. 2011 Oct;**36** (10):24–36; quiz 7.
5. Deng DY. Urinary incontinence in women. *Med Clin North Am*. 2011 Jan;**95**(1):101–9.
6. Abrams P, Cardozo L, Fall M, et al. The standardisation of terminology of lower urinary tract function: report from the Standardisation Sub-committee of the International Continence Society. *Neurourol Urodyn*. 2002;**21**(2):167–78.
7. Resnick NM. Geriatric incontinence. *Urol Clin North Am*. 1996 Feb;**23**(1):55–74.
8. Abrams P, Andersson KE, Birder L, et al. Fourth International Consultation on Incontinence Recommendations of the International Scientific Committee: evaluation and treatment of urinary incontinence, pelvic organ prolapse, and fecal incontinence. *Neurourol Urodyn*. 2010;**29**(1):213–40.
9. Danforth KN, Townsend MK, Lifford K, et al. Risk factors for urinary incontinence among middle-aged women. *Am J Obstet Gynecol*. 2006 Feb;**194**(2):339–45.
10. Auwad W, Steggles P, Bombieri L, et al. Moderate weight loss in obese women with urinary incontinence: a prospective longitudinal study. *Int Urogynecol J Pelvic Floor Dysfunct*. 2008 Sep;**19**(9):1251–9.
11. National Institute for Health and Care Excellence (NICE). *Urinary incontinence in women (CG171)*. 2nd ed. London: Royal College of Obstetricians and Gynaecologists, 2013.
12. Kadar N. The value of bladder filling in the clinical detection of urine loss and selection of patients for urodynamic testing. *Br J Obstet Gynaecol*. 1988 Jul;**95**(7):698–704.
13. Swift SE, Yoon EA. Test-retest reliability of the cough stress test in the evaluation of urinary incontinence. *Obstet Gynecol*. 1999 Jul;**94**(1):99–102.
14. Laycock J. Pelvic muscle exercises: physiotherapy for the pelvic floor. *Urol Nurs*. 1994 Sep;**14**(3):136–40.
15. Slevin ML, Plant H, Lynch D, et al. Who should measure quality of life, the doctor or the patient? *Br J Cancer*. 1988 Jan;**57**(1):109–12.
16. Bristow SE, Hilton P. Assessment and investigations for urinary incontinence. *Baillieres Best Pract Res Clin Obstet Gynaecol*. 2000 Apr;**14**(2):227–49.
17. Nager CW, Brubaker L, Litman HJ, et al. A randomized trial of urodynamic testing before stress-incontinence surgery. *N Engl J Med*. 2012 May 24;**366**(21):1987–97.
18. Weber AM, Taylor RJ, Wei JT, et al. The cost-effectiveness of preoperative testing (basic office assessment vs. urodynamics) for stress urinary incontinence in women. *BJU Int*. 2002 Mar;**89**(4): 356–63.

19. DuBeau CE, Morrow JD, Kraus SR, et al. Efficacy and tolerability of fesoterodine versus tolterodine in older and younger subjects with overactive bladder: a post hoc, pooled analysis from two placebo-controlled trials. *Neurourol Urodyn.* 2012 Nov;**31**(8): 1258–65.

20. Johnson ST. From incontinence to confidence. *Am J Nurs.* 2000 Feb;**100**(2):69–74, 76.

21. Scottish Intercollegiate Guidelines Network. Management of urinary incontinence in primary care – a national clinical guideline 2005. Available from: www.sign.ac.uk. Accessed May 1, 2015.

22. Kafri R, Shames J, Raz M, Katz-Leurer M. Rehabilitation versus drug therapy for urge urinary incontinence: long-term outcomes. *Int Urogynecol J Pelvic Floor Dysfunct.* 2008 Jan;**19**(1):47–52.

23. National Institute for Health and Care Excellence (NICE). Mirabegron for treating symptoms of overactive bladder, 2013. Available from: www.nice.org .uk/guidance/TA290. Accessed December 20, 2015.

Chapter 21

Office management of pelvic relaxation

Tristi W. Muir

Introduction

Pelvic organ prolapse (POP) is a loss of support in the vagina, which allows for descent of the pelvic organs into or through the vaginal opening. Primarily dependent upon the extent of the loss of support, POP may be asymptomatic or may produce mass symptoms (bulging at the vaginal opening, pressure) and interfere with bowel, bladder, or sexual function. The support of the vagina is described in compartments- loss of support of the anterior vaginal wall (urethrocele, cystocele), apex (enterocele or uterine prolapse), and posterior wall support (rectocele and enterocele). Loss of support at the perineal body (perineocele) or attenuation may occur.

Anatomy

Before recognizing and correct abnormal anatomy such as prolapse, the physician must understand normal anatomy. Support of the pelvic organs is provided by a complex interaction of the integrity of the vaginal tube, the connective tissue support, and muscular support of the pelvic floor. John DeLancey divided the connective tissue support of the vagina into three levels.[1] All three levels of support should be evaluated and addressed during the physical examination and in consideration of treatment options (Figure 21-1).

At level 1, the support of the uterus and the apical portion of the anterior and posterior vaginal walls is provided primarily by the cardinal-uterosacral ligaments.[2, 3] This mesentery of support originates at the sacrum and the pelvic sidewalls and inserts onto the posterior cervix and upper vagina. With normal support, the vagina is directed dorsally to lie in a horizontal fashion over the levator ani muscles. With increases in abdominal pressure, the vaginal tube is closed and is primarily supported by the pelvic floor muscles (levator ani and coccygeus muscles) rather than connective tissue.

Level 2 includes the support for the midportion of the vagina. This support is provided by the endopelvic fascia attaching the lateral anterior and posterior vaginal walls to the aponeurosis of the levator ani. The proximal half of the anterior and posterior vagina is supported by endopelvic attachment to the arcus tendineus fasciae pelvis. The lateral attachment of the posterior wall diverges dorsally from the arcus tendineus fasciae pelvis in the distal vagina.

Level 3, or distal support of the posterior vaginal wall, is primarily provided by the perineal membrane, superficial and deep perineal muscles, and perineal body. The perineal body resists caudally directed abdominal pressure and provides a physical barrier between the vagina and rectum. The perineal membrane anchors this perineal body laterally and anteriorly to the bones of the pelvis to resist downward movement of the vagina during periods of increased abdominal pressure. Separation of the perineal body from the perineal membrane results in perineal body hypermobility and defecatory dysfunction (Figure 21-2). The perineal body extends cranially to the hymenal ring and is suspended by the levator ani muscles. On magnetic resonance imaging (MRI), the perineal body descends more caudally in women with posterior wall prolapse or with levator defects than controls.[4, 5]

The levator ani muscles provide a sling of support, enclosing the genital hiatus, through which the urethra, vagina, and anorectum pass. In a woman with an intact pelvic floor, the levator ani muscles are in a chronic state of contraction, and the anterior and posterior vaginal walls are in direct apposition. During defecation the increased pressure placed on the posterior vaginal wall is equilibrated by the opposing abdominal pressure on the anterior vaginal wall. There is no stress placed on the

Office Care of Women, ed. Martin E. Olsen and Botros Rizk. Published by Cambridge University Press.

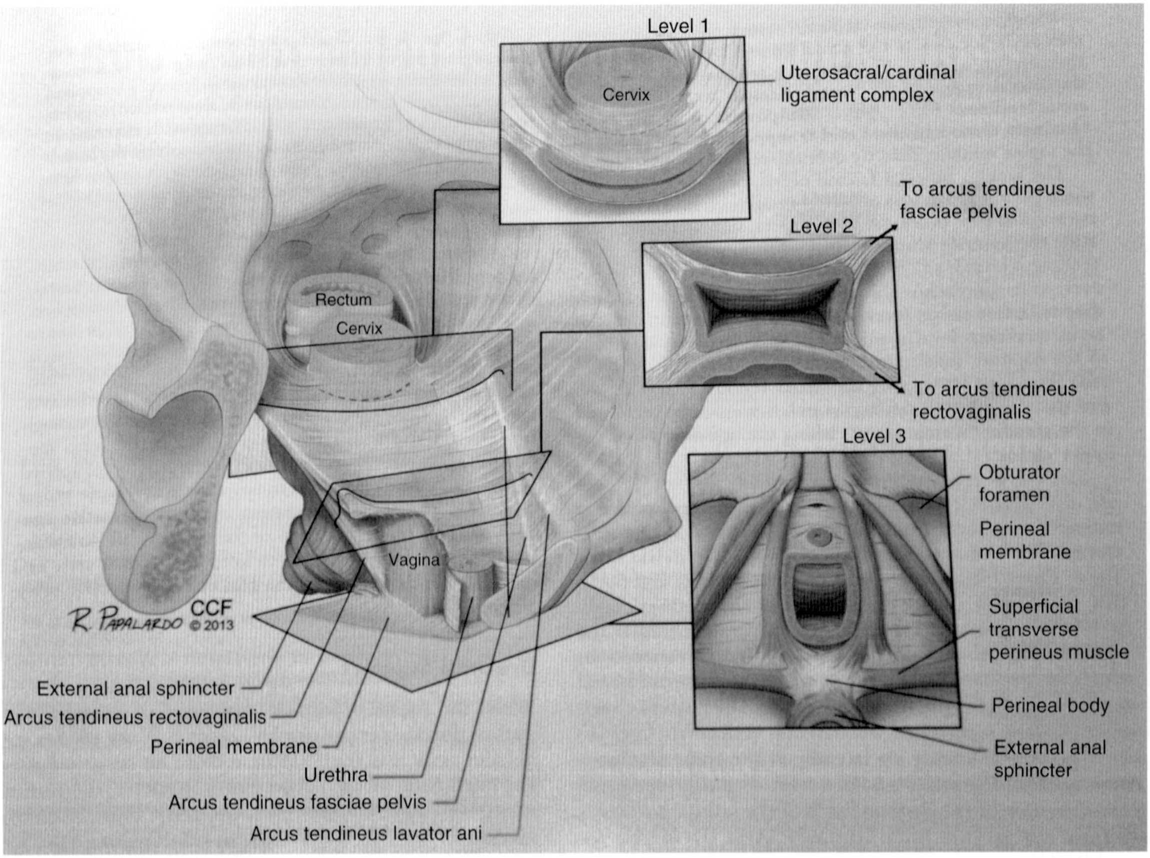

Figure 21-1 Connective tissue support of the vagina. Level 1 (suspensory support) includes the uterosacral/cardinal ligament. Level 2 support includes the lateral attachment to the levator ani muscles through the arcus tendineus fasciae pelvis and arcus tendineus rectovaginalis. Level 3 support anchors the distal support to the pelvic bone through the perineal membrane with a union of distal support at the perineal body. (Walters MD, Karram MM. *Urogynecology and Reconstructive Pelvic Surgery*. 4th Edition. Philadelphia: Elsevier, 2014; figure 2.10.)

connective tissue attachments. In the presence of muscular or neurologic damage to the pelvic floor, the levator hiatus widens and the vaginal canal opens. The increased rectal pressure and distension associated with defecation now places strain on the connective tissue attachments and the fibromuscularis of the posterior vaginal wall.

Epidemiology of pelvic organ prolapse

Some degree of POP is described in 50% of women during a vaginal examination; however, only 3%–9% of women see or feel a bulge at the vaginal opening. The incidence of POP surgery ranges from 1.5 to 1.8 per 1,000 women years with a 12.6% lifetime risk of surgery.[6, 7] The anterior vaginal wall (supporting the urethra and bladder) is the most common site for primary and recurrent pelvic organ prolapse.[6] The risk of surgery peaks in the elderly population of women aged 60–79 years.[6–8]

The US baby boomer population is entering the "elderly" classification, and the number of American women 65 years and older will more than double by 2050. In 1997, 220,000 surgeries were performed for pelvic organ prolapse in the United States.[9] It has been estimated that the workload related to pelvic organ prolapse will increase by 46%–200% by the year 2050 due to the exponential growth in the elderly population.[10]

Risk factors for pelvic organ prolapse

A number of risk factors for the development of POP have been identified. Risks can be differentiated into those that are inheritable, related to trauma, or occur with time (Table 21-1). Birth defects that damage the pelvis (such as bladder exstrophy) and structural components (e.g., collagen) can increase the attributable risk of development of POP and lower the age in which it occurs.[11, 12] Genetic linkage studies have mapped predisposition for the development of POP to the chromosomes 10 and 17.[13] Although genetic linkage studies begin to unveil an important piece of the complexity of POP, age (promotional) and vaginal delivery (trauma) are currently the most important recognized determinants of POP.[8, 14]

History

Women with POP may have symptoms related to the change in anatomy – vaginal pressure or bulging mass – or symptoms may be related to urinary, defecatory, or sexual dysfunction. The severity of prolapse does not necessarily correlate with severity of symptoms.

Most cases of POP are insidious in progression, however prolapse may be acutely identified when the prolapse is perceived to "suddenly" protrude through the vaginal opening. Women with POP frequently describe a bulging sensation that is worsened with prolonged activity in the standing position. This discomfort often improves or resolves with lying down.

Table 21-1 Risk factors for the development of pelvic organ prolapse

Inheritable	Trauma	Promotional
Genetics	Childbirth	Aging
	Pelvic surgery	Obesity
		Smoking
		Chronic cough or straining

The protrusion of the vagina beyond the vaginal opening may lead to irritation, dryness, or ulceration of the vaginal skin or cervix.

Bladder symptoms may be related to prolapse of all segments of the vagina. Loss of support at the urethra may result in alteration of the stream or urine (such as spraying) or leakage of urine with cough, sneeze, and activity; this is stress urinary incontinence. As the anterior vaginal wall loses support a mechanical kinking of the urethra may occur. This is more predominant in a setting of a combination of apical and anterior wall prolapse. This mechanical urethral kinking may hinder complete emptying of the bladder resulting in voiding dysfunction (hesitancy, straining, change of position to void), urinary retention, urinary tract infections, and overactive bladder. Digital reduction of the prolapse may be necessary to facilitate complete emptying of the bladder. The mechanical kinking of the urethra may mask symptoms of stress urinary incontinence, which may be unmasked with treatment (pessary or surgery). Posterior vaginal wall bulging (rectocele or enterocele) may additionally compress the urethra and contribute to urinary retention.

Loss of support over the rectum may lead to defecatory dysfunction. Sung et al. reported in a prospective evaluation of 160 women undergoing rectocele repair that 87% had bowel symptoms. The most common symptom was incomplete evacuation (85%) followed by straining (74%), sensation of obstructed defecation (66%) and anal incontinence (63%), and manual splinting (56%).[15] Stool may be trapped in the rectocele and increase the likelihood of fecal incontinence. Many of the defecatory symptoms may be improved with

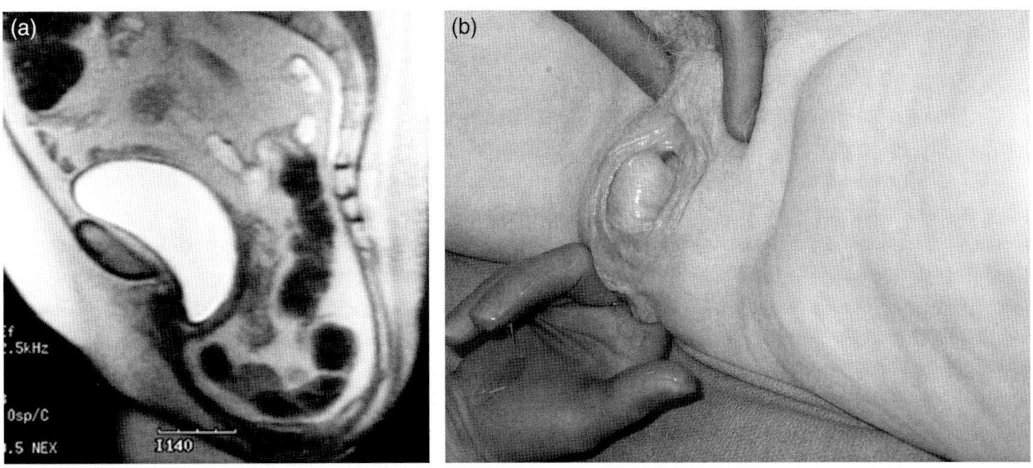

Figure 21-2 Perineal body descent. (A) Rectal examination reveals perineal body hypermobility and rectocele. (B) Sagittal MRI with large enterocele is accompanied by perineal body descent and enlarging of the levator hiatus. (A) (B)

increasing fiber or water intake. Infrequent bowel movements are *unlikely* to be related to POP and may require a transit study to evaluate for slow colonic transit.

Sexual function is multifaceted in women. This may occur in the setting of POP through an alteration of body image, loss of sensation, discomfort, or fear of urinary of fecal incontinence. Postmenopausal women may have decreased arousal due to vaginal atrophy, and heterosexual women may have partners with erectile dysfunction. A thorough understanding a woman's goals with treatment of her prolapse with regard to sexual function is important in design of treatment and specific surgical planning (i.e., if the partner has erectile dysfunction, constriction of the vaginal opening should be avoided).

Physical examination

A complete physical examination should be performed in women with POP, including evaluation of skeletal, mental, cardiovascular, abdominal and pelvic systems and organs.

Skeletal/gait

Limitations in mobility can impair a woman's ability to void or defecate on time. Kyphosis and/or loss of lumbar lordosis will increases the pressure placed on the pelvic floor and may increase the risk for development of prolapse.

Mental status

Mental status includes the degree of consciousness, orientation, comprehension, memory, and speech. Disorders impacting a woman's mental status include dementia, brain tumors, stroke, and Parkinson's disease. Mental status may have a significant impact on the ability to obtain an accurate history and limit treatment options.

Cardiovascular/lungs

Congestive heart failure may increase lower extremity edema resulting in nocturia (frequent nighttime voiding) as a woman mobilizes the fluid with her legs up in bed. A chronic cough will increase pressure on the prolapse and may increase the frequency and bother of stress urinary incontinence.

Abdominal

Prior incisions should be noted. POP is thought to be a hernia; therefore, evaluation of the abdomen should include an evaluation for umbilical, ventral, inguinal, and femoral hernias.

Pelvic

The patient is typically examined in the dorsal lithotomy or semirecumbent position. The pelvic examination should start with a thorough examination of the groin for adenopathy and skin lesions. Vulvar dermatoses, such as lichen sclerosis or lichen planus, may impact treatment choice and outcomes (whether pessary or surgical therapy is selected).

Women with neurologic disorders should undergo a focused neurologic examination of sacral nerves 2–4. The patient can be asked to discriminate between sharp and dull sensation on the perineum. Reflex testing includes the bulbocavernosus reflex and anal wink. The bulbocavernosus reflex is contraction of the bulbocavernosus muscles in response to pressure on the clitoris. The anal wink is produced with light touch of the perianal skin eliciting contraction of the external anal sphincter. These reflexes are more useful if present than reflective of neurological damage if absent. They may be difficult to evaluate and are not consistently present even in neurologically intact women.

The vaginal examination includes evaluation of the urethra, uterus, adnexa, and support and health of the vaginal tissue. Abnormal or postmenopausal vaginal bleeding may be related to the uterus (in which case an endometrial sampling may be indicated) or due to ulceration of the vaginal skin. The urethra should be palpated for the presence of a urethral mass (diverticulum, abscess, or carcinoma). Initial evaluation of stress incontinence includes observation of the urethral meatus during a cough to evaluate for leakage of urine during the pelvic examination and an observation for leakage of urine from the urethra. Size, shape, mobility of the uterus and presence of adnexal masses may be determined with a bimanual examination; this may be inaccurate, however, in overweight or obese women.

In many postmenopausal women, vaginal atrophy is present and symptomatic. Atrophy alters the function and appearance of the vaginal skin. Upon speculum examination, the vaginal tissue may appear pale, thin, friable, and display a loss of rugation. Women with symptomatic vaginal atrophy who elect to proceed with treatment of POP (pessary or surgery) should be treated with vaginal estrogen unless a contraindication is present.

Table 21-2 The POPQ system of prolapse classification*

Stage of prolapse	Extent of prolapse (in relationship to the hymen: prolapse above the hymen, negative numbers; prolapse beyond the hymen, positive numbers)
Stage 0	No prolapse (apex can descend as far as 2 cm relative to the total vaginal length)
Stage 1	The most distal portion of prolapse descends to a point less more than 1 cm above the hymen
Stage 2	Maximum descent is within 1 cm of the hymen
Stage 3	Prolapse extends more than 1 cm beyond the hymen but no more than 2 cm of the total vaginal length
Stage 4	Complete eversion of the vagina or descent within 2 cm of the total vaginal length

* Each compartment is staged, and the total stage is the most related to the highest staged compartment.

Table 21-3 Baden-Walker system of POP assessment*

Grade of prolapse	Extent of prolapse (in relation to the hymen)
Grade 0	Normal position for each site
Grade 1	Descent halfway to the hymen
Grade 2	Descent to the hymen
Grade 3	Descent halfway beyond the hymen
Grade 4	Maximum possible descent for each site

* The anterior, apical, and posterior compartments are assessed on its relationship to the hymen.

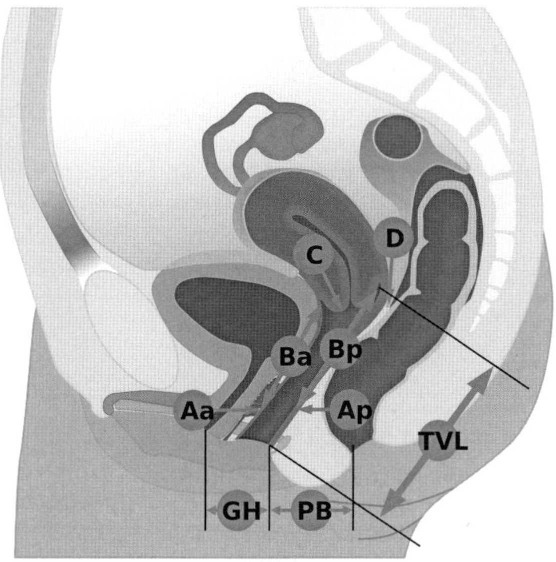

Figure 21-3 All measurements of the pelvic organ prolapse quantification system (POPQ), with the exception of total vaginal length (TVL), are performed while the patient performs the Valsalva maneuver. The anterior vaginal wall has two measurements: Aa and Ba. Point C represents the cervix or cuff. Point D is the posterior fornix when a woman has a uterus. The posterior vaginal wall has two points of measurement: Ap and Bp. All measurements inside the hymen are (–) while all points extending beyond the hymen are (+).

Support of each segment of the vagina (urethra, bladder, uterus or apex, rectum, perineal body, genital hiatus, and total vaginal length) can be evaluated through the pelvic organ prolapse quantification system (POPQ) or the Baden-Walker classification (Tables 21-2 and 21-3) (Figure 21-3).[16, 17] The POPQ system is a series of nine site-specific measurements. This system of measurement is easy to learn and has been validated and adopted internationally as a common language to convey support before and after treatment. When women perform a maximal Valsalva maneuver, there is an excellent correlation between the supine and standing positions.[16] Some women lose their ability to bear down effectively during the examination. If the patient is contracting the pelvic floor rather than pushing out, she should be directed to cough vigorously. If the examiner does not visualize the extent of prolapse that a woman describes, examining her in the standing position may allow for a more accurate determination of her prolapse (however, evaluation in this position is much more difficult to accomplish).

Pelvic floor muscle strength can be assessed by asking the woman to squeeze around exam fingers placed in the vagina (as if she is going to stop the flow of urine). Many women loose the ability to employ their pelvic floor muscles on demand, whether through loss of muscle memory or through muscular or neurologic damage to the pelvic floor. Referral to pelvic floor physical therapy should be considered in all these women.

Rectal examination can confirm the presence of a rectocele, enterocele, and determine the functional tone and squeeze of the anal sphincter. Women with an external anal sphincter defect may exhibit a "dovetail" sign, with absence of contraction of the anterior external anal sphincter and flattening of skin pucker in this area. The presence of rectal prolapse, low anal

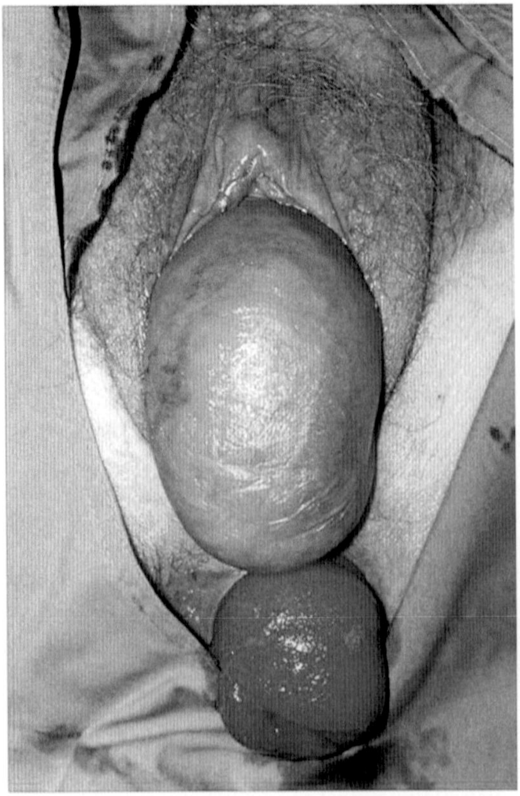

Figure 21-4 Woman with stage 4 POP and rectal prolapse. Complex pelvic relaxation may occur through a damage levator ani muscle.

mass, hemorrhoids, or fecal impaction may be identified during a rectal examination. If a woman's history or physical examination is suggestive for significant defecatory complaints or the presence of abnormal rectal anatomy, referral to a colorectal surgeon is recommended. Pelvic organ prolapse commonly coexists with rectal prolapse, likely related to the same mechanisms that cause POP (Figure 21–4).[18]

Treatment

The natural history of pelvic organ prolapse is not well understood. Recently, physical examination over a five-year period of the women participating in the estrogen plus progesterone arm of the Women's Health Initiative (WHI) Hormone Therapy Clinical Trial showed an overall increase in the rate of prolapse by 4% during this time frame.[19]

Pelvic organ prolapse is a far more common incidental physical finding than a symptomatic problem for which a woman seeks medical care. Typically, when the loss of support does not lead to bulging of the pelvic organs beyond the plane of the hymen, a woman may not have symptoms and will often choose observation. Physical therapy with pelvic floor muscle strengthening during a period of observation may decrease the need for future intervention. [20] Education on POP and pelvic floor muscle exercises is often the treatment of choice in early stage prolapse. Showing the woman the loss of support with a handheld mirror and educating her on POP symptoms can be enlightening. However, once the bulge is through the plane of the vagina and/or it affects bladder, bowel, or sexual function, she may want to proceed with treatment. A woman's treatment choice is often related to her severity of prolapse, degree of symptoms, associated urinary, defecatory and sexual function, her medical comorbidities, and her personal obligations (children, job, parental care, or spousal care).

Pessary

In the fifth century BC, Hippocrates described the first pessary placing a pomegranate in a woman's vagina for the treatment of uterine prolapse.[21]Treatment of POP has evolved, and surgical options have become available since that time; however, more than 2,000 years later, pessaries remain a viable first-line treatment option for all women with POP. Overall, in a study of more than 34,000 Medicare beneficiaries with POP in the United States, 11.6% were identified as being treated with a pessary. The prevalence of using a pessary to treat POP increases with age (4.9% in women aged 65–69 to 24.7% in women aged 85 and older).[21]

A pessary is a mechanical support device, typically made of medical grade silicone, which is fitted in the vagina to reduce the symptoms of POP. Pessaries are minimally invasive and can provide immediate relief of many of the symptoms of prolapse. A pessary may be used indefinitely or used to provide relief of symptoms prior to surgical management. A variety of shapes and sizes are available; however, there are two primary categories of pessaries: (1) support and (2) space-occupying (Figure 21–5).

The support pessaries are placed between the posterior fornix and posterior portion of the pubic bone. The ring pessary (with and without a diaphragm) is the most commonly used support pessary. The ring is bent in half and lubrication is placed at the leading edge of the pessary. While two fingers from the nondominant hand separate the labia, the ring is inserted

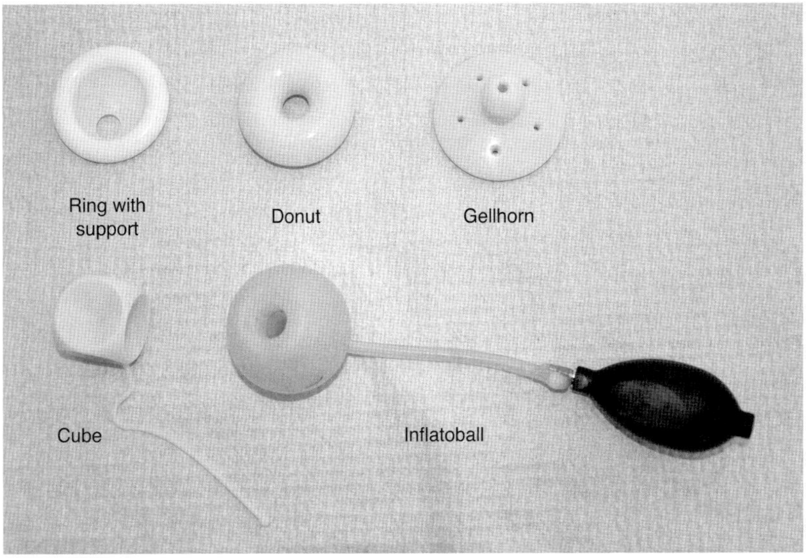

Figure 21-5 Examples of support (ring with support) and space-occupying (donut, Gellhorn, cube, and Inflatoball) pessaries.

to the apex of the vagina with the distal edge pushed up behind the pubic bone. The pessary may be rotated a quarter turn so that the collapsing portion of the ring is not in the vertical plane of the vaginal opening.

Space-occupying pessaries (i.e., Gellhorn, donut, cube, inflatoball) are typically used for high stage prolapse and/or women with a widened genital hiatus.[22, 23] The goal of treatment with a pessary is to provide support of the vagina with no discomfort.

The pessary should maintain the prolapse inside the hymen, not be expelled with Valsalva, be comfortable, and not compress the vaginal tissue excessively. Typically there should be a finger's breadth between the vaginal wall and pessary and the back of the pubic bone and pessary. More than one office visit may therefore be needed to find the pessary that is "just right." Women typically return to the office within two to four weeks of initiation of pessary treatment for evaluation of fit; comfort; effects on defecatory, urinary, and sexual function; and health of vaginal tissue. Refitting may be necessary for women who have discomfort with the original pessary or expel their pessary. Fitting is successful in approximately three-quarters of women.[23] The rate of continuation of pessary use at three months is approximately 60%.[24] A vaginal length of less than 6 cm and a widened genital hiatus have been associated with unsuccessful fittings.[23]

After a successful fitting, education on pessary care should be performed. There are no clear guidelines on pessary management, but if the woman is able to insert and remove the pessary, cleaning the pessary once a week with water or mild soap and water is recommended. Space occupying pessaries will need to be removed prior to sexual function. Women who are unable to manage their pessary care, can return for management in the clinic at an interval dependent upon the tolerance of the pessary in the vagina (generally four- to eight-week intervals). Due to an increased risk of vaginal tissue erosion, the cube and donut pessary should be removed/cleaned/replaced more frequently (nightly is preferred). Caution should be used in prescribing these pessaries in a woman who is unable to maintain pessary use herself.

The risks of pessary use include vaginal wall irritation and vaginal discharge. The vaginal discharge can be caused by a physiologic response to the friction on the vaginal walls. If the discharge is profuse and malodorous, a careful examination of the vagina for ulceration should be performed. Vaginitis is diagnosed in up to 35% of women with pessary use.[21] Bacterial vaginosis (BV) is more common in women who use a pessary.[25] This may be resolved with antibiotics (metronidazole tablet or gel). Estrogen vaginal cream use does not appear to have a protective effect on prevention of BV. The pessary may place pressure on the vaginal wall producing focal devascularization and leading to erosions. Removal, cleaning, and replacement of the pessary may change the location of pressure and decrease the risk of erosion. Reduction of a prolapsed bladder with the pessary may uncover occult urinary incontinence. Alternatively, pessary use (particularly space-occupying pessaries) may obstruct urination (causing urinary tract infections or urinary retention) or defecation. A neglected pessary (left in place for an extended period of time without removal for cleaning and replacement) may lead to more serious complications including damage to surrounding organs such as fistula or incarceration of the pessary. Nine years after pessary placement, 3% of women developed a vesicovaginal or rectovaginal fistula. [21] Protection or improvement of the health of the vaginal wall with vaginal estrogen cream is a common component of management when a pessary is used.

Surgery

Women, their family members, and even physicians exclude the option of surgical management solely based on the patient's advanced age. However, the surgical outcomes and complications in the elderly are very similar to those found in younger women. [26] The quality of life and satisfaction are both very high in the elderly population undergoing surgical repair of prolapse.[27] The elderly population is expanding rapidly; age should not be the sole factor in determining surgical eligibility.

Surgical options for management of POP depend upon many factors such as whether the prolapse is recurrent, the compartments involved, coexisting morbidities, and surgical preference of surgeon and patient. Uterine preserving options exist and should be considered for particularly for women considering future pregnancy. Evaluation of cervical length in women electing uterine preserving procedures should be performed. If the cervix is elongated, cervical shortening in women not desirous of future childbearing should be considered to decrease the risk of recurrence.

Surgery may be approached through a vaginal, abdominal, laparoscopic, or robotically assisted laparoscopic route. Anterior and posterior colporrhaphies (a plication of the native fibromuscular tissue of the vaginal wall) are effective with a low complication rate. Apical support for each compartment should be evaluated and addressed if indicated. Colpocleisis (an obliterative surgical option) is a safe, effective surgical option for women who do not desire intravaginal intercourse in their futures.

Surgical procedures that use mesh to support the vaginal may be performed from an abdominal or vaginal route. Mesh is used in an attempt to increase the durability of the repair. Complications unique to the usage of mesh include erosion or exposure of the mesh in the vagina or less commonly in the bladder or bowel. The estimated probability of mesh erosion in the extended Colpopexy and Urinary Retention Efforts (CARE) trial (at 6.18 years) was 10.5% (95% CI, 6.8%–16.1%).[27] In 2008, the Food and Drug Administration (FDA) issued a public health notification that cited more than 1,000 complications reported by the manufacturers of transvaginal POP mesh kits.[29] In 2011, the FDA issued a public health warning that complications in the use of transvaginal mesh for POP repair are not rare, and it is unclear if there is an anatomic benefit to its use.[30] Studies are underway to prospectively compare native tissue to transvaginal mesh repairs for POP.

Concluding remarks

Pelvic organ prolapse is common in women; the lifetime risk of surgical intervention is 12%. As our elderly population is expected to grow exponentially over the next 30 years, the need for health-care providers to identify and treat these women will also expand. Currently management options rely upon mechanical devices (pessaries) and surgery; however, in the future, regeneration of pelvic floor muscles and nerves may improve our ability to treat prolapse and minimize complications.

References

1. DeLancey JO. Anatomic aspects of vaginal eversion after hysterectomy. *Am J Obstet Gynecol* 1992, Jun;**166** (6 Pt 1):1717–24; discussion 1724–8.
2. DeLancey JO. Structural anatomy of the posterior pelvic compartment as it relates to rectocele. *Am J Obstet Gynecol* 1999, Apr;**180**(4):815–23.
3. Hsu Y, Lewicky-Gaupp C, DeLancey JO. Posterior compartment anatomy as seen in magnetic resonance imaging and 3-dimensional reconstruction from asymptomatic nulliparas. *Am J Obstet Gynecol* 2008;**198**(6):651.e1.
4. Lewicky-Gaupp C, Yousuf A, Larson KA, et al. Structural position of the posterior vagina and pelvic floor in women with and without posterior vaginal prolapse. *Am J Obstet Gynecol* 2010, May;**202**(5):497. e1–6.

5. Clark NA, Brincat CA, Yousuf AA, Delancey JO. Levator defects affect perineal position independently of prolapse status. *Am J Obstet Gynecol* 2010, Dec;**203**(6):595.e17–22.
6. Barber MD, Maher C. Epidemiology and outcome assessment of pelvic organ prolapse. *Int Urogynecol J* 2013, Nov;**24**(11):1783–90.
7. Wu JM, Matthews CA, Conover MM, et al. Lifetime risk of stress urinary incontinence or pelvic organ prolapse surgery. *Obstet Gynecol* 2014, Jun;**123**(6): 1201–6.
8. Samuelsson EC, Victor FT, Tibblin G, Svärdsudd KF. Signs of genital prolapse in a Swedish population of women 20 to 59 years of age and possible related factors. *Am J Obstet Gynecol* 1999, Feb;**180**(2 Pt 1):299–305.
9. Brown JS, Waetjen LE, Subak LL, et al. Pelvic organ prolapse surgery in the united states, 1997. *Am J Obstet Gynecol* 2002, Apr;**186**(4):712–16.
10. Wu JM, Hundley AF, Fulton RG, Myers ER. Forecasting the prevalence of pelvic floor disorders in US women: 2010 to 2050. *Obstet Gynecol* 2009, Dec;**114**(6):1278–83.
11. Muir TW, Aspera AM, Rackley RR, Walters MD. Recurrent pelvic organ prolapse in a woman with bladder exstrophy: a case report of surgical management and review of the literature. *Int Urogynecol J* 2004;**15**(6):436–8.
12. Fernandes NF, Schwartz RA. A “hyperextensive” review of ehlers-danlos syndrome. *Cutis* 2008, Oct;**82**(4):242–8.
13. Allen-Brady K, Cannon-Albright LA, Farnham JM, Norton PA. Evidence for pelvic organ prolapse predisposition genes on chromosomes 10 and 17. *Am J Obstet Gynecol* 2015 Jun;**212**(6):771.e1–7. doi: 10.1016/j.ajog.2014.12.037. Epub 2014 Dec 31.
14. Chow D, Rodríguez LV. Epidemiology and prevalence of pelvic organ prolapse. *Curr Opin Urol* 2013, Jul;**23**(4):293–8.
15. Sung VW, Rardin CR, Raker CA, et al. Changes in bowel symptoms 1 year after rectocele repair. *Am J Obstet Gynecol* 2012, Nov;**207**(5):423.e1–5.
16. Bump RC, Mattiasson A, Bø K, et al. The standardization of terminology of female pelvic organ prolapse and pelvic floor dysfunction. *Am J Obstet Gynecol* 1996;**175**(1): 10–17
17. Baden WF, Walker TA. Genesis of the vaginal profile: a correlated classification of vaginal relaxation. *Clin Obstet Gynecol*, 1972;**15**:1048–54.
18. Altman D, Zetterstrom J, Schultz I, et al. Pelvic organ prolapse and urinary incontinence in women with surgically managed rectal prolapse: A population-based case-control study. *Dis Colon Rectum* 2006, Jan;**49**(1):28–35.
19. Kudish BI, Iglesia CB, Sokol RJ, et al. Effect of weight change on natural history of pelvic organ prolapse. *Obstet Gynecol* 2009, Jan;**113**(1):81–8.
20. Hagen S, Stark D, Glazener C, et al. Individualised pelvic floor muscle training in women with pelvic organ prolapse (POPPY): a multicentre randomised controlled trial. *The Lancet* 2014, Mar;**383**(9919):796–806.
21. Alperin M, Khan A, Dubina E, et al. Patterns of pessary care and outcomes for Medicare beneficiaries with pelvic organ prolapse. *Female Pelvic Med Reconstr Surg* 2013;**19**(3):142–7.
22. Cundiff GW, Weidner AC, Visco AG, et al. A survey of pessary use by members of the American urogynecologic society. *Obstetrics & Gynecology* 2000;**95**(6 Pt 1):931–5.
23. Clemons JL, Aguilar VC, Tillinghast TA, et al. Risk factors associated with an unsuccessful pessary fitting trial in women with pelvic organ prolapse. *Am J Obstet Gynecol* 2004 Feb;**190**(2):345–50.
24. Cundiff GW, Amundsen CL, Bent AE, et al. The PESSRI study: symptom relief outcomes of a randomized crossover trial of the ring and gellhorn pessaries. *Am J Obstet Gynecol* 2007, Apr;**196**(4):405.e1–8.
25. Alnaif B, Drutz HP. Bacterial vaginosis increases in pessary users. *Int Urogynecol J Pelvic Floor Dysfunct* 2000;**11**(4):219–22; discussion 222–3.
26. Shah AD, Kohli N, Rajan SS, Hoyte L. The age distribution, rates, and types of surgery for stress urinary incontinence in the USA. *Int Urogynecol J Pelvic Floor Dysfunct* 2008, Jan;**19**(1):89–96.
27. Barber MD, Amundsen CL, Paraiso MF, et al. Quality of life after surgery for genital prolapse in elderly women: obliterative and reconstructive surgery. *Int Urogynecol J Pelvic Floor Dysfunct* 2007, Jul;**18**(7):799–806.
28. Nygaard I, Brubaker L, Zyczynski HM, et al. Long-term outcomes following abdominal sacrocolpopexy for pelvic organ prolapse. *JAMA* 2013;**309**(19): 2016–24.
29. FDA Public Health Notification: serious complications associated with transvaginal placement of surgical mesh in repair of pelvic organ prolapse and stress urinary incontinence. 20 October 2008. Available at: www.fda.gov/MedicalDevices/Safety/AlertsandNotices/PublicHealthNotifications/ucm061976.htm. Accessed January 11, 2015.
30. FDA Safety Communication: update on serious complications associated with transvaginal placement of surgical mesh for pelvic organ prolapse. 13 July 2011. Available at: www.fda.gov/MedicalDevices/Safety/AlertsandNotices/ucm262435.htm. Accessed January 11, 2015.

Chapter 22

Vulvovaginal disease

Christine Conageski

Introduction

"Vulvovaginitis" is a term used to describe a spectrum of disorders of the vulva and vagina that may cause discharge, odor, pruritus, pain, and/or dyspareunia. These disorders may be caused by infections, inflammation, dermatologic conditions, or changes in the normal vaginal flora.

Scope of the problem

Vulvovaginal complaints are extremely common in primary care and account for more than 10 million office visits and over $1 billion in medical expenses annually. [1] This number represents over three physician office visits per 100 women and 2% of all visits to physicians. [2] Despite a significant number of women presenting with vulvovaginal complaints, many providers fail to use simple diagnostic tests and 30% of women go without a diagnosis after initial evaluation.[3]

Approach to the patient with vulvovaginal complaints

History

Every woman who presents with vulvovaginal complaints should have a focused history, physical exam, and complete laboratory evaluation. The history should focus on symptoms including change in bleeding patterns, discharge, vaginal malodor, itching, irritation, burning, swelling, dyspareunia, and associated bowel and bladder symptoms. Questions about the location of the symptoms, duration, the relation to the menstrual cycle, response to prior treatments including over-the counter medications, and a sexual history should be obtained.

Physical exam

The physical exam should include an examination of the vulva, perineum, anus, vagina, cervix, and uterus. Many patients with vaginal complaints have concurrent vulvar manifestations of disease, and thus no portion of the exam should be excluded. The exam should focus on an evaluation for erythema, induration, fissures, ulcerations, and changes in architecture from normal anatomy. After careful visual inspection and prior to insertion of the speculum, a detailed pain exam with mapping of problem areas is performed using a cotton-tipped swab.

Following a visual inspection, speculum is inserted and discharge noted. Discharge is characterized by color, odor, consistency, adherence to the vaginal wall, and amount. Visualization of the cervix is important to rule out cervicitis as a source of abnormal vaginal discharge. Finally, a bimanual exam is performed to evaluate for cervical motion or uterine tenderness.

Laboratory analysis

Office laboratory tests are useful for diagnosing vulvovaginal complaints. Studies show that symptoms and physical exam alone are not reliable for diagnosis. [3, 4] Complete laboratory evaluation should include determination of the vaginal pH, performance of a "whiff" test and collection of samples for saline and 10% KOH microscopy. The pH is determined first. In healthy individuals, the bacterial flora is dominated by lactobacilli, which maintain the normal acidic (pH 3. 8–4.2) environment of the vagina.

Two slides for microscopy are then prepared. Samples are obtained from the posterior fornix. One specimen slide, or "wet mount," is prepared with a drop of 0.9% saline and the addition of the collected vaginal discharge. The second is prepared in a similar fashion with 10% KOH. The slide is examined immediately under a microscope at both low (10×) and high (40×) power. The whiff test is performed after the10% KOH slide is prepared and the slide is "whiffed" to determine

Office Care of Women, ed. Martin E. Olsen and Botros Rizk. Published by Cambridge University Press.

the presence of the characteristic fishy (amine) odor of bacterial vaginosis.

Each wet mount should be evaluated for the appearance of squamous epithelial cells including their size and shape, number of background lactobacilli, number of polymorphonuclear cells, presence of clue cells and trichomonads. The KOH slide is useful for identifying yeast. KOH dissolves white and red blood cells making the branching, budding, and cell walls of *Candida albicans* easier to visualize.

In selected patients, additional testing may be performed depending on suspicion for causes not seen on normal saline wet mount. Other tests may include cultures or commercially available testing for diagnosis of yeast, trichomoniasis, bacterial vaginosis, *Neisseria gonorrheae*, and *Chlamydia trachomatis*. Vaginal cultures especially for bacterial vaginosis are rarely useful.

In patients with vulvar dominant complaints, a vulvar biopsy may be necessary and is easily performed in the clinic. As with any dermatologic biopsy, the area is first cleansed and then anesthetized. Several biopsy instruments are available. The choice of biopsy is dependent on the type of abnormality or area to be sampled. The Kevorkian or Tischler forceps can be used to sample raised or warty lesions. Macular lesions are best sampled using a Keye's punch biopsy. A punch with a minimum diameter of 4 mm is necessary to remove an adequate amount of tissue. Areas of ulceration, blistering, atrophy, or scaring should be biopsied along the edge of the lesion and papular lesions, especially pigmented lesions, should be biopsied at the most abnormal area.

Differential diagnosis

The most common causes of acute vulvovaginal symptoms include bacterial vaginosis (22%–50% of symptomatic women), vulvovaginal candidiasis (17%–39%), and trichomoniasis (15%–20%).[3] In some cases, however, the etiology may be mixed and there may be more than one disease present. Chronic conditions typically include less familiar diagnoses such as contact dermatitis (21%), recurrent vulvovaginal candidiasis (20.5%), atrophic vaginitis (14.5%), and vulvar vestibulitis syndromes (12.5%).[5]

Vulvar disorders

The vulva encompasses the area between the mons pubis anteriorly and the anus posteriorly. This area includes the mons pubis, labia minora, labia majora, clitoris, vestibule, Skene glands and ducts, hymen, Bartholin glands and ducts, and urethral meatus. The vestibule has various gland openings. The Skene ducts are directly inferior and lateral to the urethra. The Bartholin glands are located along the vestibule at 5 o'clock and 7 o'clock. Vulvar abnormalities encompass a wide differential diagnosis and include cysts, ulcers, infections, vulvar dermatoses, and dysplasia.

Vulvar cysts

Vulvar cysts commonly arise from the Bartholin's glands. Cysts and abscesses are the most common disorders of these structures. They occur in 2%–3% of women. The pathophysiology of a Bartholin's cyst is related to obstruction of the gland duct; this leads to dilation of the duct proximal to the obstruction. An obstructed Bartholin's duct cyst can become infected and form an abscess. These cysts can mimic other vulvar masses including inclusion cysts, urethral diverticulums, and Gartner duct cysts. They are distinguished by their anatomic location. The most common symptom is pain. No intervention is necessary in asymptomatic women. Management of symptomatic women necessitates drainage of the cyst or abscess. Simple incision and drainage carries a high risk of recurrence. It is, therefore, recommended that these cysts be drained and a Word catheter placed.[6] For recurrent cysts, marsupialization is highly effective, carries minimal risk and offers a low recurrence rate (less than 20%). Rarely in recurrent cases, removal of the gland is required.

Vulvar ulcers

Vulvar ulcers represent a wide differential diagnosis. They commonly are associated with sexually transmitted pathogens. Less commonly vulvar ulcers are noninfectious. The etiology of noninfectious lesions is generally not understood as in Behcet's disease or aphthous ulcers. Patients typically present with painful ulcers often preceded by vague symptoms such as itching or burning in the area without obvious signs of ulcers. Women may also report dysuria or constitutional symptoms such as fever, malaise, and myalgias. This is frequently encountered in women with aphthous ulcers and primary HSV. On exam, ulcers may be singular or multiple and associated with lymphadenopathy. Diagnosis should include viral cultures of the ulcer to identify HSV. Other testing may include serologic screening for syphilis and HIV. Treatment depends on the etiology of the ulcer, but in women without an infectious etiology, treatment is generally supportive care. Some studies have shown more rapid improvement in symptoms with topical and oral steroid treatment in women with Behcet's or aphthous ulcers.

Vulvar infections

Vulvar infections can include those related to various infectious agents including viral, bacterial, and fungal organisms. Several of these are sexually transmitted (including genital herpes simplex virus, condyloma, syphilitic lesions, and chancroid) and are thus further discussed in Chapter 17 on sexually transmitted infections. Other infections are generally polymicrobial and treatment depends on the presence or absence of a vulvar abscess. In patients with abscess, the mainstay of treatment is drainage. In those women with swelling and erythema without an obvious mass, antibiotics may be the only treatment necessary. It is important to identify women at risk for necrotizing fasciitis including those that are diabetic and obese. These women present with fever, soft tissue involvement with pain out of proportion to exam and hemodynamic instability. These women must be treated with an immediate combination of debridement and aggressive antibiotic therapy.

Vulvar dermatoses

"Vulvar dermatoses" describes a number of disorders of the vulva. The most common dermatosis is vulvar *dermatitis* reported in 20%–25% of women presenting to a vulvar specialty clinic.[7] It may be found in isolation or associated with dermatitis in other areas of the body. There are two types of dermatitis: endogenous and exogenous. Endogenous dermatitis is used to describe atopic dermatitis of the vulva, whereas exogenous dermatitis results from external factors that cause a localized reaction. External factors may produce an allergic response (20%) or may trigger an irritant effect (80%).[8] Common irritants include sanitary pads or tampons, soaps, sweat, douches, vaginal hygiene products, latex, perfumes, and benzocaine.

Patients complain of chronic vulvar itching that can be intense at times. Physical exam findings may include thickened skin in areas that are chronically scratched or rubbed. The histologic changes of the dermis associated with these thickened areas is termed "lichen simplex chronicus," or "squamous cell hyperplasia." The diagnosis is made after other etiologies for itching including yeast, vulvar intraepithelial neoplasia, and other vulvar dematoses have been excluded. A biopsy can be helpful to rule out other disorders but for dermatitis is typically nondiagnostic.

The mainstay of treatment is avoidance of all irritating substances and supportive vulvar hygiene measures. The initial treatment includes application of a corticosteroid at least daily. Generally a medium potency steroid is sufficient, but in severe cases, an ultrapotent steroid may be necessary.[9] The steroid cream is generally tapered as symptoms improve and skin returns to normal.

Lichen sclerosus

Lichen sclerosus is a benign, chronic, progressive dermatologic condition characterized by marked inflammation, epithelial thinning, and distinctive dermal changes accompanied by symptoms of pruritus and pain.[10] It is typically found in prepubertal and postmenopausal women.[11] True prevalence is unknown, but estimates range from 1 in 30 in elderly women to 1 in 1,000 patients referred to dermatologists.[12] The etiology is unknown, but several mechanisms have been postulated including genetic factors, immunologic abnormalities, hormonal factors, and possible infectious etiologies.

Women with lichen sclerosus typically present with pruritus and irritation, although many women are asymptomatic. On exam, the skin has a characteristic thin, white, wrinkled appearance termed "tissue paper." In more advanced cases, the labia may become fused with a distinct loss of architecture. Lichen sclerosus can cause significant morbidity in women including detrimental effects on sexual function such as dyspareunia, apareunia, and difficulty achieving orgasm.[13]

The diagnosis of lichen sclerosus is made with biopsy. Biopsy is important to make the diagnosis and exclude vulvar squamous cell carcinoma. Women with lichen sclerosus are at increased risk of developing squamous cell carcinoma, although their risk is estimated to be less than 5%.[14]

The management of lichen sclerosus includes ensuring proper vulvar hygiene practices and topical medications. Medical management includes application of a topical ultrapotent steroid.[15] Treatment is once or twice daily application of the steroid cream until relief of symptoms is achieved. Following initial therapy, patients are transitioned to maintenance therapy, which is usually one to three times per week of an ultrapotent steroid or more frequent application of a medium potency steroid. Patients should be examined at least every six months and possibly more frequently depending on symptom control.[14]

Lichen planus

Lichen planus is an inflammatory dermatologic condition, which affects the skin, mucosa, nails, and scalp. Vulvar lichen planus is characterized by erosive or papular lesions on the vulva, with or without vaginal involvement. The incidence is not clearly established and the etiology is unknown.

Women with lichen planus are typically postmenopausal and complain of pain, burning, pruritis, soreness, or vaginal discharge.[16] Vulvar lichen planus is most commonly erosive, and the lesions appear as shiny violaceous papules or glassy, erythematous erosions.[17] Lesions may occur on the labia minora and vestibule. Vaginal lesions are common.[18] When the vagina is involved, the epithelium is friable and may show areas of inflammation with increased vaginal discharge. In severe cases, adhesions and synechiae may develop, leading to narrowing or obliteration of the vagina.

Diagnosis is primarily clinical and a biopsy obtained will rule out other diagnoses such as squamous cells cancer. Lichen planus has been associated with squamous cell carcinoma.[19]

Treatment of lichen planus is similar to the other dermatoses with a focus on education and support, vulvar hygiene, and medical therapy. First line therapy includes topical ultrapotent corticosteroids. The therapy is initiated with once or twice daily application and once symptoms improve, the therapy is tapered to a maintenance regimen of two to three times weekly.[20] Other therapies that have been studied include tacrolimus.[15] If the vagina is involved, steroid suppositories can be used directly in the vagina.[21]

Hidradenitis suppurativa

Hidradenitis suppurativa (HS) is a chronic inflammatory disease that for many patients can be disfiguring and difficult to treat. This disorder effects 1%–3% of the population. In women, its onset is typically between puberty and age 40 with the highest prevalence in the second and third decade of life.[22] The etiology of HS is not entirely understood; however, with continued research, the most likely involved structures include skin follicles with follicular occlusion, follicular rupture, and the associated immune response with that process.[23]

HS most commonly involves the groin or upper inner thigh, axilla, chest, and buttocks. Other involved areas may also include sites of skin compression and friction. HS begins with painful red nodules, which may rupture and form chronic draining sinus tracks. Less commonly, ulcers may appear. The ulcers and sinuses may heal with thick, ropelike scars eventually leading to chronic scarring. Diagnosis is made clinically. The clinical features leading to diagnosis include the presence of multiple lesions, the location of lesions within the milk line, recurrence at the same site, long duration of individual lesions (weeks to months), bacterial cultures that are either negative or demonstrate the presence of multiple bacterial species, and failure to respond quickly to antibiotic therapy.

Treatment includes a multitude of approaches; there are no high-quality studies to demonstrate superiority of one treatment over another. In general terms, medical therapy is useful for the reduction of local inflammation and surgical intervention is useful for the treatment of nodules and sinus tracks. Oftentimes a combination of therapies is necessary. As in most vulvar dermatologic conditions, the initial therapy is a combination of vulvar hygiene measures, avoidance of irritating substances and education. Topical therapies have included local clindamycin cream, intralesional steroids, systemic antibiotics, and hormonal therapy.

Vulvar dysplasia

Vulvar dysplasia is a common cause of lesions of the vulva and should always be considered when evaluating women with vulvar complaints. Incidence is increased in elderly patients. Vulvar intraepithelial neoplasia (VIN) is pathologically defined as a precancerous lesion without evidence of invasion. VIN has been divided into differentiated and usual types. Differentiated VIN arises as a result of vulvar dematoses such as lichen sclerosus, whereas usual type VIN is that caused by human papillomavirus (HPV). Rarely, VIN is defined by cells that are nonsquamous such as Paget's disease and melanoma in situ.

Usual type VIN has been further divided into low-grade (LSIL) and high-grade (HSIL) lesions as recommended by the Lower Anogenital Squamous Terminology (LAST) project in 2012.[24] Low-grade lesions are those that are not considered premalignant. HSIL lesions represent distinct precancerous lesions. There is a strong association with HPV 16 and therefore with other lower genital tract neoplasias; 22% of usual VIN patients have concurrent cervical intraepithelial neoplasias (CIN).

Up to 22% of women are symptomatic. Most commonly women report chronic vulvar itching or burning at the site of the lesion; however, there is a wide variation in symptoms. The lesions themselves have a highly variable appearance. Lesions can range from white macules to dark, pigmented papules. Many lesions are quite subtle and therefore any suspicious lesion of the vulva should be further investigated with a biopsy. Vulvar cytology is not useful for screening or diagnosis.

Treatment may include a variety of approaches but most commonly includes laser ablative therapy, excision, or medical therapy. Women should have close follow-up after treatment as these lesions have a high recurrence rate with a significant risk of future vulvar carcinoma. In one retrospective review by van de Nieuwenhof et al., the risks of progression over a 14-year period of differentiated VIN was 32.8%, whereas usual type VIN was 5.7%.[25]

Vaginal disorders

The vagina is delineated by Hart's line distally and the vaginal fornices proximally. It is characterized by stratified squamous epithelium and underlying smooth muscle. The vaginal mucosa is highly responsive to hormonal fluctuations and provides lubrication. The superficial cells continuously exfoliate and are replaced by basal cells. The basal cells then undergo keratinization. Similarly to the vulva, vaginal cysts, ulcers, dermatoses, infections, and dysplasia, can affect the vagina.

Vaginal cysts

Vaginal cysts are not as common as vulvar cysts. Differential diagnosis includes hematoma, urethral diverticulum, Skene and Bartholin cysts, and inclusion cysts. The most common vaginal cysts are Gartner duct cysts. Gartner duct cysts are embryologic remnants that infrequently cause symptoms. Most are noted incidentally during routine pelvic exam. If women become symptomatic either due to abscess formation or due to the size of the cyst, they can easily be incised and drained. There have been several reports of marsupialization of Gartner duct cysts with good response rates.

Vaginal infections

Vaginal infections encompass a wide differential and are the most frequent reason women present with vulvovaginal complaints.

Yeast vaginitis

Yeast vaginitis is commonly found in practice. More than 75% of women will have at least one episode of vulvovaginal candidiasis in their lifetime.[26] *Candida albicans* is the most frequent causative agent of vulvovaginal candidiasis. Other species which may cause yeast symptoms include *Candida glabrata, Candida parapsilosis, Candida tropicalis,* and *Candida krusei.* Some studies have shown as many as 20% of women with vulvovaginal candidiasis are caused by *Candida glabrata.*[27] Risk factors for infection include pregnancy, nulliparity, use of spermicides, and young age (the risk is highest from ages 15 to 19 years old and then decreases with time).[28] There is some evidence that choice of contraception may increase risk of vulvovaginal candidiasis, including progesterone intrauterine devices (IUD) and high dose estrogen, 75 μg –150 μg, containing birth control pills.[28, 29] Recent antibiotic use has also been shown to be a risk factor.[30]

The most common symptom for vulvovaginal candidiasis is pruritus. Less commonly women report symptoms of burning, irritation, dyspareunia, pain with urination, and thick, white discharge.[27] Physical exam findings may include erythema, induration and satellite lesions of the vulva and thick, cottage cheese–like discharge.

Diagnosis requires visualization of blastospheres or pseudohypae on saline or 10% KOH microscopy. KOH has a sensitivity and specificity of 61% and 77% with a positive predictive value of 56%.[31] The absence of yeast argues against candidiasis but does not exclude it. Therefore, in symptomatic women, it may be prudent to perform a yeast culture to not only identify the presence of yeast, but also the species.

Diagnosis should be further classified as uncomplicated or complicated (see Table 22-1). For

Table 22-1 Classification of vulvovaginal candidiasis

Uncomplicated
• Sporadic or infrequent episodes
• Mild to moderate symptoms or findings
• Suspected *Candida albicans* infection
• Nonpregnant woman without medical complications
Complicated
• Recurrent episodes (four or more per year)
• Severe symptoms or findings
• Suspected or proved non–*C. albicans* infection
• Women with diabetes, severe medical illness, immunosuppression, other vulvovaginal conditions
• Pregnancy

Source: ACOG Practice Bulletin. Clinical management guidelines for obstetrician-gynecologists, Number 72, May 2006.[82]

uncomplicated vulvovaginal candidiasis, there are several available treatment options (see Table 22-2). All available treatments have similar efficacy; therefore, treatment should be tailored to each woman taking into account patient preference, prior treatment successes or failures and prior adverse reactions. The overall cure rate ranges from 80% to 90%. Oral treatment has been shown to achieve a similar or marginally higher cure rate than vaginal preparations.[32] Women may be treated with either a single dose or multi-dose regimen. Cure rates with single dose fluconazole approached 94% compared with 97% cure rates with clotrimazole.[33]

In women with complicated infections either due to non-*albicans* species or chronic/recurrent vulvovaginal candidiasis, more aggressive therapy may be indicated. In women with recurrent or severe disease, there is benefit to repeat doses. In a randomized placebo-controlled trial of 387 women with severe or recurrent vulvovaginal candidiasis, two sequential doses of 150 mg given three days apart compared to a single 150 mg dose showed a significantly higher cure rate, 67% improved to 80%.[34] In women with frequent, recurrent vulvovaginal candidiasis (greater than four episodes per year), initial intensive therapy followed by maintenance dosing has been shown to decrease symptomatic relapse. This therapy was described by Sobel to include an initial intensive therapy with three 150 mg doses of fluconazole at 72-hour intervals followed by once weekly dosing of 150 mg fluconazole orally or placebo for six months. This therapy decreased recurrence rates significantly and showed prolonged remission in approximately 50% of women.[35]

Refractory infections may be due to non-*albicans* species or less likely azole-resistant *Candida albicans.* Non-*albicans* species are often resistant to many of the azoles. Vaginal boric acid (600 mg) prescribed in a gelatin capsule for 14 days or amphotericin B suppositories are effective for refractory cases from *Candida glabrata.*[36] In patients in whom boric acid fails, a success of 90% was achieved with a two-week course of topical 17% flucytosine (5 g intravaginal dose).[37] This therapy can be used in combination with amphotericin B. None of these therapies should be used in pregnancy.

At this time, there is no evidence that probiotics or partner treatment is effective to prevent recurrences. Patients with multiple episodes of vaginal candidiasis may benefit from evaluation for conditions associated with immunocompromised conditions such as diabetes or human immunovirus (HIV) infection.

Bacterial vaginosis

Bacterial vaginosis (BV) is a change in a woman's natural vaginal flora in which the normal vaginal lactobacilli are replaced by a variety of anaerobic bacteria and mycoplasmas. The major bacteria that have been identified include *Gardnerella vaginalis*, anaerobic gram-negative rods belonging to the genera *Prevotella*, *Porphyromonas*, and *Bacteroides*, as well as *Peptostreptococcus* species, *Mycoplasma hominis*, *Ureaplasma urealyticum*, and often *Mobiluncus* species.[38] BV is the most common cause of vaginal discharge in women of childbearing age. In the United States, the National Health and Nutrition Examination Survey estimated the prevalence of BV to be 29% in the general population of women aged 14–49.[39]

There are several risk factors for BV including sexual activity and IUD use.[39] Condoms are associated with a decreased risk of BV, as is the use of combined hormonal contraception pills.[40] The association of IUD use and BV appears to be mediated by irregular bleeding and those without irregular bleeding did have an increased risk for BV.[41] Other risk factors include douching and cigarette smoking.[42]

Table 22-2 Treatment of vulvovaginal infections

Indication	Drug	Formulation	Dosage	Duration
Uncomplicated yeast candidiasis	Butoconazole	2% cream	5 g per vagina	3 days
		2% cream Bioadhesive product	5 g per vagina	1 day
	Clotrimazole	1% cream	5 g per vagina	7–14 days
		2% cream	5 g per vagina	3 days
	Fluconazole	150 mg	150 mg oral tablet daily	1 day
	Miconazole	4% cream	5 g per vagina	7 days
		100 mg suppository	100 mg daily	7 days
		200 mg suppository	200 mg daily	3 days
	Nystatin	100,000 unit vaginal tablet	One vaginal tablet	14 days
	Terconazole	0.4% cream	5 g per vagina	7 days
		0.8% cream	5 g per vagina	3 days
		80 mg vaginal suppository	One suppository	3 days
	Tioconazole	6.5% ointment	5 g per vagina	1 day
Bacterial vaginosis	Clindamycin	2% vaginal cream	5 g per vagina nightly	7 days
		300 mg oral	300 mg twice daily	7 days
		100 mg vaginal ovules	100 mg nightly	3 days
	Metronidazole	500 mg oral tablet	500 mg twice daily	7 days
		0.75% vaginal gel	5 g per vagina daily	5 days
	Tinidazole	2 g oral tablet	2 g daily	2 days
		1 g oral tablet	1 g daily	5 days
Trichomoniasis	Metronidazole	2 g oral tablet	2 g single dose	1 day
		500 mg oral tablet	500 mg twice daily	7 days
	Tinidazole	2 g oral tablet	2 g single dose	1 day

Source: Centers for Disease Control and Prevention. *Sexually transmitted diseases treatment guidelines 2010.*[83]

The classic symptoms of BV include thin, gray, homogenous discharge that is malodorous. Other symptoms may include a yellowish discharge, abdominal pain, intermenstrual bleeding, and menorrhagia. Physical exam findings include the presence of abnormal discharge, malodorous smell, and rarely evidence of inflammation.

The gold standard for the diagnosis of BV is a Gram's stain. It is used mostly in research studies. BV is more commonly diagnosed clinically based on Amsel's criteria. Amsel's criteria requires the presence of three out of four defined criteria: abnormal gray discharge, vaginal pH greater than 4.5, a positive amine or "whiff" test, and more than 20% of the epithelial cells being clue cells on a wet mount.[43] Amsel's criteria have a sensitivity of 92% and specificity of 77%.[44]

There are several commercially available tests to aid in the diagnosis of BV when microscopy is not available. The BD Affirm VPIII test is an automated DNA probe assay for detecting *Gardeneralla vaginalis* when present at a high concentration (2×10^5 CFU/mL). It is able to detect three infectious agents – *G. vaginalis*, *Candida* species, and *Trichomonas vaginalis* – making it useful in the detection of mixed infections.[45] Another available test is the OSOM BVBlue system. This system is a chromogenic diagnostic test based on the presence of elevated sialidase enzyme activity in vaginal fluid samples. This enzyme is produced by bacterial pathogens associated with BV including *Gardenerella*, *Bacteroides*, *Prevotella*, and *Mobiluncus* species.[46, 47] There is no role in the diagnosis of BV for vaginal cultures.

In nonpregnant women, BV is associated with an increased risk of chlamydia, gonorrhea, herpes simplex virus type 2, and trichomoniasis.[48–50] BV has also shown to increase transmission rates of HIV.[51] It has been implicated in the development of pelvic inflammatory disease and post-procedural gynecologic infections.[52] In pregnant women, several studies have shown a relationship of BV infection to early miscarriage, late miscarriage, preterm labor, low birth weight, prematurity, preterm premature rupture of membranes, histologic chorioamnionitis, and postpartum endometritis.[53–55]

Currently recommended therapies for the treatment of BV are listed in Table 22-2. The listed regimens have comparable safety and efficacy and therefore treatment should be individualized.[56, 57] Topical therapy is more expensive than oral systemic therapy, although the later is associated with more gastrointestinal side effects. Short-term treatment response rates approach 84%.[56, 58] BV, however, persists or recurs in 11%–29% of women at one month and 30% of women relapse within three months. Recurrence rates may be as high as 50% within one year.[59] Standard therapy is effective for the treatment of BV in pregnant women, so those with symptomatic BV should be treated.[60]

Probiotic therapy has not yet shown a clear benefit to reduce recurrences. Studies of partner treatment have also failed to show any significant benefit.[61]

Trichomoniasis

Trichomoniasis is a common nonviral STD worldwide. The total prevalence in the female population was estimated at 3%, affecting non-Hispanic black women most frequently with a prevalence of 13.3%. Prevalence in this population increases with age. Trichomoniasis is found 18%–50% in women with vaginal complaints.[62]

Trichomoniasis is caused by a single cell, flagellated protozoan *Trichomonas vaginalis*. Coinfection with BV is common with rates as high as 60%–80%.[63] Risk factors include multiple sexual partners, low socioeconomic status, history of other sexually transmitted diseases, and lack of condom use.

Symptoms of trichomonal infections include frothy, gray or yellow-green vaginal discharge. It is often associated with pruritius, burning, dysuria, abdominal pain, post-coital bleeding, or dyspareunia. Up to 50% of women are asymptomatic.[64] Physical exam may reveal erythema or inflammation of the vulva and vagina, cervical petechiae, or strawberry cervix.[65, 66]

The diagnosis of trichomoniasis relies on the visualization of motile trichomonads on wet mount. A wet mount has only 55%–60% sensitivity in the diagnosis of trichomoniasis and depends on the experience of the technician and collection technique.[67] Other findings on wet mount that may suggest the presence of trichomonads include an elevated pH and increase in PMNs.

The gold standard for diagnosis is polymerase chain reaction (PCR). PCR is available from Gen-Probe as the APTIMA Trichomoniasis assay. This assay uses target capture and transcription mediated nucleic acid amplification testing (NAAT) to detect species specific ribosomal RNA, including *N. gonorrhea, C. trachomatis,* and *T. vaginalis*. This technology is highly sensitive (100%) and specific (99%) and can be performed on urine and self-collected samples.[68] Other commercially available tests include rapid antigen or nucleic acid probes including the BD AFFIRM VPIII and the OSOM Trichomonas Rapid Test.

Trichomoniasis has been implicated in numerous studies to increase the risk of transmission of HIV [69–71] and increase the risk of CIN.[72] It has also been shown to increase the risk of atypical PID in HIV positive women.[73] Similarly to BV, it increases the risk of posthysterectomy cuff cellulitis and abscesses.[52] In pregnant women, it is associated with an increased risk of adverse pregnancy outcomes including PPROM and preterm labor.[74]

Treatment of trichomoniasis is further discussed in the chapter on sexually transmitted diseases.

Desquamative inflammatory vaginitis

Desquamative inflammatory vaginitis (DIV) is a rare but disabling condition.[5] The prevalence of DIV is unknown, although it has been reported to be as high as 8% of a referral population to a specialty vulvovaginitis clinic.[5] Reichman and Sobel characterized the largest cohort of women with DIV and described these women as mostly Caucasian, perimenopausal, more likely to have thyroid disease and allergic diatheses, and more likely to respond to anti-inflammatory therapy.[75]

The etiology of DIV remains unknown. Possible etiologies have included vitamin D deficiency, unidentified microbial pathogen, diminished estrogen, autoimmune disorder, cell-mediated immune activation, and possible genetic link.[76] Most likely DIV represents a heterogeneous group of disorders with common clinical and microscopic characteristics.

Women with DIV report profuse, purulent vaginal discharge; DIV is very frequently associated with vulvar soreness, burning, and dyspareunia.[77] Patients may also describe itching and irritation. Almost all women are symptomatic.[78] Physical exam findings can include significant erythema with marked inflammation and even erosive findings. The visible discharge is typically purulent and without odor.

DIV is diagnosed clinically. The classic findings on microscopy include an elevated number of PMNs, predominance of parabasal cells (immature squamous cells) and vaginal pH greater than 4.5. Clinical and microscopic findings mimic those found in other conditions like trichomoniasis and vaginal atrophy. DIV is, therefore, a diagnosis of exclusion and *N. gonorrhea*, *C. trachomatis*, and *T. vaginalis* must be excluded.

Treatment for DIV is mostly derived from case reports. There are no large, randomized studies. Regimens have included intravaginal steroids either alone or in combination with clindamycin vaginal cream. Studies have shown reasonable response rates. Treatments are summarized in Table 22-3. In a small study of 51 women treated with intravaginal 2% clindamycin, the overall improvement was 90% with symptomatic relapse occurring in 29%.[79] Women are treated for two to four weeks. Given the high risk of recurrence, multiple maintenance regimens have been proposed. Consideration of twice weekly intravaginal steroids has been used for prevention of recurrences.[78]

Other disorders

Other less common disorders may also cause symptoms of vulvar and vaginal irritation and increase in vaginal discharge. In postmenopausal women, patients commonly present with atrophic vaginitis. These women report abnormal vaginal discharge, dryness, itching, burning and/or dyspareunia. Diagnosis is made on the basis of elevated pH, parabasal cells on microscopy, and negative amine test. There are no clue cells present. It is possible to have elevated polymorpholated neutrophils (PMNs) on microscopy with advance disease. Treatment consists of topical estrogen therapy and/or water based vaginal moisturizers.[80, 81]

Foreign bodies such as retained tampons may also cause an increase in vaginal discharge. These are almost always characterized by significant vaginal discharge that is reported as malodorous. It is treated simply with removal of the foreign body. Vaginal dysplasia is found less frequently than vulvar and cervical dysplasia. It is typically HPV mediated. Lesions are highly variable; therefore, any suspicious findings on exam warrant biopsy. Other even more rare disorders include group A *Streptococcus* infections, which can cause profuse vaginal irritation and purulent discharge.

Concluding remarks

Vulvovaginal disorders are prevalent among women. A complete history and physical exam is important in

Table 22-3 Treatment for desquamative inflammatory vaginitis

Topical steroids	Hydrocortisone 25 mg intravaginal suppository	Nightly for 2–4 weeks, reduce frequency for maintenance
	10% hydrocortisone foam intravaginal	2–3 times daily for 2 weeks; consider prolonged course for maintenance
Topical antibiotics	Clindamycin 200 mg intravaginal suppository	Nightly for 2–4 weeks
	2% clindamycin cream intravaginal	5 g nightly for 2–8 weeks
Combined therapy	2% clindamycin cream alternating with hydrocortisone, 25 mg suppository	Alternate nightly for 14 nights
	Hydrocortisone, 100 mg/g in clindamycin 2% cream base intravaginal	Insert 5 g every other night for 14 doses
	2% clindamycin cream (1 applicator) combined with hydrocortisone, 25 mg suppository	Insert both every other night for 14 doses
	Hydrocortisone, 100 mg/g in clindamycin 2% cream base, compounded	Insert 5 g applicator every other night for 14 doses

Source: Stockdale, C. Clinical spectrum of desquamative inflammatory vaginitis.[76]

the evaluation of the women with these symptoms. Basic clinical exam and laboratory testing will aid in the diagnosis of most of these disorders so that treatment can be tailored to the woman and her diagnosis, thereby improving clinical outcomes.

References

1. Kent HL. Epidemiology of vaginitis. *American journal of obstetrics and gynecology.* 1991;**165**(4 Pt 2):1168–76.
2. Lipsky MS, Waters T, Sharp LK. Impact of vaginal antifungal products on utilization of health care services: evidence from physician visits. *The Journal of the American Board of Family Practice /American Board of Family Practice.* 2000;**13**(3):178–82.
3. Anderson MR, Klink K, Cohrssen A. Evaluation of vaginal complaints. *JAMA: the journal of the American Medical Association.* 2004;**291**(11):1368–79.
4. Berg AO, Heidrich FE, Fihn SD, et al. Establishing the cause of genitourinary symptoms in women in a family practice. Comparison of clinical examination and comprehensive microbiology. *JAMA: the journal of the American Medical Association.* 1984;**251**(5):620–5.
5. Nyirjesy P, Peyton C, Weitz MV, et al. Causes of chronic vaginitis: analysis of a prospective database of affected women. *Obstetrics and gynecology.* 2006;**108**(5):1185–91.
6. Haider Z, Condous G, Kirk E, et al. The simple outpatient management of Bartholin's abscess using the Word catheter: a preliminary study. *The Australian & New Zealand journal of obstetrics & gynaecology.* 2007;**47**(2):137–40.
7. Ball SB, Wojnarowska F. Vulvar dermatoses: lichen sclerosus, lichen planus, and vulval dermatitis/lichen simplex chronicus. *Seminars in cutaneous medicine and surgery.* 1998;**17**(3):182–8.
8. Hoang MP, Reuter J, Papalas JA, et al. Vulvar inflammatory dermatoses: an update and review. *American journal of dermatopathology.* 2014;**36** (9):689–704.
9. Green C, Colquitt JL, Kirby J, Davidson P. Topical corticosteroids for atopic eczema: clinical and cost effectiveness of once-daily vs. more frequent use. *British journal of dermatology.* 2005;**152**(1):130–41.
10. Ridley CM, Neill SM. *The vulva.* 2nd ed. Oxford; Malden, MA: Blackwell Science; 1999. ix, 314 pp.
11. McPherson T, Cooper S. Vulval lichen sclerosus and lichen planus. *Dermatologic therapy.* 2010;**23**(5): 523–32.
12. Leibovitz A, Kaplun VV, Saposhnicov N, Habot B. Vulvovaginal examinations in elderly nursing home women residents. *Archives of gerontology and geriatrics.* 2000;**31**(1):1–4.
13. Dalziel KL. Effect of lichen sclerosus on sexual function and parturition. *Journal of reproductive medicine.* 1995;**40**(5):351–4.

14. Neill SM, Lewis FM, Tatnall FM, Cox NH, British Association of Dermatologists British Association of Dermatologists' guidelines for the management of lichen sclerosus 2010. *British journal of dermatology.* 2010;**163**(4):672–82.
15. Chi CC, Kirtschig G, Baldo M, et al. Topical interventions for genital lichen sclerosus. *Cochrane database of systematic reviews.* 2011;**12**:CD008240.
16. Kennedy CM, Galask RP. Erosive vulvar lichen planus: retrospective review of characteristics and outcomes in 113 patients seen in a vulvar specialty clinic. *Journal of reproductive medicine.* 2007;**52**(1):43–7.
17. Lewis FM, Bogliatto F. Erosive vulval lichen planus – a diagnosis not to be missed: a clinical review. *European journal of obstetrics, gynecology, and reproductive biology.* 2013;**171**(2):214–19.
18. Ridley CM. Chronic erosive vulval disease. *Clinical and experimental dermatology.* 1990;**15**(4):245–52.
19. Kennedy CM, Peterson LB, Galask RP. Erosive vulvar lichen planus: a cohort at risk for cancer? *The Journal of reproductive medicine.* 2008;**53**(10):781–4.
20. Cooper SM, Wojnarowska F. Influence of treatment of erosive lichen planus of the vulva on its prognosis. *Archives of dermatology.* 2006;**142**(3):289–94.
21. Anderson M, Kutzner S, Kaufman RH. Treatment of vulvovaginal lichen planus with vaginal hydrocortisone suppositories. *Obstetrics and gynecology.* 2002;**100**(2): 359–62.
22. Alikhan A, Lynch PJ, Eisen DB. Hidradenitis suppurativa: a comprehensive review. *Journal of the American Academy of Dermatology.* 2009;**60** (4):539–61; quiz 62–3.
23. van der Zee HH, Laman JD, Boer J, Prens EP. Hidradenitis suppurativa: viewpoint on clinical phenotyping, pathogenesis and novel treatments. *Experimental dermatology.* 2012;**21**(10):735–9.
24. Darragh TM, Colgan TJ, Thomas Cox J, et al. The Lower Anogenital Squamous Terminology Standardization project for HPV-associated lesions: background and consensus recommendations from the College of American Pathologists and the American Society for Colposcopy and Cervical Pathology. *International journal of gynecological pathology: official journal of the International Society of Gynecological Pathologists.* 2013;**32**(1):76–115.
25. Van de Nieuwenhof HP, Massuger LF, van der Avoort IA, et al. Vulvar squamous cell carcinoma development after diagnosis of VIN increases with age. *European journal of cancer.* 2009;**45**(5):851–6.
26. Foxman B. The epidemiology of vulvovaginal candidiasis: risk factors. *American journal of public health.* 1990;**80**(3):329–31.
27. Sobel JD. Vulvovaginal candidosis. *Lancet.* 2007;**369** (9577):1961–71.
28. Barbone F, Austin H, Louv WC, Alexander WJ. A follow-up study of methods of contraception, sexual activity, and rates of trichomoniasis, candidiasis, and bacterial vaginosis. *American journal of obstetrics and gynecology.* 1990;**163**(2):510–14.
29. Donders GG, Berger J, Heuninckx H, et al. Vaginal flora changes on Pap smears after insertion of levonorgestrel-releasing intrauterine device. *Contraception.* 2011;**83**(4):352–6.
30. Xu J, Schwartz K, Bartoces M, et al. Effect of antibiotics on vulvovaginal candidiasis: a MetroNet study. *Journal of the American Board of Family Medicine: JABFM.* 2008;**21**(4):261–8.
31. Abbott J. Clinical and microscopic diagnosis of vaginal yeast infection: a prospective analysis. *Annals of emergency medicine.* 1995;**25**(5):587–91.
32. Watson MC, Grimshaw JM, Bond CM, et al. Oral versus intra-vaginal imidazole and triazole anti-fungal agents for the treatment of uncomplicated vulvovaginal candidiasis (thrush): a systematic review. *BJOG: an international journal of obstetrics and gynaecology.* 2002;**109**(1):85–95.
33. Sobel JD, Brooker D, Stein GE, et al. Single oral dose fluconazole compared with conventional clotrimazole topical therapy of *Candida vaginitis. Fluconazole Vaginitis* Study Group. *American journal of obstetrics and gynecology.* 1995;**172**(4 Pt 1):1263–8.
34. Sobel JD, Kapernick PS, Zervos M, et al. Treatment of complicated *Candida* vaginitis: comparison of single and sequential doses of fluconazole. *American journal of obstetrics and gynecology.* 2001;**185**(2):363–9.
35. Sobel JD, Wiesenfeld HC, Martens M, et al. Maintenance fluconazole therapy for recurrent vulvovaginal candidiasis. *The New England journal of medicine.* 2004;**351**(9):876–83.
36. Phillips AJ. Treatment of non-*albicans Candida* vaginitis with amphotericin B vaginal suppositories. *American journal of obstetrics and gynecology.* 2005;**192**(6):2009–12; discussion 12–13.
37. Sobel JD, Chaim W, Nagappan V, Leaman D. Treatment of vaginitis caused by *Candida glabrata*: use of topical boric acid and flucytosine. *American journal of obstetrics and gynecology.* 2003;**189**(5):1297–300.
38. Hill GB. The microbiology of bacterial vaginosis. *American journal of obstetrics and gynecology.* 1993;**169**(2 Pt 2):450–4.
39. Allsworth JE, Peipert JF. Prevalence of bacterial vaginosis: 2001–2004 National Health and Nutrition Examination Survey data. *Obstetrics and gynecology.* 2007;**109**(1):114–20.
40. Fethers KA, Fairley CK, Hocking JS, et al. Sexual risk factors and bacterial vaginosis: a systematic review and meta-analysis. *Clinical infectious diseases: an official*

publication of the Infectious Diseases Society of America. 2008;**47**(11):1426–35.

41. Madden T, Grentzer JM, Secura GM, et al. Risk of bacterial vaginosis in users of the intrauterine device: a longitudinal study. *Sexually transmitted diseases.* 2012;**39**(3):217–22.
42. Ness RB, Hillier SL, Richter HE, et al. Douching in relation to bacterial vaginosis, lactobacilli, and facultative bacteria in the vagina. *Obstetrics and gynecology.* 2002;**100**(4):765.
43. Amsel R, Totten PA, Spiegel CA, et al. Nonspecific vaginitis. Diagnostic criteria and microbial and epidemiologic associations. *The American journal of medicine.* 1983;**74**(1):14–22.
44. Landers DV, Wiesenfeld HC, Heine RP, et al. Predictive value of the clinical diagnosis of lower genital tract infection in women. *American journal of obstetrics and gynecology.* 2004;**190**(4):1004–10.
45. Sheiness D, Dix K, Watanabe S, Hillier SL. High levels of *Gardnerella vaginalis* detected with an oligonucleotide probe combined with elevated pH as a diagnostic indicator of bacterial vaginosis. *Journal of clinical microbiology.* 1992;**30**(3):642–8.
46. Bradshaw CS, Morton AN, Garland SM, et al. Evaluation of a point-of-care test, BVBlue, and clinical and laboratory criteria for diagnosis of bacterial vaginosis. *Journal of clinical microbiology.* 2005;**43**(3):1304–8.
47. Myziuk L, Romanowski B, Johnson SC. BVBlue test for diagnosis of bacterial vaginosis. *Journal of clinical microbiology.* 2003;**41**(5):1925–8.
48. Wiesenfeld HC, Hillier SL, Krohn MA, et al. Bacterial vaginosis is a strong predictor of *Neisseria gonorrhoeae* and *Chlamydia trachomatis* infection. *Clinical infectious diseases: an official publication of the Infectious Diseases Society of America.* 2003;**36**(5):663–8.
49. Cherpes TL, Meyn LA, Krohn MA, et al. Association between acquisition of herpes simplex virus type 2 in women and bacterial vaginosis. *Clinical infectious diseases: an official publication of the Infectious Diseases Society of America.* 2003;**37**(3):319–25.
50. Plitt SS, Garfein RS, Gaydos CA, et al. Prevalence and correlates of *Chlamydia trachomatis, Neisseria gonorrhoeae, Trichomonas vaginalis* infections, and bacterial vaginosis among a cohort of young injection drug users in Baltimore, Maryland. *Sexually transmitted diseases.* 2005;**32**(7):446–53.
51. Martin HL, Richardson BA, Nyange PM, et al. Vaginal lactobacilli, microbial flora, and risk of human immunodeficiency virus type 1 and sexually transmitted disease acquisition. *Journal of infectious diseases.* 1999;**180**(6):1863–8.
52. Soper DE, Bump RC, Hurt WG. Bacterial vaginosis and trichomoniasis vaginitis are risk factors for cuff cellulitis after abdominal hysterectomy. *American journal of obstetrics and gynecology.* 1990;**163**(3): 1016–21; discussion 21–3.
53. Leitich H, Bodner-Adler B, Brunbauer M, et al. Bacterial vaginosis as a risk factor for preterm delivery: a meta-analysis. *American journal of obstetrics and gynecology.* 2003;**189**(1):139–47.
54. Hillier SL, Krohn MA, Cassen E, The role of bacterial vaginosis and vaginal bacteria in amniotic fluid infection in women in preterm labor with intact fetal membranes. *Clinical infectious diseases: an official publication of the Infectious Diseases Society of America.* 1995;**20**(Suppl 2):S276–8.
55. Hillier SL, Kiviat NB, Hawes SE, et al. Role of bacterial vaginosis-associated microorganisms in endometritis. *American journal of obstetrics and gynecology.* 1996;**175** (2):435–41.
56. Hanson JM, McGregor JA, Hillier SL, et al. Metronidazole for bacterial vaginosis. A comparison of vaginal gel vs. oral therapy. Journal of reproductive medicine. 2000;**45**(11):889–96.
57. Paavonen J, Mangioni C, Martin MA, Wajszczuk CP. Vaginal clindamycin and oral metronidazole for bacterial vaginosis: a randomized trial. *Obstetrics and gynecology.* 2000;**96**(2):256–60.
58. Livengood CH 3rd, Soper DE, Sheehan KL, et al. Comparison of once-daily and twice-daily dosing of 0.75% metronidazole gel in the treatment of bacterial vaginosis. *Sexually transmitted diseases.* 1999;**26**(3): 137–42.
59. Bradshaw CS, Morton AN, Hocking J, et al. High recurrence rates of bacterial vaginosis over the course of 12 months after oral metronidazole therapy and factors associated with recurrence. *Journal of infectious diseases.* 2006;**193**(11):1478–86.
60. Yudin MH, Landers DV, Meyn L, Hillier SL. Clinical and cervical cytokine response to treatment with oral or vaginal metronidazole for bacterial vaginosis during pregnancy: a randomized trial. *Obstetrics and gynecology.* 2003;**102**(3):527–34.
61. Vejtorp M, Bollerup AC, Vejtorp L, et al. Bacterial vaginosis: a double-blind randomized trial of the effect of treatment of the sexual partner. *British journal of obstetrics and gynaecology.* 1988;**95**(9):920–6.
62. Centers for Disease Control and Prevention. Sexually transmitted diseases treatment guidelines 2002. *MMWR Recommendations and reports: Morbidity and mortality weekly report recommendations and reports / Centers for Disease Control.* 2002;**51**(RR-6):1–78.
63. Sobel JD, Subramanian C, Foxman B, et al. Mixed vaginitis – more than coinfection and with therapeutic implications. *Current infectious disease reports.* 2013;**15**(2):104–8.

64. Van Der Pol B, Williams JA, Orr DP, et al. Prevalence, incidence, natural history, and response to treatment of *Trichomonas vaginalis* infection among adolescent women. *Journal of infectious diseases.* 2005;**192**(12): 2039–44.

65. Hammill HA. *Trichomonas vaginalis. Obstetrics and gynecology clinics of North America.* 1989;**16**(3):531–40.

66. Wolner-Hanssen P, Krieger JN, Stevens CE, et al. Clinical manifestations of vaginal trichomoniasis. *JAMA: the journal of the American Medical Association.* 1989;**261**(4):571–6.

67. Krieger JN, Tam MR, Stevens CE, et al. Diagnosis of trichomoniasis. Comparison of conventional wet-mount examination with cytologic studies, cultures, and monoclonal antibody staining of direct specimens. *JAMA: the journal of the American Medical Association.* 1988;**259**(8):1223–7.

68. Schwebke JR, Hobbs MM, Taylor SN, et al. Molecular testing for *Trichomonas vaginalis* in women: results from a prospective US clinical trial. *Journal of clinical microbiology.* 2011;**49**(12):4106–11.

69. Sorvillo F, Kerndt P. *Trichomonas vaginalis* and amplification of HIV-1 transmission. *Lancet.* 1998;**351**(9097):213–14.

70. Sorvillo F, Smith L, Kerndt P, Ash L. *Trichomonas vaginalis*, HIV, and African-Americans. *Emerging infectious diseases.* 2001;**7**(6):927–32.

71. McClelland RS, Sangare L, Hassan WM, et al. Infection with *Trichomonas vaginalis* increases the risk of HIV-1 acquisition. *Journal of infectious diseases.* 2007;**195** (5):698–702.

72. Zhang ZF, Begg CB. Is *Trichomonas vaginalis* a cause of cervical neoplasia? Results from a combined analysis of 24 studies. *International journal of epidemiology.* 1994;**23**(4):682–90.

73. Moodley P, Wilkinson D, Connolly C, et al. *Trichomonas vaginalis* is associated with pelvic inflammatory disease in women infected with human immunodeficiency virus. *Clinical infectious diseases: an official publication of the Infectious Diseases Society of America.* 2002;**34**(4):519–22.

74. Silver BJ, Guy RJ, Kaldor JM, et al. *Trichomonas vaginalis* as a cause of perinatal morbidity: a systematic review and meta-analysis. *Sexually transmitted diseases.* 2014;**41**(6):369–76.

75. Reichman O, Sobel J. Desquamative inflammatory vaginitis: best practice and research. *Clinical obstetrics & gynaecology.* 2014.

76. Stockdale CK. Clinical spectrum of desquamative inflammatory vaginitis. *Current infectious disease reports.* 2010;**12**(6):479–83.

77. Oates JK, Rowen D. Desquamative inflammatory vaginitis: a review. *Genitourinary medicine.* 1990;**66**(4):275–9.

78. Sobel JD, Reichman O, Misra D, Yoo W. Prognosis and treatment of desquamative inflammatory vaginitis. *Obstetrics and gynecology.* 2011;**117**(4):850–5.

79. Sobel JD. Desquamative inflammatory vaginitis: a new subgroup of purulent vaginitis responsive to topical 2% clindamycin therapy. *American journal of obstetrics and gynecology.* 1994;**171**(5):1215–20.

80. Nyirjesy P. Postmenopausal vaginitis. *Current infectious disease reports.* 2007;**9**(6):480–4.

81. Ballagh SA. Vaginal hormone therapy for urogenital and menopausal symptoms. *Seminars in reproductive medicine.* 2005;**23**(2):126–40.

82. Bulletins – Gynecology ACoP. ACOG Practice Bulletin. Clinical management guidelines for obstetrician-gynecologists, Number 72, May 2006: Vaginitis. *Obstetrics and gynecology.* 2006;**107**(5): 1195–206.

83. Katz AR, Lee MV, Wasserman GM. Sexually transmitted disease (STD) update: a review of the CDC 2010 STD treatment guidelines and epidemiologic trends of common STDs in Hawai'i. *Hawai'i journal of medicine & public health: a journal of Asia Pacific Medicine & Public Health.* 2012;**71**(3): 68–73.

Chapter 23

Office care of patients with leiomyomata of the uterus

Julie Zemaitis DeCesare and Gail Joseph

Scope of the problem

Uterine leiomyoma, also known as fibroids (because of the fibrous texture created by the increased collagen content of these tumors), fibromyoma, myofibroma, leiomyofibroma, fibroleiomyoma, myoma, fibroma, and fibroid are benign tumors of the smooth muscle cells of the uterus (Figures 23-1 and 23-2). They maintain varying amounts of fibrous connective tissue, but smooth muscle predominates. The elongated smooth muscle fibers are aggregated in bundles, but it is believed that each fibroid originates from one single cell that launches into dysplastic growth.[1] There may be hundreds of these benign tumors in various stages of growth on the uterus at the same time. Although the use of the word "tumor" tends to stir up trepidation in many patients, these tumors are readily distinguishable from their actually malignant counterparts by the absence of mitotic figures on histological staining. See Figure 23.3 for an example of a large fibroid uterus.

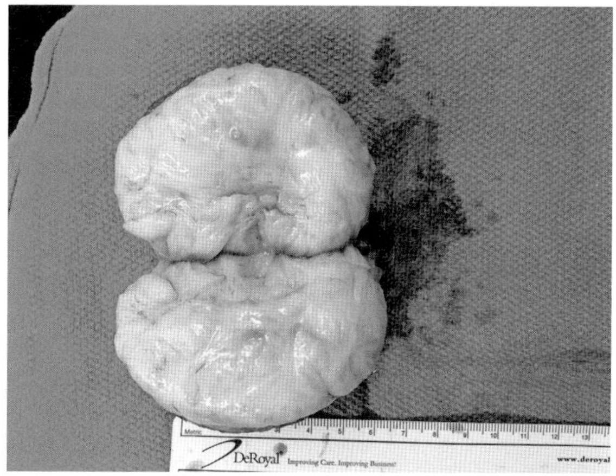

Figure 23-1 Large benign fibroid.

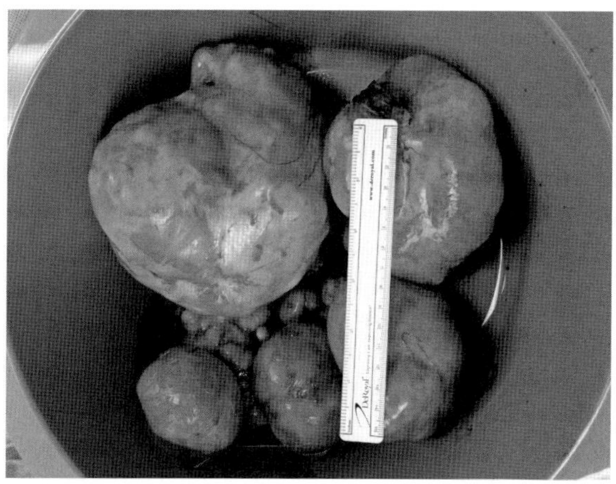

Figure 23-2 Multiple benign fibroids.

Leiomyoma are the most common tumor in women,[2] and the leading indication for hysterectomy in the United States.[3] They are responsible for one-third of all hospital admissions, with symptoms ranging from pelvic pressure and pain to severe menorrhagia requiring transfusion. Fibroids are larger in African-American women, and occur at a younger age. This racial difference, like most of the racial disparities in medicine, is as yet inexplicable. They are more common in African-America women, and have lifetime prevalence of 80% in African-American women, as compare to 70% in Caucasian women by age 50.[4] A difference of 10% may not seem very discrepant; however, African-American women suffer a disproportionate effect from these tumors, including size at presentation, growth, and symptoms.[5] The health-care costs associated with fibroids are staggering, and the annual cost to treat this condition is estimated to be \$5.9 billion–\$34.4 billion.[6] In the United States, as more preventive services are covered through the Affordable Care Act (ACA), it is a natural assumption that more fibroid tumors will be diagnosed. The

Office Care of Women, ed. Martin E. Olsen and Botros Rizk. Published by Cambridge University Press.

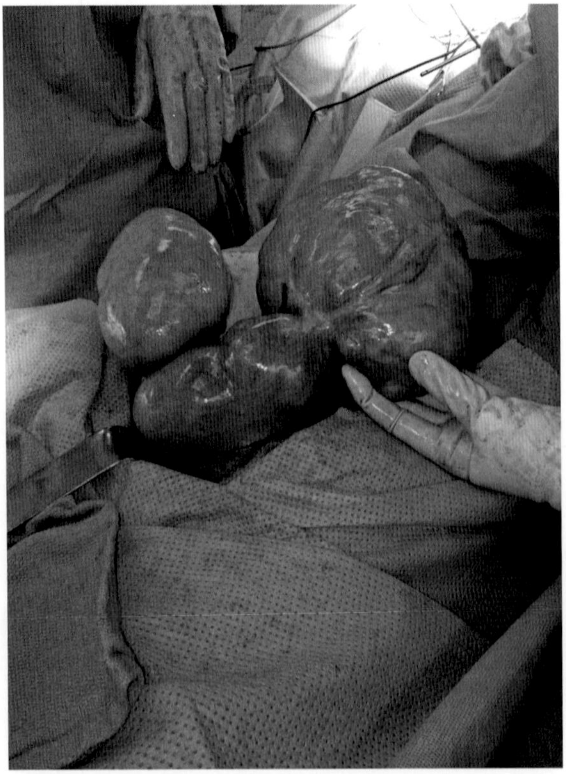

Figure 23-3 Large fibroid uterus 20 weeks size on physical exam 0700.

prudent practitioner needs to consider cost-effective and evidenced based treatment.

Fibroids are uncommon in any women before 20 years of age. The prevalence of uterine leiomyoma in women aged more than 35 years is 20%, while the prevalence increases to 51.2%–60.0% in women aged 40–50 years.[7] The incidence is noted to be the same in pre- and postmenopausal women, but the average number and size of the lesions tend to be much more significant in premenopausal women. Multiple studies have shown that despite the number estimated during the preoperative diagnosis of fibroids, the total number of fibroids found in pathological samples is consistently far greater than expected. This calls into question the ability to ever remove all the leiomyoma present on a uterus in the process of a myomectomy.

Genetics

Some characteristics of leiomyoma would seem to indicate that there is a genetic link to the disease. For example, patients with uterine leiomyoma often have a positive family history of uterine leiomyoma, with a particular correlation being noted between first-degree relatives.[8] A small subset of patients has also been noted who seem to exhibit a strong predisposition to developing profusely disseminated leiomyoma in conjunction with renal cell carcinoma. This syndrome is collectively labeled leimyomatosis and renal cell carcinoma syndrome and has been noted to have an autosomal dominant inheritance pattern. Research in this group of patients has led to the discovery of a loss of function mutation in the fumarate hydratase gene that results in loss of suppression of leiomyoma formation.[9, 10] However no specific genetic syndromes have been identified that accounts for the development of uterine fibroids alone, and even in familial settings, their occurrence seems to be multifactorial.

From a cytogenetic perspective, most leiomyoma are chromosomally normal. However, about 40%–50% of leiomyoma show karyotypically detectable chromosomal abnormalities which are most often not random, and specific to that tumor. Recent studies of the molecular genetics of leiomyoma have suggested that the process of chromothripsis (chromosomal breakage and reformation) is the key for the etiology of the fibroid tumor.[11] Additional further research on the topic has yielded the knowledge that location of leiomyoma with reference to the endometrial lining may have a relationship to the presence of cytogenetic abnormalities. One study suggested submucous myomas consistently had fewer cytogenetic abnormalities relative to intramural and subserosal fibroids. The quoted rates were 12%, 35%, and 29%, respectively.[12]

Classifications of fibroids

Leiomyoma are traditionally classified based on their anatomic location relative to the endometrial lining or serosa of the uterus, and the direction of their growth. Subserosal leiomyoma grow out of myocytes that are directly adjacent to the serosal layer of the uterus and often protrude or bulge from the surface of the uterus. Often these may become parasitic, attaching to nearby structures and harvesting from their vascular supply. Intramural leiomyoma are nestled into the myometrium of the uterus. Submucosal leiomyoma, also termed intracavitary leiomyoma, impinge on the endometrial lining of the uterus. Pedunculated fibroids may be located on the serosal layer or be classifiably submucosal; in either case they have a stalk or pedicle as the base from which they protrude. The European Society of

Hysteroscopy posits a different classification of leiomyoma, born more out of utility, and based on the percentage of the fibroid located within the myometrium. Type 0 leiomyoma are located entirely within the uterine cavity (intracavitary), type 1 leiomyoma are 50% buried into the myometrium (or 50% extending into the intramural space), and type 2 leiomyoma are less than 50% buried in the myometrium (or greater than 50% extending into the intramural space).[3] This classification system helps to predict the likelihood of successful resection by hysteroscopic methods. Reports indicate as much as 95% success rate retrospectively, in populations where the great majority of leiomyoma were type 2.[13]

History

Treatment of leiomyoma constitutes a significant realm of gynecologic care. In fact, in the years 1998–2005, up to 27% of gynecologic related admissions to hospitals were due to symptoms related to uterine leiomyoma.[14] The clinician must therefore take care to obtain a good history on any patient presenting with symptoms which may be indicative of uterine leiomyomas, as this will guide the workup and help to avoid the use of costly and redundant studies. Additionally, thorough history taking will allow the clinician to discern the urgency of treatment, and appropriately counsel the patient about treatment options.

The most common complaint of women who have symptoms from leiomyoma is abnormal uterine bleeding; thus a careful menstrual and bleeding history is key in the ambulatory gynecologic visit. The most frequent complaints are prolonged menstrual bleeding, heavier menstrual bleeds, and more painful periods. Most women still maintain the cyclic predictability of their menstrual bleeding, but as symptoms worsen this often becomes difficult as bleeding episodes may go on for more than a month, or occur multiple times per month. Menorrhagia is defined as over 80 cc of blood loss per menstrual cycle. Up to 10% of women with menorrhagia and up to 40% of women with more severe menorrhagia have fibroids.[15] It is intuitive that the larger the fibroids and hence the uterine size, the more likely the patient is to be symptomatic. It is a common clinical misperception that submucous fibroids cause more bleeding. Studies suggest that submucous fibroids are more common in women with large fibroid uterus, but it is unclear if the actual submucos fibroids themselves cause more bleeding.[16]

Pelvic pressure is also a common complaint as the leiomyoma increase in size and begin to weigh down the uterus or impinge on other pelvic structures. A significant number of women may also complain of urinary frequency and incontinence as leiomyoma begin to press on the bladder. Additionally, some may complain of chronic constipation or changes in bowel habits. These symptoms are related to the bulk of the fibroids, and usually indicate fairly large tumors. In cases of extremely large leiomyoma, the uterus may become elevated above the pelvic brim. This causes the uterus to be an abdominal organ. These women often report increased sense of abdominal pressure, bloating and increasing abdominal girth. In uteri that extend to above the umbilicus (20-week sized or greater), early satiety may be a symptom as pressure is applied to the greater curvature of the stomach.

It is also important to note that many women with leiomyoma are asymptomatic. They become aware of their fibroids in the process of being evaluated for other complaints, most commonly pelvic pain. The end result is that they tend to attribute their pelvic pain to the presence of fibroids. In reality, pain is a quite uncommon symptom of benign leiomyoma, occurring only in the settings of torsion, prolapse of the fibroid, when there is impingement of the fibroid on other pelvic structures, or when there is degeneration of the fibroid. Degeneration refers to the replacement of the muscle fibers in the tumor by various degenerative substances, and usually occurs after infarction or some other trigger of necrosis. The type of degeneration is based on the substance replacing the muscle fiber and may be fatty, carneous/red, hyaline, calcific, cystic, or myxoid.[17]

A history of recurrent pregnancy loss or infertility may be a sign of leiomyoma, particularly submucosal fibroids. The usual findings in these scenarios are fibroids which are located near and block the corneal openings, or which severely distort the endometrium creating difficulty with sperm transport or causing inflammation or vascular changes which may lead to abnormal placentation and subsequent pregnancy wastage.[18]

Physical exam

The physical exam is just as important, if not more important, than the history. Before ultrasound technology became ubiquitous, the diagnosis of

Table 23-1 Physical exam descriptions for a fibroid uterus

Uterine flexion	Shape/texture	Uterine mobility
Anteflexed	Elongated	Fixed
Anteverted	Wide	Freely mobile
Retroflexed	Heterogonous	
Retroverted	Globular	

leiomyoma was dependent on the clinician's exam. The clinician's assessment of the pelvis is often just as informative as imaging. For asymptomatic patients, the use of imaging is likely to be incidental and only beneficial in documenting the presence, location and size of the leiomyoma for future monitoring. A good bimanual exam is the most essential first step to the physical exam. This should include gauging the size of the uterus in weeks of gestational age or grams, assessment of the positioning of the uterus (midline versus lateral) and the flexion and or version of the uterus. Assessment of the shape and texture of the uterus and assessment of uterine mobility should be undertaken (Table 23-1). The usual findings include and enlarged uterus with irregularities in shape or contour. Additionally, a well-trained clinician will recognize the value of clinical pelvimetry in assessing the patient. Knowing the width and depth of the pelvic inlet and outlet with respect to the fibroid uterus can help guide the counseling regarding options and allow for an informed decision to be made with respect to treatment options.

Workup

When leiomyoma are suspected, a comprehensive differential diagnosis should be considered. In addition to fibroids, the following diagnosis should be entertained; uterine polys, endometrial hyperplasia or cancer, cervicitis, cervical dysplasia or cancer, anovulation, thyroid dysfunction, or perimenopausal bleeding. A basic workup should start with a blood count to discern the presence or absence of anemia. Additional lab tests ordered must be tailored to demonstrated symptoms. An endometrial sampling may also be indicated and should be performed liberally, especially if the heavy bleeding occurs in women with risk factors for endometrial hyperplasia such as obesity, chronic anovulation, and metabolic syndrome.

Pelvic ultrasound is generally the first imaging modality employed in women who complain of any pelvic symptoms. The utility of ultrasound in diagnosing uterine fibroids is limited and should be used in conjunction with interpretation of clinical presentation and the physical exam. The main utility is in deciphering the location of uterine leiomyoma and qualifying their appearance, especially in women who present with acute pain syndromes. Fever and elevated white blood cell counts may be indicative of a degenerating leiomyoma.[19] Each class of degenerating leiomyoma has a distinctive echogenicity pattern on ultrasound, with cystic and calciferous degenerations being the most sonographically distinctive. Calcifications have been noted to be hyperechoic and may be stippled throughout the body of the tumor, or rim the edges. Both cystic and myxoid degeneration may take on the appearance of multiple hypoechoic areas scattered throughout the body of the tumor.[20]

Saline infused sonohysterography may be employed as a diagnostic technique in any woman who presents with abnormal bleeding. This will help to define the texture and shape of the uterine cavity, elucidating polyps, submucosal leiomyoma, synechiae, or congenital malformations of the uterine cavity such as the presence of septa or multiple horns.[21] This method of evaluation may be performed concurrently with an endometrial biopsy to help rule out malignancy, particularly in obese patients and those over the age of 35, or with a Hysterosalpingogram to rule out tubal occlusion in women who present with complaints of infertility.

Computed tomography (CT) imaging is often the initial modality used to work up abdominal pain and indeed is how many uterine fibroids are brought initially to the attention of the gynecologist. However, the ability to differentiate the source of what is almost always reported as a "pelvic mass" is by ultrasound follow-up or magnetic resonance imaging (MRI). MRI has been shown to be more specific in terms of pinpointing the size, number, and location of leiomyoma when compared to other imaging modalities, especially in obese patients.[22] It is particularly important in differentiating changes in tissue texture that can help to define the origin of a mass as ovarian, versus, uterine, versus gastrointestinal and may help point the clinician in the direction of other diagnoses such as adenomyosis.

Treatment

As the growth of leiomyoma is dependent on estrogen and progesterone production, many treatment modalities focus on hormonal agents to offer symptom relief. Continuous estrogen exposure is believed to be the most important underlying risk factor in the development of leiomyoma, with most growth occurring in the reproductive years and cessation of growth with regression of ovarian estrogen secretion. This chapter will confine discussion of treatment options to nonsurgical approaches.

Oral contraceptive pills (OCPs) and nonsteroidal anti-inflammatory agents (NSAIDs) are often offered as first-line therapy for the treatment of fibroids. Data is mixed on the efficiency of either of these therapeutic agents in terms of treatment of leiomyoma. OCPs do an excellent job in control of irregular menses; however, there is no clear data on their efficacy in the treatment of fibroids. NSAIDs are useful in the treatment of menorrhagia, but the evidence suggests they are less effective on the treatment of menorrhagia associated with fibroids. A small randomized controlled trial (RCT), which only included 25 patients total (11 of whom had fibroids), demonstrated that in the presence of fibroids, NSAIDs were not efficacious on the treatment of menorrhagia.[23] As evidence for the benefit of either of these two agents is limited, one must utilize these agents with caution if the therapeutic intent is symptom reduction from leiomyoma.

Gonadotropin-releasing hormone analogues (GnRH agonists) have been proven with several RCTs to reduce both the size and the total volume of the leiomyoma.[24] This medication works by suppressing gonadotropin release, thus suppressing ovarian release of estrogen and progesterone. This therapy can cause a decrease in the patient's bleeding symptoms, which in turn will correct anemia. The biggest drawback to this therapy is the hormonal withdrawn symptoms. Side effects such as bone loss, hot flushes, vaginal dryness, and mood changes can cause this agent to be discontinued. These side effects restrict the use for a maximum six-month course. Add back hormones, most commonly in the form of a low dose OCP, can be utilized to control symptom relief. This therapy is especially useful in perimenopausal women, as it can shrink the size of her leiomyoma and control some symptoms until natural menopause occurs. These tumors naturally shrink postmenopausal, when the patient's endogenous ovarian steroid production of hormones declines.

The progesterone intrauterine device (IUD) has an indication for the treatment of menorrhagia. Its efficacy in reducing bleeding while providing contraception makes this agent a good therapeutic choice for women.[25] A comprehensive systematic review article concluded that the progesterone IUD will reduce the amount of menorrhagia in women with fibroids. However, expulsion rates may be higher in women with large fibroids or women whose fibroids may distort the uterus.[26, 27] Counseling the patient to recognize signs of IUD dislodgment or use of a postinsertion IUD may help mitigate this complication. Additional care must be taken upon insertion into a uterus with a distorted cavity to avoid uterine perforation.

Mifepristone, or RU-486, is classified as selective progesterone receptor modulators (SPRM), or antiprogesterone on the uterus. This agent has been studied in the treatment of fibroids, and has shown to have clinical efficacy rates similar to the GnRH agonists.[28, 29] These agents reduce the size of the fibroids, but not the actual uterine volume. In addition they reduce bleeding symptoms associated with fibroids and increase the hemoglobin levels in women taking this medication. Widespread use has been somewhat limited by high rates of side effects, including elevation in liver function tests and stimulation of the endometrial lining. Additionally, commercial availability is limited and often necessitates a compounding pharmacy dosing for the treatment of fibroids. This fact alone has limited the widespread use of this agent.

Another commercially available SPRM is very promising. Ulipristal acetate is available as post-coital contraception; it works by blocking the progesterone receptor, thereby delaying or inhibiting ovulation. In leiomyoma cell culture, these agents have actual proapoptotic effects. Additionally, they thin the endometrial lining, which induces amenorrhea. These actions have created an agent that appears to be efficacious and well tolerated in the treatment of fibroid tumors.[30, 31] They are currently under consideration for approval for label use in the treatment of fibroid tumors. These agents are as efficacious in treatment of bleeding and induction of amenorrhea as Lupron but are better tolerated (Table 23-2).

Tranexademic acid, an antifibrolybtic agent, is a lysine analog that binds and prevents the conversion of plasminogen to plasmin. This decreases fibrinolysis

Table 23-2 Lupron verses ulipristal acetate in treatment of fibroids [30]

	Mechanism of action	Major side effects	Average time to amenorrhea
Lupron	GnRH agonist	Menopause symptoms (40%)	21 days
Ulipristal acetate	SPRM (selective progesterone receptor modulator)	Menopause symptoms (10%–11%) Endometrial stimulation	5–7 days

and decreases the amount of menstrual blood lost each month. This agent was FDA approved in 2009 and has been available in many European countries over the counter. This drug also has indications for use in trauma and surgical patients and is being studied in postpartum hemorrhage patients. It also has utility in patients with hemophilia. Studies have shown that tranexademic acid works to decrease blood loss in women with fibroids.[32] Use of this agent with fibroids may slightly increase the chance of pain and fever from fibroid degradation and necrosis.[33] Careful counseling must be used when prescribing this medication in these patients. Another possible side effect of this medication is a slightly higher rate of deep vein thrombosis; it must be used with caution patients with this history.

Uterine artery embolization (UAE) is an outpatient procedure that treats uterine leiomyoma. This procedure is in the scope of the interventional radiologist and involves placement of microspheres into the uterine arteries and vascular structures feeding the fibroid tumor to cause involution and degradation of the fibroid tumor. Several studies have validated the efficacy of this procedure. The pivotal EMMY trial was a randomized controlled trial in which women with classic indication for hysterectomy due to symptoms of fibroid tumors were randomized to UAE verses hysterectomy.[34] Ultimately, approximately 72% of patients who were randomized to receive UAE had sufficient symptom relief that they did not undergo hysterectomy. The biggest advantage to this procedure is the quicker return to work with a less invasive approach. The complication rate is low, and major complications are reported in less than 2.9%, (hospitalization >48 hours or permanent sequelae). Common complications include vaginal discharge, fibroid expulsion, and infection.[35]

Prevention

The exact etiologic cause of fibroid formation is undetermined, making prevention of leiomyoma difficult. However, certainly hereditary factors play a role as clusters are prevalent in families.[36] Specific lifestyle factors, such as obesity, have been linked to the development of fibroids. Some data suggest that the higher the body mass index, the more likely a woman is to have fibroids. This risk declines when the weigh is lost.[37] Smoking will reduce the risk of the development of fibroids, but the biological explanation for this is uncertain.[38] The obvious harmful effects of tobacco outweigh any preventative benefits. Specific dietary links have been postulated as causes for fibroids, but there is no clear data on this topic, and specific foods cannot be blamed for causing fibroids with any certainty.

Concluding remarks

Uterine fibroids are a huge medical issue and affect thousands of women. Almost one-third of hysterectomies performed in the United States includes leiomyoma as an indication. Hysterectomy is often offered as first-line option even though there are a number of conservative options. No clear preventative strategies exist except the avoidance of obesity, and surgical intervention may not be the best option for all patients. Familiarity with the various nonsurgical management strategies described in the chapter will allow the clinician to better treat and manage the patient's symptoms in the ambulatory setting.

References

1. Walker CL, Stewart EA. Uterine fibroids: the elephant in the room. *Science* 2005 Jun; **308**(5728): 1589–92.
2. Okolo S. Incidence, aetiology and epidemiology of uterine fibroids. *Best Practice & Research Clinical Obstetrics & Gynaecology* 2008 Aug; **22**(4): 571–88.
3. American College of Obstetricians and Gynecologists. ACOG Practice Bulletin No. 96. Alternatives to Hysterectomy in the Management of Leiomyomas. *Obstet Gynecol* 2008; **112**: 201.
4. Baird D, Dunson B, Hill M, et al. High cumulative incidence of uterine leiomyoma in black and white women: ultrasound evidence. *Am J Obstet Gynecol* 2003; **188**: 100–7.

5. Eltoukhi HM, Modi MN, Weston M, et al. The health disparities of uterine fibroid tumors for African American women: a public health issue. *Am J Obstet Gynecol* 2014 Mar; **210**(3): 194–9.
6. Cardozo ER, Clark AD, Banks NK, et al. The estimated annual cost of uterine leiomyomata in the United States. *Am J Obstet Gynecol* 2012 Mar; **206** (3):211.e1–9.
7. Shen Y, Xu Q, Xu J, et al. Environmental exposure and risk of uterine leiomyoma: an epidemiologic survey. *European Review for Medical and Pharmacological Sciences* 2013; **17**: 3249–56.
8. Segars JH, Parrott EC, Nagel JD, et al. Proceedings from the Third National Institutes of Health International Congress on Advances in Uterine Leiomyoma Research: comprehensive review, conference summary and future recommendations. *Hum Reprod Update* 2014 May–Jun; **20**(3): 309–33.
9. Stewart EA, Morton CC, The genetics of uterine leiomyoma: what clinicians need to know. *Obstet Gynecol* 2006 April; **107**; 917–21.
10. Medikare V, Kandukuri LR, Ananthapur V, et al. The genetic bases of uterine fibroids: a review. *Journal Reprod Infertil* 2011 Jul/Sept; **12**(3): 181–91.
11. Mehine M, Kaasinen E, Mäkinen N, et al. Characterization of uterine leiomyomas by whole-genome sequencing. *N Engl J Med* 2013 July; **4**(369): 43–53.
12. Brosens J, Campo R, Gordts S, Brosens I. Submucous and outer myometrium leiomyomas are two distinct clinical entities. *Fertil Steril* 2003 Jun; **79**(6): 1452–4.
13. Polena V, Mergui JL, Perrot N, et al. Long-term results of hysteroscopic myomectomy in 235 patients. *Eur J Obstet Gynecol Reprod Biol* 2007 Feb;**130** (2): 232–7.
14. Whiteman MK, Kuklina E, Jamieson DJ, et al. Inpatient hospitalization for gynecologic disorders in the United States. *Am J Obstet Gynecol* 2010 Jun; **202**(6):541.e1–6.
15. Duckitt K, Collins, S. Menorrhagia. *Clinical Evidence* 2012;**01**(805): 1–69.
16. Bachmann GA, Bahouth LA, Amalraj P, et al. Uterine fibroids: correlations of anemia and pain to fibroid location and uterine weight. *J Reprod Med* 2011 Nov–Dec; **56**(11–12): 463–6.
17. Gupta S, Manyonda I. Acute complications of fibroids. *Best Pract Res Clin Obstet Gynaecol* 2009 Oct; **23**(5): 609–17.
18. Pritts EA, Parker WH, Olive DL. Fibroids and infertility: an updated systematic review of the evidence. *Fertil Steril* 2009 Apr; **91**(4): 1215–23.
19. Khan A, Shehmar M, Gupta J. Uterine fibroids: current perspectives. *Int J Womens Health* 2014 Jan; **29**(6): 95–114.
20. McLucas B. Diagnosis, imaging and anatomical classification of uterine fibroids. *Best Practice & Research Clinical Obstetrics and Gynaecology* 2008; **22**(4): 627–42.
21. Berridge B, Winter T, Saline infusion sonohysterography technique, indications, and imaging findings. *J Ultrasound Med* 2004; **23**: 97–112.
22. Dueholm M, Lundorf E, Hansen E, et al. Accuracy of magnetic resonance imaging and transvaginal ultrasonography in the diagnosis, mapping, and measurement of uterine myomas. *American Journal of Obstetrics and Gynecology* 2002 Mar; **186**(3): 409–15.
23. Ylikorkala O, Pekonen F. Naproxen reduces idiopathic but not fibromyoma-induced menorrhagia. *Obstet Gynecol* 1986 Jul; **68**(1): 10–12.
24. Lethby A, Vollenhoven, B. Evidenced based approach to hormonal therapies for premenopausal women with fibroids. *Best Practice and Research Clinical Ob and Gyn* 2008; **22**(2): 307–31.
25. Parker W. Uterine myomas: management. *Fertility and Sterility* 2007 Aug; **88**(2): 255–71.
26. Mercorio F, De Simone R, Di Spiezio Sardo A, et al. The effect of a levonorgestrel-releasing intrauterine device in the treatment of myoma-related menorrhagia. *Contraception* 2003 Apr; **67**(4): 277–80.
27. Zapata LB, Whiteman MK, Tepper NK, et al. Intrauterine device use among women with uterine fibroids: a systematic review. *Contraception* 2010 Jul; **82**(1): 41–55.
28. Carbonell Esteve JL, Acosta R, Heredia B, et al. Mifepristone for the treatment of uterine leiomyomas: a randomized controlled trial. *Obstet Gynecol.* 2008 Nov; **112**(5): 1029–36.
29. Fiscella K, Eisinger SH, Meldrum S, et al. Effect of mifepristone for symptomatic leiomyomata on quality of life and uterine size: a randomized controlled trial. *Obstet Gynecol* 2006 Dec; **108**(6): 1381–7.
30. Donnez J, Tomaszewski J, Vázquez F, et al. Ulipristal acetate versus leuprolide acetate for uterine fibroids. *N Engl J Med* 2012 Feb 2; **366**(5): 421–32.
31. Donnez J, Vázquez F, Tomaszewski J, et al. Long-term treatment of uterine fibroids with ulipristal acetate PEARL III and PEARL III Extension Study Group. *Fertil Steril* 2014 Jun; **101**(6): 1565–73.e1–18.
32. Eder S, Baker J, Gersten J, et al. Efficacy and safety of oral tranexamic acid in women with heavy menstrual bleeding and fibroids. *Womens Health* 2013 Jul; **9**(4): 397–403.
33. Ig PP, Lam KW, Cheung CL, et al. Tranexamic acid associated necrosis and intralesional thrombosis of uterine leiomyoma: a clinicopathologic study of 147 cases emphasizing the importance of drug-induced

necrosis and early infarcts in leiomyoma. *Am J of Surg Pathology* 2007 Aug; **31**(8): 1215–24.

34. Van Der Kooii SM, Hehenkamp WJ, Volkers NA, et al. Uterine artery embolization vs hysterectomy in the treatment of symptomatic uterine fibroids: 5-year outcome from the randomized EMMY trial. *Am J Obstet Gynecol* 2010 Aug; **203**(2): 105. e1–13. doi: 10.1016/j.ajog.2010.01.049. Epub 2010 Jul 1.
35. Toor S, Jaberi A, Macdonald D, et al. Complication rates and effectiveness of uterine artery embolization in the treatment of symptomatic leiomyoma: a systematic review and meta-analysis. *American Roentgen Ray Society* 2012 Nov; **199**: 1153–63.
36. Gross K. Morton C. Genetics and the development of fibroids. *Clin Obstet Gynecol* 2001; **44**: 335–49.
37. Summers W, Watson R, Wooldridge W, et al. Hypertension, obesity, and fibromyomata uteri, as a syndrome. *Arch Intern Med* 1971; **128**: 750–4.
38. E. Faerstein, M. Szklo, N. Rosenshein. Risk factors for uterine leiomyoma: a practice-based case–control study. I. African-American heritage, reproductive history, body size, and smoking. *Am J Epidemiol* 2001; **153**: 1–10.
39. Parker, W. The utility of MRI for the surgical treatment of women with uterine fibroid tumors. *American Journal of Obstetrics and Gynecology* 2012, Jan; **206**(1): 31–6.

Chapter

24

Sexual dysfunction

Joseph E. Peterson

Introduction

Many women will experience sexual dysfunction during their lifetimes. Whether a temporary problem with one partner, or a generalized long-term issue with multiple partners, sexual dysfunction can disrupt a patient's sense of well-being and ability to emotionally and physically cope with other aspects of life.

Female sexual dysfunction, chronic or acute, can occur at any point throughout the life cycle. It is generalized if it occurs at all times, with all types of stimulation, or with all partners. Situational dysfunction is unique to particular times, types of stimulation, or partners.[1]

According to the DSM-IV-TR and DSM-V, if a complaint meets the definition of a dysfunction by disrupting interpersonal relationships or causing significant distress, then it is a classifiable disorder.[1, 2] The dysfunction may be classified as:

- Low desire (hypoactive sexual desire disorder)
- Sexual arousal disorder
- Orgasmic disorder
- Sexual pain disorder (dyspareunia and vulvodynia)

There can be considerable overlap in these diagnoses and women are likely to report issues in more than one area.[3] Sexual aversion disorder, due to its rarity, has been removed from the DSM-V. The first two classifications have also been combined into disorders of either arousal or desire. However, for purposes of discussion here and in light of an expanded understanding of sexual dysfunction classification, this chapter will use the preceding categories.

The DSM-V no longer separates diagnosis into subtypes stemming from psychological, biological, or combined factors, but instead recognizes the complex interplay between all elements of a patient's well-being. However, for strict diagnostic criteria, if the disorder is accounted for by another axis 1 disorder, then it is not considered a sexual disorder. Also, though diagnosis and treatment may begin at any time, a sexual dysfunction now must be present for at least six months in order to qualify for diagnosis.[1]

Female sexual response

For practical purposes of diagnosis, it is helpful to review the stages of female sexual response. Kinsey began his study of female sexual behavior in 1953, and Masters and Johnson refined the idea of the female sexual response cycle with the publication of their book in 1966.[4, 5] The predominant model of female sexual response presented has persisted until late, consisting of a description of four distinct phases: excitement/arousal, plateau, orgasm, and resolution (Figure 24-1).

A baseline desire was believed to be necessary prior to initiation of excitement. The process of desire is not well understood but apparently involves both neurotransmitters such as dopamine as well as sex hormones.[6]

Excitement or arousal is characterized by vascular changes and autonomic sensations of excitement influenced by the noradrenergic system. The clitoris engorges, increasing exposure and sensitivity, and blood flow increases to the vulva and vagina, increasing lubrication from transudate.[6] Transitory feelings of intense pleasure occur with accompanying contractions of the muscles of the pelvic floor and release of endogenous opioids, serotonin, prolactin, and oxytocin characterize orgasm.[6]

Plateau is a heightened state of arousal below the threshold for the reflex of orgasm. It may persist until resolution, be returned to after orgasm before resolution, or be returned to multiple times after multiple orgasms.

Resolution is the period after orgasm or plateau with an accompanying increase in serotonin and a decrease in dopamine.[6]

Office Care of Women, ed. Martin E. Olsen and Botros Rizk. Published by Cambridge University Press.

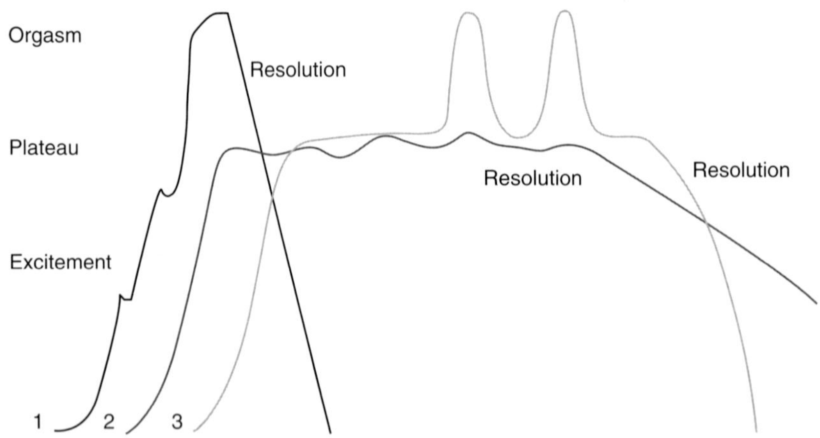

Figure 24-1 Female sexual response depicting three different women or one woman at different times.

(Linear model as researched and developed by Masters and Johnson.)

Traditionally, a woman was believed to progress sequentially through these phases. Deviations, such as a lack of progression to orgasm or orgasm without excitement was presumed dysfunctional.

This model is not inaccurate in depicting the phases that *can* be a part of sexual response. There may, however, be overlap of the stages and varying sequence which could give the appearance of dysfunction. With more recent categorization, the conceptualization of the female sexual response has been expanded to recognize this process as a cycle rather than linear. The model of sexual response was modified to integrate subjective arousal, satisfaction without orgasm, a baseline of neutral desire, and acquisition of nonsexual rewards (emotional intimacy, well-being) which then feed future arousal and motivation to begin the cycle again, more accurately reflecting the non-linear nature of female sexual response.[7]

This nonlinear model reflects the World Health Organization's definition of sexual health which states it "includes physical, mental, emotional, and social well being in all sexual behaviors and beliefs."[8] This implies that irrespective of classification system, the patient's unique sexual response and activity is not a dysfunction if it causes her no distress.

According to Basson and the efforts of the International Committee of the American Foundation of Urological Disease and the Second International Consensus of Sexual Medicine, a newer revision of the major categories of sexual dysfunction (yet to be validated) would include:[8]

- Subjective sexual arousal disorder – feelings of excitement and pleasure from stimulation are absent or diminished despite a physical response.
- Genital arousal disorder – minimal vulvar swelling or lubrication results from stimulation but subjective excitement may still be present.
- Combined sexual arousal disorder – both of the preceding disorders are present concurrently.
- Sexual desire/interest disorder – feelings of desire, fantasies, and responsiveness are absent or diminished.
- Persistent sexual arousal disorder – genital arousal is spontaneous, unsolicited and sexual desire may or may not be present; it is unrelieved by orgasm.
- Orgasmic disorder – orgasm from any kind of stimulation is absent despite arousal.
- Vaginismus – involuntary contractions of the pelvic floor muscles prevent or make difficult the entry of a penis, finger, or any object into the patient's vagina despite desire.
- Dyspareunia – persistent or recurrent pain with attempted or deep vaginal entry.

These definitions address the fact that a women's sexuality is susceptible to context. Although they still reflect the phases of sexual response, they clarify that these phases are likely to overlap. They also present a shift in focus from initial desire and note that desire *can* be triggered by arousal instead of vice versa, rather than considering this sequence dysfunctional. This system also divorces the ideas of subjective sexual arousal and objective arousal of the genitalia.[8] This more granular approach to the classifications may assist the clinician in fully understanding the patient's problem and forming a more complete treatment plan.

The potential causes for sexual dysfunction are broad and varied (Table 24-1). Regardless of the underlying cause of the distress, the clinician must

Table 24-1 Risk factors and causes of sexual dysfunction

Medical conditions

- Anemia
- Arthritis
- Cardiovascular disease
- Endocrinopathies
  - Diabetes
  - Hyperprolactinemia
  - Hypoestrogenism (menopausal)
  - Hypothyroidism
  - Premature ovarian failure
- Hyper/hypotonicity of pelvic floor muscles (vaginismus or prolapse)
- Malignancy (primary or metastatic, affecting the pelvis or abdomen)
- Neurological disease
  - Stroke
  - Spinal cord injury
  - Parkinsonism
- Urinary tract dysfunction
  - Cystitis (chronic or recurrent)
  - Incontinence
  - Urethritis

Medications

- Alkylating agents
- Anticholinergics
- Antiandrogens
- Antidepressants
- Anti-estrogens
- Antihistamines
- Antihypertensives
  - Diuretics
  - Calcium channel blockers
- Depressants
  - Alcohol
  - Hypnotics
  - Sedatives
- GnRH antagonists
- Sympathomimetic amines

Physical factors

- Atrophy
- Adenomyosis
- Bartholin's gland abnormalities (cyst or infection, chronic or recurrent)
- Condylomata
- Dermatoses
  - Lichen sclerosus

Table 24-1 (cont.)

- Dyspareunia
- Endometriosis
- Infection/inflammation (vulva, vagina, uterus, PID)
- Irritable bowel syndrome
- Pelvic adhesive disease
- Pelvic congestion
- Pelvic organ prolapse
  - Cystocele
  - Rectocele
  - Uterine prolapse

Psychological factors and interpersonal relationship disorders

- Anxiety
- Depression
- Decreased self esteem
- Educational deficit (unrealistic expectations, lack of understanding of normal anatomy or function)
- Guilt
- Inexperience
- Life stressors
- Poor body image
- Religious restrictions
- Sexual abuse
- Sexual assault
- Sexual identity conflict

Radiation

Trauma

- Accidental
- Genital surgery

Source: Adapted from information from references 20, 37, and 48.

perform a thorough exploration of the patient's history, with specific focus on the sexual history, and also seek out a broad range of psychological and physical findings that could be responsible for the dysfunction. Although the dysfunction may be the problem itself and disrupt other areas of the patient's life, it can also be a symptom of another underlying medical or psychological disorder or even such a disorder's treatment such as a medication side effect. If so, the clinician should seek to address not only the sexual dysfunction itself, but the underlying cause.

Scope

More than 40% of women have a sexually related complaint.[9, 10] However, this encompasses all

We recognize that these questions are highly personal. It is important to ask them so that your physician can provide you with the most complete care.

Are you satisfied with your current sexual functioning? Y/N

If not, how long have you been dissatisfied with your sexual functioning? ______________________

Which problem(s) do you have with your sexual functioning? (check)

___ Problem with little or no interest in sex
___ Problem with decreased genital sensations (feeling touch)
___ Problem with decreased vaginal lubrication (dry)
___ Problem with reaching orgasm
___ Problem with pain during sex
___ Other: (describe)

Please circle the problem above that is *most* bothersome to you.

Would you like to talk about this with your doctor today? Y/N

Figure 24-2 Screening questionnaire based on the Basic Sex Symptoms Checklist – Women.[13]

women with *any* complaint that does not necessarily meet criteria of a disorder or dysfunction in that the complaints are not distressing or negatively impacting interpersonal relationships. Using stricter criteria, several population surveys have found the prevalence rates to range approximately 3%–12% for the different types of dysfunction, age and sexual orientation.[10–12]

The prevalence of sexual disorders varies with age as different factors (situational, medication use, disease history) come into play. Hypoactive sexual desire disorder is the most common female sexual disorder in the United States with estimates ranging from 7.4% to 12.3%.[10] Dyspareunia and vaginismus are also common though the reported rates vary widely.[6] Female sexual arousal disorder is less common, with a national survey putting the prevalence at 3.3%–6.0%. Orgasmic disorder is less common at 3.4%–5.8%.[10]

History

Screening questionnaire

A preprinted questionnaire administered prior to the encounter may be helpful in initiating conversations regarding sexual health. The simplest would include questions that are derived from or based on the Brief Sexual Symptoms Checklist for Women, soliciting information in a non-threatening and straightforward way. The clinician is free to create one to suit the unique needs of the clinical environment (Figure 24-2).[13]

If the screening questionnaire is positive for a sexual problem and the visit was not originally scheduled to address sexual issues, a separate visit may be necessary to fully elucidate the history and extent of the problem.

Environment

The clinician must not fail to meet the patient's need by appearing uncomfortable addressing sexuality or holding biases that could lead to a lack of exploration of sexual history. Patients desire a welcoming environment with knowledgeable providers that provide personable relationships.[14] Sexual history taking can, however, be uncomfortable for both the clinician and the patient, so rapport and an empathic attitude are paramount.

It is important for the clinician to enter the encounter with no preconceived notions of the patient's sexual orientation. After eliciting a positive answer that the patient is sexual active, a simple follow-up question such as, "with men, women, or both?" portrays the clinician as nonjudgmental, normalizing, and validating the context of the patient's particular situation.

Approach

There are various models to structure the approach to the patient with a sexual complaint including the ALLOW and PLISSIT models (Figures 24-3 and 24-4).

Sub-specialization in sexuality is not required to address patient complaints adequately. Even if the

Ask (use open-ended questions)

Legitimize (reassure that concerns are important)

Limitations (assess one's own interest and ability - refer if unable to meet patient's need)

Open up for further discussion (at a future visit if necessary)

Work together (develop an appropriate treatment plan)

Figure 24-3 ALLOW model for approaching discussions of sexual activity and dysfunction.[15]

Permission (obtain permission to discuss matter of sexuality and include a normalizing/legitimizing statement "I ask all my patient's about…")

Limited Information (provide the patient with information on normal anatomy, physiology, and response as well as potential causes for the problem)

Specific Suggestions (offer strategies for management of patient's particular complaint, i.e., medication change, couple's therapy, self-stimulation)

Intensive Therapy (consider referral to subspecialist, appropriate other specialty)

Figure 24-4 PLISSIT model for approaching discussions of sexual activity and dysfunction.[46, 47]

clinician only makes it through the first three steps of the ALLOW model and refers the patient, it could be said that "ALL" has been done for the patient.[15]

The PLISSIT model also has room for referral for problems beyond the clinician's scope in the "Intensive Therapy" element of the algorithm.

Either model effectively has the clinician normalizing the discussion, legitimizing the complaint with recognition of its importance to the patient, and focusing on either referring the patient for specialist care or planning on methods of management together.

Patient perception

Asking the patient what she believes the problem to be is often helpful, particularly with psychosocial issues. A dysfunctional thought process may be revealed that would otherwise not be treated if merely the end physical symptoms were addressed. For example, consider the woman with a sexual encounter prematurely postpartum and resultant episiotomy breakdown. Avoidance of sex due to fear of pain and potential disruption of the old wound may lead to decreased desire. If this "hypoactive desire disorder" were addressed traditionally without acknowledging the fears of the sex act itself with education regarding healing and wound integrity, the problem would be unlikely to resolve. Similarly, a patient's fears of infection or pregnancy may motivate aversive behaviors that could be perceived as a lack of desire.

This direct line of questioning may also elicit detail that screening questionnaires lack. A frank answer detailing abuse or a loss of self-esteem or attraction due to weight gain could aid the clinician in a more timely diagnosis and treatment plan.

Sexual history

A standard sexual history including age at first coitus, whether the patient is currently sexually active, number of lifetime partners, number of current partner(s), sex of partner(s), sexual practices (oral, anal, vaginal as well as use of lubricants, aids, toys, etc.) and time with current partner should be elicited. If a screening survey is not used, then the sexual history should include asking an open-ended question such as, "Is there any problem with your sexual function that you would like to discuss?" Each positive answer warrants further exploration. For instance, if the patient reports pain with intercourse, it is important to determine under what conditions (position, depth of insertion, movement, etc.).

Previous sexual response/dysfunction history

It is important to assess whether the patient's problem is recent and acute versus prolonged and chronic. Does it occur only with her current partner or with other partners? If the complaint is anorgasmia, has she ever had an orgasm with self-stimulation or with a different partner? If the concern is dysfunction of desire, is there a history in this in previous relationships? Mapping the patient's own sexual response patterns aids the clinician in both fully understanding the context of this patient's problem at this point in her life as well as leading to a more effective plan for management.[7]

In addition to the standard and expanded sexual history, additional historical elements can influence the diagnosis and treatment plan. These include factors that are risks associated with sexual dysfunction as well as potential causes of dysfunction (Table 24-1).

Age

Although sexual desire and activity may decrease with age, to exclude a sexual history in patients over 70 would ignore the potential 22% that report vaginal intercourse in the past year.[16] Masters and Johnson established with their work that there is no apparent absolute age at which sexual activity ceases.[5] The clinician should not assume that sexual identity and activity has become any less important to the patient due to age alone. Instead, realize that it may be an important part of the patient's life, potentially impacting her ability to maintain healthy interpersonal relationships, self-image, and a sense of self-worth.[17]

Also important in the later years, particularly after natural or surgical menopause, is the known decrease in estrogen and the accompanying decreases in sexual desire as well as vaginal lubrication and atrophy, which may lead to dyspareunia.

Comorbid conditions and relationships

Predictable prognosticators for those with sexual dysfunction include poor general health, low mental health scores or marital difficulties.[3] In fact, a large cross-sectional population survey found the single strongest association with arousal, orgasmic, and enjoyment problems in women was marital difficulties. All women in the survey who reported a sexual problem also showed an association with anxiety and depression.[18] Patients with known depression are much more likely to experience sexual dysfunction.[19]

Although these connections with depression and anxiety may be somewhat expected, assumed positive elements in a patient's history are also found to correlate with sexual dysfunction. At least among middle-aged and older women, a higher association with sexual dysfunction can be found in those with a college degree or higher as well as those in a significant relationship.[3]

The clinician can easily draw connections between specific medical problems, such as vascular or neurogenic disease that could decrease physiologic response and contribute to a dysfunction in a patient who otherwise would have no lack of desire or ability to orgasm. Pain syndromes or musculoskeletal deformities may contribute to pain and avoidance (Table 24-1). The clinician should review the patient's medical history in detail to guide both diagnosis and treatment.

The clinician must always keep in mind the possibility that more than one of the sexual dysfunctions may exist, particularly in light of the evolving understanding of the overlap of both the phases and the dysfunctions of sexual response.[20, 7]

Medications and social history

Medications can impact sexual function through either direct physical effects or via their psychological effects or side effects (Table 24-1).

Smoking is connected to erectile dysfunction in males.[21] Due to similar vascular responses in the genitalia and the impact of atherosclerotic disease on these responses, there may be similar impact on sexual function in females who smoke.

The drug class most frequently associated with sexual dysfunction is SSRIs. These can affect the sexual response across all phases, causing difficulty with orgasm, decreased sexual desire, and decreased arousal.[19]

Pregnancy and contraception

A history of pregnancies with delivery shows a direct correlation with increased rates of sexual dysfunction long after the postpartum period. Although scarring and dyspareunia may result from episiotomy or operative delivery, these two specific elements do not impact sexual function more than those with spontaneous vaginal deliveries over intact perineums.[22]

Pregnant patients exhibit a strong desire to discuss sexual matters, with almost one-half of pregnant patients initiating the conversation themselves despite one-third reporting a reluctance to do so. Consequently, a current pregnancy may offer the clinician an increased confidence that the discussion will be well received. Seventy-six percent of pregnant patients with whom their provider never addressed sexual activity reported that they felt it *should* have been addressed.[23] The clinician who sees pregnant patients should take advantage of the increased number of encounters during the antepartum period to address sexual matters.

Patients using oral contraceptive pills for long periods may see a decrease in desire or arousal due to an increase in sex hormone binding globulin and subsequent decrease in bioavailable androgens.[24]

Abuse and violence

Because approximately 20% of women have a history of childhood sexual abuse and potentially suffer from resultant fear, shame, humiliation, guilt, self-blame, distorted self-perception, anxiety, depression, and post-traumatic stress disorder, it is important to screen each patient for abuse. Childhood sexual abuse can result in any of the disorders of desire, arousal, orgasm, or pain.[25, 26]

For patients who experiences intimate partner violence, pregnancy increases risk for more severe violence unless pregnancy motivates a cessation in the violence.[27] Intimate partner violence presents an obvious compromise to the patient's mental and physical well-being, leading to increased potential for anxiety, depression, and marital difficulties that could lead to sexual dysfunction either during the pregnancy or later.

Surgical history

Although theories have been posited as to why a simple hysterectomy could cause sexual dysfunction in a patient after surgery, both subtotal (supracervical) and total hysterectomy show no significant changes in desire, orgasms, body image and relationships with partners.[6, 28]

However, surgeries for cervical, ovarian, bladder, and rectal malignancies of the pelvis are associated with increased dysfunction of desire, arousal, orgasm, and pain.[28]

If bilateral oophorectomy is performed, then the patient would be deficient in endogenous estrogen. This would be accompanied with an increased risk of dyspareunia secondary to the resultant changes of the vaginal tissues associated with estrogen withdraw.

Detailed questionnaires

If preferred by either the patient or the clinician, validated instruments exist for further detailed examination of the multidimensional aspects of female sexual health including:

Female Sexual Function Index (FSFI) – a 19-point self-reported questionnaire.[29]

Female Sexual Distress Scale (FSDS) – a 20-point (also validated in a 12-point focused version) questionnaire to assess the level of distress a dysfunction causes.[30]

Sexual Interest and Desire Inventory – Female (SIDI-F) – a 13-point questionnaire used to explore in detail the severity of hypoactive sexual desire disorder.[31]

Physical exam

An exam that assesses systems other than the genitourinary tract may yield clues to medical diagnoses that could lead to the development of a sexual dysfunction and require treatment themselves in order to fully address the dysfunction. However, the external, speculum, and bimanual exams of the genitourinary system are of the utmost importance in the patient with sexual dysfunction.

Clinicians should examine the external genitalia for distribution and density of pubic hair that may indicate an endocrine etiology of the dysfunction. The presence of lesions or masses, obvious signs of prolapse, signs of chronic or acute irritation/inflammation/infection of the vulva/introitus/urethra/perineum/rectum, signs of atrophy, discharge, obvious skin disorders/dermatoses, and evidence of trauma to the genitals could be causes of dyspareunia. Congenital or acquired genital malformations of the clitoris, labia, and perineum could result in either pain or poor body image.

A cotton swab test can be used to map areas of pain at the introitus and in the vestibule in cases of suspected vulvodynia or vestibulitis.

A speculum exam should be used to assess the vagina and cervix for lesions, masses, or congenital or acquired deformities. A decreased vaginal depth or caliber may be found after hysterectomy, surgery for prolapse, or radiation therapy. Changes in coloration, texture, and general turgor may indicate estrogen deficiency. Difficulty with insertion of the speculum could be a sign of vaginismus.

The bimanual exam should include assessment of the urethra for pain, the muscles of the pelvic floor for hyper- or hypotonicity, the uterosacral ligaments or muscles of the pelvic floor for tenderness, and the uterus for fixed retroversion or retroflexion. A rectal exam could alert the clinician to masses, obvious constipation, or loss of sphincter tone.

One recommended adjunct to the bimanual exam in patients with dyspareunia would be the *monomanual* exam. The clinician proceeds with the vaginal portion of the bimanual exam but leaves the other hand held away from the abdomen so that no confusion is introduced as to the source of the pain.[20]

Invasive testing such as EMG, vaginal photoplethysmography, and measurements of genital blood flow, temperature, and so on have been used in the research setting but have no impact on outcomes of therapy and are unnecessary in the clinical setting.[32]

Labs

In general, most labs will not be beneficial in either determining or monitoring sexual dysfunction. Even when treated with androgens, women's sex hormone binding globulin, free and total testosterone, free and total estradiol and estrone levels showed no clear correlation with either side-effects, discontinuation rates, satisfaction, improvement in functioning or safety of short-term use. Baseline androgen levels are not necessary as they do not correlate with the level of dysfunction reported by the patient.[33]

Little is known of the potential implications for cardiovascular risk in the female patient receiving testosterone. The American Congress of Obstetricians and Gynecologists states that despite the paucity of evidence, it "seems reasonable" to monitor serum lipid levels and liver function tests in women receiving testosterone.[6]

A wet prep of any vaginal discharge may point to an infectious cause of dyspareunia. Cultures for gonorrhea and chlamydia could similarly contribute to a definitive diagnosis. However, unless the patient's history or exam warrants them, routine acquisition of these labs should not be done simply because a patient has a sexual dysfunction even if dyspareunia is the suspected cause.

If a medical condition is suspected or determined to be the underlying source of a patient's dysfunction, such as an endocrinopathy involving prolactin or thyroid hormones, then laboratory studies to confirm the diagnosis or monitor treatment would be helpful. Where the history and clinical presentation is unclear, confirmatory estrogen or anti-müllerian hormone levels might assist in determining a patient's menopausal state.

Treatment

The treatment of a sexual dysfunction will not likely be undertaken by one clinician but instead require a multidisciplinary approach. However, merely discussing the patient's complaint in an open, welcoming environment without judgment is the first step toward complete treatment. If the clinician does not feel comfortable addressing the particular psychological issue, a referral to a marriage and family counselor, sex therapist or other specialized psychiatric provider may be warranted.

All types of sexual dysfunction can see a benefit from psychotherapy.[34] Even basic education on desire, arousal, and orgasm with description of the physiologic responses can fill in a patient's knowledge gap. Using the expanded descriptions of the nonlinear model of female sexual response and its dysfunctions can help her understand what is normal.

In general, despite the impact of its absence and its position as a mainstay of treatment for female sexual dysfunction, estrogen replacement alone does not directly influence desire or arousal or overall sexual function.[35, 36] However, if a lack of desire is the result of aversion or fear of the pain of dyspareunia secondary to vaginal atrophy, or if the patient has an overall decreased quality of life from debilitating hot flushes, then estrogen could prove beneficial. In patients with signs and symptoms of natural or surgical hypoestrogenism, replacement may be of benefit regardless of classification.

As situation stressors can be a cause of decreased desire or arousal, improving the situational status of the patient is paramount. Reduction in life stressors, regular exercise, and sleep could provide benefit.[37]

Treatment of any chronic medical or gynecologic conditions may see a secondary benefit of improvement in sexual dysfunction. For instance, changing an SSRI dose may be all that is necessary to improve desire and arousal.[19]

There is a high degree of overlap in the types of disorders and the possibility of multiple dysfunctions and/or multiple causative factors within the same patient. In addition to the generally applicable treatments already described, there are type specific treatments as well.

Disorders of desire

In both naturally and surgically menopausal women, short-term use (up to 24 weeks) of androgen therapy has proven to be effective in improving desire and sexual function. A matrix patch provides 300 mcg per day.[33, 38] Side effects could include hirsutism, deepening voice, clitoromegaly, and increased muscle mass.

For premenopausal women, flibanserin, a 5-HT1Aagonist/5-HT2A antagonist, given at 100 mg qhs can provide improvement in sexual functioning and desire.[39] Androgen replacement is not as well studied as in postmenopausal women but shows similar improvement in sexual function with a testosterone spray preparation.[40]

Testosterone therapy has not been approved by the Food and Drug Administration (FDA) for use in women and use of it or analogous preparations is off-label.

Aversion may be the result of a sexual trauma with resultant depression and anxiety, or fear of pain. Consequently, treatments should be aimed at treating the underlying disorders.

Disorders of arousal

The Eros Clitoral Therapy device is available and FDA approved for improving genital arousal by increasing the blood flow to the clitoris by means of a vacuum device.[41]

Phosphodiesterase inhibitors such as sildenafil, prescribed for erectile dysfunction in men, may also impact genital engorgement in females, but they have not been consistently shown to improve sexual functioning.[42] Prescription of these medications are off-label and of unknown benefit unless the patient had specific testing that showed a lack of genital blood flow during arousal.

Twenty minutes of vigorous exercise immediately before stimulation may improve arousal in some women who are taking antidepressants.[43]

Disorders of orgasm

Any underlying disorders of arousal that may result in a lack of orgasm should be addressed. Directed masturbation with or without a partner under the guide of a therapist, cognitive behavioral therapy, and sensate focusing where the patient learns to focus on enjoyment of the sexual activity leading up to and including orgasm are otherwise the mainstays of treatment for anorgasmia.[44]

Disorders of sexual pain

It is important to treat any underlying infectious or inflammatory condition that leads to sexual pain.

In cases of atrophied tissues resulting in difficulty of either arousal or dyspareunia, topical estrogen, applied either in cream, tablets, pessaries, or ring form appear to be equally effective for addressing symptoms.[45]

Lubricants may provide benefits for patients that have an aversion to or contraindication to estrogen replacement.[6]

A recent trial looking at treatment of hot flushes in postmenopausal women with venlafaxine found a subtle decrease in sexual pain, although overall function was not impacted significantly.[35]

Teaching the patient to serially dilate the vagina alone or with her partner until passage of the penis is possible without pain may be helpful in treating vaginismus. This combined with cognitive behavioral therapy appears to have the best results.[6]

Treatment for vestibulodynia is similar for other chronic pain syndromes that are believed to stem from stress-induced dysregulation of the central nervous system and includes psychotherapy. Surgery may also offer improvement in select cases.[34]

Concluding remarks

Female sexual dysfunction is a complex, multifaceted phenomenon that warrants awareness and attention by the clinician as patients may be reluctant to volunteer discussion. Although problems of this nature are distressing for the patient and potentially the clinician, finding the path to treatment and a return to gratifying sexual encounters is possible by utilizing open-ended questions, a welcoming, accepting environment, and attention to all aspects of the patient's emotional, mental, and physical care.

References

1. American Psychiatric Association. *Diagnostic and statistical manual of mental disorders* (5th edition). Arlington, VA: American Psychiatric Publishing; 2013.
2. American Psychiatric Association. *Diagnostic and statistical manual of mental disorders* (4th edition, text rev.). Arlington, VA: American Psychiatric Publishing; 2000.
3. Addis I, Van Den Eeden S, Wassel-Fyr C, et al. Sexual activity and function in middle-aged and older women. *Obstetrics and Gynecology* 2006;**107**(4):755–64.
4. Kinsey A, Pomeroy W, Martin C, Gebhard P. *Sexual Behavior in the Human Female.* Philadelphia: Saunders; 1953.
5. Masters W, Johnson V. *Human Sexual Response.* Boston, MA: Little, Brown; 1966.
6. American College of Obstetricians and Gynecologists. Practice Bulletin 119, April 2011 (Reaffirmed 2013).
7. Basson R. Women's sexual dysfunction: revised and expanded definitions. *Canadian Medical Association Journal* 2005;**172**(10):1327–33.

8. World Health Organization. *Defining Sexual Health: Report of a Technical Consultation on Sexual Health*, January 28–31, 2002. Geneva, Switzerland: World Health Organization; 2006, 1–35.
9. Laumann E, Paik A, Rose R. Sexual dysfunction in the United States: prevalence and predictors. *Journal of the American Medical Association* 1999;**281**(6):537–44.
10. Shifren J, Monz B, Russo P, et al. Sexual problems and distress in United States women: prevalence and correlates. *Obstetrics and Gynecology* 2008;**112**(5): 970–8.
11. Spector I, Carey M. Incidence and prevalence of the sexual dysfunctions: a critical review of the empirical literature. *Archives of Sexual Behavior* 1990;**19**(4):389–408.
12. Simons J, Carey M. Prevalence of sexual dysfunctions: results from a decade of research. *Archives of Sexual Behavior* 2001;**30**(2):177–219.
13. Hatzinchristou D, Rosen R, Derogatis L, et al. Recommendations for the clinical evaluation of men and women with sexual dysfunction. *Journal of Sexual Medicine* 2010;7(1 Pt 2):337–48.
14. Murtagh J. Female sexual function, dysfunction, and pregnancy: implications for practice. *Journal of Midwifery and Women's Health* 2010; **55**(5):438–46.
15. Sadovsky R. The role of the primary care clinician in the management of erectile dysfunction. *Reviews in Urology* 2002;**4**(Suppl 3):S54–63.
16. National Survey of Sexual Health and Behavior (NSSHB). Findings from the National Survey of Sexual Health and Behavior, Centre for Sexual Health Promotion, Indiana University. *Journal of Sexual Medicine* 2010;7(Suppl 5):243–373.
17. Bauer M, McAuliff L, Nay R. Sexuality, health care and the older person: an overview of the literature. *International Journal of Older People Nursing* 2007;**2**(1):63–8.
18. Dunn K, Croft P, Hackett G. Association of sexual problems with social, psychological, and physical problems with men and women: a cross-sectional population survey. *Journal of Epidemiology and Community Health* 1999;**53**(3):144–8.
19. Kennedy S, Rizvi S. Sexual dysfunction, depression, and the impact of antidepressants. *Journal of Clinical Psychopharmacology* 2009;**29**(2):157–64.
20. Phillips N. Female sexual dysfunction: evaluation and treatment. *American Family Physician* 2000 Jul 1;**62**(1):127–36.
21. McVary K, Carrier S, Wessells H. for the Subcommittee on Smoking and Erectile Dysfunction Socioeconomic Committee, Sexual Medicine Society of North America. Smoking and erectile dysfunction: evidence based analysis. *Journal of Urology* 2001;**166**(5):1624–32.
22. Botros S, Abramov Y, Miller J, et al. Effect of parity on sexual function: an identical twin study. *Obstetrics and Gynecology* 2006;**107**(4):765–70.
23. Bartellas E, Crane JM, Daley M, et al. Sexuality and sexual activity in pregnancy. *BJOG: An International Journal of Obstetrics and Gynaecology* 2000;**107**(8): 964–8.
24. Sanders S, Graham C, Bass J, Bancroft J. A prospective study of the effects of oral contraceptives on sexuality and well-being and their relationship to discontinuation. *Contraception* 2001;**64**(1):51–8.
25. Adult manifestations of childhood sexual abuse. Committee Opinion No. 498. *Obstetrics and Gynecology* 2011;**118**:392–5.
26. Tjaden P, Thoennes N. *Prevalence, Incidence, and Consequences of Violence against Women: Findings from the National Violence against Women Survey. Research in brief.* Washington DC: US Department of Justice, Office of Justice programs 1998. Available at www.ncjrs.gov/pdffiles/172837.pdf. Accessed December 11, 2015.
27. Brownridge D, Taillieu T, Tyler K, et al. Pregnancy and intimate partner violence: risk factors, severity, and health effects. *Violence against Women* 2011;**17**(7): 858–81.
28. Raina R, Pahlajani G, Khan S, et al. Female sexual dysfunction: classification, pathophysiology, and management. *Fertility and Sterility* 2007;**88**(5):1273–84.
29. Rosen R, Brown C, Heiman J, et al. The Female Sexual Function Index (FSFI): a multidimensional self-report instrument for the assessment of female sexual function. *Journal of Sex and Marital Therapy* 2000;**26**(2):191–208.
30. Derogatis L, Rosen R, Leiblum S, et al. The Female Sexual Distress Scale (FSDS): initial validation of a standardized scale for assessment of sexually related personal distress in women. *Journal of Sex and Marital Therapy* 2002;**28**(4):317–30.
31. Clayton A, Segraves R, Leiblum S, et al. Reliability and validity of the Sexual Interest and Desire Inventory-Female (SIDI-F), a scale designed to measure severity of female hypoactive sexual desire disorder. *Journal of Sex and Marital Therapy* 2006;**32**(2):115–35.
32. Latif E, Diamond M. Arriving at the diagnosis of female sexual dysfunction. *Fertility and Sterility* 2013;**100**(4):898–904.
33. Davis S, Moreau M, Kroll R, et al. Testosterone for low libido in postmenopausal women not taking estrogen. APHRODITE Study Team. *New England Journal of Medicine* 2008;**359**(19):2005–17.
34. Basson R. Sexuality and sexual disorders. *ACOG Clinical Update in Women's Health Care* 2014; **XIII**(2):1–110.
35. Reed S, Mitchell C, Joffe H, et al. Sexual function in women on estradiol or venlafaxine for hot flushes:

a randomized controlled trial. *Obstetrics and Gynecology* 2014;**124**(2 Part 1);233–41.

36. Hays J, Ockene J, Bruner R, et al. for the Women's Health Initiative Investigators. Effects of estrogen plus progestin on the health-related quality of life. *New England Journal of Medicine* 2003;**348**(19): 1839–54.
37. Frank J, Mistretta P, Will J. Diagnosis and treatment of female sexual dysfunction. *American Family Physician* 2008;**77**(5):635–42.
38. Buster J, Kingsberg S, Aguirre O, et al. Testosterone patch for low sexual desire in surgical menopausal women: a randomized trial. *Obstetrics and Gynecology* 2005;**105**(5 Part 1):944–52.
39. Thorp J, Simon J, Dattani D, et al. on behalf of the DAISY trial investigators. Treatment of hypoactive sexual desire disorder in premenopausal women: efficacy of flibanserin in the DAISY study. *Journal of Sexual Medicine* 2012;**9**(3):793–804.
40. Davis S, Papalia M, Norman R, et al. Safety and efficacy of a testosterone metered-dose transdermal spray for treating decreased sexual satisfaction in premenopausal women: a randomized trial. *Annals of Internal Medicine* 2008;**148**(8):569–77.
41. Billups K, Berman L, Berman J, et al. A new non-pharmacological vacuum therapy for female sexual dysfunction. *Journal of Sex and Marital Therapy* 2001;**27**(5):435–41.
42. Basson R, McInnes R, Smith M, et al. Efficacy and safety of sildenafil citrate in women with sexual dysfunction associated with female sexual arousal disorder. *Journal of Women's Health and Gender Based Medicine* 2002;**11**(4):367–77.
43. Lorenz T, Meston C. Acute exercise improves physical sexual arousal in women taking antidepressants. *Annals of Behavioral Medicine* 2012;**43**(3):352–61.
44. Laan E, Rellini A, Barnes T. Standard operating procedures for female orgasmic disorder: consensus of the International Society for Sexual Medicine. *Journal of Sexual Medicine* 2013;**10**(1):74–82.
45. Suckling J, Kennedy R, Lethaby A, Roberts H. Local oestrogen for vaginal atrophy in postmenopausal women. *Cochrane Database of Systematic Reviews* 2006;**4**:CD001500. Available at: www.ncbi.nlm.nih.gov/pubmed/17054136. Accessed December 11, 2015.
46. Annon J. The PLISSIT Model: a proposed conceptual scheme for the behavioural treatment of sexual problems. *Journal of Sex Education and Therapy* 1976;**2**(1):1–15.
47. Sexual Health Fundamentals for Patient Care Initiative Report of a US Consensus Process. Association of Reproductive Health Professionals (ARHP) March 2010. www.arhp.org/uploadDocs/SHF_meetingreport.pdf. Accesed December 11, 2015.
48. McVary K. Sexual dysfunction. In: Longo D, Fauci A, Kasper D, Hauser S, Jameson J, Loscalzo J. eds. *Harrison's Principles of Internal Medicine*, 18th edition. New York: McGraw-Hill; 2012, chapter 67.

Chapter 25

Office management of endometriosis

Juan Garcia-Velasco

Introduction

Endometriosis has been traditionally defined as an ectopic implantation of viable endometrial cells outside the uterine cavity.[1] It now has a broader definition, described as an estrogen-dependent inflammatory disease with the presence of endometrium-like tissue in sites outside the uterine cavity, primarily on the pelvic peritoneum and ovaries.[2] It is a major contributor to pelvic pain and subfertility. This disease affects approximately 6%–10% of women of reproductive age and up to 50% of women with infertility. It is an incurable disease and often presents as a diagnostic challenge.

Frequently delay exists in the initial diagnosis of endometriosis – often 7–12 years elapse from onset of symptoms to definitive diagnosis. Making an early diagnosis is important for it may help avoid or reverse complications from this chronic disease such as infertility.

A wide variety of clinical practices exist in the management of endometriosis. This represents a problem because endometriosis poses a major burden on different aspects of women's life:

- It has a significant effect on social, sexual, work, and study life.
- The partner's life can also be affected to some degree and directly related to the impact on sexuality and infertility.
- Endometriosis is an economic burden. It has been reported that the annual cost in Europe for treating endometriosis could be between EUR 0.8 million and EUR 12.5 billion.[3, 4]

Health professionals should optimize the management of women with endometriosis in order to achieve certain goals:

- improve diagnosis
- improve endometriosis care
- reduce personal costs
- reduce societal costs

Etiology and pathophysiology of endometriosis

Pathogenesis

Many theories have been proposed to explain the pathogenesis of endometriosis; they still remain to be conclusively confirmed. These are the several theories that have been proposed:

- retrograde menstruation
- metaplasia
- hormones
- oxidative stress and inflammation
- immune dysfunction
- apoptosis suppression and alteration of endometrial cell fate
- genetics
- stem cells

This diversity of theories points toward a complex and multifactorial etiology of endometriosis.

Pathophysiology of ovarian endometriosis

Ovarian endometriomas may result from the invagination of the ovarian cortex after accumulation of menstrual debris coming from active endometriotic lesions.[5] In women with endometriosis, between 17% and 40% will present with an ovarian endometrioma.[6]

Clinical data supports the fact that an endometrioma may cause damage to healthy ovarian tissue, independent of the mechanical stretching and its size. The damage caused by the endometrioma results in several morphological and functional changes compared to healthy ovarian tissue. The fluid of an

Office Care of Women, ed. Martin E. Olsen and Botros Rizk. Published by Cambridge University Press.

BOX 25-1 Genesis of pain: suggested mechanisms

- The production of substances such as cytokines and growth factors by macrophages and other cells related to the endometriotic implants
- Direct and indirect effects of active bleeding from the implants
- Irritation of pelvic floor nerve fibers or direct invasion of those nerves by the implants

endometrioma (or chocolate cyst, as it is commonly known) contains many inflammatory molecules, free iron, reactive oxygen species (ROS), cellular damage-mediating factors, and proteolytic enzymes. These molecules are present in higher concentrations compared to those in serum or other types of benign cysts; some even appear to be in the same range as found in malignant tumors. Because of this fluid, the endometriotic cells that surround the cyst are subject to certain changes ranging from gene expression modifications to genetic mutations. Additionally, the thin barrier that surrounds the cyst is composed of ovarian cortex or fibroreactive tissue. ROS and other molecules from the cyst fluid may permeate to surrounding tissues and may cause the substitution of normal ovarian cortex with fibrous tissue. This fibrous reaction is also associated with smooth muscle metaplasia with intraovarian vascular injury and follicular loss. It is not clear, however, whether this damage is acute or progressive over time.

Pathophysiology of pain in endometriosis

Generally speaking, there is no established relationship between the extent of disease and symptoms, but the location and type of disease can impact pelvic pain.

The most common suggested mechanisms by which endometriosis causes pain are described in Box 25-1. It may be possible that all these mechanisms operate individually or together.

Estrogens and progesterone may also have an impact on pain. Estrogens increase pain associated with endometriosis by directly stimulating the lesions. Progesterone also has an impact by a dampening effect on neuronal activity. The endometriotic lesions present variable levels of estrogen and progesterone receptors (ER and PR, respectively) and hormonal responsiveness. This correlates with worsening pain symptoms in women of reproductive age and an improvement in hypoestrogenic states and menopause.

Additionally, although endometriosis is usually considered a progressive disease, it may also remain static and even regress without treatment.

Risk factors of endometriosis

Risk factors include obstruction of menstrual outflow, exposure to diethylstilbestrol in utero, short menstrual cycles, low birth weight, prolonged exposure to endogenous estrogen (situations such as early menarche, late menopause, or obesity), and exposure to endocrine-disrupting chemicals. A genetic component has been proposed derived from twin and family studies.

Endometriosis is also associated with an increased risk of autoimmune diseases and ovarian endometrioid and clear-cell cancers, as well as melanoma and non-Hodgkin's lymphoma.

Protective factors against endometriosis include prolonged lactation and multiple pregnancies.

Diagnosis of endometriosis

The average delay in the diagnosis of endometriosis has been reported to be 9.3 years.[7] Early detection is of significant importance because many complications of this chronic disease, such as infertility, may be reversed or treated earlier.

The causes of this diagnostic delay appear to be multifactorial, beginning with oral contraceptive use for years, examinations that are nondiscriminatory, misdiagnosis, and diverse attitudes toward menstruation and the normalization of pain.[8] Refining the knowledge in clinicians and the general public may help decrease this delay with the resultant improvement of quality of life in women with endometriosis.

The diagnosis of endometriosis is first suspected based upon the medical history and then corroborated by the physical examination, next through imaging techniques, and finally proven by histological examination obtained during laparoscopy.[8]

The gold standard of diagnosis continues to be the combination of visualization of lesions during laparoscopy and histological verification of endometrial glands outside the uterine cavity. The revised scoring system of the American Society for Reproductive Medicine (ASRM) is used to define the disease stage depending on location, extent, and depth of endometriotic implants; presence and severity of adhesions and the presence and size of ovarian endometriomas. Although useful for determining the burden of disease as well as management, the scoring system does not correlate with the severity of pain or predict the response to therapy for pain or infertility.

Differential diagnosis of endometriosis

Other different conditions of the reproductive tract can cause chronic pelvic pain such as adenomyosis, pelvic adhesions, pelvic inflammatory disease, congenital anomalies of the reproductive tract, and ovarian or tubal masses. It may also be related to other non-gynecologic conditions such as irritable bowel syndrome, interstitial cystitis, fibromyalgia, and other musculoskeletal disorders. A thorough evaluation should be carried out in order to exclude other causes of pain and specially in those women that have not responded with conventional therapy.

Symptoms of endometriosis

Many symptoms are associated with endometriosis, ranging from pelvic and intestinal complaints to referred pain. The clinician should always suspect endometriosis when any of the following signs are reported by women of reproductive age:

- Pelvic symptoms: dysmenorrhea, dyspareunia, cyclical pelvic pain, dyschezia, infertility, fatigue, and weariness
- Intestinal complaints: periodic bloating, diarrhea, and constipation (these are commonly unrecognized symptoms)
- Referred pain: legs, back (specially in adolescents), and shoulder

The most severe forms of dyschezia and dyspareunia are associated with deep endometriosis of the rectovaginal septum.

Some studies have aimed at identifying the symptoms that are most predictive of endometriosis. Abdominopelvic pain, dysmenorrhea, heavy menstrual bleeding, infertility, dyspareunia, postcoital bleeding, diagnosis of ovarian cyst, irritable bowel syndrome, and pelvic inflammatory disease are all predictive of endometriosis. Menstrual dyschezia strongly predicts it.

Medical literature does not well correlate the prediction of endometriosis with specific symptoms. Nonetheless, the condition should be suspected and the clinician should explore the diagnosis when the following gynecological symptoms appear: dysmenorrhea, noncyclical pelvic pain, deep dyspareunia, infertility, and fatigue in the presence of any of the above. Suspicion should arise also when dyschezia, dysuria, hematuria, rectal bleeding, and shoulder pain are suffered by the patient.

Pain assessment

Measuring pain is not an easy task, for it is very subjective. Questionnaires and quality-of-life scales may be utilized. They may help to assess the impact of pain and treatment response.

Clinical examination in the diagnosis of endometriosis

Clinical examination is aimed at facilitating diagnosis and treatment of the disease. Although exam has limitations, it is low cost. Reliability of pelvic endometriosis detection is improved during menstruation. The physical examination should include:

- inspection of the vagina with a speculum
- bimanual palpation
- rectovaginal palpation
- inspection and palpation of the abdomen

As an important reminder, clinical examination may be inappropriate in some patients (adolescents, sexual abuse victims, certain religious beliefs) and could be very painful in some women. Other technologies could be of help in these situations. In some cases where vaginal exploration cannot be performed, rectal examination may be helpful.

The clinician should consider the diagnosis of deep endometriosis when finding a painful induration and/or nodules of the rectovaginal wall, or when there are visible nodules in the posterior vaginal fornix.

An ovarian endometrioma should be considered when adnexal masses are found during the physical examination.

The evidence in the medical literature is weak for diagnosing pelvic endometriosis with physical examination. Ultrasound and magnetic resonance imaging (MRI) technologies are more accurate at diagnosing ovarian and/or deep endometriosis.

Medical technologies for the diagnosis of endometriosis

Endometriosis is initially suspected on the patient's history, then corroborated by physical examination and imaging technologies. The final diagnosis is proven by histological examination of tissue samples.

Laparoscopy for the diagnosis of endometriosis

Laparoscopy affords the opportunity to visualize endometriotic lesions and to obtain tissue samples for analysis. The gold standard of endometriosis diagnosis is still considered to be the combination of laparoscopy and histological confirmation of endometrial glands and/or stroma.

Controversy exists concerning whether laparoscopy should be performed in all patients when endometriosis is suspected. It could be argued that empirical treatment can be started without a definitive diagnosis, especially in young women or those who are not in need of diagnosis confirmation. Many women will not want to go through surgery if medical treatment relieves the pain.[9] Conversely, arguments to perform a laparoscopy include the patient's wish to have a definitive diagnosis or advanced disease (such as deep endometriosis).

In cases of infertility and ovarian endometriosis, laparoscopy should be approached with caution for the procedure may change from a diagnostic tool into an operative event. Surgery, especially before ART treatment, should be envisioned only in specific circumstances. Surgery may have a detrimental effect on ovarian reserve; this will be covered in more depth later in the chapter.

A lack of consensus in the medical literature exists about the value of a positive laparoscopy (visualizing lesions) without histologic confirmation. See Table 25-1. Conversely, a woman with a negative laparoscopy (no visualized lesions) can be reassured without the need for further testing, for negative laparoscopy is highly reliable for the exclusion of endometriosis.

Table 25-1 Endometriosis Diagnosis

Head	Head	Head
Positive laparoscopy	Negative histology	Diagnosis of endometriosis should not be excluded (it may still be present)
Negative laparoscopy	No tissue samples obtained	Reassuring (highly reliable and no need for further testing)

The diagnosis of endometriosis should not be excluded even with a negative histologic result, for the negative result may be caused by lack of the clinician's knowledge or by bad sampling and wrong sample locations. The final result of the procedure of laparoscopy will always depend on the ability and experience of the surgeon performing it.

Ultrasound examination

Transvaginal ultrasound appears to be an effective investigation tool to confirm or rule out the diagnosis of an endometrioma, in a patient with an adnexal mass. This conclusion was reached by a systematic review that evaluated transvaginal and transabdominal ultrasound for the accurate diagnosis of pelvic endometriosis.[10]

The characteristics for diagnosis of an endometrioma are best described by Van Holsbeke, et al.[11] The optimal rule to detect endometriomas in a clinical setting according to this study was an adnexal mass in a premenopausal patient with ground glass echogenicity of the cyst fluid, one to four locules, and no papillations with detectable blood flow. Interestingly, CA-125 serum levels were not of value in distinguishing endometriomas from tumors. Of importance, masses in postmenopausal women whose cystic contents have a ground glass appearance have a high risk of malignancy.

If a patient is diagnosed with ovarian endometriosis, deep infiltrating disease should be investigated.

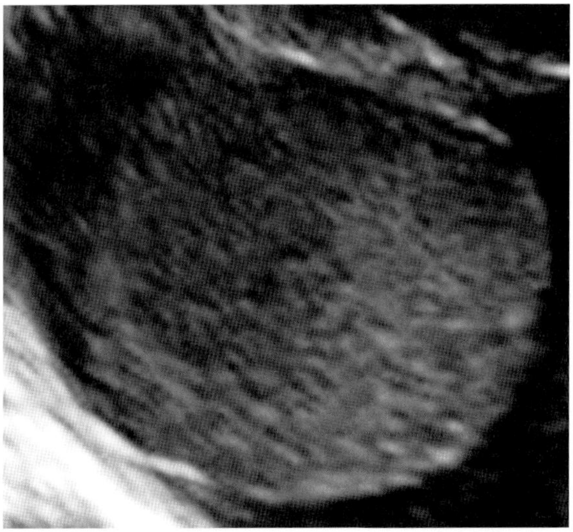

Figure 25-1 Typical appearance of an endometrioma with "ground glass" echogenicity.

Women with an endometrioma tend to have more pelvic and intestinal areas invaded by endometriosis compared to women without ovarian endometriosis. An endometrioma is a soft marker for detecting the presence of deep endometriosis. Once detected, the patient should be managed by a specialized multidisciplinary team.

Transvaginal sonography for the diagnosis of rectal endometriosis

A recent systematic review related to use of transvaginal sonography (TVS) for the diagnosis of bowel endometriosis reported a positive predictive value of 98% and a negative predictive value of 95%. TVS therefore appears to be useful for identifying and ruling out rectal endometriosis, but should be performed by clinicians that are highly experienced in TVS.

Magnetic resonance imaging

MRI is a useful technology for the diagnostic workup of ovarian and deep endometriosis, especially when there is suspicion (based on history or physical examination) of ureter or bowel involvement.

Laparoscopy may have blind spots and this is where MRI can have a key role. MRI can help to visualize those areas that may have escaped the laparoscopic field of view. Such areas include the retroperitoneal space or lesions obscured by dense adhesions. MRI may also be helpful to assess response to treatment and the recurrence of disease.

A major limitation is the diagnosis of peritoneal implants. The usefulness of MRI for diagnosis of peritoneal endometriosis is not well established. A promising breakthrough for MRI technology could be the concomitant use of a specific contrast agent called gadofosveset-trisodium. Because this agent extravasates from hyperpermeable vessels more easily than from mature vessels, it can detect angiogenesis more efficiently. It has been demonstrated that endometriotic lesions show formation of new vessels on histologic examination. The signal from those angiogenic spots have proven to be enhanced at least in an animal model. Schreinemacher, et al. recently described this potential application.[12]

Imaging technologies: specific considerations in deep infiltrating disease

Bladder involvement can be suspected from patient history, and TVS is helpful for corroborating the diagnosis. The usefulness of 3D ultrasound for diagnosing rectovaginal endometriosis is not well established.[13] The accuracy of barium enema for diagnosing bowel wall involvement is impossible at present to confirm.

Biomarkers

Many studies have focused on identifying biomarkers on blood or urine samples. May, et al. in a comprehensive two article review cover many molecules that have been studied as potential biomarkers.[14, 15] It is not recommended at present to clinically use biomarkers for the diagnosis of endometriosis.

Table 25-2 presents a list of the most common types of peripheral biomarkers that have been studied and those biomarkers assessing endometrial alterations. By far the most studied potential marker has been CA-125. A relationship exists between this marker and the presence of endometriosis. It may not be accurate in early stages of disease to distinguish between presence and absence of disease, but it may have higher accuracy at later stages.[16, 17] It also appears to be more commonly elevated with the presence of an endometrioma, but it is still not currently used to diagnose endometriosis. One potential future use may be for treatment monitoring.

Table 25-2 Peripheral and endometrial biomarkers

Peripheral biomarkers	Endometrial biomarkers
Cytokines	Endometrial cytokines
Antibodies	Immunology
Cell populations	Hormones and steroids
Glycoproteins	Growth factors and cell adhesion molecules
Cell adhesion molecules	Tissue remodeling
Growth factors	Angiogenesis and apoptosis
Proteomics	Reactive oxygen species
Hormones	Genetic studies
Other factors	Proteomics: menstrual and endometrial fluid analysis
	Histology

Endometrial biomarkers

Because of the ease of obtaining samples in the office setting without the need for anesthesia, endometrial tissue differences in endometriosis have been considered as potential diagnostic tools.

Certain molecules, such as cell adhesion molecules and angiogenesis factors, have the potential for future use as markers for endometriosis. The current recommendation, however, is that endometrial samples are not a diagnostic tool for endometriosis.

Treatment of pain in endometriosis

Patients with chronic pelvic pain associated with endometriosis require long-term treatment that involves repeated courses of medical and/or surgical therapy. In many cases the pain recurs within 6–12 months after completion of the treatment.[18] There are no studies that directly compare the effectiveness of medication versus surgery, so it is not possible to draw conclusions about the superiority of one over the other. Medical treatment is usually the initial choice because of the lower costs and lower risks.

Medical treatment

Because endometriosis is an estrogen-mediated condition, all medical treatments block ovarian function, but they do so in different ways. The hormonal medications used for treating endometriosis include gonadotropin-releasing hormone (GnRH) agonists, oral contraceptives, danazol, progestogens, and antiprogestogens. Pain relief is also a part of the medical treatment. These medications are effective for alleviating pain and also reduce the risk of recurrence after surgery. Because medical treatments block ovarian function, these medications are not indicated for treating infertile patients who also have endometriosis.

A brief description of the different kinds of medications used for treating pain in endometriosis is provided in the following sections.

Nonsteroidal anti-inflammatory drugs

Nonsteroidal anti-inflammatory drugs (NSAIDs) are usually the first line of treatment for pain. They seem to be effective for the treatment of primary dysmenorrhea, but a recent Cochrane analysis did not find enough evidence to show that they significantly reduce pain in endometriosis.[19]

Combined hormonal contraceptives

Combined hormonal contraceptives have been used in a continuous or cyclic manner to treat endometriosis symptoms. The proposed mechanism of action is that of decidualization followed by atrophy of the endometrium. Oral contraceptives (OC) appear to be more effective at alleviating symptoms after surgical treatment if used in a continuous fashion compared to cyclic administration. OC with desogestrel are equally effective as the traditional ones containing the more androgenic progestagens, such as 19-nortestosterone derivatives.

Progestagens

Progestagens are also commonly used and seem to be effective in reducing pain. The mechanism of action is similar to OC, with the addition of suppression of matrix metalloproteinases (important for the growth and implantation of ectopic endometrium) and inhibition of angiogenesis. The most common types include medroxyprogesterone acetate (MPA) and 19-nortestosterone derivatives. The levonorgestrel-releasing intrauterine device also appears to improve the symptoms of dysmenorrhea.

GnRH agonists

GnRH agonists bind to GnRH receptors in the pituitary resulting in a down-regulation of the pituitary-ovarian axis. Their mode of action is also related to the induction of amenorrhea and endometrial atrophy. Commonly used GnRH agonists are leuprolide, goserelin, buserelin, and triptorelin. They are usually administered in a depot formulation by injection every one to three months, but there is also short-acting presentations. Another option is a nasal spray presentation (nafarelin).

GnRH agonists are effective in alleviating symptoms in women with endometriosis, and no route of administration appears superior to another, according to a recent systematic review.[20]

Important side effects include the hypoestrogenic symptoms (hot flushes, vaginal dryness, decreased libido, headache, mood swings, and bone loss). They are usually not administered for more than six months because of these side effects, including the risk of osteopenia. To reduce the side effects and to allow longer treatment periods, an "add-back" therapy has been advocated. This treatment consists of norethindrone or a combination of estrogens and progestogens. It should be started at the same time of agonist administration. It has been show that this approach can decrease bone loss and reduces the severity of the side effects.[21]

Danazol

Danazol is a derivative of 17 alpha-ethinyl testosterone . Its mode of action is related to the inhibition of the luteinizing hormone (LH) surge and by increasing free testosterone levels. It is generally administered orally although there are different presentations. Danazol appears to relieve symptoms of endometriosis, but hyperandrogenic effects are common (acne, weight gain, hirsutism, and deepening of the voice). These significant side effects limit its clinical usefulness.

Aromatase inhibitors

Because of the increased activity of aromatase in the endometriotic tissue, aromatase inhibitors (AI) have been used as therapy. They seem to be an effective option for the treatment of pelvic pain in endometriosis, although they have not been approved for this indication specifically.

It must be mentioned that AI can increase follicle-stimulating hormone (FSH) levels in premenopausal women, leading to multifollicular development. They should therefore be used in combination with other agents such as OC, GnRH-a, or progestogens.

Gestrinone

Gestrinone is an antiprogestational steroid that inhibits ovarian steroidogenesis. It is administered orally. Anti-estrogenic and androgenic side effects have been described. It has been shown to be as effective as danazol and GnRH agonists. It is not currently available in the United States but is in use in Europe.

Other molecules

Several other options are under investigation. These include mifepristone, selective PR and ER modulators, GnRH antagonists, agents that inhibit angiogenesis and the effects of TNF-alpha, matrix metalloproteinases, and pentoxifylline.

Adjuvant therapy

Acupuncture and Chinese herbal remedies have been studied, and both seem to significantly relieve pain.

Since chronic pelvic pain may cause musculoskeletal pain derived from muscle contractures, referral to a physiotherapist may prove to be beneficial in relieving part of the pain. A mental health professional may add benefit because of the psychological stress and depression that come with chronic pelvic pain. Additionally, a pain management specialist may help to guide the analgesic treatment.

Surgical treatment

Surgical treatment consists of eliminating endometriotic lesions, division of adhesions (to restore pelvic anatomy), and interruption of nerve pathways (with the intention of improving pain control). Surgical treatment may be recommended to treat endometriotic lesions at the time of the diagnostic laparoscopy. It has been observed that treatment with laparoscopic surgery in endometriosis appears to alleviate symptoms and promote disease improvement. Practically, the presence of pain strongly weighs in favor of surgery at the time of diagnostic laparoscopy.

Pain recurrence after primary surgery ranges between 20% and 40%; this is similar after repeat surgery because of recurrent disease.

Laparoscopic uterosacral nerve ablation, presacral neurectomy, and hysterectomy

Currently, laparoscopic uterosacral nerve ablation does not seem to offer any added benefits to conservative surgery. Rare complications have been described such as uterine prolapse and transection of the ureter.

Presacral neurectomy is a technically challenging procedure associated with significant risk of bleeding. Although it has been proposed to treat midline pain associated with menstruation, its effects on other types of pain are inconsistent.

Hysterectomy with bilateral salpingo-oophorectomy (BSO) is usually the procedure of last resort. It is reserved for women with incapacitating symptoms related to endometriosis that have completed childbearing and in whom other therapies have failed. Hysterectomy without BSO is commonly less effective as recurrence rates are higher. Combined hormonal therapy (estrogen-progesterone) is the usual regimen for treating women after hysterectomy and BSO. Although hormonal therapy always carries the risk of disease recurrence, unopposed estrogens might be more likely to promote it. Hormonal therapy should always be used with caution due to therapeutic risks.

Adjuvant medical treatment after surgery

In women with advanced disease, moderate-to-severe dysmenorrhea and noncyclic pelvic pain, postoperative medical therapy may improve pain management.

It appears that the return of symptoms is a significantly longer time interval with adjuvant medical therapy after surgery.

Medical treatment of ovarian endometriosis

Endometriomas do not usually respond well to medical treatment, and surgical resection is a very common procedure around the world either to overcome infertility or to relieve pain. Resection of such an endometrioma, however, is not based on solid clinical evidence.

Medical therapy may cause a temporary reduction in size of the cyst, but not complete resolution. The simple drainage of endometriomas is associated with a high recurrence rate within 6 months; it is therefore not recommended as definitive therapy.

Endometriosis and infertility

There is good correlation between the amount, type, and location of endometriotic lesions and the pain encountered.[22] On the other hand, the relationship between endometriosis and infertility is less clear, although the association is clinically recognized.[23] The current vision today is that infertility in endometriosis is multifactorial.[24] Of course when infertility is present, both the female and male partner should undergo a full evaluation.

Treatment of infertility

Before contemplating surgery, certain factors must be considered. If the ovarian reserve is altered, or the patient is older than 38 years of age or if infertility is longstanding, ART procedures should be offered initially. If tubal or sperm status is altered, then the option also is to go straight to ART. Another factor to consider is the availability of time, for many women desire to achieve pregnancy as soon as possible.

When semen parameters and tubal status are not an issue, the usefulness of middle-ground treatment (such as intrauterine insemination) is of questionable value in patients with endometriosis. They do not seem to be better than a wait-and-see approach with natural conception. Until more data is available, it is not recommended to use this middle-ground approach in women with endometriosis, either before or after surgery.[25]

Although success rates of ART procedures such as in vitro fertilization (IVF) appear to be diminished in women with endometriosis (compared to women with tubal factor infertility), IVF can maximize cycle fecundity.

If a patient goes through surgery then it is advisable to wait at least one year for natural conception to happen. If this is not achieved, then ART procedures should be offered.

It should be emphasized that the patient needs to have all the pertinent information, with advantages and disadvantages of surgery and the availability of ART. A valid option is to go directly to ART procedures if the couple being treated for infertility decides to avoid surgery.

In certain cases the main reason for choosing surgery or ART procedures comes from the primary activity of the health professional that is being initially consulted; the best interests of the patient would be a better approach.

In principle, surgery performed immediately before ART is of little help.[24] The exception could be pelvic pain, hydrosalpinges, and large endometriomas. Hydrosalpinges are important to consider, for they reduce the outcome of ART almost by 50%; surgery should also be envisioned in patients with severe pain, because pain by itself can be associated with infertility.

Information about the value of surgery improving the chances of natural conception is complex. Confusion exists because there are different forms of endometriosis (superficial, deep infiltrating, and endometriomas), different types of surgery, and different modes of assessing fertility (natural or in vitro). There is some evidence weighing in favor of surgery for superficial lesions to improve fertility.[26] At least one year is needed as sufficient time to maximize the chances of a natural pregnancy. Women treated surgically for any stage of endometriosis have an approximately 50% chance of spontaneous conception one to two years after the procedure.[24] This increase is seen irrespective of disease stage. On the other hand, surgery for deep infiltrating disease is usually for alleviating pain and data in relation to improving fertility after surgery is still unclear.

Surgical removal of endometriomas in infertility

Surgery should be approached with caution in women with endometriomas. Regardless of the type of surgical procedure used for removal of the endometrioma, it seems to cause some damage to healthy ovarian tissue with consequences on the ovarian reserve. This has an even more deleterious effect for bilateral endometriomas; a potential risk of premature ovarian failure exists after the procedure.

When infertility is present, sparing the surgical procedure and proceeding directly to ART reduces the time to achieve a pregnancy. Surgery should be performed only during specific circumstances, such as pelvic pain, difficult access to the follicles during oocyte retrieval and risk of malignancy. It has also been seen that excision of an endometrioma does not appear to have any additional benefits on ART outcomes. Garcia-Velasco, et al. in a case-control study of surgery for ovarian endometriosis showed no outcome improvement for ART versus expectant management.[27] Some authors have argued that keeping endometriomas in place could increase the risk of infection during oocyte retrieval, but this has not been confirmed.

Medical pretreatment before ART

Ovarian suppression with GnRH agonists appears to have favorable effects on ART outcome in women with endometriosis.[28] The optimal duration of this pretreatment is still unknown, but a meta-analysis confirmed the benefit of a three- to six-month period of GnRH agonists before commencing ART.[29] The mechanism by which this pretreatment improves ART outcome is uncertain, but it could be related to correcting endometrial alterations and because of this possibly amplifying receptivity for embryo implantation.

Concluding remarks

Endometriosis is a chronic disease that causes significant morbidity in women's lives. A lifelong management plan is beneficial. Medical therapy is usually the initial approach and surgical support may eventually be required. Assisted reproductive technologies are an option for overcoming infertility. Endometriosis continues to be a challenging disease not only to diagnose but also to treat. In order to obtain more specific diagnostic tools and treatment options, research must continue to improve our understanding of the pathogenesis of endometriosis.

References

1. Sampson JA. Peritoneal endometriosis due to menstrual dissemination of endometrial tissue into the peritoneal cavity. *Am J Obstet Gynecol* 1927;**14**:422–69.
2. Giudice LC, Kao LC. Endometriosis. *Lancet* 2004;**364**: 1789–99.
3. Nnoaham KE, Hummelshoj L, Kennedy SH, et al. and World Endometriosis Research Foundation Women's Health Symptom Survey C. Developing symptom-based predictive models of endometriosis as a clinical screening tool: results from a multicenter study. *Fertil Steril* 2012;**98**:692–701.
4. Simoens S, Dunselman G, Dirksen C, et al. The burden of endometriosis: costs and quality of life of women with endometriosis and treated in referral centres. *Hum Reprod* 2012;**27**:1292–9.
5. Brosens IA, Van Ballaer P, Puttemans P, Deprest J. Reconstruction of the ovary containing large endometriomas by an extraovarian endosurgical technique. *Fertil Steril* 1996;**66**:517–21.
6. Vercellini P, Chapron C, DeGiorgi O, et al. Coagulation or excision of ovarian endometriomas? *Am J Obstet Gynecol* 2003;**188**:606–10.
7. Gupta S, Agarwal A, Sekhon L, et al. Serum and peritoneal abnormalities in endometriosis: potential use as diagnostic markers. *Minerva Ginecol.* 2006;**58** (6):527–51.
8. Dunselman GA, Vermeulen N, Becker C, et al. ESHRE guideline: management of women with endometriosis. *Hum Reprod* 2014;**29**(3):400–12. doi: 10.1093/humrep/det457. Epub 2014 Jan 15.
9. Kennedy S. Should a diagnosis of endometriosis be sought in all symptomatic women? *Fertil Steril* 2006;**86**:1312–13; discussion 1317.
10. Moore J, Copley S, Morris J, et al. A systematic review of the accuracy of ultrasound in the diagnosis of endometriosis. *Ultrasound Obstet Gynecol* 2002;**20**: 630–4.
11. Van Holsbeke C, Van Calster B, Guerriero S, et al. Endometriomas: their ultrasound characteristics. *Ultrasound Obstet Gynecol* 2010;**35**:730–40.
12. Schreinemacher MH, Backes WH, Slenter JM, et al. Towards endometriosis diagnosis by gadofosveset-trisodium enhanced magnetic resonance imaging. *PLoS One* 2012;7(3):e33241. doi: 10.1371/journal.pone.0033241. Epub 2012 Mar 22.
13. Pascual MA, Guerriero S, Hereter L, et al. Diagnosis of endometriosis of the rectovaginal septum using introital three-dimensional ultrasonography. *Fertil Steril* 2010;**94**:2761–5.
14. May KE, Conduit-Hulbert SA, Villar J, et al. Peripheral biomarkers of endometriosis: a systematic review. *Hum Reprod Update* 2010;**16**:651–74.
15. May KE, Villar J, Kirtley S, et al. Endometrial alterations in endometriosis: a systematic review of putative biomarkers. *Hum Reprod Update* 2011;**17**: 637–53.

16. Maiorana A, Cicerone C, Niceta M, Alio L. Evaluation of serum CA 125 levels in patients with pelvic pain related to endometriosis. *Int J Biol Markers* 2007;**22**: 200–2.
17. Mol B, Bayram N, Lijmer J, et al. The performance of CA-125 measurement in the detection of endometriosis: a meta-analysis. *Fertil Steril* 1998;**70**:1101–8.
18. Giudice LC. Clinical practice: endometriosis. *N Engl J Med* 2010;**362**(25):2389–98. doi: 10.1056/NEJMcp 1000274.
19. Allen C, Hopewell S, Prentice A, Gregory D. Nonsteroidal anti-inflammatory drugs for pain in women with endometriosis. *Cochrane Database Syst Rev* 2009;**2**:CD004753.
20. Brown J, Pan A, Hart RJ. Gonadotrophin-releasing hormone analogues for pain associated with endometriosis. *Cochrane Database Syst Rev* 2010; **12**: CD008475.
21. Practice Committee of the American Society for Reproductive Medicine. Treatment of pelvic pain associated with endometriosis: a committee opinion. *Fertil Steril* 2014;**101**(4):927–35. doi: 10.1016/j.fertnstert.2014.02.012. Epub 2014 Mar 13.
22. Bulun SE. Endometriosis. *N Engl J Med* 2009;**360**: 268–79.
23. Gupta S, Goldberg JM, Aziz N, et al. Pathogenic mechanisms in endometriosis-associated infertility. *Fertil Steril* 2008;**90**(2):247–57. doi: 10.1016/j.fertnstert.2008.02.093.
24. De Ziegler D, Borghese B, Chapron C. Endometriosis and infertility: pathophysiology and management. *Lancet* 2010;**376**(9742):730–8. doi: 10.1016/S0140-6736(10)60490-4.
25. Omland AK, Tanbo T, Dale PO, Abyholm T. Artificial insemination by husband in unexplained infertility compared with infertility associated with peritoneal endometriosis. *Hum Reprod* 1998;**13**:2602–5.
26. Jacobson TZ, Duffy JM, Barlow D, et al. Laparoscopic surgery for subfertility associated with endometriosis. *Cochrane Database Syst Rev* 2010;**1**:CD001398.
27. Garcia-Velasco JA, Mahutte NG, Corona J, et al. Removal of endometriomas before in vitro fertilization does not improve fertility outcomes: a matched, case-control study. *Fertil Steril* 2004;**81**:1194–7.
28. Surrey ES, Silverberg KM, Surrey MW, Schoolcraft WB. Effect of prolonged gonadotropin-releasing hormone agonist therapy on the outcome of in vitro fertilization-embryo transfer in patients with endometriosis. *Fertil Steril* 2002;**78**:699–704.
29. Sallam HN, Garcia-Velasco JA, Dias S, Arici A. Long-term pituitary down-regulation before in vitro fertilization (IVF) for women with endometriosis. *Cochrane Database Syst Rev* 2006;**1**:CD004635.
30. ACOG. Practice bulletin no. 114: management of endometriosis. *Obstet Gynecol* 2010;**116**(1):223–36. doi: 10.1097/AOG.0b013e3181e8b073.
31. Garcia-Velasco JA, Somigliana E. Management of endometriomas in women requiring IVF: to touch or not to touch. *Hum Reprod* 2009;**24**:496–501.
32. Leyland N, Casper R, Laberge P, Singh SS; SOGC. Endometriosis: diagnosis and management. *J Obstet Gynaecol (Can)* 2010;**32**(7 Suppl 2):S1–32.
33. Practice Committee of the American Society for Reproductive Medicine. Endometriosis and infertility: a committee opinion. *Fertil Steril* 2012;**98**(3):591–8. Epub 2012 Jun 15.

Chapter 26

Outpatient evaluation of the infertile couple*

Spiros A. Liatsikos and Geeta Nargund

Introduction

Subfertility is a common problem in the modern world, affecting about one out of six couples. Recent advances in the management of such a problem have resulted in an increased number of couples seeking help. Appropriate management of the patient/couple can be offered only after an accurate diagnosis of the problem has been established. This in turn requires taking a thorough medical history from both partners, performing a physical examination, and arranging a number of investigations, including biochemical, hormonal, genetic, imaging and in some cases more invasive studies (Table 26-1). The modern couple wants to know why they have not conceived, the available treatment options, and the chances of success with each option.

The aim of this chapter is to provide an overview of the approach to the outpatient evaluation of the infertile couple. This evaluation can be offered on a "one-stop" basis. Female investigation is enhanced with the availability of high-quality ultrasound (u/s) equipment with Doppler and preferably three-dimension (3D) facilities. Male investigation can run in parallel; ideally a semen analysis result should be available for the consultation. Such an approach is more time- and cost-effective.

Medical history

Understanding the length of subfertility is quite important. Traditionally it has been recommended that a couple should have infertility investigations if no conception has occurred after one year of frequent

Table 26-1 Outpatient evaluation of the infertile couple

Medical history	General Gynecological Andrological
Physical examination	General Female (pelvic) Male (in case of repeat abnormal semen analysis)
Biochemical, hormonal, genetic tests	For female partner: AMH, FSH, LH, estradiol, progesterone, testosterone, sex hormone binding globulin (SHBG), TSH, prolactin For male partner: semen analysis In case of severe oligospermia/azoospermia: FSH, LH, testosterone, prolactin, chromosome analysis, Y-chromosome deletions, cystic fibrosis mutations
Imaging	Fertility ultrasound scan (ideally with Doppler and 3D facilities) Hydrosonography Hysterosalpingo-contrast sonography (HyCoSy)
Endoscopy	Outpatient hysteroscopy, diagnostic and/or operative (if required)

* The authors are grateful to Professor Stuart Campbell (CREATE Fertility, London, UK), who generously offered representative ultrasound images from his collection.

Office Care of Women, ed. Martin E. Olsen and Botros Rizk. Published by Cambridge University Press.

unprotected sexual intercourse. However individual circumstances should also be considered, such as advanced female age, irregular menstrual cycles, history of pelvic surgery, or history of recurrent miscarriages. For these diagnoses, earlier investigation is in general recommended.

Details of any previous pregnancies as well as of previous fertility investigations or treatment should be recorded. A brief description of current or previous symptoms, illnesses, or surgery can help the diagnosis. Dysmenorrhea and pelvic pain could indicate endometriosis. Previous pelvic surgery or pelvic infections from chlamydia or ureoplasma increase risk for peritubular adhesions and tubal occlusion. Menopausal symptoms, such as hot flushes, could raise the suspicion of premature ovarian failure. A detailed menstrual history including the duration and the frequency of the cycle and the duration of menstruation can help the diagnosis of ovulation disorders which are common in women with subfertility. Oligomenorrhea and hirsutism commonly occur in women with polycystic ovarian syndrome (PCOS).

Lifestyle must be assessed. Smoking can affect female fecundity and also increases the risk of miscarriage.[1] On the other hand the evidence relating to alcohol consumption with subfertility is conflicting. [2, 3] Due to the unquestionable detrimental effect of alcohol consumption on embryonic development, it is advisable for preconception patients to keep alcohol intake to a minimum (1–2 units/week). Female body mass index (BMI) should be calculated as the association between obesity and ovulatory disorders has been well established.[4] Women with BMI above normal range (19 kg/m^2–25 kg/m^2) should be encouraged to lose weight; this can restore normal ovulation, but it also may increase the chance of success if assisted conception treatment is eventually required. Similarly, underweight women need to be encouraged to increase their BMI to the normal range, especially if they are amenorrheic.

Finally, history of early menopause in the patient's female ancestors could raise the suspicion of premature ovarian failure as there is evidence of familial predisposition.[5]

Although a semen analysis is the most informative investigation for male partners' fertility potential, a brief medical history for males could also provide useful information. This should focus on previous pregnancies fathered, genitourinary infections, maldescent of testes in childhood, testicular surgery (including vasectomy), postpubertal mumps infection with associated orchitis, sexual function, neurologic conditions, prescription drugs intake, possible use of anabolic steroids, smoking, alcohol consumption, and any history of subfertility among the male members of the family.

Physical examination

A thorough physical examination of the prospective mother is traditionally recommended. If an overview of physical characteristics reveals short stature, webbed neck, and undeveloped breasts, these findings suggest Turner's syndrome. Hirsutism and severe acne are usually the result of androgen excess, and the most common reason for that is PCOS. Absent or scanty pubic hair may be the result of either gonadotrophin deficiency (Kallmann's syndrome or androgen insensitivity syndrome) or impaired sex steroid production (as in Turner's syndrome). Neck palpation may raise the suspicion of thyroid dysfunction; the presence of galactorrhea suggests hyperprolactinemia. Surgical scars and pelvic masses are identified with abdominal examination and palpation.

Congenital anomalies of the lower genital tract, such as imperforate hymen, vaginal septa, agenesis of the vagina (which is commonly accompanied with agenesis of the uterus in Mayer-Rokitansky-Kuster-Hauser syndrome), and a double cervix (common feature of a didelphys uterus) can easily be recognized with pelvic examination. The position, shape, size, and mobility of the uterus can be assessed with a bimanual palpation; bimanual is also important for the recognition of any large ovarian masses. Discomfort during the examination and/or palpation of nodules along the uterosacreal ligaments may suggest endometriosis.

Speculum examination can provide information on the appearance of the cervix. It also allows for a Pap smear to be taken (if needed), as well as for a cervical culture for chlamydia and a vaginal culture of any abnormal discharge.[6] The usefulness of pelvic examination in asymptomatic women (excluding the Pap smear) has recently been debated, with the American College of Physicians developing a guideline against it. [7] Much of the information gained by pelvic examination can be obtained by a detailed ultrasound scan which will be subsequently described.

Male physical examination is indicated in cases of repeat abnormal semen analysis results and should ideally be offered by a specialist urologist/andrologist.

Investigations

Biochemical, hormonal, genetic

Hormonal profile of female infertility patients

Plasma levels of gonadotrophins, sex steroids, thyroid-stimulating hormone (TSH), prolactin and anti-müllerian hormone (AMH) could provide potentially useful information about the normal function of the menstrual cycle. However, none of those tests is absolutely necessary to establish a diagnosis and can be omitted or postponed during the "one-stop" fertility assessment.

High follicular-stimulating hormone (FSH) and luteinizing hormone (LH) levels and low estradiol level in the first days of the cycle as well as low AMH level at any time of the cycle suggest low ovarian function and diminished ovarian reserve. This can be confirmed with an ultrasound scan, which could show reduced volume, absent or few antral follicles, and low stromal blood flow velocity in the ovaries. High testosterone level, especially when combined with low sex hormone binding globulin (SHBG) level (high free androgen index), in a woman with polycystic ovaries (PCO) and anovulation suggests PCOS. However, hirsutism is considered a good marker of hyperandrogenemia for the diagnosis of PCOS in the presence of PCO or anovulation.[8] TSH and prolactin blood tests are not routinely recommended in the presence of normal ovulation. It is advisable, however, that women who plan to start treatment have these tests. There is evidence that suboptimal levels of those hormones are related with an adverse reproductive outcome following in vitro fertilization (IVF).[9, 10]

A woman with a regular menstrual cycle should be ovulating normally. This can be confirmed with a midluteal serum progesterone measurement. The appropriate time for this test is a week before the expected onset of menses (e.g., day 21 for a normal 28-day cycle), otherwise the interpretation is difficult. The precise level of the hormone above which ovulation is expected to have occurred is controversial, however a value exceeding 32 nmol/L is recommended by the European Society of Human Reproduction and Embryology (ESHRE).[11] A progesterone test as an indicator of ovulation is not absolutely necessary as this can be suggested by the presence of a dominant, peri ovulatory follicle in a mid-cyclical ultrasound scan or the presence of a corpus luteum, secretory endometrium, and free fluid in the pouch of Douglas in a luteal-phase scan. Alternatively, blood or urine measurements of the LH hormone to detect a surge provide an indirect method to predict ovulation.

Semen analysis, hormonal and genetic profile of male partners

The main investigation for male partners is a semen analysis, which should ideally be performed after two to five days of abstinence. The World Health Organization (WHO) criteria of normal semen values are widely accepted.[12] A normal semen analysis is shown in Figure 26-1. Common abnormal findings in the semen analysis involve low sperm count (oligospermia), low progression (asthenospermia), and low normal forms (teratospermia). If the initial semen analysis is found to be abnormal, a repeat one is recommended a few weeks later, as temporary fluctuation in semen parameters may occur.[13] Further investigation is indicated in case the repeat semen analysis is also abnormal.

Plasma levels of FSH, LH, testosterone, and prolactin should be measured in cases of total absence of live spermatozoa (azoospermia) or severe oligospermia. Normal volume ejaculate (>1 mL) from a man with high FSH, high or normal LH, and normal or low testosterone suggests testicular failure. Such cases should be further investigated with a chromosome analysis in order to exclude Klinefelter's syndrome or other chromosomal abnormalities. Low levels of FSH, LH, and testosterone indicate hypogonadotropic hypogonadism; Kallman's syndrome, hyperprolactinemia, or other acquired causes would then be assessed. Causes of nonobstructive azoospermia or severe oligospermia include Y-chromosome deletions of the azoospermia factor region (AZF), translocations, and chromosomal abnormalities (such as Klinefelter's syndrome). Diagnosis of obstructive azoospermia is increased in the presence of normal hormonal levels and normal testicular size. A common genetic cause of obstructive azoospermia is inheritance of cystic fibrosis genes, which results in vasal aplasia. Fertilization is possible for men with azoospermia or severe oligospermia by means of testicular biopsy and intracytoplasmic sperm injection (ICSI).

Low volume ejaculate (<1 mL) from a man with azoospermia or oligoasthenospermia, normal FSH level and normal testicular size suggests ejaculatory duct obstruction. A referral to a specialist urologist is indicated in such cases.

SEMEN ANALYSIS REPORT

Patient's Name			
Patient's D.O.B			
Partner's Name			
Partner's D.O.B			
Date of Analysis	26-08-2014	Period of abstinence	2 Days
Time of production	14:44	Time of analysis	14:45
Place of production	Create Clinic	Analysed by:	

SAMPLE INFORMATION		
	Sample Parameters (Actual Result)	WHO Parameters 2010 (Reference values)
Volume ml	1.80	≥1.5 ml
pH	7.50	7.2-8.0
Appearance	Normal	Normal
Viscosity	Normal	Normal
Liquefaction	Complete	Complete within 20 Minutes
Density $x10^6$/ml	90.00	$\geq 15x10^6$/ml
Total count $x10^6$	162.00	$\geq 39x10^6$
Motility %		
Progressive	61.0	≥ 32% (≥40%)
Non progressive	8.0	(≥40%)
Immotile	31.0	≤ 60%
Normal forms %	8.00	≥ 4%
Other Parameters		
Agglutination	NIL	
Aggregation	NIL	
Round Cells ($x10^6$/ml)	None	
Debris	None	

Conclusions:

Normozoospermia. All parameters above the lower reference limits, therefore this sample is suitable for any form of treatment.

Figure 26-1 Report of a normal semen analysis according to the WHO criteria.

Increased levels of antisperm antibodies (ASAs) IgA and IgG have been associated with male factor subfertility. Antisperm antibodies reduce the sperm progression through the cervical mucus and the zona pellucida. However, the exact role of ASAs, the level that is clinically significant and the management of the affected couples are still unclear.[14]

The fertility ultrasound scan

An accurate, noninvasive assessment of the female pelvic organs has become feasible due to recent advances in u/s technology. The scan performed for the evaluation of subfertility is called a fertility scan. As opposed to other types of scans (such as the gynecological or the early pregnancy scans), a fertility scan is focused on specific aspects related to the female fertility potential.

An advanced fertility scan requires high-resolution equipment with sensitive color and spectral Doppler modalities. Although a 3D facility is not absolutely necessary, it is desirable as it can eliminate the need for additional tests such as hydrosonography or hysteroscopy. Precise imaging of the female pelvic organs requires the scan to be performed transvaginally.

A fertility scan can provide different but useful information when performed in different times of the menstrual cycle. Traditionally it was recommended that fertility scans should be arranged in the beginning of the cycle, most studies suggesting day 2 or 3 for a more accurate assessment of ovarian reserve. A mid-cycle scan, however, could provide information on the dominant follicle and the quality of the endometrium. A scan in the luteal phase of the cycle can reveal the presence of a corpus luteum as a proof of ovulation. It is clear that some compromise has to be made for the timing of the scan. However, we believe that it is quite important to determine whether a "good quality" dominant follicle is present and also to assess the endometrial response to follicular development. For women with a regular 28- to 30-day cycle, these assessments would prerequisite a scan ideally on day 10, 11, or 12. A comprehensive fertility scan should include all the data shown in Table 26-2.

Table 26-2 Features assessed with a comprehensive fertility scan (day 10–12 of a regular, 28-day menstrual cycle)

Uterus	Position Mobility Dimensions Identification of fibroids or adenomyosis Uterine arteries Doppler assessment (peak systolic velocity, pulsatility index) Congenital malformations (mainly with a 3D scan)
Endometrium	Thickness Morphology Identification of polyps Doppler assessment Assessment of cavity with hydrosonography
Ovaries	Position Mobility Morphology Accessibility for oocyte retrieval Dimensions, volume Identification of cysts (simple, endometriotic, dermoid, complex, etc.) Antral follicle count Stromal blood flow Doppler assessment Identification of a dominant follicle, its dimensions, and the perifollicular blood flow
Fallopian tubes	Identification of hydrosalpinx Assessment of patency with HyCoSy
Pouch of Douglas	Presence of free fluid Identification of masses

Uterus

The scan should ideally show an anteverted uterus, measuring about 75 mm in length (from fundus to cervix) with a normal myometrium. Good diastolic velocities with a mean pulsatility index (PI) <3 in the blood flow of uterine arteries are favorable signs. Abnormal findings consist of large intramural fibroids (especially in close proximity to the endometrium), submucous fibroids, excessive adenomyosis (especially close to the endometrium), and high-resistance uterine artery blood flow.

Transverse imaging of the uterus could raise the suspicion of an arcuate, subseptate, bicornuate, or didelphys uterus. If 3D facilities are available, such an investigation would help with high accuracy to confirm or exclude those anomalies and also to differentiate between each other (Figure 26-2). Otherwise, an outpatient hysteroscopy will need to be added in the evaluation of the woman in order to understand the degree to which such abnormalities will affect her fertility potential and if there is need for further management. It's our policy to perform as a routine a 3D scan to obtain a coronal plane of the uterus, not only to identify such congenital malformations but also to demonstrate the precise position of any submucous fibroids (Figure 26-3) and to assess the appearance of the junctional zone between the endometrium and the myometrium in cases of suspected adenomyosis (Figure 26-4).

Endometrium, receptivity

A day 10–12 scan should normally demonstrate a triple layer endometrium with a thickness greater than 7 mm. A clear layer of mucus might also appear in the cervical canal. Vessels (spiral arteries) extending into the triple layer should appear after applying color Doppler (Figure 26-5). A thin or echogenic endometrium and the presence of an endometrial polyp greater than 5 mm in diameter are not favorable signs.

Although the endometrial scan can usually raise the suspicion of a polyp, sometimes it is difficult to differentiate whether that is actually a polyp (especially if it's less than 10 mm in size) or an endometrial fold or even a small submucous fibroid. A 3D scan can contribute

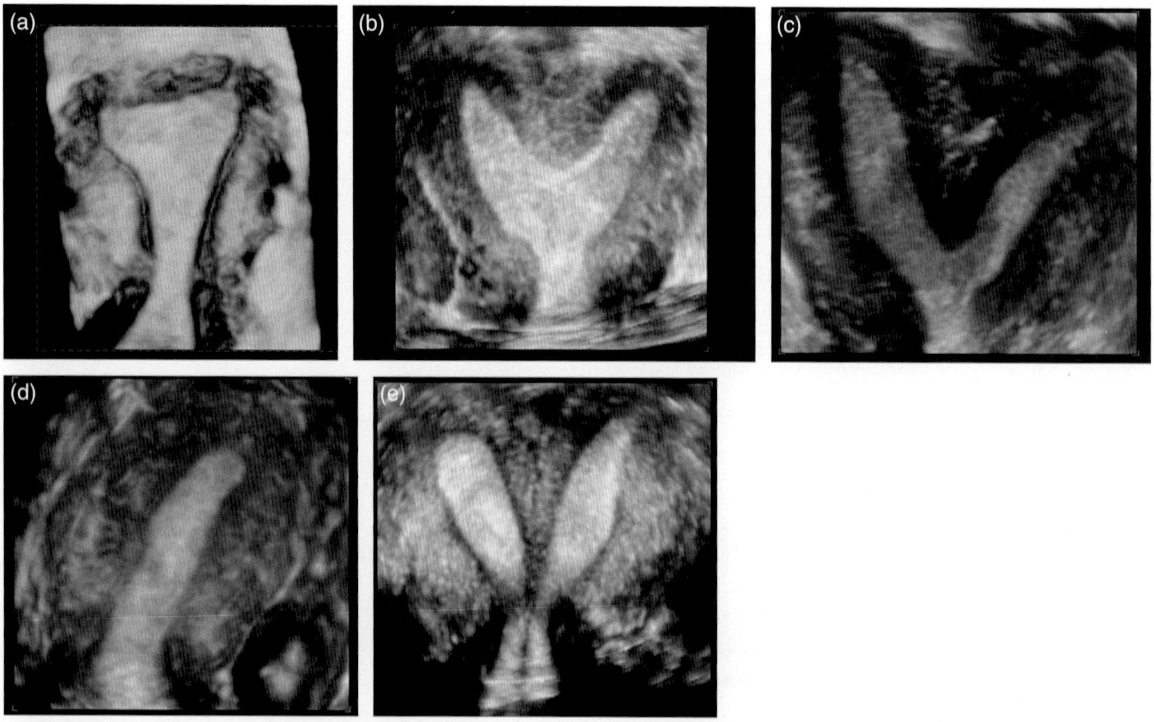

Figure 26-2 3D transverse coronal u/s view of the cavity of: (a) a normal; (b) an arcuate; (c) a subseptate; (d) a unicornuate; (e) a didelphys uterus.

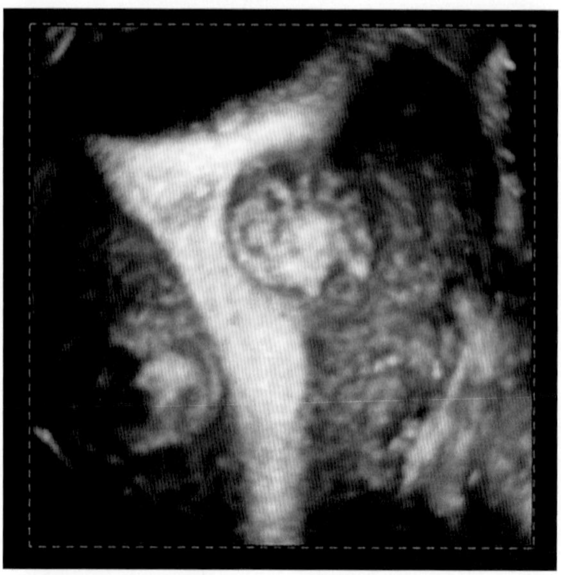

Figure 26-3 3D transverse coronal u/s view of the cavity of a uterus with a submucous fibroid.

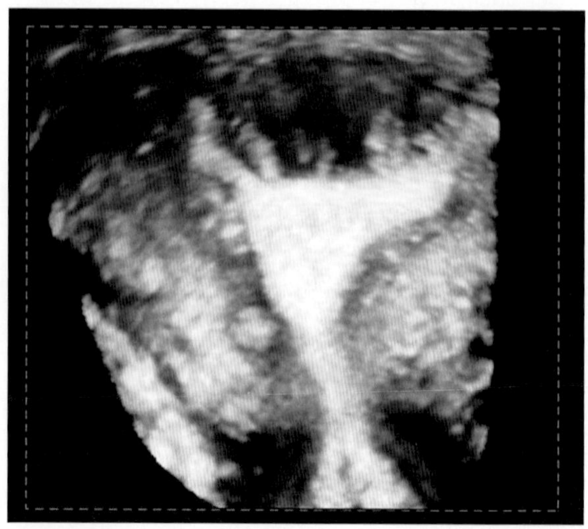

Figure 26-4 3D transverse coronal u/s view of a uterus with severe adenomyosis.

toward such a clarification; however, in order to achieve a more accurate diagnosis in cases of suspected intrauterine adhesions, sonohysteroscopy is usually recommended. Sonohysteroscopy is a simple technique, performed with the infusion of a negative contrast (saline) into the uterine cavity through a catheter during vaginal ultrasound; it can easily be performed at the same time as the tubal patency test (HyCoSy) or

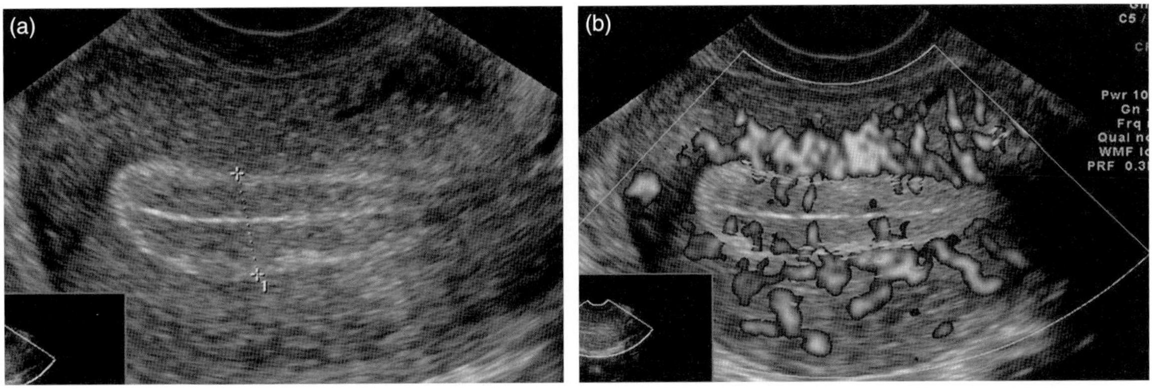

Figure 26-5 (A) u/s view of a mid-cycle receptive endometrium; (B) color Doppler depicts spiral arteries extending into the triple layer.(A)(B)

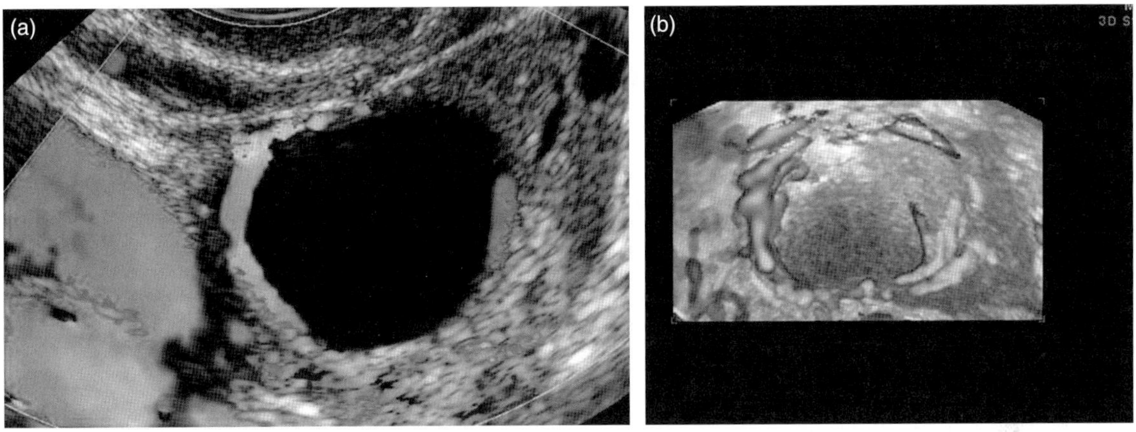

Figure 26-6 Ring of blood vessels around a dominant follicle as demonstrated with (A) color Doppler and (B) 3D scan.(A)(B)

independently in cases where it is decided that a HyCoSy is not necessary. Alternatively, outpatient hysteroscopy would easily establish the diagnosis of an endometrial polyp, submucous fibroid, or Asherman's syndrome. It is recommended that big endometrial polyps (greater than 5 mm), submucous fibroids and endometrial adhesions may require hysteroscopic removal before any type of fertility treatment begins.

Assessing endometrial receptivity is an important aspect of fertility investigation. Ultrasound scanning assessment is based on endometrial thickness and morphology in conjunction with an estimation of the blood flow velocities in the uterine arteries using Doppler. An endometrial thickness of 7 mm or more, a triple layer appearance and a uterine artery pulsatility index (PI) <3 are considered reliable markers of adequate receptivity. More recently, the visualization of the spiral arteries extending into the layer of the endometrium has been correlated with good receptivity. Older methods of endometrial assessment including endometrial biopsy for analysis and correlation with various molecular and biochemical markers can be abandoned due to low specificity and the invasive nature of technique.

Ovarian reserve assessment

The volume of each ovary is calculated by measuring the organ in three dimensions. There should be five or more antral follicles (mean diameter 2 mm–9 mm) scattered in the stroma of each one of the ovaries. Ideally, the stromal blood flow velocity should be 6 cm–12 cm/sec. On the day 10–12 scan, a dominant follicle should normally be present in one of the ovaries, with a mean diameter of 16 mm–18 mm and with a ring of blood vessels around the follicle demonstrated with color Doppler (Figure 26-6). The perifollicular peak systolic velocity (PSV) at this stage is expected to be 5 cm–10 cm/sec. The mobility of each ovary in relation to the uterus can be assessed in response to abdominal palpation.

Abnormal findings consist of the presence of ovarian cysts (simple, endometriotic, dermoid, complex), a polycystic appearance of the ovaries, absence of a dominant follicle, low ovarian volume (less than 3 mL for the non-dominant ovary), less than four or five antral follicles and low velocity in stromal blood flow (PSV less than 6 cm/sec). Ovarian cysts may have to be removed before starting fertility treatment, especially if they are large and complex cysts. Small simple cysts usually do not require surgery. The evidence on whether the endometriotic cysts should be removed is controversial. For endometriomas measuring less than 5 cm, especially with previous surgery to the ovaries or in a woman with low ovarian reserve or over the age of 40 it would be wiser to proceed with no delay to fertility treatment.

The prevalence of polycystic ovaries in the population of women with subfertility is around 33% (though many women remain asymptomatic) and is the most common cause of anovulatory subfertility. Polycystic ovaries can be easily differentiated from normal ovaries with the day 8–10 scan. By definition, they are larger and each has more than 12 small follicles.[15]

The fertility scan should be able to determine if the PCO is ovulatory or anovulatory. Moreover, women with PCOS are known to exhibit an excessive response to ovarian stimulation with gonadotrophins; they are at an increased risk of ovarian hyperstimulation syndrome (OHSS).[16] Lower doses of gonadotrophins may be considered. PCO patients with higher ovarian stromal blood flow velocities may be experiencing over response to low dose gonadotrophins thus increasing their risk of OHSS.[17, 18]

An increasing number of women delay conception until their late thirties or even early forties. This has resulted in a significant increase in subfertility, which is due to aging of oocytes and lower ovarian reserve. Thus, assessing a woman's ovarian reserve is an important aspect of the evaluation in fertility investigation. The role of u/s scan in such an assessment is widely recognized.[19] Ovarian volume, antral follicle count (AFC), and ovarian stromal flow are the main parameters that reflect ovarian reserve and response. Ovarian volume less than 3 mL or less than 5 antral follicles in total suggests diminished ovarian reserve. The standard 2D measurement of the AFC is considered accurate. Doppler measurement of PSV in one or two stromal vessels is a simple technique that can provide complementary information when assessing ovarian response.[20] Difficulty in visualizing stromal vessels or PSV less than 6 cm/sec suggests low ovarian reserve.[21]

Ovarian reserve has been traditionally assessed with an FSH blood test at the beginning of the menstrual cycle, but this is an indicator with low sensitivity. More recently, the blood test for AMH has been introduced in the evaluation of the subfertile woman. The AMH blood test can be performed on any day of the cycle and is considered as an accurate indicator of ovarian reserve. It is not clear so far if a hormonal assessment is absolutely necessary in the evaluation of ovarian reserve, especially if advanced u/s facilities are available to an experienced clinician.[22, 23] In our practice, we have found u/s parameters accurate and predictive of ovarian response for women undergoing treatment. However, for women over 35 years old with a suspected low ovarian reserve we recommend an AMH blood test in order to confirm (or refute) the findings from ultrasound.

The lack of a dominant follicle on the day 10–12 scan usually suggests ovarian dysfunction. But even if a dominant follicle with appropriate size is present, it doesn't necessarily mean that it contains a "good quality" oocyte. Perifollicular vascularity is an important indicator of the oocyte quality. Optimal peri-follicular flow as demonstrated with color or power Doppler (more than 50% of the follicular perimeter) and an adequate PSV in the peri-follicular vessels (more than 10 cm/sec) have been associated with the production of "good quality" oocytes and embryos.[24, 25]

Tubal patency assessment

Assessment of the fallopian tube patency in the outpatient evaluation of the infertile couple is quite important, as tubal problems are present in about 30% of the subfertile patients.[26] Fallopian tubes are not normally visible with u/s imaging. Hydrosalpinges on the other hand are generally easily visible even by operators with moderate experience.

A tubal patency test can be avoided in cases of obvious bilateral hydrosalpinges, low ovarian reserve, and severe male factor problem. IVF tends to be the only treatment option in such cases, and the result of a tubal patency test would not change the management of the situation.

The most widely used technique to assess tubal patency is x-ray hysterosalpingography (HSG), which also offers the added advantage of evaluating the uterine cavity for defects like fibroids and polyps. Alternatively, laparoscopy with chromopertubation can be used for tubal patency assessment. Laparoscopy can additionally provide information about other pelvic pathology, such as endometriosis and peritubular adhesions, but there is growing evidence against performing laparoscopy as a routine for tubal patency due to its high cost and morbidity. Some abnormalities detected at the time of laparoscopy, however, can also be treated during the procedure.

Although HSG has been the gold standard for confirmation of tubal patency, its use for the outpatient evaluation of the couple is restricted by the demand of x-ray facilities. The development of HyCoSy has offered an alternative to HSG, as it seems to provide similar information regarding tubal patency and the uterine cavity.[27] HyCoSY can be combined with the fertility scan and performed following the sonohysteroscopy. From the patient's perspective, HyCoSy seems to be a more acceptable technique compared to HSG, with significantly less total pain scores.[28]

The original HyCoSy technique consists of injecting 10 mL of a positive contrast (Echovist, Schering AG, Berlin, Germany) into each fallopian tube through a balloon catheter, in order to demonstrate fill of the tubes and spill of medium into the peritoneal cavity. Its main risks involve infection and allergic reaction to the contrast medium. For this reason it is carried out under antibiotic prophylaxis and is not offered to patients with a known allergy to the medium. The authors have adapted the original technique by injecting less Echovist (only 2–5 mL) slowly into each tube and by using a fine intrauterine insemination catheter instead of the balloon catheter. Those modifications have helped to eliminate side effects and reduce patient discomfort without compromising effectiveness.

Outpatient hysteroscopy

Routine hysteroscopy in subfertility cases has little benefit, especially if high-resolution u/s equipment with advanced 3D technology is available for use by an experienced clinician. Sonohysteroscopy in combination with a 3D scan can accurately give the diagnosis in most cases of uterine-factor subfertility Assessment of endometrial polyps, submucous fibroids, endometrial adhesions, and congenital malformations of the uterus, including arcuate, subseptate, and bicornuate can be performed. However, hysteroscopy is the only diagnostic tool that allows a direct, panoramic visualization of the uterine cavity. It is very important for the diagnosis of uterine abnormalities when a 3D scan is not available and for confirmation and mapping of any filling defects identified previously by sonohysteroscopy, HyCoSy, or HSG.

Outpatient hysteroscopy involves the use of miniaturized endoscopic equipment to examine the uterine cavity without the need for general anesthesia. Outpatient hysteroscopy can be successfully completed within 15–30 minutes; recent advances in endoscopic technology and equipment have enabled the development of operative hysteroscopic procedures in an outpatient setting. Minor procedures such as endometrial polypectomy, removal of small submucous fibroids, and endometrial adhesiolysis can be performed at the same time as a diagnostic study.[29]

Office hysteroscopy is considered a safe, convenient, well-tolerated, and cost-effective diagnostic tool. Variations in the equipment, adaptations in the technique, and pharmacological agents have been advocated in order to minimize patient discomfort and pain. It allows for more rapid mobilization and recovery of the patient as well as for high and equivalent levels of patient satisfaction compared to the traditional day-case hysteroscopy under general anesthesia.[30] It can be performed in an appropriately sized, fully equipped multipurpose office examination room. The clinician should have the necessary skills and expertise to carry out such a procedure. With the patient in dorsal lithotomy position, the hysteroscope is introduced into the vagina and the cervix. The panoramic view of the uterine cavity is achieved if the hysteroscope is placed at the junction of the upper cervical canal and the lower uterine segment. It can then be advanced into the cavity for a closer view.

Routine administration of opiate analgesia before the procedure should be avoided as it has been related to adverse effects, such as nausea, vomiting, and bradycardia.[31] Women could instead be advised to take standard doses of nonsteroidal anti-inflammatory agents (NSAIDs), such as ibuprofen or diclofenac, about one hour before their scheduled appointment in order to reduce the pain in the post-operative period.[32]

Outpatient diagnostic hysteroscopy is performed with miniature hysteroscopes, which help to reduce the patient's discomfort (2.7 mm with a 3 mm–3.5 mm sheath). Hysteroscopes could be equipped with 0° or fore-oblique optical lenses; 0° hysteroscopes are more intuitive, facilitating entry through the cervical canal and thus minimizing discomfort and the risk of uterine trauma. On the other hand, offset distal lenses (e.g., 12°, 25°, 30°) offer a wider field of view, enabling visualization of the tubal ostia with minimal external movement of the hysteroscope. There is not sufficient evidence to recommend 0° or fore-oblique lenses for routine diagnostic hysteroscopy, and the choice of the equipment is left to the discretion of the operator.[33, 34] Fore-oblique lenses seem to be advantageous for operative hysteroscopy as they facilitate visualization of the ancillary instrumentation. There is also not enough evidence to support the use of either the rigid or flexible hysteroscope for routine outpatient hysteroscopy. The flexible one is associated with less pain and discomfort for the patient. The rigid is associated with less failed procedures and reduced cost. It may provide better images and is easier to sterilize and maintain.[35]

Proper distension of the endometrial cavity is very important for a successful hysteroscopy. Carbon dioxide has traditionally been used as distension medium, but more recently tends to be replaced by normal saline. Neither seems to be superior in reducing pain, but normal saline appears to reduce the incidence of vasovagal episodes and also reduces the total time needed for the procedure and provides improved image quality.[36, 37] Use of bipolar electrosurgery in the context of hysteroscopy requires normal saline to act both as distension and conducting medium.

The most serious complication of hysteroscopy is uterine trauma, mainly laceration of the cervix and uterine perforation. Factors related to uterine trauma involve blind dilatation of the cervical canal, cervical stenosis, and a deviated uterine cavity. Prostaglandin or misoprostol administration has been suggested to reduce cervical resistance and the need for cervical dilatation when hysteroscopy is performed under general anesthesia. However, routine cervical preparation with such drugs before outpatient hysteroscopy should be avoided due to the absence of any evidence of benefit in reducing pain or the risk of uterine trauma.[38]

Blind dilatation of the cervix in order to facilitate the insertion of the hysteroscope is unnecessary in the majority of the cases of office hysteroscopy and therefore should be avoided. Dilatation of the cervix in a conscious woman causes pain and discomfort; if needed, it will general require administration of local anesthetics. Routine administration of local anesthetics should be offered when there is a need for larger hysteroscope to be used (diameter of outer sheath greater than 5 mm). Use of thinner hysteroscopes and wider use of the vaginoscopic technique may diminish the need for any local anesthesia. Conscious sedation does not seem to offer any benefit in terms of pain control and patient satisfaction compared to local anesthesia.[39] As conscious sedation carries risks, it is not recommended in the routine practice of outpatient hysteroscopy.

Vaginoscopy refers to the "no touch" approach for hysteroscopy, where the hysteroscope is introduced into the vagina, the cervical canal, and the uterine cavity without need of a vaginal speculum. It helps to reduce the pain and discomfort caused by the procedure and should be offered as a routine, especially if the insertion of a speculum is expected to be difficult or extremely painful for the patient.[40] In addition, vaginoscopy allows increased external movement of the hysteroscope.

Concluding remarks

A complete evaluation of the infertile couple includes the availability of high technology ultrasound equipment and facilities for semen analysis. A medical and gynecological history and a physical examination initiate the evaluation; biochemical, hormonal, and genetic blood tests are ordered as indicated by the history and exam findings.

A detailed fertility ultrasound scan is essential for many patients. This scan will exclude gross abnormalities of the uterus and the ovaries and provide valuable information about ovarian reserve and endometrial receptivity. If needed, it is also possible to assess patency of the fallopian tubes at the same time. Three-dimensional ultrasound can replace diagnostic hysteroscopy, as it provides accurate imaging of anatomical factors distorting the endometrial cavity, like polyps, fibroids, and septa.

Outpatient hysteroscopy may be needed in the absence of a 3D scan, or in selected cases to provide a direct visualization of the endometrial cavity. Operative hysteroscopy in an office setting has enabled minor procedures to be performed at the same time as the diagnostic evaluation.

Even after a complete investigation, a proportion of the subfertile couples will be labeled as having "unexplained infertility." The cause for this is considered to be a subtle, unknown factor of infertility, not diagnosed with the conventional investigations.

References

1. Hughes EG, Brennan BG. Does cigarette smoking impair natural or assisted fecundity? *Fertil Steril* 1996; **66**(5): 679–689.
2. Grodstein F, Goldman MB, Cramer DW. Infertility in women and moderate alcohol use. *Am J Public Health* 1994; **84**(9): 1429–1432.
3. Zaadstra BM, Looman CW, te Velde ER, et al. Moderate drinking: no impact on female fecundity. *Fertil Steril* 1994; **62**(5): 948–954.
4. Friedman CI, Kim MH. Obesity and its effect on reproductive function. *Clin Obstet Gynecol* 1985; **28**(3): 645–663.
5. Persani L, Rossetti R, Cacciatore C. Genes involved in human premature ovarian failure. *J Mol Endocrinol* 2010; **45**(5): 257–279.
6. Hillis SD, Joesoef R, Marchbanks PA, et al. Delayed care of pelvic inflammatory disease as a risk factor for impaired fertility. *Am J Obstet Gynecol* 1993; **168**(5): 1503–1509.
7. Bloomfield HE, Olson A, Greer N, et al. Screening pelvic examinations in asymptomatic, average-risk adult women: an evidence report for a clinical practice guideline from the American College of Physicians. *Ann Intern Med* 2014; **161**(1): 46–53.
8. Fauser BC, Tarlatzis BC, Rebar RW, et al. Consensus on women's health aspects of polycystic ovary syndrome (PCOS): the Amsterdam ESHRE/ASRM-Sponsored 3rd PCOS Consensus Workshop Group. *Fertil Steril* 2012; **97**(1): 28–38.
9. Fumarola A, Grani G, Romanzi D, et al. Thyroid function in infertile patients undergoing assisted reproduction. *Am J Reprod Immunol* 2013; **70**(4): 336–341.
10. Bahceci M, Sismanoglu A, Ulug U. Comparison of cabergoline and bromocriptine in patients with asymptomatic incidental hyperprolactinemia undergoing ICSI-ET. *Gynecol Endocrinol* 2010; **26**(7): 505–508.
11. The ESHRE Capri Workshop. European Society for Human Reproduction and Embryology. Infertility revisited: the state of the art today and tomorrow. *Hum Reprod* 1996; **11**(8): 1779–1807.
12. World Health Organization. *WHO laboratory manual for the examination and processing of human semen*. 5th ed. Geneva: World Health Organization, 2010.
13. Schwartz D, Laplanche A, Jouannet P, David G. Within-subject variability of human semen in regard to sperm count, volume, total number of spermatozoa and length of abstinence. *J Reprod Fertil* 1979; **57**(2): 391–395.
14. Hjort T. Antisperm antibodies. Antisperm antibodies and infertility: an unsolvable question? *Hum Reprod* 1999; **14**(10): 2423–2426.
15. Rotterdam ESHRE/ASRM-Sponsored PCOS Consensus Workshop Group. Revised 2003 consensus on diagnostic criteria and long-term health risks related to polycystic ovary syndrome. *Fertil Steril* 2004; **81**(1): 19–25.
16. Engmann L, Maconochie N, Sladkevicius P, et al. The outcome of in-vitro fertilization treatment in women with sonographic evidence of polycystic ovarian morphology. *Hum Reprod* 1999; **14**(1): 167–171.
17. Zaidi J, Jacobs H, Campbell S, Tan SL. Blood flow changes in the ovarian and uterine arteries in women with polycystic ovary syndrome who respond to clomiphene citrate: correlation with serum hormone concentrations. *Ultrasound Obstet Gynecol* 1998; **12**(3): 188–196.
18. Zaidi J, Campbell S, Pittrof R, et al. Ovarian stromal blood flow in women with polycystic ovaries–a possible new marker for diagnosis? *Hum Reprod* 1995; **10**(8): 1992–1996.
19. Sharara F, Scott RJ, Seifer D. The detection of diminished ovarian reserve in infertile women. *Am J Obstet Gynecol* 1998; **179**: 804–812.
20. Engmann L, Sladkevicius P, Agrawal R, et al. Value of ovarian stromal blood flow velocity measurement after pituitary suppression in the prediction of ovarian responsiveness and outcome of in vitro fertilization treatment. *Fertil Steril* 1999; **71**(1): 22–29.
21. Younis JS, Haddad S, Matilsky M, et al. Undetectable basal ovarian stromal blood flow in infertile women is related to low ovarian reserve. *Gynecol Endocrinol* 2007; **23**(5): 284–289.
22. Hendricks DJ, Mol EW, Banksi LF, et al. Antral follicle count in the prediction of poor ovarian response and pregnancy after invitro fertilisation; a meta analysis and comparison with basal follicle stimulating hormone level. *Fertil Steril* 2005; **83**(2): 291–301.
23. McIlveen M, Skull JE, Ledger WL. Evaluation of the utility of multiple endocrine and ultrasound measures of ovarian reserve in the prediction of cycle cancellation in a high risk IVF population. *Hum Reprod* 2007; **22**(3): 778–785.
24. Nargund G, Bourne T, Doyle P, et al. Ultrasound derived indices of follicular blood flow before HCG administration and the prediction of oocyte recovery

and pre-implantation embryo quality. *Hum Reprod* 1996; **11**: 2512–2517.

25. Bhal P. Pugh N, Chui DK, et al. The use of transvaginal power Doppler ultrasonography to evaluate the relationship between perifollicular vascularity and outcome of in-vitro fertilisation treatment cycles. *Hum Reprod* 1999; **14**(4): 919–945.
26. Campbell S, Bourne TH, Tan SL, Collins WP. Hysterosalpingo contrast sonography (HyCoSy) and its future role within the investigation of infertility in Europe. *Ultrasound Obstet Gynecol* 1994; **4**(3): 245–253.
27. Strandell A, Bourne T, Berg C, et al. The assessment of endometrial pathology and tubal patency: a comparison between the use of ultrasonography and X-ray hysterosalpingography for the investigation of infertile patients. *Ultrasound Obstet Gynecol* 1999; **14**(3): 200–204.
28. Ghazeeri G, Kutteh W, Ke R. Sonohysterography (SHG); a prospective study to determine patient acceptability of SHG over hysterosalpinography (HSG) in the assessment of uterine structural abnormalities and tubal patency. *Fertil Steril* 1974; **1** (Suppl): 234–235.
29. Litta P, Cosmi E, Saccardi C, et al. Outpatient operative polypectomy using a 5 mm hysteroscope without anaesthesia and/or analgesia: advantages and limits. *Eur J Obstet Gynecol Reprod Biol* 2008; **139**: 210–214.
30. Kremer C, Duffy S, Moroney M. Patient satisfaction with outpatient hysteroscopy versus day case hysteroscopy: randomised controlled trial. *BMJ* 2000; **320**: 279–282.
31. Floris S, Piras B, Orrù M, et al. Efficacy of intravenous tramadol treatment for reducing pain during office diagnostic hysteroscopy. *Fertil Steril* 2007; **87**: 147–151.
32. Tam WH, Yuen PM. Use of diclofenac as an analgesic in outpatient hysteroscopy: a randomized, double-blind, placebo-controlled study. *Fertil Steril* 2001; **76** (5): 1070–1072.
33. Campo R, Molinas CR, Rombauts L, et al. Prospective multicentre randomized controlled trial to evaluate factors influencing the success rate of office diagnostic hysteroscopy. *Hum Reprod* 2005; **20**: 258–263.
34. Rullo S, Sorrenti G, Marziali M, et al. Office hysteroscopy: comparison of 2.7 and 4 mm hysteroscopes for acceptability, feasibility and diagnostic accuracy. *J Reprod Med* 2005; **50**: 45–48.
35. Unfried G, Wieser F, Albrecht A, et al. Flexible versus rigid endoscopes for outpatient hysteroscopy: a prospective randomized clinical trial. *Hum Reprod* 2001; **16**: 168–171.
36. Shankar M, Davidson A, Taub N, Habiba M. Randomised comparison of distension media for outpatient hysteroscopy. *BJOG* 2004; **111**: 57–62.
37. Cooper NA, Smith P, Khan KS, Clark TJ. A systematic review of the effect of the distension medium on pain during outpatient hysteroscopy. *Fertil Steril* 2011; **95**: 264–271.
38. Cooper NA, Smith P, Khan KS, Clark TJ. Does cervical preparation before outpatient hysteroscopy reduce women's pain experience? A systematic review. *BJOG* 2011; **118**(11): 1292–1301.
39. Guida M, Pellicano M, Zullo F, et al. Outpatient operative hysteroscopy with bipolar electrode: a prospective multicentre randomized study between local anaesthesia and conscious sedation. *Hum Reprod* 2003; **18**: 840–843.
40. Cooper NA, Smith P, Khan KS, Clark TJ. Vaginoscopic approach to outpatient hysteroscopy: a systematic review of the effect on pain. *BJOG* 2010; **117**: 532–539. Erratum in: BJOG 2010; **117**: 1440.

Chapter 27

Outpatient infertility management

Botros Rizk, Ibrahim El-Masri, and Rola Turki

Introduction

One in seven couples seeking to have a family will encounter infertility as a result of female problems, male problems, or both. For approximately 20% of those families seeking help for their fertility, the problem will be due to anovulation. The clinical manifestation of anovulation is oligomenorrhea where the cycle exceeds 35 days, or amenorrhea where the menstrual period occurs every six or more months apart. The evaluation of patients with anovulation has been discussed Chapter 26. Approximately 80% of patients with anovulation are normogonadotropic normoestrogenic with normal levels of follicle-stimulating hormone (FSH), luteinizing hormone (LH), and estradiol. Approximately 10% will be diagnosed with hypogonadotropic hypogonadism with low FSH and LH levels. Less than 10% will have high FSH and LH with low estradiol as a result of imminent ovarian failure.

The majority of anovulatory patients who are normogonadotropic normoestrogenic have polycystic ovarian syndrome (PCOS). The National Institutes of Health (NIH) defined PCOS based on the combination of anovulation and hyperandrogenism (Figure 27-1). More recently, the European Society of Human Reproduction and Embryology (ESHRE)/American Society of Reproductive Medicine (ASRM) Rotterdam consensus criteria (RCC) define PCOS as the presence of two of the three main features: anovulation, hyperandrogenism, and polycystic ovaries.[1, 2] The Androgen Excess Society (AES) stresses that the presence of hyperandrogenism or hirsutism as the key component of PCOS (Figure 27-1).

This chapter will cover the office management of infertility secondary to ovulatory problems. Complication of ovarian hyperstimulation will also be described.

The goal of primary treatment for patients presenting with anovulation and infertility is restoration of the normal ovarian physiology that results in selection of a single dominant follicle and subsequent mono-ovulation. The treatment is usually referred to as ovulation induction. The ovarian stimulation that is used in assisted conception such as in vitro fertilization or intrauterine insemination is usually referred to as controlled ovarian hyperstimulation.

Lifestyle modification

Lifestyle modifications such as overweight reduction, exercise, and smoking cessation are recommended. These interventions may improve insulin sensitivity and decrease androgen excess, which therefore normalizes the patient's endocrinology.

Weight reduction

Permanent weight reduction may lead to ovulation and subsequent pregnancy. A wide array of treatment strategies has been used to achieve weight reduction including behavioral counseling lifestyle, therapy pharmacological treatment and bariatric surgery (see Chapter 39). No randomized trials compare these treatments benefits in the area of infertility management. Fertility guidelines in some European countries recommend withholding treatment in all obese women with a body mass index (BMI) above 35 kg/m^2 until weight is normalized.[3, 4] Women who are overweight benefit from reduction of the glycemic load by alleviating hyperinsulinemia and its metabolic consequences.[5] The effect of different diets on PCOS patients has been studied in two randomized control trials.[6, 7] Neither specific type was superior to the other in weight loss and outcome.

Office Care of Women, ed. Martin E. Olsen and Botros Rizk. Published by Cambridge University Press.

• Chronic anovulation • Hyperandrogenemia and/or hirsutism • PCO on ultrasound	+ + +	+ + −	− + +	+ − +
NIH	✓	✓	×	×
RCC	✓	✓	✓	✓
AES	✓	✓	✓	×

Figure 27-1 NIH vs. RCC vs. AES criteria for PCOS.

Exercise

The combination of diet and exercise has proven efficacy;[8] there are no available studies that evaluate exercise alone.

Smoking cessation

Smoking accelerates follicular depletion and increases serum FSH concentrations in young smokers versus nonsmokers. Smoking may also increase spontaneous miscarriage and ectopic pregnancy. Every effort should be made to encourage patient before fertility treatment is started (see Chapter 40).

Ovulation induction in hypogonadotropic hypogonadism

Anovulation in hypogonadotrpic hypogonadism results from hypothalamic-pituitary problems. A gonadotropin-releasing hormone (GnRH) stimulation test can make the distinction between pituitary and hypothalamic etiologies. The administration of GnRH agonist will be successful in increasing the serum gonadotropins only if the pituitary gland is functional. If anovulation is related to significant weight loss, restoration of the normal weight will eventually result in return of regular ovulatory cycles.[9] A pulsatile GnRH agonist pump could achieve safe and successful outcomes in patients with functional pituitary problems. The use of the pulsatile pump restores the secretion of LH and FSH, which in turn will induce ovarian induction. If no pregnancy occurs after using the GnRH agonist pump, the next step is stimulation with gonadotropins for follicular growth and ovulation. After conception, luteal phase support using human chorionic gonadotropin or progesterone should be considered until HCG production is provided by the pregnancy.[10]

Ovulation induction in normogonadotropic induction

Multiple options exist for the treatment of anovulatory infertility patients with normogonadotropic laboratory findings. Medications include clomiphene citrate, tamoxifen, metformin, aromatase inhibitors and gonadotropins as will be discussed. Typically, anovulatory polycystic ovarian patients are started on clomiphene citrate as first line. If treatment fails or is resistant to clomiphene citrate, gonadotropins are to be used (Figure 27-2).

Anti-estrogens

Clomiphene citrate

Clomiphene citrate has been the first line treatment of anovulation since the early 1930s, as this medication is effective, safe, and inexpensive.[11]

Mechanism of action

Clomiphene citrate is a nonselective estrogen receptor antagonist that interferes with the endogenous estrogen feedback in the hypothalamic-pituitary level. Gonadotropin released by the pituitary gland is enhanced and ovarian stimulation follows.

Plan of treatment

Clomiphene citrate is started on day 3 of the menstrual cycle whether it starts spontaneously or after

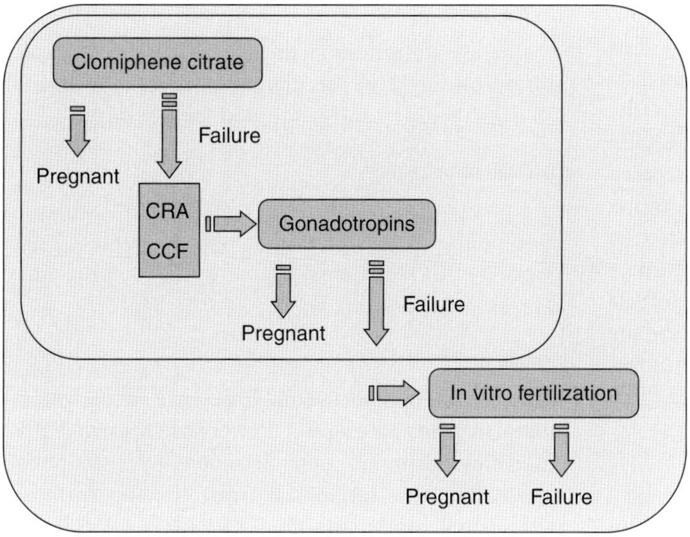

Figure 27-2 Treatment of anovulatory polycystic ovarian patients.

progesterone withdrawal. Typically the starting dose of clomiphene citrate is 50 mg/day for five days. If the patient fails to ovulate, the dose will be increased to a maximum of 150 mg/day. The starting day of clomiphene citrate has varied between the United States and Europe. When clomiphene citrate treatment was started on day 5 instead of day 1, ovulation rate and pregnancy rate were lower.[12] Routine addition of metformin to clomiphene citrate does not increase pregnancy rate.[13, 14] Also, routine addition of dexamethasone to clomiphene citrate does not increase the pregnancy rate. Estrogen vaginal cream may be useful if the endometrium is thin during the follicular phase and vaginal progesterone gel may be added when necessary.

Outcome of treatment

Ovulation is restored in approximately 80% of anovulatory patients and cumulative live births vary from 40% to 60%.[15, 16] Most pregnancies occur in the first six ovulatory cycles. Continuation of treatment to more than six cycles yields very low success.

Complications

Hot flashes and nausea may occur but are uncommon side effects. Visual problems occur in 1.5% of patients. Multiple follicular developments occur in 2%–10% of cycles. The use of clomiphene citrate for longer than 10 months has been considered a potential risk factor for ovarian cancer.[17] Severe ovarian hyperstimulation syndrome has not been reported after the use of clomiphene citrate by the preceding protocol.[18] The rate of twinning is approximately 6%.

Tamoxifen citrate

Tamoxifen is less commonly used than clomiphene citrate for ovulation induction and is not licensed by the manufacturer for the indication of ovulation induction. It has less anti-estrogenic effect on the endometrium and cervical mucus.[19]

Mechanism of action

Tamoxifen is a nonselective estrogen receptor modulator that is widely used in breast cancer treatment.

Plan of treatment

Tamoxifen is typically started on day 3 of menstrual bleeding at a dose of 20 mg/day and continued for five days. If anovulation persists, it may be increased to 40 mg/day then to 60 mg/day. In a prospective randomized controlled trial, comparing clomiphene citrate and tamoxifen citrate showed no significant change in the pregnancy rate.

Complications

The complications of tamoxifen are similar to clomiphene citrate.

Metformin

Metformin may normalize ovarian response to FSH and promote ovulation by lowering insulin resistance and hyperandrogenism.[20]

Mechanism of action

Metformin is an insulin sensitizer that reduces hepatic gluconeogenesis and insulin concentrations. It is currently used to treat patients with diabetes. Insulin resistance plays an important role in the pathogenesis of anovulation in PCOS patients. Hyperinsulinemia increases ovarian androgen production and at the same time decreases sex hormone binding globulin serum concentration. The net effect is an increased bioavailability of androgens.[21] Further more, hyperinsulinemia promotes excessive estrogen response during ovarian stimulation, which induces an early drop in the FSH.[22] This may cause follicle growth arrest in the early follicular phase showing the classic polycystic appearance of the ovaries on ultrasonography.[20]. Metformin therefore reduces these effects of hyperinsulinemia.

Plan of treatment

Metformin is started with two or three tablets of 500 mg to a maximum daily dose of 5,000 mg/day.

Outcome of treatment

First-line treatment using metformin is not superior to clomiphene citrate.[13, 23, 24] Furthermore, routine combined use of metformin and clomiphene citrate is not superior to clomiphene citrate alone. But, for second-line treatment of patients presenting with clomiphene citrate resistant anovulation and a BMI more than 35 kg/m^2, Legro, et al. found that the addition of metformin to clomiphene citrate results in 50% ovulation rate.[14] Therefore the use of metformin is recommended in patients with documented glucose intolerance.[20]

Complications

Common side effects are gastrointestinal complaints such as nausea, vomiting, and diarrhea. Lactic acidosis is very rare and has only been reported in patients with renal insufficiency or liver disease. Metformin may reduce the risk of gestational diabetes and may be safe during pregnancy.[25]

Aromatase inhibitors

Aromatase inhibitors block estrogen synthesis in the ovary and therefore stimulate gonadotropin release. They are widely used for the treatment of breast cancer. Aromatase inhibitors do not have an anti-estrogen effect on endometrium and uterus as is seen with clomiphene citrate. Inhibition of aromatase enzyme activity in granulosa cells decreases the conversion of androgen to estrogen and stops the negative feedback of estrogen on the hypothalamic-pituitary pathway.[26]

Mechanism of action

Aromatase inhibitors such as letrozole are typically started on day 3 of the menstrual cycle at a dose of 2.5 mg–5 mg/day and continued for five days.

Outcome of treatment

In a prospective randomized control trial comparing clomiphene citrate 100 mg/day and letrozole 2.5 mg/day in 74 PCOS patients, similar ovulation pregnancy rates were reported.[27]

Complications

Tulandi, et al. reported no difference of congenital malformations among 911 newborns conceived after infertility treatment with letrozole or clomiphene citrate.[28] This large trial from Canada contrasts with a small study, also from Canada, on 150 babies following treatment with letrozole demonstrating potential cardiac malformations. The second study was an oral presentation at the American Society for Reproductive Medicine annual meeting in Canada that resulted in an official warning by the manufacturer Novartis Pharmaceutical that letrozole should not be used for ovulation induction.

Gonadotropin

Patients who fail to conceive with clomiphene citrate and letrozole, or patients who are resistant to clomiphene citrate may benefit from gonadotropins (Figure 27-2). Gonadotropins are glycoproteins composed of alpha and beta subunits (Figure 27-3). The glycosylation of the gonadotropins secreted by

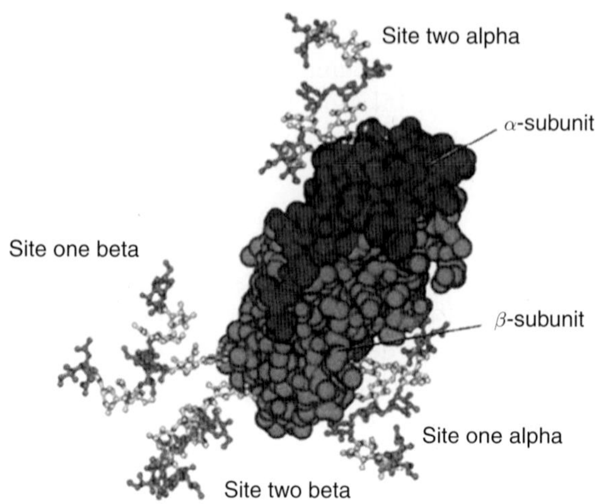

Figure 27-3 Gonadotropin composition.

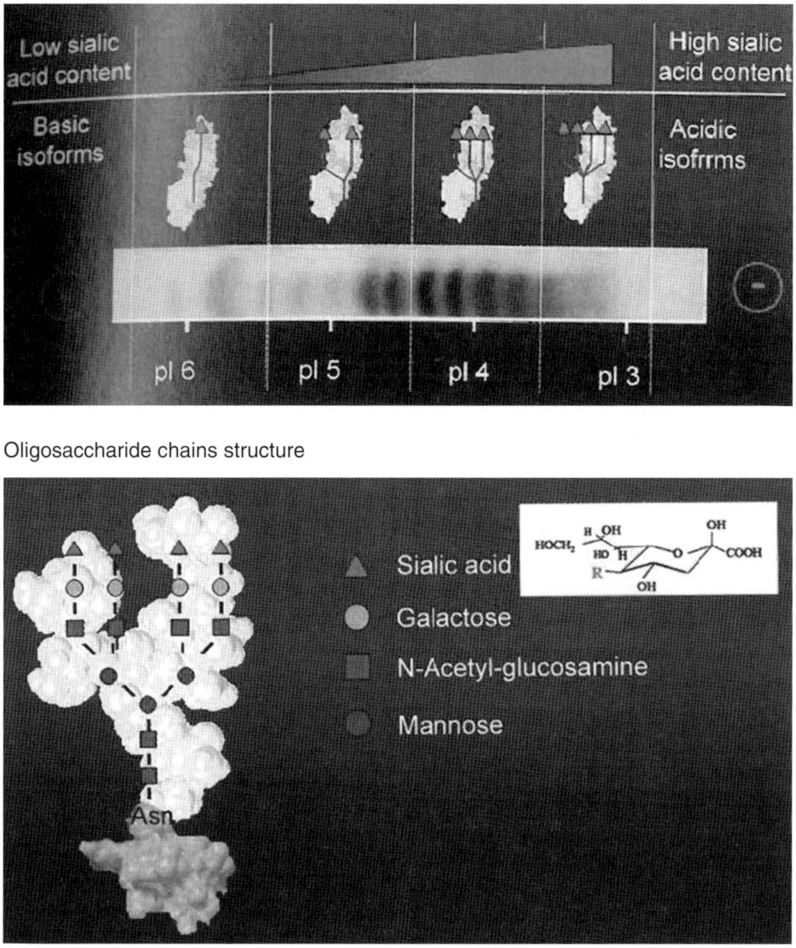

Figure 27-4 Human FSH is a mix of isoforms.

the pituitary gland vary among women of different ages and also during different times within the menstrual cycle (Figure 27-4). They have been used since the early 1960s. Initially, gonadotropins were extracted from urine of postmenopausal women, and then the urine proteins were removed which resulted in highly purified gonadotropins (Figure 27-5). FSH was then purified alone (Figure 27-6). The large number of postmenopausal women required for the extraction process, combined with the increased demand worldwide, stimulated research in an effort to produce recombinant FSH. Modern recombinant preparations improved purity, consistency and at the same time lead to less variability. Recombinant FSH has now been used worldwide for the last decade even though pregnancy outcomes are comparable between the urinary and recombinant FSH.[29]

Mechanism of action

Follicle-stimulating hormone stimulates follicular growth in ovaries. Luteinizing hormone accomplishes the resumption of meiosis. In the ovarian theca cells, the LH promotes the conversion of cholesterol to androstenedione and testosterone. Follicle-stimulating hormone then induces aromatization of these androgens in granulosa cells to estrone and estradiol, respectively. The use of gonadotropins in an anovulatory patient therefore promotes the development of follicles mainly by the FSH followed by the release of the oocytes and resumption of meiosis mainly by the LH. The two hormones work in synergy to achieve the goal of ovulation in anovulatory patients or controlled superovulation in assisted reproduction. Human chorionic gonadotropin is used in place of LH to trigger ovulation (Figure 27-7).

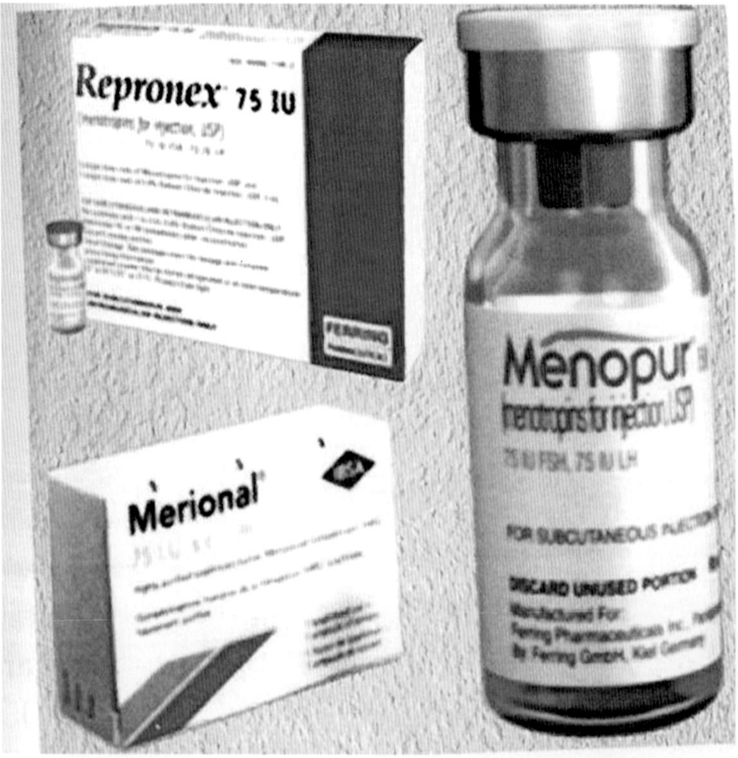

Figure 27-5 Purified gonadotropins.

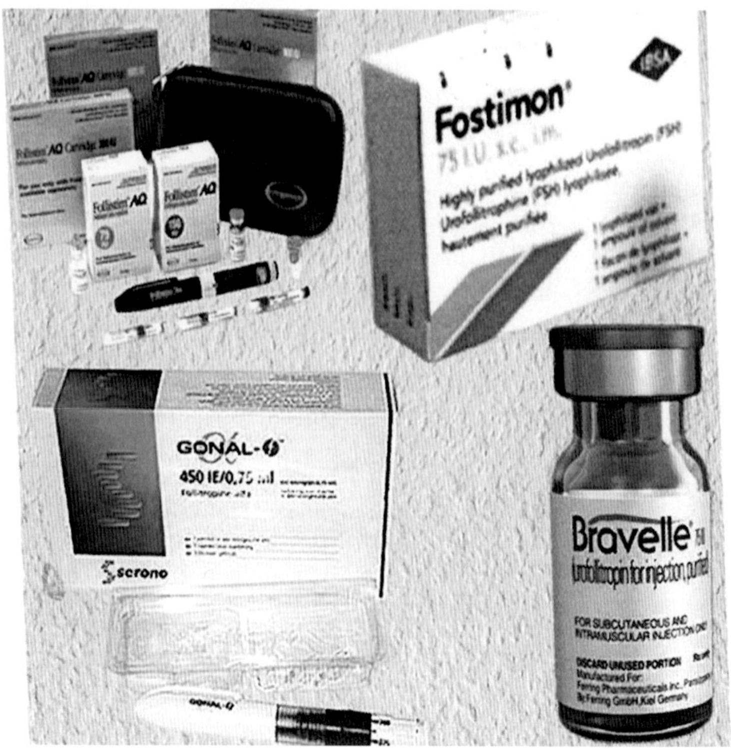

Figure 27-6 Highly purified FSH and recombinant FSH.

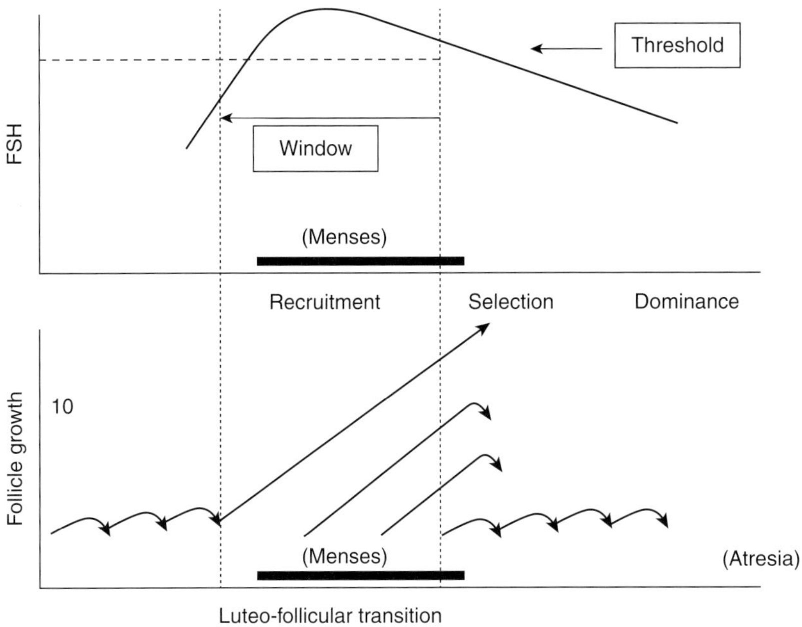

Figure 27-7 Human chorionic gonadotropin.

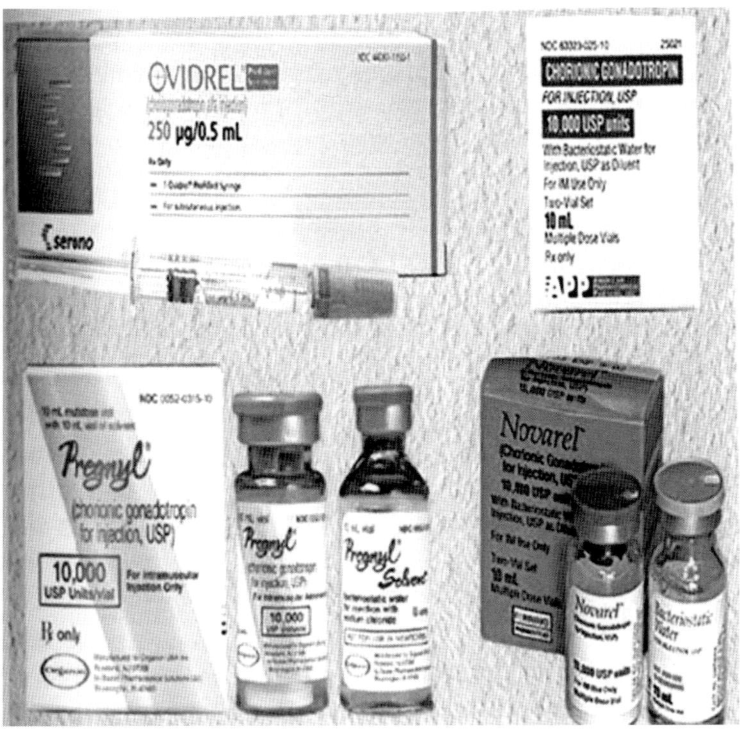

Figure 27-8 Step-up and step-down protocol.

Plan of treatment

Van Santbrink and Fauser discussed the two main protocols for ovarian stimulation, namely step-up and step-down protocol (Figure 27-8).[20] The step-up protocol is aimed at increasing low FSH doses by small increments of 37.5 IU/day until the FSH threshold is surpassed resulting in continued follicular growth and ovulation. In contrast, the step-down

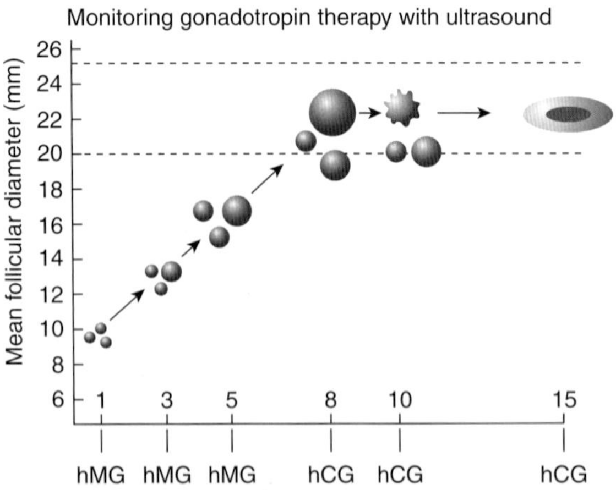

Figure 27-9 Monitoring gonadotrophin therapy with ultrasound.

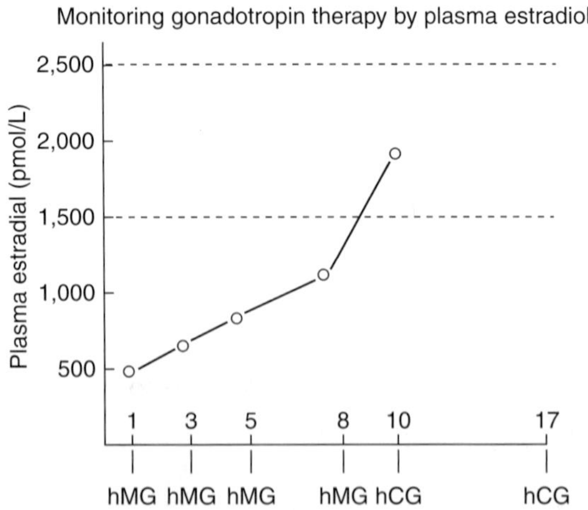

Figure 27-10 Monitoring gonadotrophin therapy by plasma estradiol.

protocol is aimed at starting a dose of FSH that is equal to the response dose,[20] and then the daily FHS dose may be decreased to 37.5 UI/day resulting in development of a single dominant follicle. Van Santbrink and Fauser noted that whereas the step-down protocol mimics the physiologic serum FSH response, the dominant follicle dose develops more quickly resulting in less ovarian hyper response and cancellation. They recommend the termination of the individual FSH dose using a step-up protocol and then consecutive treatment cycles may be performed according to the step-down protocol.[20] In case the starting dose is equal to the response dose; a fixed dose regimen could be utilized. Monitoring is performed using ultrasound and serum estradiol (Figures 27-9 and 27-10). Human chorionic gonadotropin can then be used to trigger ovulation when at least one follicle is 16 mm–18 mm in diameter. Cancellation is recommended if more than three follicles are larger than 14 mm (Figure 27-11). Luteal phase may be supported with progesterone (Figure 27-12).

Outcome of treatment

Using gonadotropins can lead to an ovulation rate of over 80% and a pregnancy rate of 60% with 45% of single live birth rate and 5%–8% in multiple birth rate.[30]

Complications

The two main complications of gonadotropins are ovarian hyperstimulation syndrome and multiple gestation pregnancy (Figure 27-13).

Ovarian hyperstimulation syndrome

Ovarian hyperstimulation remains the most serious complication of ovulation induction with gonadotropins. [33–35] Ovarian hyperstimulation syndrome (OHSS) is characterized by bilateral multiple follicular and theca lutein cysts with acute shift in body fluid distribution resulting in ascites and pleural effusion. [36] The incidence of OHSS has been estimated at 20%–33% for mild cases, 3%–6% for moderate cases, and 0.1%–2% for severe cases.[37] Mild OHSS is of no serious clinical relevance. However, severe OHSS, characterized by massive ovarian enlargement, ascites, pleural effusion, oliguria, hemoconcentration and thromboembolic phenomena, is a life-threatening complication.[37–39]

OHSS may be mild, moderate, or severe depending on the time of onset and on its spontaneous or iatrogenic etiology.[39, 40] Early OHSS presents three to seven days after ovulatory dose of HCG, whereas late OHSS presents at 12–17 days after ovulatory dose of HCG.[41, 42] Early OHSS is related to excessive response to ovulation stimulation. Conversely, late OHSS is dependent on pregnancy initiation because the stimulation comes from the HCG that is coming from the trophoblast. The majority of OHSS cases are iatrogenic following stimulation. Very rarely, OHSS may be spontaneous as a result of FSH receptor mutation resulting in the stimulation of the FSH receptors by HCG that is abundant in early pregnancy.

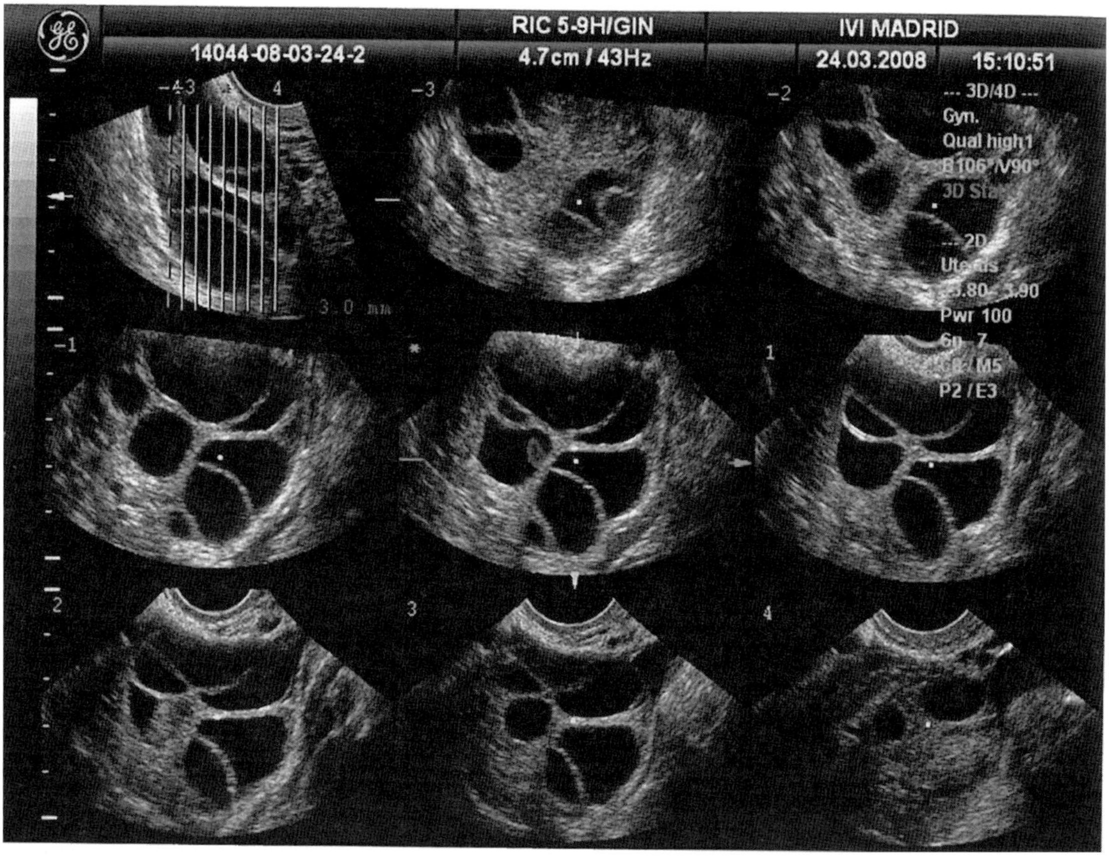

Figure 27-11 Hyperstimulated ovary.

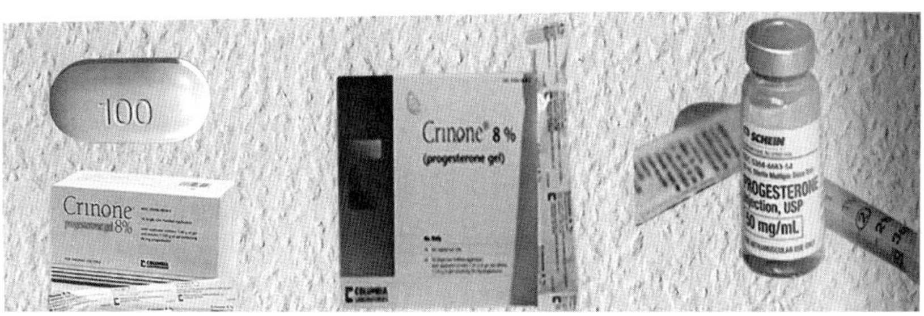

Figure 27-12 Progesterone.

Prediction of OHSS is the cornerstone of successful prevention and management (Table 27-1). OHSS can be predicted by transvaginal ultrasound and estradiol to monitor follicular development during ovarian stimulation. OHSS is managed in the office as an outpatient in its mild, moderate, and some cases of the severe form. The management is mainly by using anticoagulants, transvaginal ultrasound guided aspiration of ascitic fluid and repletion of intravascular volume (Figure 27-14).

Multiple gestation pregnancy

Families who have undergone assisted reproductive technology (ART) frequently meet the diagnosis of

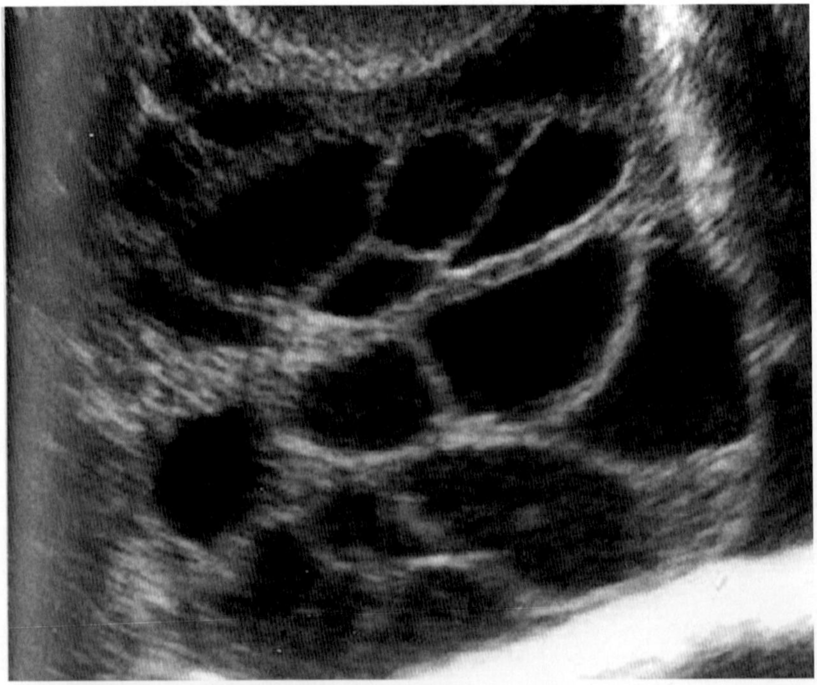

Figure 27-13 Image of a 39-year-old with PCOS after ovarian hyperstimulation.

Table 27-1 Prediction of ovarian hyperstimulation syndrome

History and physical	1. OHSS in a previous cycle 2. Polycystic ovarian syndrome 3. Young patients 4. Low body mass index 5. Hyperinsulinism 6. Allergies
During ovarian stimulation	1. High serum estradiol, rapid slope of E2, and absolute value 2. Ultrasonography a. Baseline PCO pattern b. PCO pattern of response to GnRH before gonadotropins c. Large number of follicles: >20 on each ovary 3. Doppler low intraovarian vascular resistance
Outcome of ART cycles	1. Conception cycles 2. Multiple pregnancy

multiple gestation pregnancy with joy (Figure 27-15). This happiness must be tempered by the realization that this diagnosis places the mother and fetuses at significant risk. The incidence of twin pregnancy in United States has been increasing. It has been estimated that the chance of multiple gestation pregnancy is increased by twenty-fold for twin gestation and by forty-fold for triplets/quadruplets following ART. The majority of twinning occurs after ovulation induction and intrauterine insemination; in vitro fertilization is another potential cause. A multiple gestation pregnancy causes a significant increase in both morbidity and mortality to the mother and the fetus. Congenital anomalies, preterm birth, low birth weight, cerebral palsy, intracranial hemorrhage, blindness, and chronic pulmonary disease are among many complications.

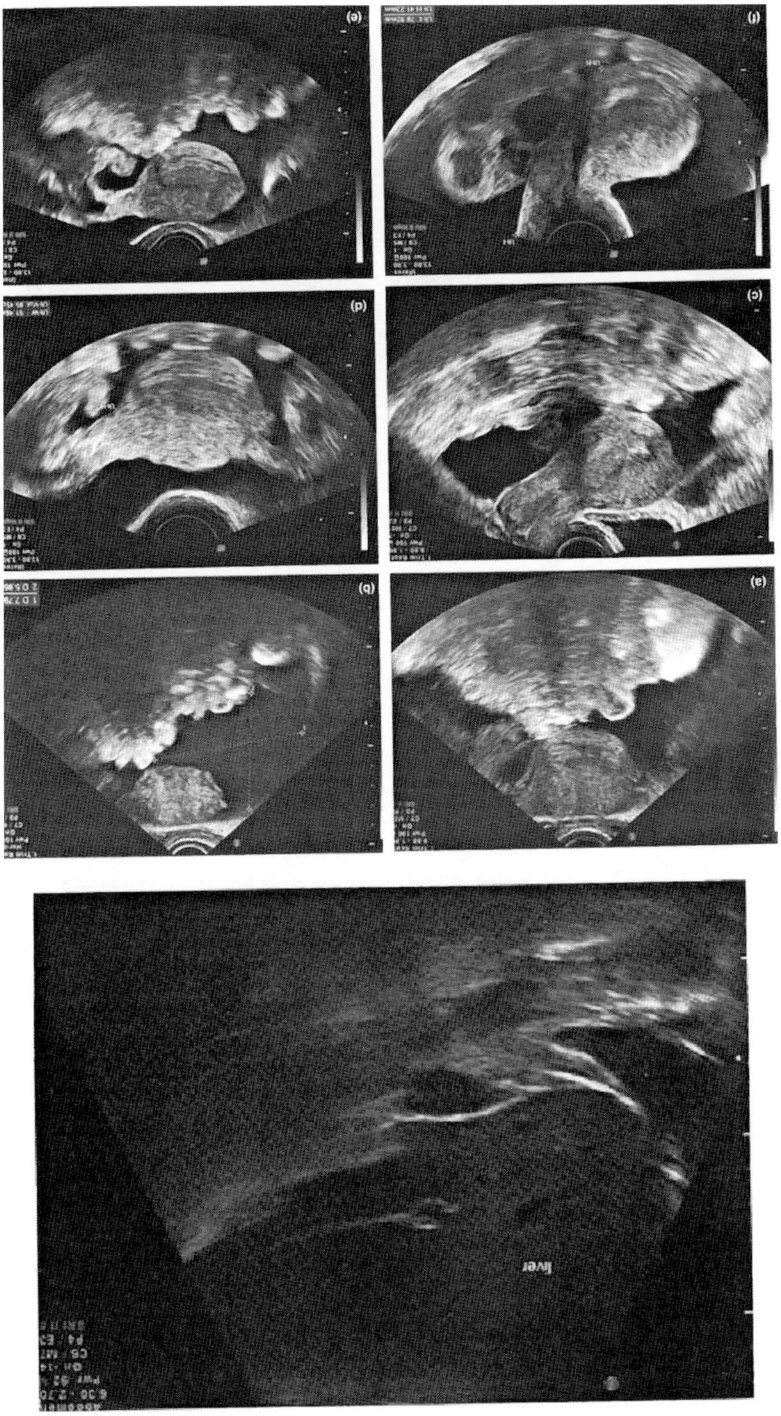

Figure 27-14 Ovarian hyperstimulation syndrome.

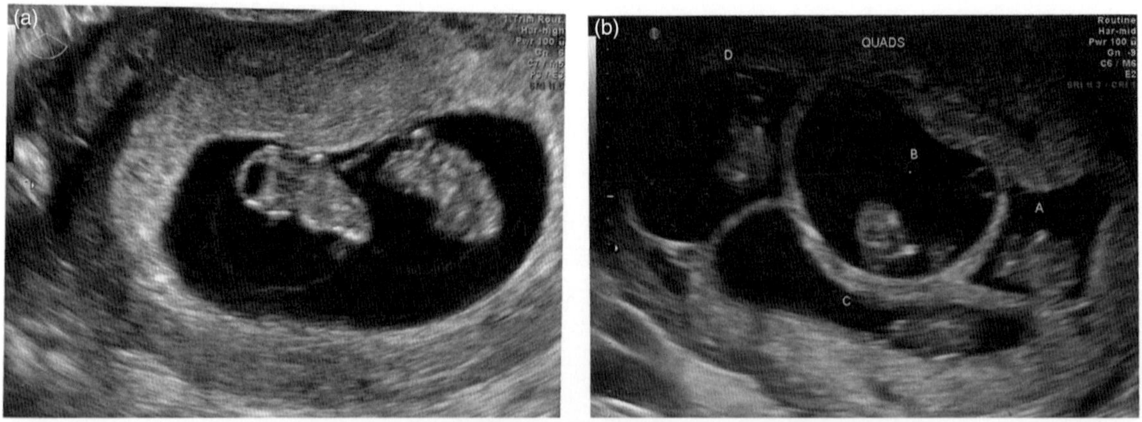

Figure 27-15 Multiple gestation pregnancy: (A) monozygotic twins, (B) quadruplet pregnancy.(A)(B)

Rizk, et al. reported that 23% of multiple pregnancy rates with 961 babies were conceived by in vitro fertilization from the birth of Louise Brown in 1978 until 1997.[43] Twins were present in 19% and triplets were present in 4% with no quadruplet or higher order multiple pregnancy. Overall, 32% were categorized with low birth weight and 6% with very low birth weight. The perinatal mortality rate was two- to threefold higher than that of infants born in England or Wales. The congenital malformation rate was in the expected range of 2.5%. Tan, et al. reported the obstetric outcome from similar series and highlighted the increase incidence from placenta previa, preeclampsia, and cesarean section.[44] Today, most IVF programs transfer only two embryos to the majority of their patients. There has also been an increased tendency toward selective single embryo transfer among IVF programs.[46]

Concluding thoughts

Infertility management is a critical contribution to the happiness and life satisfaction of the families who experience this condition. Lifestyle modifications may have important benefits for selected patients. Clomiphene citrate is the most commonly used treatment for anovulation-associated infertility. GnRH agonist pump is very useful in patients with hypogonadotropic hypogonadism. Metformin should be used only in patients with insulin resistance. The use of gonadotropins should be reserved for reproductive endocrinology specialists because of the necessity to closely monitor patients due to the risks of multiple pregnancy and ovarian hyperstimulation syndrome.

References

1. PCOS consensus. The Rotterdam ESHRE/ASRM-Sponsored PCOS consensus workshop group. Revised 2003 consensus on diagnostic criteria and long-term health risks related to polycystic ovary syndrome (PCOS). *Hum Reprod* 2004; **19**: 41–47.
2. PCOS consensus. The Rotterdam ESHRE/ASRM-Sponsored PCOS consensus workshop group. Revised 2003 consensus on diagnostic criteria and long-term health risks related to polycystic ovary syndrome (PCOS). *Fertil Steril* 2004; **81**: 19–25.
3. Balen AH, Dresner M, Scott EM, et al. Should obese women with polycystic ovary syndrome receive treatment for infertility? *BMJ* 2006; **332**: 434–435.
4. Nelson SM, Fleming RF. The preconceptual contraception paradigm: obesity and infertility. *Hum Reprod* 2007; **22**: 912–915.
5. Reaven GM. The insulin resistance syndrome: definition and dietary approaches to treatment. *Annu Rev Nutr* 2005; **25**: 391–406.
6. Moran LJ, Noakes M, Clifton PM, et al. Dietary composition in restoring reproductive and metabolic physiology in overweight women with PCOS. *J Clin Endocrinol Metab* 2003; **88**: 812–819.
7. Stamets K, Taylor DS, Kunselman A, et al. A randomized trial of the effects of two types of short-term hypocaloric diets on weight loss in women with PCOS. *Fertol Steril* 2004; **81**: 630–637.
8. Crosignani PG, Colombo M, Vegetti W, et al. Overweight and obese anovulatory patients with polycystic ovaries: parallel improvements in anthropometric indices, ovarian physiology and fertility rate induced by diet. *Hum Reprod* 2003; **18**: 1928–1932.

9. Wiksten-Almstromer M, Hirschberg AL, Hagenfeldt K. Prospective follow-up of menstrual disorders in adolescence and prognostic factors. *ACTA Obstet Gynecol Scan* 2008; **87**: 1162–1168.
10. Beckers NG, Platteau P, Eijkemans R, et al. The early luteal phase administration of estrogen and progesterone does not induce premature luteolysis in normo-ovulatory women. *Eu J Endocrinol* 2006; **155**: 355–363.
11. Pildes RB. Induction of ovulation with clomiphene. *Am J Obstet Gynecol* 1965; **15**: 466–479.
12. Dehbashi S, Vafaei H, Persanezhad M, et al. Time of initiation of clomiphene citrate and pregnancy rate in polycystic ovary syndrome. *Int J Gynaecol Obstet* 2006; **93**: 44–48.
13. Moll E, Bossuyt PM, Korevaar JC, et al. Effect of clomiphene citrate plus metformin and clomiphene citrate plus placebo on induction of ovulation in women with newly diagnosed PCOS: randomised double-blind clinical trial. *BMJ* 2006; **332**: 1485.
14. Legro RS, Barnhart HX, Schlaff WD, et al. Clomiphene, metformin, or both for Infertility in the PCOS. *N Engl J Med* 2007; **356**: 551–566.
15. Koustra E, White DM, Franks S. Modern use of CC in induction of ovulation. *Hum Reprod Update* 1997; **3**: 359–365.
16. Imani B, Eijkemans MJ, te Velde ER, et al. Predictors of patients remaining anovulatory during clomiphene citrate induction of ovulation in normogonadotropic oligoamenorrheic infertility. *J Clin Endocrinol Metab* 1998; **83**: 2361–2365.
17. Rossing MA, Daling JR, Weiss NS, et al. Ovarian tumors in a cohort of infertile women. *N Engl J Med* 1994; **33**: 771–776.
18. Homburg R. Clomiphene citrate-end of an era? A mini review. *Hum Reprod* 2005; **20**: 2043–2051.
19. Roumen FJ, Doesburg WH, Rolland, R. Treatment of infertile women with a deficient postcoital test with two antiestrogens: clomiphene and tamoxifen. *Fertility and Sterility* 1984; **41**: 237–243.
20. Van Santbrink EJ, Fauser BC. Urinary follicle-stimulating hormone for normogonadotropic clomiphene-resistant anovulatory infertility: prospective, randomized comparison between low-dose step-up and step-down dose regimens. *J Clin Endocrinol Metab* 1997; **82**: 3597–3602.
21. LaMarca A, Morgante G, Palumbo M, et al. Insulin-lowering treatment reduces aromatase activity in response to follicle-stimulating hormone in women with PCOS. *Fertil Steril* 2002; **78**: 1234–1239.
22. Coffler MS, Patel K., Dahan MH, et al. Enhanced granulosa cell responsiveness to FSH during insulin infusion in women with PCOS treated with pioglitazone. *J Clin Endocrinol Metab* 2003; **88**: 5624–5631.
23. Lord JM, Flight IH, Norman RJ. Metformin in polycystic ovary syndrome: systematic review and meta-analysis. *BMJ* 2003; **327**: 951–953.
24. Legro RS, Zaino RJ, Demers LM, et al. The effects of metformin and rosiglitazone, alone and in combination, on the ovary and endometrium in PCOS. *Am J Obstet Gynecol* 2007; **196**: 402–410.
25. Glueck CJ, Goldenberg N, Pranikoff J, et al. Height, weight and motor-social development during the first 18 months of life in 126 infants born to 109 mothers with polycystic ovary syndrome who conceived on and continued metformin through pregnancy. *Hum Reprod* 2004; **19**: 1323–1330.
26. Garcia-Velasco JA, Moreno L, Pacheco A, et al. The aromatase inhibitor letrozole increases the concentration of intraovarian androgens and improves in vitro fertilization outcome in low responder patients: a pilot study. *Fertil Steril* 2005; **84**: 82–87.
27. Bayar U, Basaran M, Kiran S, et al. Use of an aromatase inhibitor in patients with polycystic ovary syndrome: a prospective randomized trial. *Fertil Steril* 2006; **86**: 1447–1451.
28. Tulandi T, Martin J, Al-Fadhli R, et al. Congenital malformations among 911 newborns conceived after infertility treatment with letrozole or clomiphene citrate. *Fertil Steril* 2006; **85**: 1761–1765.
29. Bayram N, van Wely M, van Der Veen F. Recombinant FSH versus urinary gonadotrophins or recombinant FSH for ovulation induction in subfertility associated with polycystic ovary syndrome. *Cochrane Database Syst Rev* 2001; **2**:CD002121.
30. Mulders AG, Eijkemans MJ, Imani B, et al. Prediction of chances for success or complications in gonadotrophin ovulation induction in normogonadotrophic anovulatory infertility. *Reprod BioMed Onl* 2003; **7**: 48–56.
31. Zawadski JK, Dunaif A. Diagnostic criteria for polycystic ovary syndrome: towards a rational approach. In: Dunaif A, Givens JR, Haseltine F, eds. *Polycystic Ovary Syndrome.* Boston: Blackwell Scientific, 1992: 377–384.
32. Azziz R, Carmina E, Dewailly D, et al. Position statement: criteria for defining PCOS as a predominantly hyperandrogenic syndrome: an androgen excess society guideline. *J Clin Endocrinol Metab* 2006; **91**: 4237–4245.
33. Rizk B, Aboulghar M. Modern management of ovarian hyperstimulation syndrome. *Hum Reprod* 1991; **6**: 1082–1087.
34. Rizk B, Smitz J. Ovarian hyperstimulation syndrome after superovulation for IVF and related procedures. *Hum Reprod* 1992; **7**: 320–327.

35. Rabau E, Serr DM, David A, et al. Human menopausal gonadotrophin for anovulation and sterility. *Am J Gynecol* 1967; **98**: 92–98.
36. Rizk B, Aboulghar MA. Classification, pathophysiology and management of ovarian hyperstimulation syndrome. In: Brinsden P, ed. *A Textbook of In-vitro Fertilization and Assisted Reproduction, Second Edition*. Carnforth-Lancs, UK: The Parthenon Publishing Group, 1999: 131–155.
37. Rizk B. Ovarian hyperstimulation syndrome: epidemiology, pathophysiology. In: *Prevention and Management*. Cambridge: Cambridge University Press, 2006.
38. Rizk B, Aboulghar MA, Smitz J, RonEl R. The role of vascular endothelia growth factor and interleukins in the pathogenesis pf severe ovarian hyperstimulation syndrome. *Hum Reprod Update* 1997; **3**: 255–266.
39. Rizk B. Complications of ovulation induction II Ovarian hyperstimulation syndrome. In Dickey RP, Brinsden PR, Pyrzak R, eds. *Manual of Intrauteine Insemination and Ovulation Induction*. Cambridge: Cambridge University Press, 2010: 152–160.
40. Rizk B, Aboulghar M. Ovarian hyperstimulation syndrome. In: Rizk B, Aboulghar M, eds. *Ovarian Stimulation*. Cambridge: Cambridge University Press, 2011: 111–137.
41. Mathur RS, Akande AV, Keay SD, et al. Distinction between early and late ovarian hyperstimulation syndrome. *Fertil Steril* 2000; **73**: 901–907.
42. Lyons CA, Wheeler CA, Frishman GN, et al. Early and late presentation of the ovarian hyperstimulation syndrome: two distinct entities with different risk factors. *Hum Reprod* 1994; **9**: 792–799.
43. Rizk B, Doyle P, Tan SL, et al. Perinatal outcome and congenital malformations in in-vitro fertilizatioin babies from the Bourn-Hallam group. *Human Reprod* 1991; **6**(9): 1259–1264.
44. Tan SL, Doyle P, Campbell S, et al. Obstetric outcome of in-vitro fertilization pregnancies compared to naturally conceived pregnancies. *Am J Obstet and Gynecol* 1992; **167**(3): 778–784.
45. Hole J, Porter KB, Taylor SK, et al. Multiple pregnancy following IVF. In: Rizk B, ed. *Ultrasonography in Reproductive Medicine and Infertility*. Cambridge: Cambridge University Press, 2010: 291–296.
46. Jauniaux ERM, Rizk B. *Pregnancy After Assisted Reproductive Technology*. Cambridge: Cambridge University Press, 2011: 1–3.

Chapter 28

Polycystic ovary syndrome

Theodore Tsaltas and Meshell Stokes

Introduction

Polycystic ovary syndrome (PCOS) is an endocrine disorder characterized by disruption of the normal cyclic function of the hypothalamic-pituitary-ovarian axis. PCOS patients present to all types of women's health-care providers with various gynecologic complaints, including menstrual irregularities, infertility, and hirsutism. PCOS, however, also has significant systemic medical effects that must be considered in evaluation and management. The frequency and potential severity of PCOS make understanding the condition important for all women's health-care providers.

Scope of the problem

PCOS is poorly defined. The original report, by Stein and Leventhal in 1935, described seven women with amenorrhea, hirsutism, and enlarged, polycystic ovaries.[1] They coined the term "polycystic ovary syndrome" to describe these patients, whom they treated by ovarian wedge resection.

The variation in clinical findings in PCOS makes definition difficult. The National Institutes of Health (NIH) convened a conference in 1990 to provide expert opinion consensus for PCOS definition. The NIH criteria required hyperandrogenism, as manifested by hirsutism or serologic values, and oligomenorrhea. These criteria did not recognize ultrasound findings, and the Rotterdam criteria added polycystic ovaries on ultrasound to hyperandrogenism and oligomenorrhea, with any two of the three establishing the diagnosis. The Androgen Excess Society (AES) criteria require hyperandrogenism plus either polycystic ovaries or oligomenorrhea.[2–4]

The prevalence of PCOS depends both on definitional criteria and the population examined. Reported prevalence ranges from 1.5% to 20%, although most reports find a prevalence of 4%–5%.[5, 6] Most of these reports are from referral populations. Since there is a distinct bias in the severity of disease and distribution of symptoms in a referral population, the generalization of referral population data to the general population is difficult and potentially misleading.[7] The true population prevalence is unknown; the only large, population-based report showed a prevalence of 1.5%.[8]

Definitional criteria affect prevalence as well. The Rotterdam criteria do not require hyperandrogenism, and so produce a higher prevalence that does not reflect the pathophysiology of PCOS. The AES criteria, on the other hand, give ultrasound findings equal diagnostic weight with oligomenorrhea; in the authors' opinion, this is not well supported by the extant literature.

Given the variable criteria and presentations, PCOS should be considered as a diagnosis in the evaluation of women with oligomenorrhea and manifestations of hyperandrogenism such as acne or hirsutism, and/or infertility. The diagnosis is most strictly applied to women who have hyperandrogeniism (as manifested by either hirsutism or blood tests) and also oligomenorrhea.

Physiology of normal ovulation

PCOS involves disturbances in ovulation; it is therefore important to understand normal ovarian function. The ovarian follicles contain the oocytes and granulosa cells, along with the stroma which supports follicular function. The stromal cells produce androgens, mainly testosterone and androstenedione. These androgens are transported to the follicles where the granulosa cells convert the androgens to estrogens by aromatization.

There is a feedback loop between follicle-stimulating hormone (FSH) from the pituitary and

Office Care of Women, ed. Martin E. Olsen and Botros Rizk. Published by Cambridge University Press.

estrogens from the ovary. For most of the cycle it is a negative feedback system in which FSH stimulates the production of estradiol. This in turn reduces the production of FSH. At mid-cycle, however, this feedback loop changes to a positive one, resulting in a surge in luteinizing hormone (LH) and to a lesser extent of FSH. The LH surge is an important part of ovulation.

FSH stimulates the production of the enzyme aromatase, which is required to convert androgens to estrogens. LH stimulates the stromal theca cells to produce androgen. Thus estradiol production goes up under the stimulation of FSH and LH.

The development of the ovarian follicles does not rely on FSH until they reach about 10 mm in size. For each cycle approximately 12–20 follicles become "recruited"; they end dormancy and begin development and growth. Only one of these follicles will typically ovulate in any cycle. The rest undergo atresia and resorption. Once the follicles reach 10 mm in size, their further development is dependent upon FSH. This raises an immediate paradox. How does one follicle continue to develop while FSH levels decline? This is achieved by intra-follicular changes and intra-ovarian paracrine regulation.

FSH induces its own receptors on the granulosa cells. In this way, sensitivity to FSH increases even as levels decrease. One follicle will be more sensitive than others, and this is the one that becomes the dominant follicle. The increased sensitivity to FSH allows the dominant follicle to produce more estradiol even as FSH levels decline and the other follicles undergo atresia. The differential sensitivity of each follicle is determined by the local hormonal and paracrine environment.

Sensitivity to FSH is modulated by two hormones with antithetical functions, activin and inhibin. These are named for their effects on FSH. These peptides act both as hormones and as paracrine (i.e., is, local acting substances) ovarian regulators. As hormones, inhibin decreases FSH synthesis and secretion while activin increases FSH synthesis and secretion. activin's paracrine role increases FSH receptor binding, and induces LH receptors and aromatization within the follicle. Ovulation is then triggered by the rapid increase in estradiol and the induction of LH receptors. The exact mechanism of conversion of the negative feedback loop to a positive one is unclear; however, activin and inhibin play a significant role in the selection and promotion of the dominant follicle.

Emergence of the dominant follicle is established by day 5–7 of the cycle (where day 1 is the first day of menstrual bleeding). Although the feedback loop from ovary to pituitary is an essential part of that process, the emergence of any particular follicle as the dominant one is achieved primarily through the local factors previously described. Fundamentally the high androgen local environment converts to a high estrogen one as aromatase increases. It follows then that PCOS involves disruption and dysfunction of one or more parts of the process of follicular recruitment and development. Such a problem may involve the feedback loop, but often involves intra-ovarian functions.[9]

Pathophysiology of PCOS

The essence of PCOS is the alteration of a naturally cyclic rhythm into a steady state, the conversion of a dynamic process into a static one. Like any rhythmic function, disruption may originate from various sources and in various parts of the cycle.[10]

There may be central interruption of gonadotropin-releasing hormone (GnRH) pulsatility from the hypothalamus, such as occurs with hyperprolactinemia, stress, or anorexia. The feedback loop may be disrupted by peripheral estrogen production, as in obese patients, or from stress.

Obesity plays an important role in PCOS. Fat contains aromatase, and peripheral conversion of androgens to estrogens occurs in the peripheral fat. This estrogen production is steady, not cyclic, and may interfere in the delicate cyclic signaling between ovary and pituitary. As ovulation is impaired the ovary no longer converts androgens to estrogens, and the increased androgenic environment reduces sex hormone binding globulin (SHBG), increasing free androgen and further worsening the peripheral production of estrogens.

Androgen changes within the ovary are a critical part of the pathology of PCOS. As androgen production increases 5-alpha reduction begins to occur, producing the potent androgen dihydrotestosterone. This androgen inhibits aromatase production directly, which in turn prevents production of estradiol upon which further activin and FSH activity depend. Without activin-mediated induction of the FSH receptor, aromatase levels decline and a hyperandrogenic microenvironment is formed and perpetuated.

The androgen production of the ovary leads to increases in circulating androgens. Although testosterone is the most potent circulating androgen, it is not active in the skin. The skin is responsive to dihydrotestosterone, produced by the activity of the enzyme 5-alpha reductase (5aR) in the skin; 5aR activity produces the hirsutism and acne characteristic of PCOS.

An increased amount of circulating insulin is also an important part of PCOS in both obese and non-obese patients. Insulin acts independently of insulin-like growth factors (IGF) 1 and 2 in the ovary to increase androgen production. In the absence of sufficient FSH stimulation and ovarian aromatase activity this produces an androgen dominant micro-environment hostile to follicular development. Two conditions demonstrate the important role of hyperinsulinemia in the pathology of PCOS. Firstly, PCOS patients whose ovarian androgen production is suppressed by GnRH agonists continue to have elevated insulin levels. If, however, hyperinsulinemia is corrected, then ovarian androgen production normalizes.[11, 12]

Presentation

PCOS presents with varying combinations of four main symptoms: oligomenorrhea, hyperandrogenism, infertility, and obesity/glucose intolerance.[13] Efforts have been made to separate phenotypes for differential management. This has been unrewarding, and in the typical practice setting unnecessary.

The majority of women with PCOS will present with varying forms of menstrual irregularity; 20%–50% of women with PCOS have amenorrhea (defined as no menses for three consecutive regular cycles or six months), but 30% will have polymenorrhea or menometrorrhagia. Overall nearly 80% of women with PCOS have menstrual irregularities. Despite the frequency of menstrual disorders in PCOS it is important to remember that 20% of women with PCOS have normal menses.

Hyperandrogenism is another common presenting complaint; 70% of patients with PCOS will complain of cosmetically significant hirsutism or acne.[14] Infertility is the other major presenting symptom of PCOS.

Metabolic syndrome is a specific presentation and sequelae of PCOS.[15] It is characterized by central obesity, glucose intolerance, and hyperlipidemia. Although presentation with a primary complaint of diabetes or obesity is uncommon, both are important associated findings. Nearly 70% of PCOS patients are obese, but it is not a universal feature of PCOS.

Table 28-1 Criteria for metabolic syndrome [15]

BP	≥130/85
Waist circumference	≥35 inches
Fasting blood sugar	≥100 mg/dL
HDL (high-density lipoprotein)	≤50 mgs/dL
Triglycerides	≥150 mgs/dL

Approximately one-third of PCOS patients have a normal body mass index (BMI). The diagnostic criteria for metabolic syndrome are listed in Table 28-1. Note that patients may have metabolic abnormalities, notably glucose intolerance, or obesity, and not fulfill criteria for the diagnosis of metabolic syndrome.[16]

Infertility is common in women with PCOS secondary to anovulation. PCOS accounts for approximately three-fourths of anovulatory infertile women. Although most PCOS patients will be diagnosed from their menstrual and other symptoms, some will receive their diagnosis when presenting with infertility.

Evaluation and diagnosis

PCOS is a diagnosis of exclusion. Other readily identifiable causes of anovulation or hyperandrogenism must be eliminated before applying the term PCOS. These potential diagnoses include late-onset congenital adrenal hyperplasia, thyroid disease, hyperprolactinemia, along with adrenal and central nervous system tumors.

Patient history details are important. These include age at menarche and the sequence of pubertal events, as well as the time of onset of irregular menses and hirsutism. PCOS patients commonly have menstrual irregularities from the time of menarche, rather than later acquired abnormalities. Details of hirsutism should be elicited, with appropriate sensitivity to the personally troublesome nature of the finding. The frequency of shaving and plucking of hair, as well as the spread of affected areas and associated acne, are all significant. In contrast to the menstrual irregularities of PCOS, manifestations of hyperandrogensim are typically slowly progressive through the teen years into the early twenties. Rapid and sudden onset of hirsutism is suggestive, although not diagnostic, of either a tumor or exogenous androgen exposure. The patient's weight history must also be obtained. A history of nipple discharge is significant. Patients should be screened for depression and anxiety due to the association of these problems with PCOS.

Examination and assessment for hyperandrogenism and adrenal disease is important. Waist circumference should be measured for evaluation of truncal obesity. Moon facies and striae may suggest Cushing's disease, although this diagnosis is exceptionally rare.[17] Acanthosis nigricans, a darkening and thickening of skin folds, is a nonspecific finding seen with hyperandrogensim and insulin resistance. It may be found in any skin folds, but most commonly in the posterior folds of the neck, in the groin creases, and beneath the breasts. Breast examination should include attempts to elicit expressible galactorrhea.

Table 28-2 Examination considerations for patients with suspected PCOS

Blood pressure
Weight/BMI
Abdominal circumference
Acanthosis nigricans
Hirsutism
Acne
Moon facies
Striae

Hirsutism is quantified using the Ferriman-Gallwey score. See Figure 29-2 in Chapter 29, which shows how this score is calculated.[18] A score of >8 is diagnostic of hirsutism. The presentation of hirsutism is, however, dependent on ethnicity and local custom. Although men and women have the same number of hair follicles, the number of follicles varies substantially by ethnicity. Broadly, Asians have the fewest hair follicles, whereas southern Europeans have the most. Genetic hair distribution (familial hypertrichosis) must be differentiated from androgen dependent hair. The Ferriman-Gallwey score is quite helpful in this regard, counting only hair in androgen-dependent areas, but the practitioner must still be sensitive to the ethnic variations in hirsutism.[19] What is normal in a European woman may be marked hirsutism in an Asian woman. Finally, shaving and other depilatory practices may complicate diagnosis, and the skin must be carefully evaluated for stubble, follicles, and darkening.

Significant examination considerations for patients with suspected PCOS are listed in Table 28-2.

Ultrasound of the ovaries is indicated for all patients where PCOS is suspected. Contrary to common conceptions of PCOS, it is not overt ovarian "cysts" that are significant on ultrasound, nor the "string of pearls" array of cortical cysts. Rather, it is the number of pre-antral follicles seen on ultrasound.

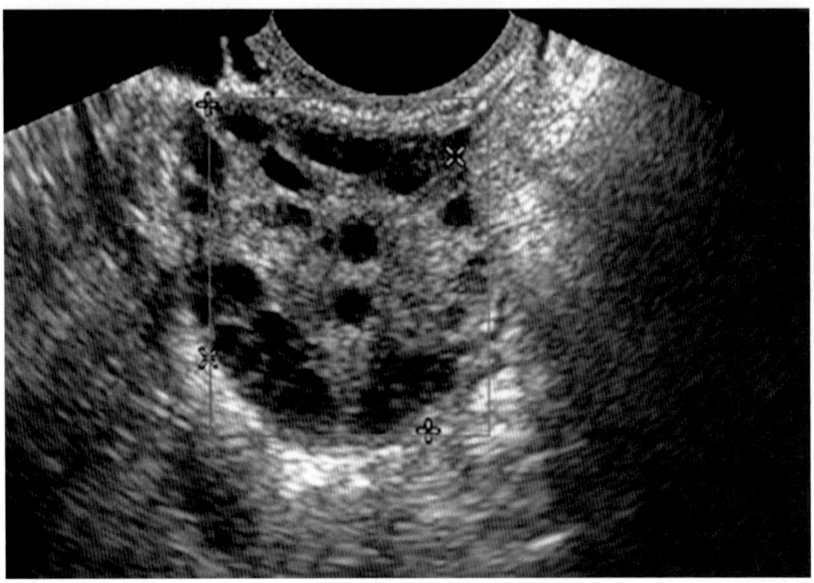

Figure 28-1 Ultrasound of a polycystic ovary.

Table 28-3 Blood tests considered for evaluation of PCOS

Labs fasting, day 3–5 of cycle (any day if amenorrheic)
Serology
FSH
LH
TSH
Prolactin
Testosterone (free)
17-OH progesterone
Fasting blood sugar
Cholesterol/HDL/LDL/triglycerides
Liver function tests
If hirsute or suspected adrenal disease, add:
0800 cortisol
DHEAS
Androstenedione
If suspected metabolic syndrome, add:
2-hour oral glucose tolerance test

This is consistent with the pathophysiology of the disorder as previously detailed. Pre-antral follicles are those less than 10 mm in size. Often these are not even reported, let alone counted, and so ultrasound evaluation should be performed by someone well versed in ob/gyn sonography and the diagnostic criteria for PCOS. A patient with 12 or more pre-antral follicles in one ovary meets the sonographic criteria for PCOS. Figure 28-1 is an example of an ovary with the sonographic criterion for PCOS.

Despite the popularity of ultrasound in making a diagnosis of PCOS, it is an unreliable single criterion; 36% of normally cycling women meet the strictest ultrasound criterion for PCOS, whereas 34% of PCOS patients have sonographically normal ovaries.[20]

Blood testing is an essential part of PCOS evaluation. Hyperandrogenism can be evaluated with a free testosterone level. Although this test is much more expensive than a total testosterone, it accounts for the decrease in SHBG seen in PCOS. This decrease can artifactually reduce total testosterone into the normal range in women. If the patient is hirsute or there is suspected adrenal disease, then androstenedione and dehydroepiandrosterone sulfate (DHEAS) should also be measured. Although dihydrotestosterone is the most potent androgen its effects are purely local within the ovary and the hair follicles. It circulates in negligent amounts, and is therefore not required.[21]

FSH and LH should be measured. There is no specific ratio which is perfectly diagnostic; however, there is typically FSH:LH inversion (i.e., LH is higher than FSH). These hormones should be measured on day 3–5 of the menstrual cycle. If the patient is amenorrheic, they may be measured at any time. Although the ratio is not predictive of PCOS, it is relevant in evaluation and management of infertility.[21]

TSH and prolactin should be measured to exclude thyroid disease and hyperprolactinemia, respectively. Mild elevations of prolactin are common in PCOS, and these should not be confused with significant hyperprolactinemia. Subclinical hypothyroidism is also much more common in patients with PCOS.[22] A simple and adequate screening for adult-onset congenital adrenal hyperplasia is 17-hydroxy progesterone. ACTH stimulatory testing is not indicated. The incidence of Cushing's disease is approximately 1:1,000,000, making suppressive adrenal testing similarly unwarranted.[17]

The metabolic problems associated with PCOS have multisystem implications, as detailed in the next section. Evaluation must therefore include screening for diabetes, hypertension, and hyperlipidemia. A summary of testing recommendations is listed in Table 28-3.

After exclusion of other causes of amenorrhea and hirsutism, the diagnosis of PCOS is based on one of two sets of criteria: the Rotterdam criteria or the Androgen Excess Society (AES) criteria. These are listed, along with the 1990 NIH criteria, in Table 28-4.[2–4]

Research into anti-müllerian hormone (AMH) has shown promise for diagnosis of PCOS. One paper suggests that a cut-off of 20 pgs/mL for AMH is as effective as measurement of androgens, sonography, or clinical examination.[23]

Long-term and other consequences of PCOS

PCOS is a systemic disorder and has multiple non-gynecologic consequences. All women's health

Table 28-4 Diagnostic criteria for PCOS

Clinical finding	NIH 1990	Rotterdam 2003	AES 2007
Hyperandrogenism*	Required	Any 2 of 3 criteria	Required
Oligomenorrhea**	Required		Any 1 of 2 criteria
Polycystic ovaries***	*Not included*		

* Ferriman-Gallwey score ≥8 OR elevated free or total testosterone
** <6–9 menses yearly or oligo ovulation
*** ≥12 pre-antral follicles in one ovary OR ovarian volume ≥10 cc

practitioners must be aware of these and provide appropriate screening and follow-up for them.

Protracted exposure to a high estrogen environment increases the risk of endometrial hyperplasia and cancer. Screening by ultrasound assessment of the endometrial stripe or endometrial biopsy is appropriate in high-risk individuals.

Diabetes is significantly more common in women with PCOS with or without Metabolic Syndrome. Approximately 7% of women with PCOS have abnormal glucose tolerance tests (GTTs) at presentation; 12% more develop abnormal glucose tolerance over six years, and one-third of PCOS patients with abnormal glucose tolerance at presentation will progress to overt type 2 diabetes within six years.[24] The lifetime risk of type 2 diabetes in PCOS is seven- to tenfold higher than in controls. Regular diabetic screening is an essential part of long-term management of PCOS.[25]

Hypertension is found in 19% of PCOS patients compared to 12% of controls.[26] Long-term observation of blood pressure and medical control is indicated. The hyperlipidemia and hyperandrogenism of PCOS is reflected in a higher risk of cardiovascular events beyond age 65.[27] The relative risk of cardiovascular events in this age group was 12.9. Even for the lowest risk subgroup, the relative risk was 2.6, making PCOS an important risk factor for cardiovascular disease.[28] Such increased risk has not been demonstrated for women under age 65, although carotid plaque deposition is increased in PCOS patients in their forties.[29]

Among women with irregular menses and elevated androgens, the incidence of elevated liver function tests (LFTs) was 15%. Among those with persistently elevated liver function tests, all biopsies showed nonalcoholic steatotic hepatitis (NASH).[30] On this basis it is reasonable and desirable to check liver function tests on all women with PCOS. It is cheap – and the patients in any event must have lab work drawn – and will exclude a serious condition that can affect surgery and pregnancy. Patients with elevated LFTs require ongoing evaluation and referral as appropriate.

Psychiatric disorders are more prevalent among women with PCOS. These include social anxiety and depression. Ongoing screening for emotional symptoms is appropriate.[31] The incidence of depression and other psychiatric disorders was not increased among slender women with PCOS. It thus appears that the psychiatric associations of PCOS are not caused by an endocrine derangement but rather by the negative social and personal judgments made on obesity and hirsutism in women.[32]

Pregnancy outcomes are substantially worse in PCOS patients.[33] Miscarriage rates are increased, presumably because of luteal phase defects in oligo-ovulatory women.[34] The risk of gestational diabetes is greatly increased. Low APGAR scores and low birth weight are also more common in PCOS patients treated for infertility than in women with tubal infertility.[35]

Management and outcomes

Although management of menstrual irregularities is one important part of treatment of PCOS, it is by no means sufficient to consider only the woman's menstrual cyclicity in treatment. The management of PCOS requires consideration of multiple medical issues and the individual's goals. This is consistent with the multiorgan system involvement of PCOS.

PCOS management will depend on its presentation and the goals of the patient. A woman desiring childbearing who has amenorrhea must be considered differently from a woman with regular menses but hirsutism and abnormal lipids. Broadly speaking the goals of treatment are:

- regulation of menses
- prevention of endometrial disease
- pregnancy (when desired)
- reduction in diabetes and cardiovascular risk
- reduction in circulating androgens

All aspects of management are best achieved by weight loss.[36] Modest weight loss is more effective than clomiphene for induction of ovulation, and is effective in reduction of circulating androgens and improvement of lipids and blood sugars. One study found no higher an incidence of metabolic syndrome in PCOS patients than in obese women without PCOS, suggesting that obesity itself predisposes to metabolic syndrome, rather than PCOS.[37] Weight loss is thus an integral part of all aspects of PCOS management. However, given the difficulties of long-term lifestyle modification and weight loss, other medical modalities are typically required.

Menstrual regulation

It is necessary for patients to have a withdrawal bleed at least once every three months to prevent risk of endometrial hyperplasia. Thus, women who have regular or semi-regular withdrawal bleeds that are of normal intensity do not require medical regulation of their menses. Medical control is needed for prevention of endometrial hyperplasia in women who have irregular, prolonged and/or heavy bleeding. For management purposes this bleeding is defined as lasting more than seven days at a time or in one month; bleeding less than every three months or at least four times yearly; passage of clots; need for combined pads and tampons; or soiling of bedding or clothes.

Pelvic ultrasound is an essential part of management of menstrual bleeding in PCOS. The thickness and character of the endometrial stripe must be documented. Recommendations for management based on endometrial stripe thickness vary. Hyperplasia can occur in women less than 35 years old with an endometrial stripe less than 15 mm. A stripe thickness less than 5 mm assures absence of endometrial cancer or hyperplasia. If the stripe is greater than 12 mm, or bleeding has been heavy and prolonged, then endometrial biopsy is the best way to exclude endometrial pathology before beginning treatment.[10, 13]

The optimum medication for bleeding control in women not desiring pregnancy is unclear. Despite the frequency of bleeding as a symptom there is very little data on the superiority of one management over another. Oral contraceptive pills reduce endometrial cancer rates, but this is true of all women, not merely women with PCOS.[38] Oral contraceptives offer many benefits. They not only regulate menses but they provide for contraception. Oral contraceptive pills also decrease LH stimulation of the ovarian stroma, thereby reducing androgen production. They additionally reduce 5aR in the hair follicles, further reducing androgen activity in the skin. Additional non-contraceptive benefits include a reduction in risk of ovarian cancer and endometrial hyperplasia.

Oral contraceptives may be started at any time in a woman with amenorrhea, provided a urine pregnancy test is negative. If the endometrial stripe is thin (less than 5 mm) then priming with estrogens for 5–10 days will reduce the incidence of breakthrough bleeding in the first few cycles of use. Conjugated equine estrogens 1.25 mgs twice daily or micronized estradiol 2 mgs daily is adequate. Alternatively the same management may be used only if breakthrough bleeding occurs.

Progestational agents are an alternative for induction of regular menses and prophylaxis against endometrial hyperplasia. Medroxyprogesterone acetate 10 mgs daily for 10–14 days every three months is sufficient protection against endometrial hyperplasia. The same medication may also be used monthly for those desiring monthly bleeding as a reassurance. Depot preparations provide very effective contraception and also will suppress LH and ovarian androgen production, at the expense of a higher incidence of breakthrough bleeding.

The lifetime risk of endometrial hyperplasia and cancer in these women make regular vaginal sonography an important tool. Periodic biopsy is invasive and painful and not warranted as a routine screening measure, although it is indicated in selected, symptomatic patients.

Induction of ovulation

PCOS patients vary markedly in the ease of ovulation induction. Successful management requires more than clomiphene citrate. The success of ovulation induction is strongly associated with metabolic syndrome. Fertile PCOS patients had an 11.5% incidence of metabolic syndrome, as opposed to 23.1% in clomiphene-responding PCOS patients, and 41.4% in clomiphene-resistant patients.[39] Higher day 3 baseline FSH values are associated with lower rates of

Table 28-5 Effects of aldactone and oral contraceptives

Medication	Effect
Aldactone	Decrease 5aR activity
Oral contraceptives	Decrease testosterone substrate for 5aR
	Competitive substrate for 5aR

clomiphene success, and PCOS is associated with higher rates of multifetal pregnancy on clomiphene.

Metformin has been used for ovulation induction. It is not more successful than clomiphene used as a single agent. Metformin and clomiphene used together have mixed results, but the preponderance of trials does not show added benefit for two drug management. There does appear to be benefit to adding metformin to clomiphene for patients who have failed clomiphene alone.[40–43] Two large reviews comprehensively address the use of metformin in PCOS-associated infertility as well as its use in other PCOS settings.[44, 45]

Given the potential for multifetal pregnancy and the high rate of failure, ovulation induction in PCOS patients may be best done by physicians with significant specialized endocrine training.

Hirsutism

Manifestations of hyperandrogenism are some of the most troubling symptoms for PCOS patients.[14] Hirsutism and obesity both are more strongly associated with emotional and psychiatric sequelae of PCOS than is PCOS itself.[31, 32] Managing hyperandrogenic symptoms is thus of great personal meaning to the patient. The mainstays of hirsutism management are oral contraceptives and spironolactone. These medications have three synergistic effects that ultimately reduce the amount of dihydrotestosterone.

Spironolactone acts in the skin to reduce the activity of 5aR. Oral contraceptives reduce ovarian androgen production, thus reducing available testosterone as substrate for 5aR. The progestational component of oral contraceptives also serves as a competitive substrate for 5aR. These effects are summarized in Table 28-5.

Patients who either cannot or do not wish to take oral contraceptives can use progestational agents successfully. Daily medroxyprogesterone 2.5 mg–5 mg is effective in conjunction with spironolactone.[10, 13, 46]

Other medications for control of hirsutism include finasteride and flutamide. These medications are both effective in suppression of 5aR activity. Side effects of finasteride are uncommon, although it can produce anomalies in male fetuses. Flutamide has the potential for significant liver toxicity, although this is typically reversible with discontinuation of the medication.[46] Both these medications are infrequently used because of the ready availability and familiarity of oral contraceptives and spironolactone. They are further limited by insurance coverage and pharmacy availability.

Control of hirsutism is a slow process dependent on the life cycle of the hair follicle. All interventions affect new hair growth, not the existing hairs. If the hair growth cycles rapidly and grows quickly, the patient will see the impact of treatment much faster than if the growth cycle is slower. Patients with marked hirsutism will see effects much more quickly than those with limited hirsutism. The first manifestation of successful intervention is typically a reduction in the frequency of shaving and depilation. A visible effect should not be expected before three to six months, and full effect of treatment cannot be assessed for one year. Acanthosis can take even longer to improve. Patients should be clearly warned about the slow pace of treatment to avoid despondency and non-compliance. See Chapter 29 for a thorough discussion of hirsuitism.

Metabolic syndrome

Metabolic syndrome is the most important long-term problem associated with PCOS. It is metabolic syndrome that transforms an otherwise purely gynecologic condition into one with whole body and whole life implications. Metabolic syndrome may require follow-up with providers of many types for the associated medical complications of metabolic syndrome.

The incidence of type 2 diabetes is sufficiently high that women with metabolic syndrome should have glucose tolerance testing (GTT) periodically throughout their lives.[25, 47] The recommended frequency of screening for diabetes is unclear; for women with metabolic syndrome, which already involves a degree of glucose intolerance, yearly screening is not unreasonable, but admittedly is burdensome for the patient.

Screening requires a fasting blood sugar and two-hour GTT with a 75 gm load. Fasting blood sugar, hemoglobin A1c, and insulin levels have all been demonstrated to be inadequate screening tools for PCOS patients.[48]

Dyslipidemia is a common problem in women with metabolic syndrome, and is at least in part a result of the hyperandrogenism of PCOS. Lipids screening should occur yearly.[27] Hyperlipidemia is discussed in Chapter 43.

There is a clear increase in cardiovascular events in PCOS women older than 65 years.[28, 29] Despite concern for and suggestion of risk for earlier cardiovascular events, such risk has not been demonstrated. Screening for cardiovascular morbidity is reasonable in women with metabolic syndrome. The timing and nature of such screening is unclear, and no single comprehensive recommendation is possible. Rather, screening should depend on the patient's presentation and family history.

Metformin has been proposed as a single agent management for metabolic syndrome. The efficacy of this has not been confirmed in larger trials, and the weight of clinical opinion is against its routine use.[44, 45]

The single best management component for metabolic syndrome is weight reduction and exercise. [36, 41] Efficacy has been repeatedly and clearly demonstrated, with reduction in androgens, return of ovulatory cycles, and improvement in glucose intolerance. Obesity is discussed in Chapter 39. Implementation of weight loss regimens remains difficult and largely unsuccessful. There is much resistance from society at large, and a tacit social acceptance of obesity and inactivity in media portrayals exists. Individual resistance to the effort and dietary changes needed for successful weight reduction is common. Some physicians have difficulty dealing with the embarrassment and demoralization engendered in discussing weight with an obese and hirsute woman. Although weight reduction and exercise are the single best management options available, they must be offered delicately, without judgment, and in a supportive and encouraging manner.

Concluding remarks

PCOS is a common gynecologic disorder that will be seen by all providers who care for women. It is an endocrine condition with multiple systemic manifestations and implications. It is used too frequently as a diagnosis without appropriate evaluation or follow-up. Appropriate use of diagnostic criteria and follow-up examinations can greatly improve outcomes.

References

1. Stein IF, Leventhal ML. Amenorrhea associated with bilateral polycystic ovaries. *Am J Obstet Gynecol* 1935;**29**:181.
2. Rotterdam ESHRE/ASRM-Sponsored PCOS Consensus Workshop Group. Revised 2003 consensus on diagnostic criteria and long-term health risks related to polycystic ovary syndrome. *Fertil Steril* 2004 Jan;**81**(1):19–25.
3. Balen AH, Laven JS, Tan SL, Dewailly D. Ultrasound assessment of the polycystic ovary: international consensus definitions. *Hum Reprod Update* 2003 Nov–Dec;**9**(6):505–14.
4. Azziz R, et al. for the Androgen Excess Society. Positions statement: criteria for defining polycystic ovary syndrome as a predominantly hyperandrogenic syndrome: an Androgen Excess Society guideline. *J Clin Endocrinol Metab* 2006 Nov;**91**(11):4237–45.
5. Knochenhauer ES1, Key TJ, Kahsar-Miller M, et al. Prevalence of the polycystic ovary syndrome in unselected black and white women of the southeastern United States: a prospective study. *J Clin Endocrinol Metab* 1998 Sep;**83**(9):3078–82.
6. Li R, Zhang Q, Yang D, et al. Prevalence of polycystic ovary syndrome in women in China: a large community-based study. *Hum Reprod* 2013 Sep;**28**(9): 2562–9.
7. Ezeh U, Yildiz BO, Azziz R. Referral bias in defining the phenotype and prevalence of obesity in polycystic ovary syndrome. *J Clin Endocrinol Metabol* 2013 Jun; **98**(6):E1088–96.
8. Okoroh EM, Hooper WC, Atrash HK, et al. Prevalence of polycystic ovary syndrome among the privately insured, United States, 2003–2008. *Am J Obstet Gynecol* 2012 Oct;**207**(4):299.e1–7.
9. Speroff L, Fritz MA. *Clinical Gynecologic Endocrinology and Infertility, 7th edition*. Philadelphia: Lippincott Williams & Wilkins, 2005; chapter 6, pp 187–231.
10. Speroff L, Fritz MA. *Clinical Gynecologic Endocrinology and Infertility, 7th edition*. Philadelphia: Lippincott Williams & Wilkins, 2005; chapter 12, pp 465–98.
11. Nestler JE, Powers LP, Matt DW, et al. A direct effect of hyperinsulinemia on serum sex hormone-binding globulin levels in obese women with the polycystic ovary syndrome. *J Clin Endocrinol Metab* 1991 Jan; **72**(1):83–9.
12. Dunaif A, Green G, Futterweit W, Dobrjansky A. Suppression of hyperandrogenism does not improve peripheral or hepatic insulin resistance in the polycystic ovary syndrome. *J Clin Endocrinol Metab* 1990 Mar;**70**(3):699–704.

13. ACOG. Practice Bulletin 108: polycystic ovary syndrome. October 2009.
14. Quinn M, Shinkai K, Pasch L, et al. Prevalence of androgenic alopecia in patients with polycystic ovary syndrome and characterization of associated clinical and biochemical features. *Fertility Steril.* 2014 Apr;**101** (4):1129–34.
15. Grundy SM, Cleeman JI, Daniels SR, et al. Diagnosis and management of the metabolic syndrome: an American Heart Association/National Heart, Lung, and Blood Institute Scientific Statement. *Circulation* 2005 Oct 25;**112**(17):2735–52.
16. Ehrmann DA, Liljenquist DR, Kasza K, et al. Prevalence and predictors of the metabolic syndrome in women with polycystic ovary syndrome. *J Clin Endocrinol Metab* 2006 Jan;**91**(1):48–53.
17. Karaca Z, Acmaz B, Acmaz G, et al. Routine screening for Cushing's syndrome is not required in patients presenting with hirsutism. *Eur J Endocrinol* 2013 Mar;**168**(3):379–84.
18. Yildiz BO. Assessment, diagnosis and treatment of a patient with hirsutism. *Nat Clin Pract Endoc* 2008;**4**:294–300.
19. Wang S, Alvero R. Racial and ethnic differences in physiology and clinical symptoms of polycystic ovary syndrome. *[Review] Semin Reprod Med* 2013 Sep;**31**(5): 365–9.
20. Clayton RN, Ogden V, Hodgkinson J, et al. How common are polycystic ovaries in normal women and what is their significance for the fertility of the population? *Clin Endocrinol* 1992 Aug;**37**(2):127–34.
21. Robinson S, Rodin DA, Deacon A, et al. Which hormone tests for the diagnosis of polycystic ovary syndrome? *Br J Obstet Gynaecol* 1992 Mar;**99**(3):232–8.
22. Morgante G, Musacchio MC, Orvieto R, et al. Alterations in thyroid function among the different polycystic ovary syndrome phenotypes. *Gynecol Endocrinol* 2013 Nov;**29**(11):967–9.
23. Eilertsen TB, Vanky E, Carlsen SM. Anti-mullerian hormone in the diagnosis of polycystic ovary syndrome: can morphologic description be replaced? *Hum Reprod* 2012 Aug;**27**(8):2494–502.
24. Celik C, Tasdemir N, Abali R, et al. Progression to impaired glucose tolerance or type 2 diabetes mellitus in polycystic ovary syndrome: a controlled follow-up study. *Fertil Steril* 2014 Apr;**101**(4):1123–8.
25. Legro RS, Kunselman AR, Dodson WC, Dunaif A, Prevalence and predictors of risk for type 2 diabetes mellitus and impaired glucose tolerance in polycystic ovary syndrome: a prospective, controlled study in 254 affected women. *J Clin Endocrinol Metab* 1999 Jan;**84** (1):165–9.
26. Shi Y, Cui Y, Sun X, et al. Hypertension in women with polycystic ovary syndrome: prevalence and associated cardiovascular risk factors. *Eur J Obstet Gynecol Reprod Biol* 2014 Feb;**173**:66–70.
27. Legro RS, Kunselman AR, Dunaif A. Prevalence and predictors of dyslipidemia in women with polycystic ovary syndrome. *Am J Med* 2001 Dec 1;**111**(8):607–13.
28. Mani H, Levy MJ, Davies MJ, et al. Diabetes and cardiovascular events in women with polycystic ovary syndrome: a 20-year retrospective cohort study. *Clin Endocrinol* 2013 Jun;**78**(6):926–34.
29. Guzick DS, Talbott EO, Sutton-Tyrrell K, et al. Carotid atherosclerosis in women with polycystic ovary syndrome: initial results from a case-control study. *Am J Obstet Gynecol* 1996 Apr;**174**(4):1224–9.
30. Setji TL, Holland ND, Sanders LL, et al. Nonalcoholic steatohepatitis and nonalcoholic fatty liver disease in young women with polycystic ovary syndrome. *J Clin Endocrinol Metab* 2006 May;**91**(5):1741–7.
31. Sahingoz M, Uguz F, Gezginc K, Korucu DG. Axis I and Axis II diagnoses in women with PCOS. *Gen Hospit Psychiat* 2013 Sep–Oct;**35**(5):508–11.
32. Milsom SR, Nair SM, Ogilvie CM, et al. Polycystic ovary syndrome and depression in New Zealand adolescents. *J Pediat Adolesc Gynecol* 2013 Jun;**26**(3): 142–7.
33. Boomsma CM, Eijkemans MJ, Hughes EG, et al. A meta-analysis of pregnancy outcomes in women with polycystic ovary syndrome. *Hum Reprod Update* 2006 Nov–Dec;**12**(6):673–83.
34. Rai R, Backos M, Rushworth F, Regan L. Polycystic ovaries and recurrent miscarriage – a reappraisal. *Hum Reprod* 2000;**15**(3):612–15.
35. Grigorescu V, Zhang Y, Kissin DM, et al. Maternal characteristics and pregnancy outcomes after assisted reproductive technology by infertility diagnosis: ovulatory dysfunction versus tubal obstruction. *Fertil Steril* 2014 Apr;**101**(4):1019–25.
36. Knowler WC, et al. for the Diabetes Prevention Program Research Group. Reduction in the incidence of type 2 diabetes with lifestyle intervention or metformin. *N Engl J Med* 2002 Feb 7;**346**(6):393–403.
37. Panidis D, Tziomalos K, Macut D, et al. Age- and body mass index-related differences in the prevalence of metabolic syndrome in women with polycystic ovary syndrome. *Gynecol Endocrinol* 2013 Oct;**29**(10):926–30.
38. Vessey M, Painter R. Oral contraceptive use and cancer. Findings in a large cohort study, 1968–2004. *Br J Cancer* 2006;**95**:385–89.
39. Verit FF. The prevalence of metabolic syndrome in clomiphene citrate resistant polycystic ovary syndrome. *Gynecol Endocrinol* 2012 May;**28**(5):365–9.

40. Creanga AA, Bradly HM, McCormick C, Witkop CT. Use of metformin in polycystic ovary syndrome. *Obstet Gynecol* 2008;**111**(4): 959–68.
41. Mathur R, Alexander CJ, Yano J, et al. Use of metformin in polycystic ovary syndrome. *Am Obstet Gynecol* 2008 Dec;**199**(6): 596–609.
42. Nestler JE, Jakubowicz DJ, Evans WS, Pasquali R. Effects of metformin on spontaneous and clomiphene-induced ovulation in the polycystic ovary syndrome. *New Engl J Med* 1998 Jun 25;**338**(26): 1876–80.
43. Velazquez E, Acosta A, Mendoza SG. Menstrual cyclicity after metformin therapy in polycystic ovary syndrome. *Obstet Gynecol* 1997 Sep;**90**(3):392–5.
44. Marshall JC, Dunaif A. Should all women with PCOS be treated for insulin resistance? *Fertil Steril* 2012 Jan;**97**(1):18–22.
45. Palomba S, Falbo A, Zullo F, Orio F. Evidence based and potential benefits of metformin in the polycystic ovary syndrome: a comprehensive review. *Endocr Rev* 2013 July;**30**(1):1–50.
46. Swiglo BA, Cosma M, Flynn DN, et al. Clinical review: antiandrogens for the treatment of hirsutism: a systematic review and metaanalyses of randomized controlled trials. *J Clin Endocrinol Metab* 2008 Apr; **93**(4):1153–60.
47. Pasquali R, Gambineri A. Glucose intolerance states in women with the polycystic ovary syndrome. *[Review] J Endocrinol Invest* 2013 Sep;**36**(8):648–53.
48. Lerchbaum E, Schwetz V, Giuliani A, Obermayer-Pietsch B. Assessment of glucose metabolism in polycystic ovary syndrome: HbA1c or fasting glucose compared with the oral glucose tolerance test as a screening method. *Hum Reprod* 2013 Sep;**28**(9): 2537–44.

Chapter 29

Hyperandrogenism

Eduardo Lara-Torre and Amanda B. Murchison

Introduction

Hyperandrogenism is defined as the clinical manifestation of excess levels of androgens in women.[1] The most common cause of hyperandrogenism in reproductive age women is polycystic ovarian syndrome (PCOS), which is discussed in Chapter 28.

Hyperandrogenism is described by its clinical manifestations. Each of these is associated with different levels of testosterone and the origin of the over production of androgens differs. The two most common clinical presentations are:

- hirsutism, defined as the male pattern distribution of excess hair, with conversion of vellus hair to terminal hair, and
- virilization, defined as the masculinization of women with a marked increase in testosterone levels.

In addition to hirsutism, patients with hyperandrogenism typically present with clitoral enlargement, temporal balding, deepening of the voice, and remodeling of the limb-shoulder girdle.

To understand the different entities associated with hyperandrogenism, a brief review of the normal androgen metabolism is needed.[2] Androgen production results from the metabolism of cholesterol (Figure 29-1). Androgens are produced in the adrenal glands and ovaries, and each androgen has a different potency as well as individual characteristics. Dehydroepiandrosterone (DHEA), a weak androgen, is produced mostly in the adrenal gland (90%). Its more stable and longer acting form is dehydroepiandrosterone sulfate (DHEAS), which is the most commonly measured adrenal androgen. Androstenodione is produced in the ovary (50%) and the adrenal gland (50%) and is also considered a weak androgen. Most androgens circulate in their most effective clinical form of testosterone. The ovarian and adrenal androgen production accounts for about 50% of circulating androgens, whereas production elsewhere in the body accounts for the remaining 50%. Testosterone is distributed throughout the body, mostly bound to albumin and sex hormone binding globulin (SHBG). This binding makes most of the circulating testosterone clinically inactive. Only between 1% and 3% of circulating testosterone travels unbound (free) and is biologically active. For this reason, total circulating testosterone does not reflect the true amount of active hormone. Testosterone can be aromatized to estrone in adipose tissue while free testosterone is converted to a more potent form, dihydrotestosterone (DHT), at the tissue level (hair follicles and within genital skin) via 5α-reductase.[2] This conversion is responsible for constitutional effects of the hormone, including increased hair growth, acne, and the physical changes associated with virilization.

Adrenal androgen production is controlled by adrenocorticotropic hormone (ACTH). As just described, the main androgen produced is DHEA, and its final active form is DHEAS. With hyperandrogenism, enzyme deficiencies in the androgen production and metabolism pathway lead to precursor molecules such as DHEA and DHEAS accumulation, which can be measured to determine the origin of the hyperandrogenism. DHEA can further be metabolized to androstenedione and testosterone.

Ovarian androgen production (mainly testosterone and some androstenedione) is stimulated by luteinizing hormone (LH) secretion from the pituitary gland. Extraglandular testosterone production occurs in adipocytes and depends on the magnitude of adrenal and ovarian androstenedione production. Obesity increases the conversion of androstenedione to testosterone.

Office Care of Women, ed. Martin E. Olsen and Botros Rizk. Published by Cambridge University Press.

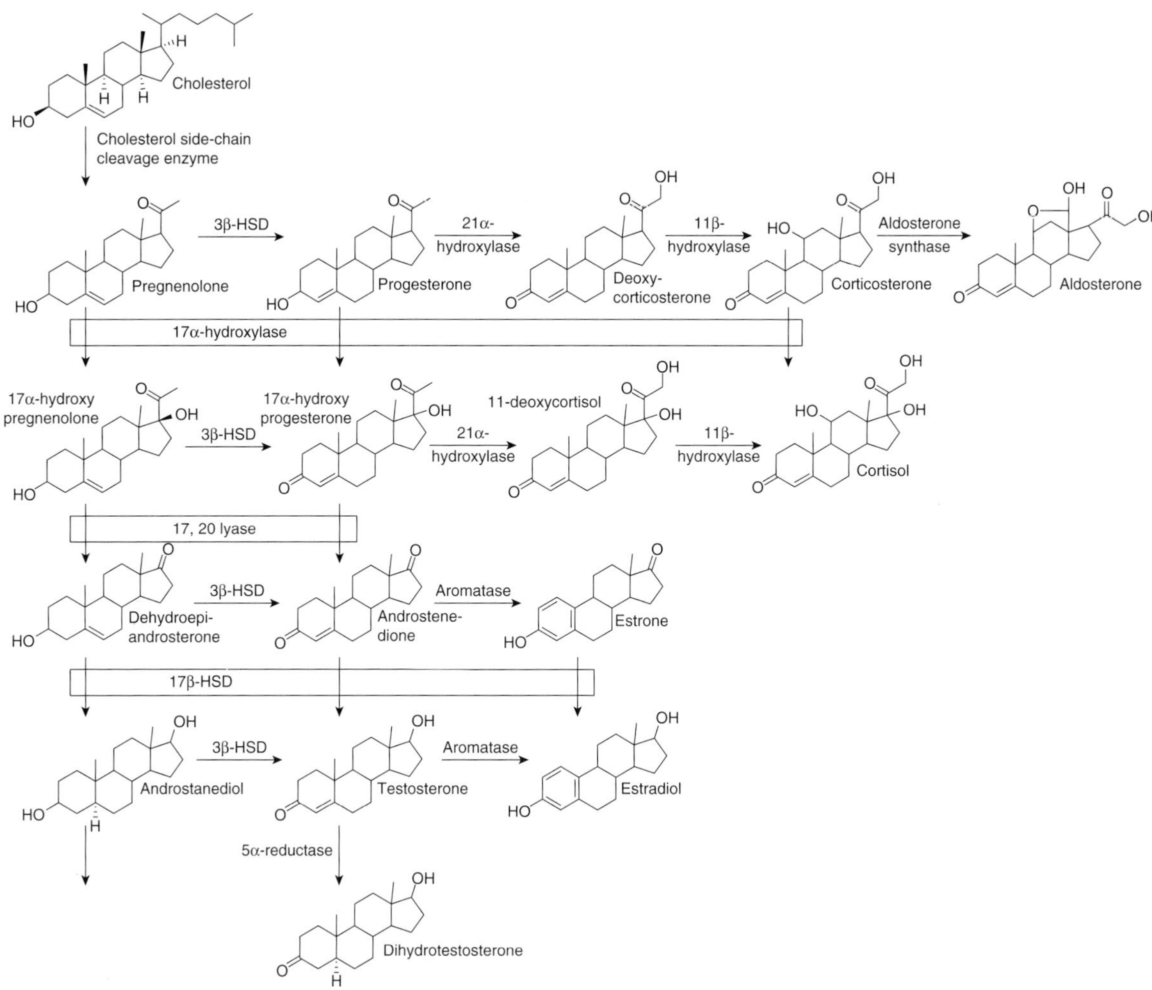

Figure 29-1 Steroidogenesis pathway. *(From David Richfield under the GNU Free Documentation License.)*

Scope of the problem

Hyperandrogenism, given the variety of etiologies associated with increased androgens in blood, has a significant impact on the population. The number of patients affected by this condition reaches significance secondary to varying causes such as androgen producing tumors, PCOS, to neonatal deficiencies in enzymes such as in congenital adrenal hyperplasia (CAH), the number of patients affected by this condition reaches significance. Many, if not most of the patients with clinical manifestations of increased androgens, seek treatment. Treatment of unwanted hair (hirsutism), acne, and clitoromegaly become as important as treating the original condition. The effects on body image and self-esteem are an integral part of the management of these conditions.

History

As described earlier, hyperandrogenism will present generally one of two ways. Patients may present with hirsutism, alopecia, and acne. They may also present with full virilization signs that include the preceding findings, as well as deepening of the voice, clitoromegaly, and changes in muscle mass distribution. Because of the disruption in ovulation created by high androgen levels, most of these patients will also have some type of menstrual dysfunction including amenorrhea, oligomenorrhea, or irregular menses.

Family history and ethnicity are important factors to consider in these patients. Individuals of Mediterranean ancestry have an increase in concentration of hair follicles, compared to their northern European counterparts. And those of Asian descent have less concentration of hair follicles, and thus are less likely to manifest complaints of hirsutism. These differences can account for the normal variation between ethnicities and do not necessarily signify hyperandrogenism. There are also genetic differences in the sensitivity of follicles to DHT and 5α-reductase that are not necessarily pathologic, and symptomatic patients can display normal androgen levels.[5]

Rapid progression of symptoms is generally indicative of a hormone-producing tumor, either ovarian or adrenal. Symptoms such as abdominal pain, bloating, and back pain could be present. However, most patients with these tumors do not have such symptoms; indeed these tumors are typically diagnosed because the systemic effects of the hormone initiated an evaluation before tumor size contributed to patient complaints.

Some conditions that cause hyperandrogenism can have severe metabolic effects; for example, newborn hypotension is associated with CAH. These conditions can also affect sexual development. Babies with CAH and male pseudohermaphroditism will typically be born with ambiguous genitalia. Teens with male pseudohermaphroditism will often present with virilization symptoms during puberty.

Personal history of hypothyroidism or symptoms such as weight gain, hair loss, central obesity, and anovulation are symptoms of hypothyroidism. If hypothyroidism is confirmed, this diagnosis may be the cause for increased hair growth. Galactorrhea, as a sign of elevated prolactin, has also been associated with hyperandrogenism via an increase in the secretion of adrenal androgens secondary to the stimulation of prolactin receptors in the adrenal gland. Moon facies, abdominal striae, central fat distribution, proximal muscle weakness, and easy bruising are associated with Cushing's syndrome and should raise suspicion for this condition.

Medication history is important, as some drugs have been identified as contributors to hirsutism even though they may not necessarily cause elevated circulating androgens, but rather have a direct effect on testosterone receptors. These drugs include phenytoin, corticosteroids, danazol, diazoxide, minoxidil, anabolic steroids, and androgens (used by some athletes).[2] Conditions that increase the secretion of LH by the pituitary gland, such as stress, can also lead to an increase in androgen production from the ovarian theca cells and lead to hyperandrogenism and its manifestations.[3]

Physical exam

In this section the different clinical findings associated with elevated androgen will be defined and their clinical assessment will be described.

Hirsutism

Hirsutism is defined as coarse, dark hair distributed in a male pattern. This is different than hypertrichosis, which is lanugo-type hair rather than terminal hair, which is associated with some malignancies and certain medications. The Ferriman-Gallwey scoring system was created as a tool to objectively quantify the degree of hirsutism. This tool has been widely used in research to standardize results on studies, but it is not used commonly in the clinical setting because of its complexity and length. Modified versions have been used in the clinical setting, but most practitioners use a mild, moderate, and severe scale to describe the amount of hair present (Figure 29-2).[6] When evaluating patients for hirsutism, it is important to ask the patients about their hair management habits such as frequency of shaving, plucking, and use of depilatory creams. This information is important because the degree of hirsutism may not be easily appreciated if these techniques are routinely used.

Acne

Acne is caused by an increase in sebaceous gland activity leading to inflammation. The most common areas affected are the face, upper back, and upper torso. An increase in circulating androgens leads to the increased conversion of testosterone to its active metabolite DHT and in turn stimulates the receptors to produce sebum. Long-standing inflammation leads comedone formation, infection with bacteria such as *Propionibacterium acnes*, and if untreated, could lead to scarring. Most patients can be classified into mild, moderate, or severe depending on the extent of the lesions and the amount of inflammation, comedone formation, and scarring present.[7]

Alopecia

Alopecia is defined as changes in the nonandrogen-dependent hair that lead to balding or thinning of the hair follicles. Patients generally present with thinner or absent scalp hair especially in the crown area, while their frontal hair line is preserved.[8] The degree of alopecia may not necessarily correlate with the levels of androgen in blood.

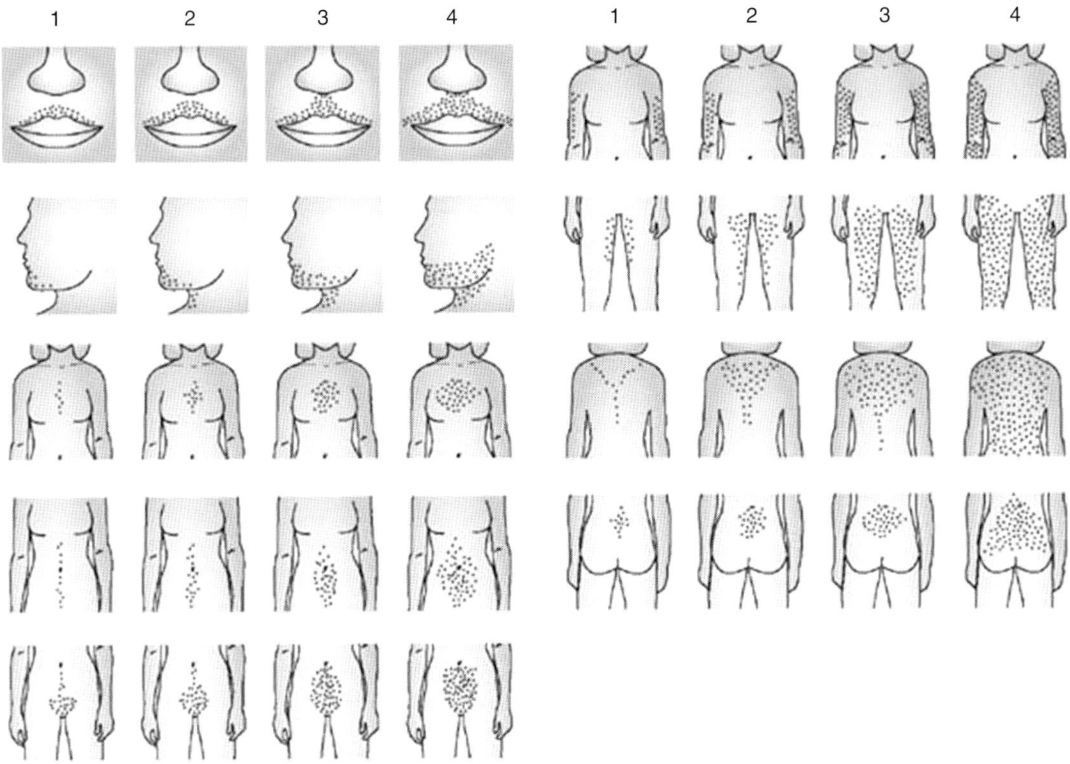

Figure 29-2 The Ferriman-Gallwey scoring system (with permission from Lara-Torre E, Hertweck PS. Medical management of gynecological problems in the pediatric and adolescent patient. In: Bieber EJ, Sanfilippo JS, Horowitz IR, Shafi MI (eds.). *Clinical Gynecology*, 2nd edition. Philadelphia: Cambridge Press 2015; figure 36.11, pp 515).

Clitoromegaly

The normal size of the clitoris has previously been defined as a width of <5 mm, with most normal adult females having a width somewhere between 2 mm and 4 mm in the non-erect state. Patients with a width of 10 mm or greater are considered to have significant virilization. Normal length of the clitoris is 16 mm ±4.3 mm (including glans and body). The normal clitoral index of 18.5 mm^2 (product of the glans width times the glans length) has also been reported. [9]

Other signs of virilization can be seen in patients with a significant increase in the amount of active circulating androgens. These include *changes in muscle mass distribution*, from a female to a male pattern, resulting in an increase in total muscle mass and a broadening of the shoulders. A *deepening of the voice* and *decrease in breast size* may also be noted.

Some other physical findings would be dependent on the underlying cause for the increase in androgens. For example, a pelvic mass would be found in patients with an androgen producing ovarian tumor or galactorrhea may be noted on breast exam in those with hyperprolactinemia. Changes associated with Cushing's and CAH were previously described.

Laboratory analysis

The initial laboratory evaluation of patients should include a baseline assessment of testosterone (free or total), DHEAS, and thyroid-stimulating hormone (TSH), given some of the symptoms of hypothyroidsm are subtle and similar to those of hyperandrogenism. In patients who also present with menstrual irregularities such as oligomenorrhea, adding prolactin, follicle-stimulating hormone (FSH), and human chorionic gonadotropin (hCG) is of value to identify other less common causes such as intersex disorders and prolactinomas, and to rule out pregnancy. Patients with abnormal values in these tests should be managed accordingly; the specific management for each disorder is beyond the scope of this chapter.

The routine measurement of 17-OH progesterone (17-OHP) is not done in every setting, and should only

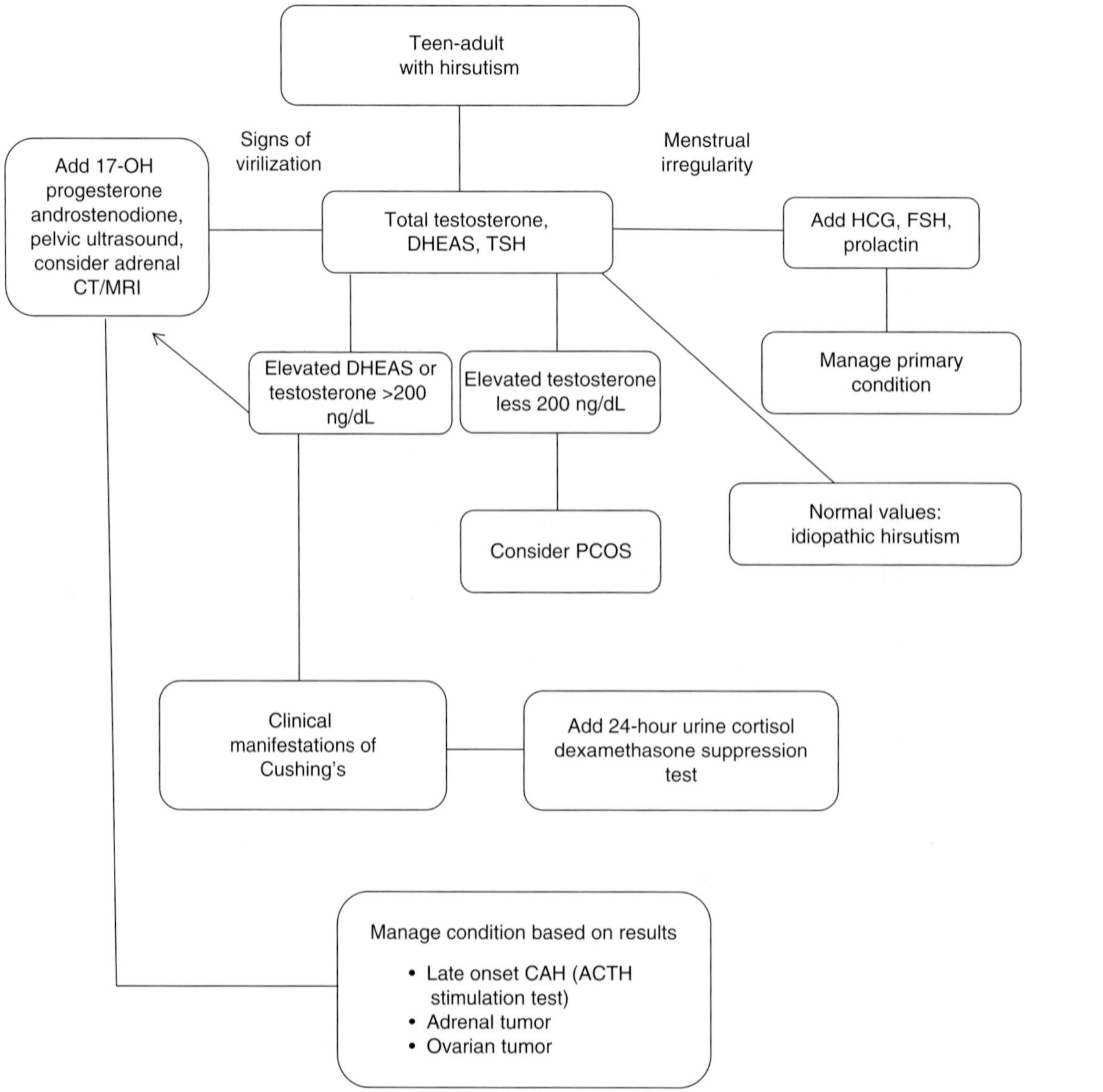

Figure 29-3 Diagnostic algorithm for patients with hirsutism. Patients who underwent 17-OHP testing with results below 200 ng/dL are unlikely to have CAH and require no further testing.[11] If the levels are above 1,000 ng/dL, then the diagnosis of 21-hydroxylase deficiency can be made. If the levels are between 200 ng/dL and 1,000 ng/dL, an ACTH stimulation test is needed to confirm the diagnosis. Patients with clinical manifestations of Cushing's as described in the chapter should undergo a 24-hour urine free cortisone and creatinine determination followed by a dexamethasone suppression test.[12]

be collected if other signs of virilization are also present or the screening DHEAS is elevated. Measurement of androstenedione may also be indicated in patients with elevation of total testosterone or DHEAS or if there is suspicion for a tumor.

Once the initial results are obtained, these will dictate further steps that need to be undertaken (Figure 29-3). Normal values of all androgens can be seen in some patients with hirsutism. This is referred to as idiopathic hirsutism and is the second most common cause. Total testosterone values over 200 ng/dL, DHEAS values higher than 600 μg/dL–700 μg/dL, or androstenedione of 500 ng/dL are associated with tumors.[10] Imaging of the ovaries with ultrasound (elevated testosterone) and/or adrenal glands with CT/MRI (elevated DHEAS, androstenedione) is indicated. Levels of androgens that fall above the normal range but below the levels just mentioned are unlikely to be associated with tumors, so imaging may not be of benefit. Most of these patients will be ultimately diagnosed with PCOS (see Chapter 28).

Treatment

Treatment of hyperandrogenism depends on the etiology of the condition. Based on the diagnosis made, specific management of not only the primary condition, but the resulting androgenic effects on the body is important. Regardless of the original cause, effects already created by the long-term exposure to androgens are not reversible and may need individual directed therapy (as described in the following sections). The main purpose of treatment is not only to correct the disorder, but to prevent new effects secondary to the increased amount of androgens circulating.

Patients with hypothyroidism, hyperprolactinemia, drug exposure, and disorders of sex differentiation should be managed for those conditions; this will lead to the resolution of hyperandrogenism.

Ovarian neoplasms

As mentioned earlier, testosterone levels above 200 ng/dL should raise suspicion for an ovarian hormone–producing tumor. Hormonally active tumors are uncommon, occurring in 1 in 500 hirsute women. Sertoli-Leydig cell tumors (androblastoma, arrhenoblastoma) are ovarian neoplasms that secrete testosterone and generally present with rapid onset (<6 months) of acne, severe hirsutism (75% of patients), amenorrhea (30% of patients), and other virilizing signs.[13] There should be no delay in surgical removal of the involved ovary to maximize regression of symptoms. During surgery, the contralateral ovary should be inspected and if enlarged, it should be bisected for gross inspection and possible biopsy. If the clitoris has become enlarged, it does not revert back to its original size, so clitoral reduction may be necessary to obtain an appropriate cosmetic result. Terminal hair in a sexual distribution will not revert to vellus hair, and patients may need mechanical or chemical removal of excess hair.

Gynandroblastoma is quite rare and has elements of both granulosa cell and arrhenoblastoma. Virilization is a predominant clinical feature. Estrogen production may simultaneously produce endometrial hyperplasia and irregular uterine bleeding. Treatment involves surgical resection.[14]

Lipid (lipoid) cell tumors contain sheets of round, clear, pale-staining cells, and virilization or defeminization can occur. Hilar cell tumors are typically found in postmenopausal women with virilization; both of these conditions resolve with surgical removal of the affected gonad.[15]

Adrenal disorders

In patients with CAH, an inborn glandular enzymatic deficiency results in precursor (substrate) excess, and leads to an overproduction of steroids. The most common enzyme deficiency, affecting 2% of the population, is 21-hydroxylase deficiency. An alteration in chromosome 6, which contains the genes for 21-hydroxylase, leads to the disorder. This enzyme catalyzes the conversion of progesterone and 17α-hydroxyprogesterone to deoxycorticosterone and compound S (see Figure 29-1). A deficiency leads to accumulation of progesterone and 17α-hydroxyprogesterone. As previously described, the classic form manifests with a virilized newborn female infant, with ambiguous genitalia as well as a life-threatening salt wasting condition with hypotension. Nonclassic forms are more common and can appear at puberty or in adulthood (late onset CAH). In general, these patients present with an increase in terminal body hair, acne, subtle alterations in menstrual cycles, and infertility. If CAH presents during puberty, adrenarche may precede thelarche. Other less common enzyme deficiencies such as 11β-hydroxylase deficiency may also occur, and their clinical presentation is more mild. The treatment goal is to restore normal cortisol levels. In high-grade enzymatic blocks there are inadequate amounts of glucocorticoids and mineralocorticoids produced, resulting in salt loss, which can be life-threatening. Nonclassic CAH can be managed by supplementing glucocorticoids (e.g., prednisone 2.5 mg daily). With therapy, facial acne improves and ovulation is restored. No new terminal hair growth occurs.[16]

As with other causes of hyperandrogenism, medical therapy for adrenal and ovarian disorders does not resolve hirsutism; it only suppresses new hair growth. Terminal hair in a sexual distribution will not revert to vellus hair and may need mechanical or chemical removal.

Cushing's syndrome

Cushing's syndrome is an adrenal disease producing hormone excess (either from an adrenal neoplasm or an ACTH-producing tumor). Adrenal neoplasms, characterized by a rapid increase in hair growth associated with severe acne, amenorrhea, and sometimes virilization, should be treated with surgical removal of the ACTH-producing pituitary or adrenal tumor. In certain cases, the exposure to external steroids is the cause of the disease, and discontinuation of these substances is the indicated approach.

Idiopathic hirsutism (constitutional, familial)

Idiopathic hirsuitism is the second most common cause of hirsutism after PCOS. During clinical and laboratory evaluation, no cause of hirsutism can be found. These patients usually present with mild to moderate hirsutism and normal circulating levels of androgens, and they usually have regular menstrual cycles. Management is once again focused on the androgenic changes in the skin.

Pharmacologic treatment of hirsutism

Multiagent therapy works best to treat patients with hirsutism. Although medications that increase SHBG and inhibit androgen synthesis are efficient in preventing new hair and acne from forming, chemical and mechanical hair removal is needed for the terminal hair that is already present. The maximum effect of most therapy to decrease hirsutism is generally not seen until after 6–12 months of continuous therapy.

Systemic treatments

Combination oral contraceptive pills

Two benefits are seen with the use of combination oral contraceptive (COC) pills. First there is a decrease in ovarian production of androgens, and second there is an increase in circulating SHBG because of the estrogenic effect in the liver. This leads to less available bioactive free testosterone and the resulting anti-androgenic effect. As many of these patients with hyperandrogenism also present with menstrual irregularities, COC provides effective menstrual regulation and as well as contraception.

Androgen receptor antagonist

Although not approved in the United States by the FDA for this indication, androgen receptor antagonist are commonly used for hirsutism and work by competing for the androgen receptor and binding to it. These antagonists will suppress future hair growth, but do not immediately cause the existing hair to disappear. Patients on androgen antagonists should be on concomitant contraception secondary to the potential teratogenicity and the demasculinizing effects of these medications on a male fetus. In addition to androgen receptor agonists, the use of COC (as the contraceptive of choice) is recommended, as it not only provides patients with regular menses and contraception, but also provides anti-androgen effects (as already described).

Androgen receptor antagonists include:

- Spironolactone 100 mg–200 mg/day: This is the most common drug used in the United States for the treatment of hirsutism. It binds to the androgen receptors and inhibits testosterone production by the ovary. It also decreases 5α-reductase activity. Given its potassium-sparing diuretic effect patients should be counseled on the use of other medications that increase potassium concentration in the blood, such as nonsteroidal anti-inflammatory drugs (NSAIDs). Serum potassium levels may need to be monitored if any of these drugs are used concomitantly.
- Flutamide: Available in the United States as an anti-androgen for the treatment of prostate cancer, flutamide is effective though rarely used because of the significant risk of hepatotoxicity.
- Cyproterone acetate: Available in Europe, Mexico, and Canada mostly as a contraceptive agent, is effective and commonly used instead of spironolactone, as it combines both the benefit of contraception, as well as the receptor antagonist properties. This medication is currently not available in the United States.[17]
- 5α-reductase inhibitors: Finasteride is currently used in the United States for the treatment of prostate cancer (5 mg/day) or male alopecia (1 mg/day). It is effective in blocking the conversion of testosterone to DHT and has been used in the management of hirsutism in women (5 mg/day). As with androgen inhibitors, concurrent use of COC is recommended.[18]

Local treatments

Eflornithine hydrochloride

This topical cream is an irreversible inhibitor of L-ornithine decarboxylase. This enzyme is needed for the normal cell division and function of the hair follicle and its blockade slows hair growth. It is applied to the face twice daily and its effect is generally seen after four to eight weeks of treatment.[19]

Depilation

This process describes separation of the hair from the skin surface. Shaving is the most commonly used method. Contrary to general belief, it does not increase hair thickness nor does it make hirsutism worse. Additionally, products containing calcium thioglycolate are widely available in the form of gels, creams and other mediums, which breaks the disulfide bonds between the hair proteins allowing it to easily separate from the skin.

Epilation

This technique removes the whole hair follicle, including the root. Multiple techniques are available including waxing, threading, plucking, electrolysis, and laser therapy. Electrolysis uses electric current to treat each individual hair follicle and destroy the hair. It is slow and more painful than other methods, and could lead to scarring. Laser treatment uses specific wavelengths to target the hair only and minimizes local spread. It tends to be more effective in patients with fair-colored skin and dark hair. It generally is better tolerated and faster, as larger areas can be treated at once. Unfortunately, the cost associated with this effective, more permanent therapy may be out of reach for many patients.

Treatment of acne

Patients with moderate and severe acne may be treated with systemic and local therapy to maximize the effect. Like patients with hirsutism who benefit from COC and anti-androgens, patients with acne also benefit from these therapies. Given the inflammatory nature and potential super infection of lesions, topical and systemic antibiotics (such as clindamycin and doxycycline) are of benefit. Local antiseptic and anti-inflammatory agents such as benzoyl peroxide are available as topical formulations for acne. Local retinoids such as tretionin derived from vitamin A are effective, because of their anti-inflammatory properties and regulation of the desquamation process. Systemic retinoids (isotretinoin) have significant teratogenicity and are therefore used only in cases that are severe and unresponsive to other therapy. The use of this medication requires patients to also be on reliable and effective contraception during treatment.[20]

Screening/prevention

No specific prevention protocol exists for patients with hyperandrogenism. Newborn screening for CAH is mandatory in all states in the United States as part of the hospital collected panel prior to hospital discharge. [21] Patients having home births and non-hospital deliveries should obtain newborn screening when visiting their pediatrician's office. This test is not routinely done in other countries, and patients with this condition can present to practitioners' offices when they immigrate to the United States. A normal newborn screen does not rule out late onset CAH and this can still present during puberty or later.

Concluding remarks

Hyperandrogenism is a condition that manifests secondary to multiple etiologies. Although PCOS and idiopathic hirsutism are the most common conditions encountered, serious life threatening conditions such as CAH, Cushing's, and ovarian or adrenal tumors can also present with an increase in androgen levels. Management of the underlying medical cause for the androgen increase must be addressed, as well as the nonreversible body image effects caused by exposure to high androgen levels.

References

1. Azziz R. The evaluation and management of hirsutism. *Obstet Gynecol.* 2003;**101**:995–1007.
2. Hoffman BL, Schorge JO, Schaffer JI, et al. Polycystic ovarian syndrome and hyperandrogenism. In: Hoffman BL, Schorge JO, Schaffer JI, et al., eds. *Williams Gynecology*, 2nd ed. New York: McGraw-Hill; 2012. http://accessmedicine.mhmedical.com/content.aspx?bookid=399&Sectionid=41722306. Accessed August 26, 2014.
3. Emans SJ. Androgen abnormalities in the adolescent girl. In: Emans SJ, Laufer MR, Goldstein DP, eds. *Pediatric and Adolescent Gynecology*, 5th ed. Philadelphia: Lippincott Williams & Wilkins; 2005: pp 296–325.
4. Archer JS, Chang RJ. Hirsutism and acne in polycystic ovary syndrome. *Best Pract Res Clin Obstet Gynaecol.* 2004;**18**:737–54.
5. Fritz MA. Hirsutism. In: Fritz MA, Speroff L, eds. *Clinical Gynecologic Endocrinology and Infertility*, 10th ed. Philadelphia: Lippincott Williams & Wilkins; 2011: pp 533–66.

6. Hatch R, Rosenfield RL, Kim MH, Tredway D. Hirsutism: implications, etiology, and management. *Am J Obstet Gynecol.* 1981;**1**(140):815–30.
7. Purdy S, de Berker D. Acne. *BMJ.* 2006;**333**:949–53.
8. Cela E, Robertson C, Rush K, et al. Prevalence of polycystic ovaries in women with androgenic alopecia. *Eur J Endocrinol.* 2003;**149**:439–42.
9. Verkauf BS, Von Thron J, O'Brien WF. Clitoral size in normal women. *Obstet Gynecol.* 1992;**80**:41–4.
11. Azziz R, Zacur HA. 21-Hydroxylase deficiency in female hyperandrogenism: screening and diagnosis. *Clin Endocrinol Metab.* 1989;**69**:577–84.
12. Nieman LK, Biller BM, Findling JW, et al. The diagnosis of Cushing's syndrome: an Endocrine Society clinical practice guideline. *J Clin Endocrinol Metab.* 2008;**93**:1526–40.
13. Borer JG, Tan PE, Diamond DA. The spectrum of Sertoli cell tumors in children. *Urol Clin North Am.* 2000;**27**:529–41.
14. Chivukula M1, Hunt J, Carter G, et al. Recurrent gynandroblastoma of ovary-A case report: a molecular and immunohistochemical analysis. *Int J Gynecol Pathol.* 2007;**26**:30–3.
15. Padilla SL. Androgen-producing tumors in children and adolescents. *Adolesc Pediatr Gynecol.* 1989;**2**:135–42.
16. Speiser PW, White PC. Congenital adrenal hyperplasia. *N Engl J Med.* 2003 Aug 21;**349**(8):776–88.
17. Van der Spuy ZM, le Roux PA. Cyproterone acetate for hirsutism. *Cochrane Database Syst Rev.* 2003;**4**: CD001125.
18. Moghetti P1, Castello R, Magnani CM, et al. Clinical and hormonal effects of the 5 alpha-reductase inhibitor finasteride in idiopathic hirsutism. *J Clin Endocrinol Metab.* 1994;**79**:1115–21.
19. Balfour JA1, McClellan K. Topical eflornithine. *Am J Clin Dermatol.* 2001;**2**:197–201
20. Zaenglein AL1, Thiboutot DM. Expert committee recommendations for acne management. *Pediatrics.* 2006;**118**:1188–99.
21. State-specific testing for congenital disorders, available at www.babysfirsttest.org/newborn-screening/states. Accessed August 26, 2014.

Chapter 30

Hyperprolactinemia*

Jessica T. Servey

Introduction

Hyperprolactinemia is the most common pituitary abnormality seen in women. It is the term simply given to having an elevated serum prolactin. Prolactin is made and stored from lactotroph cells in the pituitary gland. The control of prolactin is mainly inhibitory, with a few stimulating factors. Thyroid-releasing hormone (TRH) directly stimulates prolactin release. Estrogen can increase prolactin levels as well by augmenting TRH. The pituitary is inhibited by the neurotransmitter dopamine. Dopamine primarily controls release. Serotonin has been hypothesized to increase prolactin, but this has not been substantiated.[1] Prolactin can also come from decidualized stroma; such is not regulated by the pituitary.

The principal function of prolactin is to stimulate growth of mammary tissue, and subsequently to produce and secrete milk. Its secretion fluctuates over the course of the day, and is highest during sleep and lowest while awake. This is thought to be related to a person's circadian rhythm.[3] For this reason the most common timeframe for checking prolactin levels is first thing in the morning. In women, levels additionally fluctuate throughout the menstrual cycle with the peak in mid-cycle.

The prevalence and incidence of hyperprolactinemia varies depending on the population. In the general population, the prevalence of prolactinomas ranges from 6% to 50%.[4, 5] The prevalence of hyperprolactinemia has been reported at 90 per 100,000 in women with the peak age at 25–34 years old.[6] When special populations are defined the incidence is higher. Hyperprolactinemia can occur in 15.7% of women seeing an infertility specialist.[7] In women with a combination of oligomenorrhea or amenorrhea with galactorrhea, 75%–84% had hyperprolactinemia.[8] Specifically, in adolescents and young women with oligomenorrhea or amenorrhea, up to 13.8% were noted to have hyperprolactinemia, but in all women presenting with amenorrhea 30% may have prolactinemia.[9] For women who have abnormal uterine bleeding in the third decade of life, 9.4% have hyperprolactinemia.[10] Hyperprolactinemia can occur in men, but some estimate up to 10 times more women have this condition prior to menopause then men over a lifetime. After menopause the incidence of hyperprolactinemia is equal between men and women.

Clinical presentation

Multiple clinical symptoms and physical signs are related to hyperprolactinemia. Resulting decreases in the secretion of gonadotropin-releasing hormone and the subsequent effects on other stimulating sex hormones cause many of the clinical symptoms. Hyperprolactinemia not only suppresses release of lutenizing hormone, but has direct effects on the ovary, thereby affecting both estrogen and progesterone production.[11] Galactorrhea, amenorrhea, and infertility are the three most common presenting complaints. The symptoms otherwise vary depending on the age of the woman and the size of any adenoma. Infertility can occur even with normal menstrual cycles. Hyperprolactinemia may lead to shortened luteal phase and insufficient progesterone. If the hyperprolactinemia coexists with polycystic ovarian syndrome, there can be a delay in diagnosis unless the patient has galactorrhea. In adolescents there can be a delay in puberty.[12] Additionally subtle psychologic symptoms have been noted to

* Disclaimer: The opinions herein reflect only the author's. These are not the opinions of the Uniformed Services University, the United States Air Force, or the Department of Defense.

Office Care of Women, ed. Martin E. Olsen and Botros Rizk. Published by Cambridge University Press.

occur with hyperprolactinemia.[13] In women of all ages decreased libido may occur.

Large adenomas can cause mass effects such as visual changes and headaches. The visual symptoms are variable and can include classic bi-temporal hemianopsia to small partial defects to scotomatas.[14] In addition 10% of tumors may invade the cavernous sinus with subsequent cranial nerve palsies.[15] Postmenopausal women tend to present later in the course as the typical menstrual abnormalities are not symptoms; they tend to present with visual symptoms, headaches, or late galactorrhea with larger prolactinomas. In a study of fourteen women in three countries diagnosed from age 54 to 75, thirteen of the fourteen had macroprolactinomas, with eight of them having suprasellar extension. The mean prolactin level was 1,783 and significantly higher than in premenopausal women.[16] It seems that women have a higher risk of macroprolactinomas as they get older.[17] They can also have sexual dysfunction. These symptom are similar to the ones seen when men present with hyperprolactinemia.

Newer data confirms that hyperprolactinemia increases risk for osteoporosis and fractures. In a study of 78 women aged 20–81, 33.3% had osteopenia and 23.1% had osteoporosis. This was significantly higher than the control subjects. In the same study the vertebral fracture rate was higher in women with hyperprolactinemia and independently associated with the duration of the disease.[18] Another study looking at women with forearm and spine fractures found the effect on the bone greater in the spine which had a 25% decrease in density compared with controls. Unfortunately, even after treatment for the hyperprolactinemia, bone density was not restored.[19] At this time, hyperprolactinemia is not part of the workup for pathologic fractures, but could be a presenting sign especially in the postmenopausal woman.

Table 30-1 Medications that can cause hyperprolactinemia

Antipsychotics	Phenothiazines Haloperidol Risperidone Butyrophenones Clozapine
Antidepressants	Tricyclics Monamine oxidase inhibitors Selective serotonin reuptake inhibitors
Anti-emetics	Metoclopramide Domperidone
Antihypertensives	Verapamil Methyldopa Reserpine
Opiates	Morphine Methadone
Others	Estrogens Cocaine Cimetidine

Causes of hyperprolactinemia

Some normal physiologic causes of hyperprolactinemia exist such as pregnancy, lactation, exercise, or periods of stress. Nipple stimulation outside of pregnancy and breastfeeding does not cause hyperprolactinemia.[20] Transient hyperprolactinemia has been associated with both generalized and partial seizures.[21] This transient hyperprolactinemia after a seizure resolves within an hour. Medication induced hyperprolactinemia is found with many antipsychotics, antidepressants, estrogen, opiods, and some antihypertensives and gastrointestinal drugs (see Table 30-1). Primary hypothyroidism may cause hyperprolactinemia due to stimulation of TRH. Chronic renal failure can also cause hyperprolactinemia secondary to impaired renal degradation. Infiltrative disorders of the pituitary such as sarcoidosis increase prolactin levels. Chest wall injuries can induce hyperprolactinemia as well. The single most common cause of hyperprolactinemia is a prolactin adenoma accounting for 60% in some studies.[1, 12] See Table 30-2 for a complete list of causes.

Other associated disorders are seen with hyperprolactinemia. It can coexist with polycystic ovarian syndrome;[22] there is significant overlap in symptoms between these conditions, making it challenging to discern if one causes the other or they merely coexist frequently. Many rheumatologic disorders can coexist with hyperprolactinemia including systemic lupus erythematosus, rheumatoid arthritis, and systemic sclerosis. Cranial abnormalities associated with hyperprolactinemia include empty sella syndrome, many infiltrative diseases, radiation to the pituitary area, and trauma.[1, 12] Prolactinomas have also been associated with multiple endocrine neoplasia type I.[23]

Table 30-2 Causes of hyperprolactinemia

Physiological	Pregnancy Lactation Stress Exercise Post-ictal
Infiltrative conditions	Sarcoidosis Tuberculosis Histiocytosis X Metastasis
Pituitary adenomas	Prolactinomas Mixed growth hormone and prolactin adenomas Mixed adrenocorticotrophic and prolactin adenomas
Other pituitary tumors	Craniopharyngioma Germinomas Meningiomas
Miscellaneous	Trauma to the pituitary Irradiation to the pituitary Lymphocytic hypophysitis Empty sella syndrome

Natural history

Microprolactinomas have not been shown to have significant growth over time with the longest study having an eight-year follow-up. Note that in these studies, newer imaging such as advanced computed tomography (CT) was not available and magnetic resonance imaging (MRI) capability was rare.[24] In a study of 38 untreated patients over 31 months of follow-up, there was no significant changes in tumor size.[25] In a retrospective study of 70 patients with hyperprolactinemia, excluding macroadenomas, three out of ten normalized prolactin with no treatment over time. In those women with a pregnancy, 35% normalized requiring no further treatment versus 14% who did not have a pregnancy (P <0.05).[26] In women there is a 45% chance of normalization of prolactin levels after menopause.[27] Therefore, it seems that a percentage of women with idiopathic hyperprolactinemia and those with microadenomas have the potential for spontaneous resolution over time. There are no specific studies following the long-term natural history of macroprolactinomas.

Recent improved imaging shows many prolactinomas have had hemorrhage. In a study of 368 patients, the overall prevalence of hemorrhage was 6.8%. However, there was a significant difference in the rate of hemorrhage between macroadenomas and microadenomas at 20.3% and 3.1%, respectively. In this study, 87% of patients with hemorrhage resolved over time with dopamine agonist treatment.[28]

Diagnostic workup

Laboratory testing is the key to the initial diagnosis of hyperprolactinoma. Any woman with the combination of galactorrhea and amenorrhea or oligomenorrhea should be tested for hyperprolactinemia. Normal ranges vary slightly by lab but tend to be <25 mcg/L in women. There is a phenomenon known as the "hook effect" when the prolactin clumps and causes a falsely lower prolactin level compared with the adenoma size seen in imaging. Current guidelines recommend a single serum measurement of prolactin for diagnosis. There is a recommendation against dynamic testing of prolactin. In general the level of prolactin matches the size of the adenoma. This is not precise, but it is accepted that levels greater than 500 mcg/L are diagnostic of a macroadenoma.[2]

After the initial elevated lab test, causes of hyperprolactinemia that could be reversible must be excluded. This would include checking TRH, checking for renal abnormalities, and a thorough medication review. There is some evidence to support serum testing for the larger prolactin molecules. This is not clearly defined. If hyperprolactinoma is felt to be drug induced, removal of the offending agent should occur for three days with repeat prolactin serum testing. Current consensus is to avoid treating asymptomatic drug-induced hyperprolactinemia.[2] Additional testing of the pituitary as a whole is recommended by some, and may be warranted when the prolactin is very high or other symptoms are present.

Radiographic features of prolactinomas are best seen on gadolinium enhanced MRI; this is considered the imaging of choice. Patients with visual symptoms or severe headaches may receive urgent CT first. If this is done, an MRI should be performed to complete the imaging workup. In one recent guideline, however, specific radiologic testing of all patients with hyperprolactinemia was not mentioned.[2]

At the time of initial diagnosis, patients may be divided into subsets based on the size of the prolactinoma. Microadenomas are defined as prolactinomas less than 1 cm in size, and macroadenomas are greater than 1 cm. Giant prolactinomas are a special higher risk subset of prolactinomas. These adenomas are larger than 4 cm and/or demonstrate more than 2 cm of suprasellar extension. These tumors tend to cause more visual symptoms.

Treatment and follow-up

The treatment of hyperprolactinemia in women varies based on the etiology, the patient's desire to conceive, symptoms present, and the size or expansion of any adenoma. If the hyperprolactinemia is drug induced, the offending agent should be discontinued. If for some reason the drug cannot be stopped, a dopamine agonist may be started to treat symptoms. Current recommendations state that a patient with asymptomatic drug-induced hyperprolactinemia does not require treatment.[2]

Women with hyperprolactinemia who do not want to conceive and have no neurologic symptoms can choose to have no treatment. Additionally, the presence of a microadenoma does not require treatment unless symptoms are present.[2] If no treatment is started, periodic prolactin levels should be performed; the consensus periodicity is annual. If at any time the patient develops symptoms, treatment with a dopamine agonist is started. If a microadenoma enlarges (even without symptoms), treatment should be started.

Any woman who desires pregnancy or has a macroadenoma at the time of diagnosis should be treated with a dopamine receptor agonist. Both bromocriptine and cabergoline are available for use. Pergolide is an older drug and no longer available. Quinagolide is used in Europe but is not available in the United States.

Bromocriptine is an ergot derivative developed and approved in 1967 for the treatment of hyperprolactinemia. It is the best studied option in all age groups and during pregnancy. It has a half-life of 7–14 hours thus requiring twice daily dosing. The typical starting dose is 2.3 mg per day in divided dose and increased to a maximum of 15 mg per day. The incidence of adverse effects is 69%, with nausea, headaches, and dizziness being the most common. Many patients discontinue use secondary to the side effects. Side effects are more common when the drug is initiated and increased. Titrating slowly may therefore be effective.[29] Another potential side effects is postural hypotension.[30] Two rare adverse effects are pain in the digits related to vasospasm that occurs in response to cold,[31] and precipitation of psychotic episodes.[32] Nonsurgical cerebrospinal fluid (CSF) rhinorrhea is sometimes seen as the medication shrinks the tumor; this often resolves spontaneously.[29]

Bromocriptine is an effective medication to treat hyperprolactinemia. Early trials in the 1980s demonstrated normalization of prolactin, decreased tumor size, and visual field improvements.[33] Bromocriptine has had studies with the longest follow-up reaching 10 years. A recent meta-analysis of 39 trials further defined the effectiveness of bromocriptine. Combining the data, there was a median of 68% of patients having normalization of prolactin, and 62% having tumor shrinkage. Clinical symptoms including galactorrhea, amenorrhea, infertility, and visual field defects improved by 85%, 78%, 67%, and 53%, respectively.[34]

Cabergoline is a longer acting dopamine agonist used to treat hyperprolactinemia. Its long half-life of 65 hours allows for twice weekly or even weekly dosing. The starting dose is 0.25 mg twice weekly. The standard schedule includes an increase every four weeks. The standard dose ranges from 0.5 mg to 2.0 mg per week. Compared with bromocriptine, there are fewer total side effects. The most common side effects are nausea, headache, and dizziness. Databases report 2% of patients will discontinue the drug due to side effects. The once weekly dosing can improve patient compliance.[35] In a study of 162 patients, 85% had normalization of prolactin levels, and more than 90% of both amenorrheic and oligomenorrheic women resumed normal menstrual cycles. Only 3% of these patients discontinued use due to side effects.[36]

Cabergoline has recently been viewed as the drug of choice. It is more effective in normalizing prolactin, shrinking adenomas, and avoiding secondary procedures compared to bromocriptine.[2] One study compared the extent of tumor size reduction and prolactin level normalization among 110 patients with macroprolactinomas. Of these 110 patients, 26 were drug naïve, 19 were intolerant of other dopamine agonists, 47 were resistant to other dopamine agonists, and 28 were responsive to other dopamine agonists but no longer using them due to poor compliance or drug unavailability. The prolactin normalization in the 19 patients intolerant of other agonists was 94.7%. The prevalence of macroprolactinoma shrinkage was greatest among drug-naïve subjects at 92.3%. However, significant tumor shrinkage (>50%) still occurred in the intolerant and resistant groups, with a rate of 42.1% and 30.3%, respectively. Importantly this study demonstrated that patients who were intolerant or resistant to other dopamine agonist may respond to cabergoline when the dose was increased to 3 mg–3.5 mg weekly.[37] In another study of macroprolactinomas and resistance, 122 patients were enrolled; 72 of them were women. Normalization of prolactin levels occurred on 83% with doses of cabergoline less than 1.5 mg per week. Patients were considered partially resistant if higher doses were used. By increasing the dose to 3.5 mg per week, 94% of patients had normalization. Those patients who required a higher dose were more likely to be men or have cavernous sinus invasion.[38] Further evidence for the use of cabergoline at high doses was conducted in single-arm prospective study of 150 patients, consisting of both men and women. These patients included those resistant or intolerant to other dopamine agonists. Prolactin levels were normalized in 99.3% (149) of patients within one year using an individualized treatment protocol with higher doses of cabergoline up to 5 mg per week. There were no dropouts due to side effects.[39] These studies are the evidence behind the current recommendations that if bromocriptine does not work, a switch to cabergoline should be made. Furthermore, if standard dosing does not seem to induce normal prolactin levels, higher doses of cabergoline should be used.[2]

When bromocriptine and cabergoline have been studied together, cabergoline has demonstrated superior results with fewer side effects. In a multicenter, prospective randomized comparative trial conducted in 459 hyperprolactinemic women (279 microadenomas, 3 macroadenomas, 167 idiopathic hyperprolactinemia, 10 other), of those women treated with cabergoline, 83% achieved normoprolactinemia, 72% resumed ovulatory cycles, and 3% discontinued the medication because of adverse effects. Of the women treated with bromocriptine, 59% achieved normoprolactinemia, 52% resumed ovulatory cycles, and 12% stopped the drug because of adverse effects.[40] Additionally in a meta-analysis including six observational studies and three randomized trials, cabergoline was more effective than bromocriptine. Specifically bromocriptine was less effective in reducing persistent hyperprolactinemia, galatorrhea, and amenorrhea.[34] A more recent meta-analysis confirmed these results.[41] These studies confirmed that cabergoline is the drug of choice for hyperprolactinemia.

Cabergoline appears to have increased effectiveness, but concerns exist regarding valvular heart disease. A large amount of data shows increased prevalence of valvular heart disease in Parkinson's patients using dopamine agonists.[42] The most recent review pooled data from multiple observational studies showed significant increased risk (RR = 6.38 [3.17–12.81]) of developing moderate to severe aortic regurgitation.[43] Doses of dopamine agonists in Parkinson's are higher than those used in hyperprolactinemia. The evidence for valvular disease in patients being treated for hyperprolactinemia has been conflicted until recently.[44–47] Recent agreement is that there is no significant risk of valvular heart disease with routine dosages for hyperprolactinemia.[48–50] Further study is needed concerning the higher doses of cabergoline used in resistant adenomas.

A small group of patients will be resistant to treatment with dopamine agonists. Approximately 80% of this group who do not respond to treatment with bromocriptine will respond to cabergoline.[51] Complete resistance to cabergoline is extraordinarily uncommon, and most "partial" resistance can often be overcome by increasing the dose. One study of 150 patients found that all but one patient could get normalization of prolactin with increased doses of cabergoline.[39]

A small subset of patients can discontinue the medication once the tumor shrinks and/or normal prolactin levels are achieved. The exact reason this occurs is unclear. In a study of 89 patients who were treated with either bromocriptine of cabergoline for several years and then after withdrew from treatment, 36% remained in remission beyond one year.[52] In that study, there was no difference between the two medications. Other studies demonstrated rates of recurrence at one year from 36% to 60%.[53–55] After review of these studies, it is reasonable to give patients a trial of dopamine agonists after several years of prolactin normalization and tumor shrinkage. Since the return to hyperprolactinemia may occur as early as three months after medication termination, periodic prolactin levels should be considered. No consensus exists for the frequency of prolactin levels follow-up.

There are very few studies defining the optimal management of giant prolactinomas. Often a combination of treatment is used with cabergoline being the medication of choice.[56] A series of 68 patients with invasive prolactinomas were managed with a combination of treatments, with 33 having medical treatment with bromocriptine initially and the other

35 with surgical treatment first. Many required adjunct treatment after the initial treatment for complete management.[57] Another series of patients with parasellar extension demonstrated this feature of a macroprolactinoma may predict resistance to dopamine agonist therapy.[58]

Surgery is typically reserved for those with one of the following issues: rapid visual loss, failure of medical therapy to normalize prolactin levels and improve symptoms of hypogonadism, failure of medical therapy to slow tumor growth, tumor expansion during pregnancy not controlled with medication, and preconceptionally in a woman with problems during a prior pregnancy. Surgical options have specific risks and benefits. Transphenoidal surgical approaches are most common and have demonstrated remission rates up to 90%.[59, 60] In a recent series of 138 women under the age of 40, initial cure rate for macroadenomas was 95%. Over time there were some recurrences for a final longer-term cure for macroadenomas of 89%. Macroadenomas without invasion were more likely to have a cure.[61] The surgical approach is individualized because there are no randomized controlled trials of the surgical approach. Mortality following surgery is reported as 1%. Pituitary failure and diabetes insipidus occur in up to 20% of patients. More uncommon complications include infection, CSF leaks, visual loss, and hypothalamic injuries.[62] Endoscopic procedures and intraoperative MRI are gaining recognition but are in early stages of development. Fractionated guided radiotherapy and Gamma Knife stereotactic radiosurgery have been reserved for recalcitrant cases. Most studies include all pituitary tumors. In one study of 33 tumors (8 prolactinomas), morbidity included visual field defects and hypopituitarism.[63]

Hyperprolactinemia and pregnancy

Prolactin levels steadily increase throughout pregnancy and reach a peak in the first week postpartum. [64] There is no recommendation to follow the level periodically because of limited diagnostic value in pregnancy.[2]

Medical therapy during pregnancy is individualized. Both bromocriptine and cabergoline are known to cross the placenta.[65] As with most medication use in pregnancy, there have been no randomized placebo controlled trials. However numerous case reports and other cohort studies demonstrate the safety of both of these medications in pregnancy. Bromocriptine has been used to return ovulation in women; pregnancies have thus been exposed to bromocriptine for the first four to six weeks without any subsequent ill effects on the mother or the fetus.[66] Molitch looked at the effect of cabergoline use in more than 800 women in the beginning of pregnancy and determined no increased risk of spontaneous abortion.[67] In a series of 100 pregnancies followed to delivery, including women who needed to restart cabergoline, there was no increased risk of congenital malformations.[68] In a study comparing pregnancy outcomes in women taking dopamine agonists through various times in pregnancy (6,239 treated with bromocriptine and 789 treated with cabergoline), there were no increases in spontaneous abortion, preterm deliveries, or congenital malformations. [67] The safety for bromocriptine and cabergoline during pregnancy does not extend to quinagolide. Quinagolide does seem to cause increased risk of spontaneous abortion and malformations.[69]

Some concerns exist about the effects on fetal dopamine and subsequent neurocognitive development. In a study of 83 children followed up to 12 years, there were no noted physical or developmental abnormalities.[70] A survey completed in France following children up to nine years after exposure to bromocriptine showed normal development. [71] An additional series of 10 women with continuous use of bromocriptine during pregnancy with up to six years of follow-up had showed developmental issues.[72] In a study of 57,408 women, of which 183 had a dopamine agonist at some point in pregnancy, there was no associated psychomotor developmental delay noted.[73] Overall, these results do not show clinically significant increases in developmental concerns with the use of either dopamine agonist.

When decisions are made on continuing a dopamine agonist, the risk of enlargement is a special consideration. Multiple meta-analyses were completed over the past decades, but many of the earlier ones were completed with old technology and may have missed the enlargement that current MRIs would have detected. In the largest compilation of women with microadenomas to date, clinically important tumor growth occurs 2.7% of the time. In macroadenomas it can be 22.9% of the time if the woman had no prior ablative treatment, and 4.8% with prior ablative treatment.[67] The effect of pregnancy and lactation on the hyperprolactinemic women and adenomas is questionable. In a recent study of 104 pregnancies, 41% of those demonstrated a normal prolactin level without medical treatment for up to 22 months. A notable decrease in adenoma size was seen in many; an association with prepregnancy size exists.[74]

All dopamine agonists should be stopped once pregnancy has been confirmed. Exceptions are made for macroprolactinomas, giant prolactinomas, and those invading the optic chiasm.[2, 65] If a woman develops clinical symptoms such as headache or visual changes during pregnancy, visual field testing and an MRI without gadolinium should be considered.[2] Simultaneous initiation of a dopamine agonist is also needed. If a dopamine agonist is needed throughout pregnancy, bromocriptine is the drug of choice, since there is more experience with this drug.[2, 65] This may change over the next several years as outside of pregnancy cabergoline is the drug of choice. More experience in pregnancy may influence these recommendations.

After pregnancy, women are counseled on the effects of hyperprolactinemia, prolactinomas, and dopamine agonist use in lactation. Lactation itself has never been studied as a cause for increased adenoma growth. Both bromocriptine and cabergoline are considered safe in lactation. However, these medications have the potential to decrease a woman's milk supply as they can be used to stop lactation.[75, 76]

Concluding remarks

Overall hyperprolactinemia is a common problem in women, especially during the reproductive years. It is often diagnosed early due to the menstrual abnormalities and infertility. Many cases are easily treated with cabergoline or bromocriptine. Patients with rapid onset or worsening symptoms may need to be counseled for potential surgery. Many women with infertility can conceive starting medication, which will need to be discontinued. With follow-up patients with hyperprolactinemia will have no significant long-term effects on their health.

References

1. Molitch ME. Prolactinoma. In: Melmed S, ed. The Pituitary, 3rd ed. Waltham, MA: Academic Press; 2011: 475–531.
2. Melmed S, Casanueva FF, Hoffman AR, et al. Diagnosis and treatment of hyperprolactinemia: an Endocrine Society clinical practice guideline. *J Clin Endocrinol Metab.* 2011 Feb;**96**(2):273–88.
3. Waldstreicher J, Duffy JF, Brown EN, et al. Gender differences in the temporal organization of prolactin (PRL) secretion: evidence for a sleep independent circadian rhythm of circulation PRL levels – a clinical research center study. *J Clin Endocrinol Metab.* 1996;**81**:1483–7.
4. Daly AF, Rixhon M, Adam C, et al. High prevalence of pituitary adenomas: a cross-sectional study in the province of Liege, Belgium. *J Clin Endocrinol Metab.* 2006;**91**:4769–75.
5. Fernandez A, Karavitaki N, Wass JA. Prevalence of pituitary adenomas: a community-based, cross-sectional study in Banbury (Oxfordshire, UK). *Clin Endocrinol (Oxf).* 2010;**72**:377–82.
6. Kars M, Souverein PC, Herings RM, et al. Estimated age- and sex-specific incidence and prevalence of dopamine agonist-treated hyperprolactinemia. *J Clin Endocrinol Metab.* 2009;**94**:2729–34.
7. Thirunavakkarasu K, Dutta P, Sridhar S, et al. Macroprolactinemia in hyperprolactinemic infertile women. *Endocrine.* 2013 Dec;**44**(3):750–5.
8. Molitch ME, Reichlin S. Hyperprolactinemic disorders. *Dis Mon.* 1982;**28**:1–58.
9. Schlechte J, Sherman B, Halmi N, et al. Prolactin secreting pituitary tumours in amenorrheic women: a comprehensive study. *Endocr Rev.* 1980;**1**:295–308.
10. Lee D, Oh Y, Yoon B, et al. Prevalence of hyperprolactinemia in adolescents and young women with menstruation related problems. *Am J Obstet Gyneco.* 2012;**206**:213 e1–5.
11. Demura R, Ono M, Demura H, et al. Prolactin directly inhibits basal as well as gonadotropin-stimulated secretion of progesterone and 17 beta-estradiol in the human ovary. *J Clin Endocrinol Metab.* 1982;**54**:1246–50.
12. Prabhakar VK, Davis JR. Hyperprolactinaemia. *Best Pract Res Clin Obstet Gynaecol.* 2008 Apr;**22**(2):341–53.
13. Sobrinho LG. Emotional aspects of hyperprolactinaemia. *Psychother Psychosom.* 1998;**67**:133–9.
14. Melen O. Neuro-ophthalmologic features of pituitary tumors. *Endocrinol Metab Clin North Am.* 1987;**16**:585–608.
15. Cottier JP, Destrieux C, Brunereau L, et al. Cavernous sinus invasion by pituitary adenoma: MR imaging. *Radiology.* 2000;**215**:463–9.
16. Shimon MD, Bronstein J, Shapiro G, et al. Women with prolactinomas presented at the postmenopausal

period. *Endocrine*. 2014;**47**(3):889–94. First online 8 April 2014.

17. Maor Y, Berezin M. Hyperprolactinemia in postmenopausal women. *Fertil Steril*. 1997;**67**:693–6.
18. Delgrange E, Raverot G, Bex M, et al. Giant prolactinomas in women. *Eur J Endocrinol*. 2013 Nov 22;**170**(1):31–8.
19. Schlechte J, el-Khoury G, Kathol M, Walkner L. Forearm and vertebral bone mineral in treated and untreated hyperprolactinemic amenorrhea. *J Clin Endocrinol Metab*. 1987;**64**:1021–6.
20. Jarrell J, Franks S, McInnes R, et al. Breast examination does not elevate serum prolactin. *Fertil Steril*. 1980;**33**:49–51.
21. Luef G. Horrmonal alterations following seizures. *Epilepsy Behav*. 2010 Oct;**19**(2):131–3.
22. Bracero N, Zacur HA, Polycystic ovary syndrome and hyperprolactinemia. *Obstet Gynecol Clin North Am*. 2001;**28**:77–84.
23. Prosser PR, Karam JH, Townsend JJ, Forsham PH. Prolactin-secreting pituitary adenomas in multiple endocrine adenomatosis, type I. *Ann Intern Med*. 1979;**91**(1):41–4.
24. Schlechte J, Dolan K, Sherman B, et al. The natural history of untreated hyperprolactinemia: a prospective analysis. *J Clin Endocrinol Metab*. 1989;**68**:412–8.
25. Sisam DA, Sheehan JP, Sheeler LR. The natural history of untreated microprolactinomas. *Fertil Steril*. 1987;**48**:67–71.
26. Jeffcoate WJ, Pound N, Sturrock ND, Lambourne J. Long-term follow-up of patients with hyperprolactinaemia. *Clin Endocrinol (Oxf)*. 1996;**45**:299–303.
27. Karunakaran S, Page RC, Wass JA. The effect of the menopause on prolactin levels in patients with hyperprolactinaemia. *Clin Endocrinol (Oxf)*. 2001;**54**:295–300.
28. Sarwar KN, Huda MS, Van de Velde V, et al. The prevalence and natural history of pituitary hemorrhage in prolactinoma. *J Clin Endocrinol Metab*. 2013 Jun;**98** (6):2362–7.
29. DailyMed. Bromocriptine. Available at: http://dailymed.nlm.nih.gov/dailymed/drugInfo.cfm?setid=93a0696b-b261-4262-9e06-f3180b419f8f. Accessed 8 July 2014.
30. Webster J. A comparative review of the tolerability profiles of dopamine agonists in the treatment of hyperprolactinaemia and inhibition of lactation. *Drug Saf*. 1996;**14**:228–38.
31. Wass JA, Thorner MO, Besser GM. Letter: digital vasospasm with bromocriptine. *Lancet*. 1976;**1**:1135.
32. Turner TH, Cookson JC, Wass JA, et al. Psychotic reactions during treatment of pituitary tumours with dopamine agonists. *Br Med J (Clin Res Ed)*. 1984;**289**:1101–3.
33. Molitch ME, Elton RL, Blackwell RE, et al. Bromocriptine as primary therapy for prolactin-secreting macroadenomas: results of a prospective multicenter study. *J Clin Endocrinol Metab*. 1985;**60**:698–705.
34. Wang AT, Mullan RJ, Lane MA, et al. Treatment of hyperprolactinemia: a systematic review and meta-analysis. *Syst Rev*. 2012;**1**:33.
35. DailyMed. Cabergoline. Available at: http://dailymed.nlm.nih.gov/dailymed/drugInfo.cfm?setid=e563bf14-daca-9bfb-f324-1d243150528e. Accessed 8 July 2014.
36. Webster J, Piscitelli G, Polli A, et al. The efficacy and tolerability of long-term cabergoline therapy in hyperprolactinaemic disorders: an open, uncontrolled, multicentre study: European Multicentre Cabergoline Study Group. *Clin Endocrinol (Oxf)*. 1993 Sep;**39** (3):323–9.
37. Colao A, Di Sarno A, Landi ML, et al. Macroprolactinoma shrinkage during cabergoline treatment is greater in naive patients than in patients pretreated with other dopamine agonists: a prospective study in 110 patients. *J Clin Endocrinol Metab*. 2000;**85**:2247–52.
38. Delgrange E, Daems T, Verhelst J, et al. Characterization of resistance to the prolactin-lowering effects of cabergoline in macroprolactinomas: a study in 122 patients. *Eur J Endocrinol*. 2009;**160**:747–52.
39. Ono M, Miki N, Kawamata T, et al. Prospective study of high-dose cabergoline treatment of prolactinomas in 150 patients. *J Clin Endocrinol Metab*. 2008;**93**:4721–7.
40. Webster J, Piscitelli G, Polli A, et al. A comparison of cabergoline and bromocriptine in the treatment of hyperprolactinemic amenorrhea: Cabergoline Comparative Study Group. *N Engl J Med*. 1994;**331**:904–9.
41. Nunes V, El Dib R, Boguszewski C, et al. Cabergoline versus bromocriptine in the treatment of hyperprolactinemia: a systematic review of randomized controlled trials and meta-analysis. *Pituitary*. 2011:**14**;3:259–65.
42. Zanettini R, Antonini A, Gatto G, et al. Valvular heart disease and the use of dopamine agonists for Parkinson's disease. *N Engl J Med*. 2007; **356**:39.
43. Rasmussen VG, Østergaard K, Dupont E, Poulsen SH. The risk of valvular regurgitation in patients with

Parkinson's disease treated with dopamine receptor agonists. *Mov Disord*. 2011 Apr;**26**(5):801–6.

44. Kars M, Delgado V, Holman ER, et al. Aortic valve calcification and mild tricuspid regurgitation but no clinical heart disease after 8 years of dopamine agonist therapy for prolactinoma. *J Clin Endocrinol Metab*. 2008;**93**:3348–56.
45. Colao A, Galderisi M, Di Sarno A, et al. Increased prevalence of tricuspid regurgitation in patients with prolactinomas chronically treated with cabergoline. *J Clin Endocrinol Metab*. 2008; **93**:3777–84.
46. Halperin I, Aller J, Varela C, et al. No clinically significant valvular regurgitation in long-term cabergoline treatment for prolactinoma. *Clin Endocrinol (Oxf)*. 2012 Aug;77(2):275–80.
47. Tan T, Cabrita IZ, Hensman D, et al. Assessment of cardiac valve dysfunction in patients receiving cabergoline treatment for hyperprolactinaemia. *Clin Endocrinol (Oxf)*. 2010 Sep;**73**(3):369–74.
48. Vallette S, Serri K, Rivera J, et al. Long-term cabergoline therapy is not associated with valvular heart disease in patients with prolactinomas. *Pituitary*. 2009;**12**:153–7.
49. Auriemma RS, Pivonello R, Perone Y, et al. Safety of long-term treatment with cabergoline on cardiac valve disease in patients with prolactinomas. *Eur J Endocrinol*. 2013 Aug 28;**169**(3):359–66.
50. Delgado V, Biermasz NR, van Thiel SW, et al. Changes in heart valve structure and function in patients treated with dopamine agonists for prolactinomas, a 2-year follow-up study. *Clin Endocrinol (Oxf)*. 2012 Jul;**77**(1):99–105.
51. Colao A, Di Sarno A, Sarnacchiaro F, et al. Prolactinomas resistant to standard dopamine agonists respond to chronic cabergoline treatment. *J Clin Endocrinol Metab*. 1997;**82**:876–83.
52. Biswas M, Smith J, Jadon D, et al. Long-term remission following withdrawal of dopamine agonist therapy in subjects with microprolactinomas. *Clin Endocrinol (Oxf)*. 2005;**63**:26–31.
53. Colao A, Di Sarno A, Cappabianca P, et al. Withdrawal of long-term cabergoline therapy for tumoral and nontumoral hyperprolactinemia. *N Engl J Med*. 2003;**349**:2023–33.
54. Kharlip J, Salvatori R, Yenokyan G, Wand GS. Recurrence of hyperprolactinemia after withdrawal of long-term cabergoline therapy. *J Clin Endocrinol Metab*. 2009;**94**:2428–36.
55. Anagnostis P, Adamidou F, Polyzos SA, et al. Long term follow-up of patients with prolactinomas and outcome of dopamine agonist withdrawal: a single center experience. *Pituitary*. 2012 Mar;**15**(1):25–9.
56. Moraes AB, Silva CM, Vieira Neto L, et al. Giant prolactinomas: the therapeutic approach. *Clin Endocrinol (Oxf)*. 2013 Oct; **79**(4):447–56.
57. Wu ZB, Su ZP, Wu JS, et al. Five years follow-up of invasive prolactinomas with special reference to the control of cavernous sinus invasion. *Pituitary*. 2008;**11**:63–70.
58. Delgrange E, Duprez T, Maiter D. Influence of parasellar extension of macroprolactinomas defined by magnetic resonance imaging on their responsiveness to dopamine agonist therapy. *Clin Endocrinol (Oxf)*. 2006;**64**:456–62.
59. Faria MA, Tindall GT. Transsphenoidal microsurgery for prolactin-secreting pituitary adenomas. *J Neurosurg*. 1982;**56**:33–43.
60. Thomson JA, Davies DL, McLaren EH, et al. Ten year follow up of microprolactinoma treated by transsphenoidal surgery. *BMJ*. 1994;**309**:1409–10.
61. Ikeda H, Watanabe K, Tominaga T, Yoshimoto T. Transsphenoidal microsurgical results of female patients with prolactinomas. *Clin Neurol Neurosurg*. 2013 Sep;**115**(9):1621–5.
62. Buchfelder M, Schlaffer S. Surgical treatment of pituitary tumors. *Best Pract Res Clin Endocrinol Metab*. 2009 Oct;**23**(5):677–92.
63. Sun DQ, Cheng JJ, Frazier JL, et al. Treatment of pituitary adenomas using radiosurgery and radiotherapy: a single center experience and review of literature. *Neurosurg Rev*. 2011;**34**:181–9.
64. Rigg LA, Lein A, Yen SS. Pattern of increase in circulating prolactin levels during human gestation. *Am J Obstet Gynecol*. 1977;**129**:454–6.
65. Glezer A, Bronstein M. Prolactinomas, cabergoline and pregnancy. *Endocrine*. 2014;**47**:64–9.
66. Krupp P, Monka C. Bromocriptine in pregnancy: safety aspects. *Klin Wochenschr*. 1987;**65**:823–7.
67. Molitch ME. Prolactinoma in pregnancy. *Best Pract Res Clin Endocrinol Metab*. 2011 Dec; **25**(6):885–96.
68. Lebbe M, Hubinont C, Bernard P, et al. Outcome of 100 pregnancies initiated under treatment with cabergoline in hyperprolactinaemic women. *Clin Endocrinol*. 2010;**73**:236–42.
69. Webster J. A comparative review of the tolerability profiles of dopamine agonists in the treatment of hyperprolactinaemia and inhibition of lactation. *Drug Saf*. 1996;**14**:228–38.
70. Colao A, Abs R, Barcena DG, et al. Pregnancy outcomes following cabergoline treatment: extended results from a 12-year observational study. *Clin Endocrinol (Oxf)*. 2008;**68**:66–71.

71. Raymond JP, Goldstein E, Konopka P, et al. Follow-up of children born of bromocriptine-treated mothers. *Horm Res.* 1985;**22**:239–46.

72. Konopka P, Raymond JP, Merceron RE, et al. Continuous administration of bromocriptine in the prevention of neurological complications in pregnant women with prolactinomas. *Am J Obstet Gynecol.* 1983;**146**:935–8.

73. Hurault-Delarue C, Montastruc J-L, Beau A-B, et al. Pregnancy outcome in women exposed to dopamine agonists during pregnancy: a pharmacoepidemiology study in EFEMERIS database. *Arch Gynecol Obstet.* 2014;**23**(6):586–94.

74. Domingue ME, Devuyst F, Alexopoulou O, et al. Outcome of prolactinoma after pregnancy and lactation: a study of 73 patients. *Clin Endocrinol (Oxf).* 2014 May;**80**(5):642–8.

75. TOXNET databases. LactMed: Cabergoline. Available at: http://toxnet.nlm.nih.gov/cgi-bin/sis/search2/r?dbs±lactmed:@or±%28@na±%22CABERGOLINE%22±%29. Accessed 8 July 2014.

76. TOXNET databases. LactMed: Bromocriptine. Available at: http://toxnet.nlm.nih.gov/cgi-bin/sis/search2/r?dbs±lactmed:@term±@na±Bromocriptine. Accessed 8 July 2014.

Chapter 31

Menopausal syndrome

Julia V. Johnson

Introduction

Menopause is the physiologic cessation of menses. Menopause is defined as the absence of menses for 12 months without a pathologic cause. The absence of menses is caused by the loss of ovarian response to follicle-stimulating hormone (FSH). Estrogen and progesterone production by the ovary becomes absent. The menopause transition, referred to as perimenopause, results in menstrual irregularity and potential vasomotor symptoms. Perimenopausal symptoms are related to an intermittent decrease in estradiol and progesterone production. Menopausal symptoms are primarily related to the loss of estradiol from the ovary. Women commonly present with perimenopausal and menopausal symptoms to seek medical advice and potential treatment.

Menopausal transition

The menstrual cycle begins and ends with oligoovulation and irregular menses. The Stages of Reproductive Aging Workshop describes the normal transition (Figure 31-1).[1] Studies define the early menopausal transition as a variable length of menses with a persistent change in cycle duration of more than seven days compared to previous menses. It is common for the follicular phase to shorten in response to elevated FSH levels leading to shortened cycles.[2] Typically there are limited vasomotor symptoms in early perimenopause, although they are more common in late perimenopause.[3] Because the FSH levels vary during the early perimenopausal period, this stage of the menopausal transition is diagnosed by symptoms. An elevated cycle day 3 FSH and decreased levels of anti-müllerian hormone levels have been used to confirm the diagnosis.[4] In addition, there is a normal decrease in the number of antral follicles seen on ultrasound which demonstrates the decrease in ovarian activity.[5] Ultrasound demonstrates a near absence of antral follicles. Because of the variation in the duration of the early stage of the menopausal transition, it is not possible to advise patients on the length of this stage.[6]

The late menopausal transition is defined as more than 60 days between menses. These extended periods of amenorrhea identify that the woman is oligoovulatory, and toward the end of the transition they are anovulatroy. The ovary is no longer consistently responsive to FSH; follicular development, ovarian hormone production, and ovulation are not predictable. It is of note that the menstrual cycles can vary with a mixture of regular, shortened cycles and prolonged cycles. The hormone production is decreased, even in ovulatory cycles, whereas the gonadotropin levels increase.[7] When ovulation does not occur, the ovary does not enter the luteal phase and progesterone is not produced. Unopposed estrogen stimulates endometrial development, and without progesterone stabilizing the growth of the endometrium, patients are at risk for menorrhagia. Perimenopausal menorrhagia, related to unopposed estrogen, occurs in women during the menopausal transition.[6] As the transition continues, estradiol production decreases and menses become lighter (Figure 31-2).

Eventually the ovary does not respond to gonadotropins, there is no estradiol or progesterone production, and menses cease. The definition of menopause, absence of menses for 12 months, indicates that the duration between menses can be up to one year during perimenopause.

During late perimenopause, hormonal testing is more reliable.[6] An elevated FSH during the early follicular phase, with levels >25 mIU/mL, indicates late perimenopause, although the levels are still variable. The duration of the late menopausal transition is more predictable; women with menses more than three months apart go through menopause within four

Office Care of Women, ed. Martin E. Olsen and Botros Rizk. Published by Cambridge University Press.

Menarche (at stage −5); FMP (0) (between stages −1 and +1a)

Stage	−5	−4	−3b	−3a	−2	−1	+1a	+1b	+1c	+2
Terminology	REPRODUCTIVE				MENOPAUSAL TRANSITION		POSTMENOPUSE			
	Early	Peak	Late		Early	Late	Early			Late
					Perimenopause					
Duration	*Variable*				*Variable*	1–3 years	2 years (1+1)		3–6 years	*Remaining lifespan*
PRINCIPAL CRITERIA										
Menstrual cycle	Variable to Regular	Regular	Regular	Subtle changes in flow/ strength	*Variable length:* Persistent ≥7-day difference in length of consecutive cycles	Interval of amenorrhea of ≥60 days				
SUPPORTIVE CRITERIA										
Endocrine FSH AMH Inhibin B			Low Low	Variable* Low Low	↑ Variable* Low Low	↑ >25 IU/L• Low Low	↑ Variable Low Low		Stabilizers Very low Very low	
Antral follide count			Low	Low	Low	Low	Very low		Very low	
DESCRIPTIVE CHARACTERISTICS										
Symptoms						Vasomotor symptoms *Likely*	Vasomotor symptoms *Most likely*			*Increasing* symptoms of urogenital strophy

Arrow: elevated; FMP: final menstrual period; FSH: follicle-stimulating hormone; AMH: anti-müllerian hormone.
* Blood draw on cycle days 2 to 5.
• Approximate expected level based on assays using current international pituitary standard.

Reproduced with permission from: Harlow SD, Gass M, Hall JE, et al. Executive Summary of the Stages of Reproductive Aging Workshop + 10: Addressing the Unfinished Agenda of Staging Reproductive Aging, *J Clin Endocrinol Metab* 2012. Copyright © 2012 The Endocrine Society.

Figure 31-1 The Stages of Reproductive Aging Workshop + 10 staging system for reproductive aging in women.

years.[8] In addition to irregular menses, women in late perimenopausal may have vasomotor symptoms. The most marked are hot flushes the year before the last menses and the two years following menopause.

Menopause

The average age of menopause is 51, although the age varies from 42 to 57. Women often ask when they will go through menopause, but there is no predictor for the age of menopause. There is no influence in the age of menarche, pregnancies, or use of hormonal medications. Women who are smokers or have had a hysterectomy have earlier menopause. The best predictor is the age of menopause of the patient's mother and older sisters. Premature menopause, before age 40, occurs in 1% of women.[9] The term "postmenopausal" has been used to define the years following menopause.

Women who have had a hysterectomy do not have cessation of menses to define menopause. Because 80% of women have vasomotor symptoms, this is the best indicator that the ovaries no longer produce estradiol. Hormonal contraceptives can also impair the diagnosis of menopause. Women on birth control

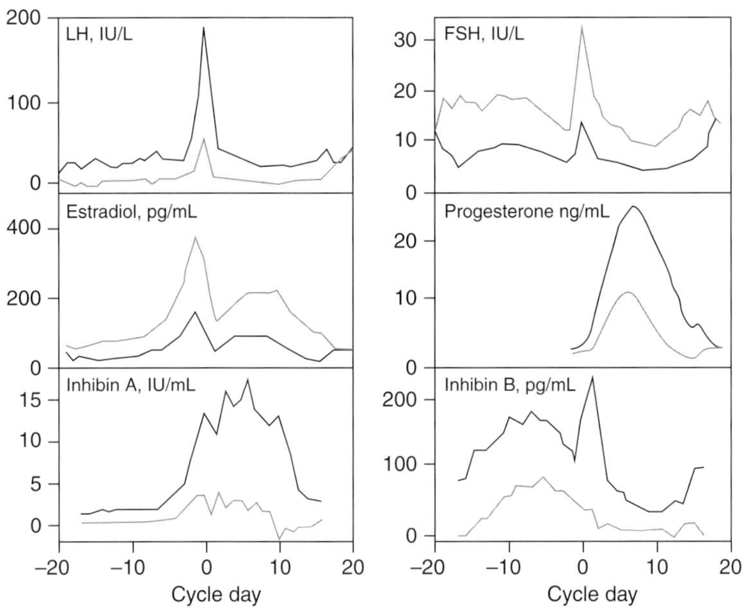

Figure 31-2 Hormone levels: older and younger reproductive age. Mean daily levels of gonadotropins, sex steroids, and inhibins in older (ages 35–46 years; $n = 21$), indicated by the dark line, and younger women (ages 20–34 years; $n = 23$), indicated by the light gray line.

(Adapted from Welt CK, McNicholl DJ, Taylor AE, Hall JE. Female reproductive aging is marked by decreased secretion of dimeric inhibin. J Clin Endocrinol Metab *1999; 84: 105.)*

pills will continue to have menses even when the ovaries do not produce hormones. And progestin contraceptives, given by injection, implant, pill, and intrauterine device, cause endometrial suppression and can stop menstruation. Although women need to use contraception until one year without menses, fertility is markedly decreased during perimenopause. Changing to nonhormonal contraceptives will allow women to know when they are menopausal.

Treatment

Irregular menses

A common symptom for perimenopausal patients is irregular menses.[1] Women can be advised that they are expected to have shorter cycles and longer cycles with heavier or lighter bleeding. There are other potential anatomic causes of menorrhagia that are common in women during their perimenopausal years, such as uterine fibroids, endometrial polyp, and endometrial hyperplasia. If bleeding is prolonged, excessive, or occurs between menses, evaluation is indicated. A transvaginal ultrasound and possible endometrial biopsy should be considered. In addition, endocrine evaluation should be considered with thyroid-stimulating hormone (TSH), as hypothyroidism can cause oligomenorrhea and menorrhagia.

If the bleeding is bothersome, it can be controlled with hormonal contraceptives, cyclic progestin, or continuous progestin. Women with heavy menses may benefit from the use of oral contraceptives, which will lighten and regulate menses. In addition, oral contraceptives manage vasomotor symptoms. With extended cycles, women can use cyclic oral progestin to make menses more predictable. Continuous progestin, by tablet, injection, implant, or intrauterine device, can be provided to minimize bleeding during the menopause transition. The progestin IUD, which lasts for five years, can be used to manage perimenopausal menorrhagia and then be removed following one year without menses.[10]

Vasomotor symptoms

Hot flushes and night sweats occur in 80% of women during late perimenopause and menopause.[2] The sudden increase in core body temperature extends from chest to neck and face, results in sweating, and may cause significant tachycardia. When the body temperature drops, women commonly become chilled. In addition to the disruption by the heat, sweating, and shivering, women may feel anxiety during and following the hot flush.

The severity and duration of these common symptoms are variable. The frequency and duration of vasomotor symptoms are variable.[11] Although most women have vasomotor symptoms, most have a significant decrease in frequency and intensity within four to five years. Interestingly, women may have vasomotor symptoms into their seventies, with 9% reporting ongoing hot flushes.

Typically vasomotor symptoms are more frequent during sleep and may disturb sleep. Sleep disruption can have a serious adverse effect on perimenopausal and menopausal women. Almost half of women have difficulty sleeping in their late perimenopause and early postmenopausal years.[12] The sleep disturbance can lead to decreased cognitive function, mood changes, and decreased overall quality of life.

Although severe hot flushes and night sweats may adversely affect the quality of life, many postmenopausal women do not require medical treatment. Since these symptoms decrease over time, women may consider no therapy for mild and moderate hot flushes. Unfortunately, methods of stress reduction, such as exercise, have not been shown to lessen vasomotor symptoms.[13] Studies examining alternative therapy, such as black cohosh, show very minimal effect when compared to a placebo. Phytoestrogens, such as isoflavones found in soy products and lignans found in flaxseed, are weak estrogens with limited effect on hot flushes. Systematic reviews have shown no significant improvement with plant estrogens.[14] Although the effectiveness of stress management, over-the-counter herbal medications, and phystoestrogens has been shown to have minimal effect on hot flushes, women commonly try these treatments.[15] It is important for health-care providers to inform patients of the ineffectiveness of these treatments and offer medical options for treatment of moderate and severe vasomotor symptoms.

The standard treatment for vasomotor symptoms continues to be hormone therapy. Estrogen (± progestin) is highly effective at lessening these symptoms. Three-fourths of women have marked reduction or elimination of hot flushes and night sweats on hormone therapy, and the remainder have some reduction.[11] No treatment has been shown to be more effective than hormone therapy for vasomotor symptoms. All forms of hormone therapy, including low doses of oral and transdermal estradiol, are effective. The current FDA recommendation is to use the lowest dose for the shortest time required to manage symptoms.

Other treatments, including selective serotonin reuptake inhibitors (SSRIs), gabapentin, clonidine, and progestins, have been used with moderate success for control of vasomotor symptoms (Figure 31-3). One SSRI, paroxetine at 7.5 mg qhs, is now FDA approved for the treatment of hot flushes with minimally increased effectiveness as compared to the placebo.[16] Other SSRIs and serotonin-norepinephrine reuptake inhibitors (SNRIs) have also been shown to have a modest effect compared to placebo, including fluoxetine, sertaline, venlafaxine, escitalopram, and desvenlafaxine. Although the effectiveness, as compared to a placebo, is modest, these are medications to consider for women who are not candidates for hormone therapy. Some caution should be made when prescribing SSRIs or SRNIs for women with breast cancer who are using tamoxifen, as these medications may lower the availability of the active metabolite of tamoxifen. This is described in a black box warning for the use of paroxetine for vasomotor symptoms.

Gabapentin has been shown to be moderately effective in reducing vasomotor symptoms. Although not FDA approved for this use, studies suggest that a significant reduction in night sweats occurs when taken at bedtime.[17] Typical doses are 900 mg, although the medication is often started at 300 mg and slowly increased. The side effects, including dizziness and fatigue, can be problematic. When compared to conjugated equine estrogen, gabapentin was equivalent, but at a high doses. As with SSRIs and SSNIs, this is a reasonable alternative therapy.

Clonidine effectively prevents tachycardia associated with temperature elevation and in some studies decreases hot flushes, although studies have been inconsistent.[18] However, because of side effects such as dizziness and dry mouth, this medication may not be tolerated. The patch form can be considered for extended effect.

Progestins alone are less effective than estrogens at decreasing hot flushes, but can reduce hot flushes in high doses. Both norethindrone acetate and depo-medroxyprogesterone acetate in high doses significantly decrease hot flushes.[19] Megestrol acetate, which has been used to treat breast cancer, has also shown to reduce hot flushes.[20] This medication stimulates appetite and can be associated with weight gain.

In summary, vasomotor symptoms are common with 80% of women reporting these symptoms. Most women can tolerate hot flushes, although they are debilitating for about 10% of women.[11] For women with significant sleep disturbance or hot flushes that impact their quality of life, estrogen or estrogen + progestin are the most effective therapy. Overtime, the dose can be reduced and eventually discontinued. When hormone therapy is not an option, SSRIs and gabapentin can be considered.

Vaginal/vulvar atrophy

The external genitalia and vaginal tissue will atrophy in the absence of estradiol from the ovary. There is a thinning of the vulva and a decrease in the elasticity. The urethra may change position with a decrease in vaginal muscular, and the anterior vaginal wall may prolapse, leading to a cystocele. The posterior vaginal wall may also have decreased muscular tone that leads to a rectocele. The thinned vaginal tissue loses its rugae, and there is a decrease in natural lubrication. There is an increased risk of uterine prolapse or development of an enterocele. Unlike vasomotor symptoms, these changes worsen over time.

Common symptoms include dryness and dyspareuenia. Many women note severe dryness, although only 25% seek therapy.[21] Women may have discomfort when physically active. Severe atrophy can cause bleeding when sexually active. There is an increased risk for bladder infections and stress incontinence. Rectal incontinence is also increased in menopausal women.

Some women have effective treatment with lubricants alone. This is a reasonable therapy for women with dryness alone, but it will not be effective for women with atrophy.

The most effective treatment of marked atrophy is systemic or vaginal estradiol in low dose. For women with vasomotor symptoms, the systemic hormone therapy is typically effective for vaginal atrophy. For women without hot flushes, vaginal estrogen alone is indicated. This medication comes in the form of a tablet, cream, and ring; all methods have been shown to improve atrophy.[22, 23] There is a minimal effect on serum estradiol levels with topical vaginal and vulvar treatment and no effect on endometrial development.[24] However, there is little data of the effect on estrogen-sensitive cancers. It is important to inform patients that very low doses are required for effective improvement in atrophy.

Vaginal estrogen is highly effective for atrophy, but it has not been shown to improve stress incontinence. It will not correct vaginal or uterine prolapse. For these conditions, surgical intervention may be indicated.

Sexual function

The effect of atrophy on dysparuenia has a direct effect on sexual function. Women with atrophy are likely to avoid sexual activity. With very severe atrophy, the vulvar tissue is friable and can be injured. In addition, there can be constriction of the vaginal vault, which prevents intercourse.[25] The treatment of vaginal atrophy can markedly decrease pain with intercourse and improve sexual function. In addition to vaginal estrogen, physical therapy may be required for women to resume sexual activity.

Sexual function may be impacted by an adverse effect of severe vasomotor symptoms on the quality of life, especially if normal sleep is adversely impacted. However, the direct effect of steroid hormones on sexual function, aside from the influence on vaginal atrophy and night sweats, is unclear.

Limited research has shown an improvement in sexual function of women on estrogen use.[26] Testosterone, given with estradiol in women with oophorectomy, has been shown to increase sexual interest and sexual activity.[27] The Cochrane Database identified that there is limited data to support the use of testosterone, but the long-term risk is not clear.[28] Currently, in the United States there is no form of testosterone that is FDA approved for sexual dysfunction, although methyltestosterone plus esterified estrogen are available for the treatment of vasomotor symptoms.

Before considering hormonal therapy, it is critical to consider relationship issues. Even women in stable relationships can benefit for therapy. Studies support the effectiveness of behavioral therapy for sexual dysfunction.[29] The most effective therapy for many women may be counseling by a skilled therapist.

Memory/cognitive dysfunction

Decreased estrogen levels have a measurable effect on short-term memory and verbal memory.[30] In addition, women who suffer from night sweats and subsequent sleep disturbance will experience a decrease in cognitive function. Data suggests that the use of estrogen improves cognitive function in menopausal women.[31] However, there is conflicting data on the effect of hormone therapy on cognitive function.[32] The WHIMS trial demonstrated a decrease in testing for older women placed on hormone therapy.[33] Based on the current data, hormone therapy should not be used to prevent dementia.

Mood disorders

Women experience major mood disorders throughout their lifetime. When caring for perimenopausal and postmenopausal women, it is critical for providers to consider the risk of mental health illnesses in all women, especially depression and anxiety disorders, which are the most common. Research has determined that when compared to premenopausal women, there is a 2.5-fold increase in women transitioning into menopause.[34] Limited studies have suggested that estrogen use may improve depressive symptoms, although the effectiveness of antidepressants has been clearly demonstrated.[35] It is important for mental health professionals who care for menopausal and perimenopausal women to be aware that new onset of mood disorders may be related to these conditions.

Long-term health issues

Decreased bone density

The loss of estrogen results in bone loss and increases the risk of osteopenia and osteoporosis. Trabecular bone is dependent on estrogen to maintain osteoblastic activity; there is a rapid decrease in bone density early in menopause.[36] Although this effect is less rapid later in menopause, women continue to lose bone. In addition, a loss of bone with aging contributes to the risk of osteoporosis. Other contributing risk factors for osteoporosis include ethnicity, smoking, poor diet, limited exercise, and certain medications. It is currently recommended that women undergo bone density evaluation at age 65 or sooner if there are one or more risk factors, such as family history and personal history of fractures.

Osteoporosis can be delayed with treatments to decrease bone loss. Calcium intake at 1,000 mg daily and vitamin D at 600 IU are reasonable. Women can increase weight-bearing exercise, quit smoking, and limit alcohol intake to decrease their risk. Unfortunately, these lifestyle changes will slow, but not prevent, bone loss.

Treatment for osteoporosis includes estrogen, bisphosphonates, SERMS, parathyroid hormone, calcitonin, and denosumab. All these treatment have their limitations, but the mortality associated with osteoporotic fractures is high.[37] Treatment is indicated for a bone density ≤2.0. See Chapter 44 for a detailed discussion of osteoporosis and osteopenia.

Cardiovascular disease

Women have an increased risk of heart and vascular disease after menopause. It is critical to optimize heart health by increasing exercise, optimizing diet, and maintaining a normal body mass index (BMI). Women at increased risk have common medical disorders such as diabetes, obesity, and hypertension. All postmenopausal women should be screened for these disorders and have lipid profiles evaluated.

The effect of hormone therapy on cardiovascular health is controversial. The Women's Health Initiative (WHI) demonstrated that women under the age of 60 or within 10 years of menopause did not have an increase in cardiovascular events when taking hormone therapy.[38] There is a suggestion that estrogen may be protective against heart disease, but there may be adverse effects with use into the sixties and seventies.[39] The limitations of the WHI, including the enrollment of older women, diminish our understanding about cardiovascular risk for older postmenopausal women. However, there is no increased risk for younger menopausal women.[40]

Because of the high risk of heart disease to women, it is critical for providers to monitor them for risk factors. Statins are the standard treatment for hyperlipidemia. Interestingly, estrogen also lowers total cholesterol levels, while risking HDL levels. However, hormone therapy is not recommended for prevention of heart disease. In conclusion, women are at an increased risk of long-term diseases, including osteoporosis and heart disease, following menopause. Providers need to screen for these common disorders and consider effective treatment options.

Concluding remarks

Menopause is a natural event that is defined as the absence of menses for 12 months without underlying cause. Most women who experience menopause have other symptoms including hot flushes and vaginal atrophy. When these symptoms adversely affect the quality of life, treatment is indicated. The most effective treatments are hormone therapy. There are alternate therapies that can be considered, although complementary and alternative therapies are typically not effective. The long-term health issues, specifically osteoporosis and cardiovascular disease, are increased for women after menopause. All healthcare providers should counsel women about these increased risks, test appropriately, and consider effective therapy.

References

1. Harlow SD, Gass M, Hall JE, et al. Executive summary of the Stages of Reproductive Aging Workshop + 10: addressing the unfinished agenda of staging

reproductive aging. *J Clin Endocrinol Metab* 2012; **97**: 1159–68.

2. Van Voorhis BJ, Santoro N, Harlow S, et al. The relationship of bleeding patterns to daily reproductive hormones in women approaching menopause. *Obstet Gynecol* 2008; **112**:101–8.
3. Randolph JF Jr, Sowers M, Bondarenko I, et al. The relationship of longitudinal change in reproductive hormones and vasomotor symptoms during the menopausal transition. *J Clin Endocrinol Metab* 2005; **90**:6106–12.
4. Broer SL, Eijkemans MJ, Scheffer GJ, et al. Anti-mullerian hormone predicts menopause: a long-term follow-up study in normoovulatory women. *J Clin Endocrinol Metab* 2011; **96**:2532–9.
5. Broer SL, Willem B, Hendriks D, et al. Then role of antimullerian hormone in prediction of outcome after IVF - comparison with the antral follicle count. *Fert Steril* 2009; **91**:705–14.
6. Burger HG, Hale GE, Dennerstein L, Robertson DM. Cycle and hormone changes during perimenopause: the key role of ovarian function. *Menopause* 2008; **15**: 603–12.
7. Hee J, MacNaughton J, Bangah M, Burger HG. Perimenopausal patterns of gonadotrophins, immunoreactive inhibin, oestradiol and progesterone. *Maturitas* 1993; **18**:9–20.
8. Ahmed Ebbiary NA, Lenton EA, Cooke ID. Hypothalamic-pituitary ageing: progressive increase in FSH and LH concentrations throughout the reproductive life in regularly menstruating women. *Clin Endocrin* 1994; **41**:199–206.
9. Santoro N, Brockwell S, Johnston J, et al. Helping midlife women predict the onset of the final menses: SWAN, the Study of Women's Health across the Nation. *Menopause* 2007; **14**:415–424.
10. Luborsky JL, Meyer P, Sowers MF, et al. Premature menopause in a multi-ethnic population study of the menopause transition. *Hum Reprod*; **18**:199–206.
11. Marret H, Fauconnier A, Chabbert-Buffet N. Clinical practice guidelines on menorrhagia: management of abnormal uterine bleeding before menopause. *Eur J Obstet Gynecol* 2010; **152**:133–7.
12. Stearns V, Ulmer L, Lopez JF, et al. Hot flushes. *Lancet* 2002; **360**:1851–61.
13. Kravitz HM, Ganz PA, Bromberger J, et al. Sleep difficulty in women at midlife: a community survey of sleep and the menopausal transition. *Menopause* 2003; **10**:19–28.
14. Nedrow A, Miller J, Walker M, et al. Complementary and alternative therapies for the management of menopause-related symptoms: a systematic evidence review. *Arch Intern Med* 2006; **166**:1453–65.
15. Newton KM, Reed SD, LaCroix AZ, et al. Treatment of vasomotor symptoms of menopause with black cohosh, multibotanicals, soy, hormone therapy, or placebo: a randomized trial. *Ann Intern Med* 2006; **145**: 869–79.
16. Taylor HS, Manson JE. Update in hormone therapy use in menopause. *J Clin Endocrinol Metab* 2011; **96**: 255–64.
17. Simon J, Portman DJ, Kaunitz AM, et al. Low-dose paroxetine 7.5 mg for menopausal vasomotor symptoms: two randomized controlled trials. *Menopause* 2013; **20**:1027–35.
18. Reddy SY, Warner H, Guttuso T, et al. Gabapentin, estrogen, and placebo for treating hot flushes: A randomized controlled trial. *Obstet Gynecol* 2006; **108**:41–8.
19. Nagamani M, Kelver ME, Smith ER. Treatment of menopausal hot flashes with transdermal administration of clonidine. *Am J Obstet Gynecol* 1987; **156**:561–5.
20. Bertelli G, Venturini M, Del Mastro L, et al. Intramuscular depot medroxyprogesterone versus oral megestrol for the control of postmenopausal hot flashes in breast cancer patients: a randomized study. *Ann Oncol* 2002; **13**:883–8.
21. Loprinzi CL, Michalak JC, Quella SK, et al. Megestrol acetate for the prevention of hot flashes. *N Engl J Med* 1994; **331**:347–52.
22. Studee DW, Panay N. Recommendations for the management of postmenopausal vaginal atrophy. *Climacteric* 2010; **13**:509–22.
23. Suckling J, Lethaby A, Kennedy R. Local oestrogen for vaginal atrophy in postmenopausal women. *Cochrane Database Syst Rev* 2003; **4**:CD001500.
24. Weisberg E, Ayton R, Darling G, et al. Endometrial and vaginal effects of low-dose estradiol delivered by vaginal ring or vaginal tablet. *Climacteric* 2005; **8**:83–93.
25. Simon J, Nachtigall L, Ulrich LG, et al. Endometrial safety of ultra-low-dose estradiol vaginal tablets. *Obstet Gynecol* 2010; **116**:876–83.
26. Barlow DH, Cardozo LD, Francis RM, et al. Urogenital ageing and its effect on sexual health in older British women. *Br J Obstet Gynaecol* 1997; **104**:87–91.
27. Cayan F, Dilek U, Pata O, Dilek S. Comparison of the effects of hormone therapy regimens, oral and vaginal estradiol, estradiol + drospirenone and tibolone, on sexual function in healthy postmenopausal women. *J Sex Med* 2008; **5**:132–8.
28. Shifren JL, Braunstein GD, Simon JA. Transdermal testosterone treatment in women with impaired sexual function after oophorectomy. *N Engl J Med* 2000; **343**: 682–6.

29. Somboonporn W, Bell RJ, Davis SR. Testosterone for peri and postmenopausal women. *Cochrane Database Syst Rev* 2005 Oct 19; **4**:CD004509.

30. Sarwer DB, Durlak JA. A field trial of the effectiveness of behavioral treatment for sexual dysfunctions. *J Sex Marital Ther* 1997; **23**:87–97.

31. Greendale GA, Derby CA, Maki PM. Perimenopause and cognition. *Obstet Gynecol Clin North Am* 2011; **38**: 519–35.

32. Shaywitz SE, Shaywitz BA, Pugh KR, et al. Effect of estrogen on brain activation patterns in postmenopausal women during working memory tasks. *JAMA* 1999; **281**:1197–202.

33. Lethaby A, Hogervorst E, Richards M, et al. Hormone replacement therapy for cognitive function in postmenopausal women. *Cochrane Database Syst Rev* 2008 Jan 23; **1**:CD003122.

34. Rapp SR, Espeland MA, Shumaker SA, et al. Effect of estrogen plus progestin on global cognitive function in postmenopausal women: the Women's Health Initiative Memory Study: a randomized controlled trial. *JAMA* 2003; **289**:2663–72.

35. Avis NE, Brambilla D, McKinlay SM, Vass K. A longitudinal analysis of the association between menopause and depression. Results from the Massachusetts Women's Health Study. *Ann Epidemiol* 1994; **4**:214–20.

36. Freeman EW, Sammel MD, Lin H, Nelson DB. Associations of hormones and menopausal status with depressed mood in women with no history of depression. *Arch Gen Psychiatry* 2006; **63**:375–82.

37. Recker R, Lappe J, Davies K, Heaney R. Characterization of perimenopausal bone loss: a prospective study. *J Bone Miner Res* 2000; **15**: 1965–73.

38. Panula J, Pihlajamäki H, Mattila VM, et al. Mortality and cause of death in hip fracture patients aged 65 or older: a population-based study. *BMC Musculoskelet Disord* 2011; **12**:105.

39. Rossouw JE, Prentice RL, Manson JE, et al. Postmenopausal hormone therapy and risk of cardiovascular disease by age and years since menopause. *JAMA* 2007; **297**:1465–77.

40. Santen RJ, Allred DC, Ardoin SP, et al. Postmenopausal hormone therapy: an Endocrine Society scientific statement. *J Clin Endocrinol Metab* 2010; **95**:s1–s66.

Chapter 32

Selected endocrine disorders

Theodore Tsaltas

Thyroid disease

Thyroid disorders may present with several common gynecologic complaints. An understanding of the presentation, diagnosis, and management of thyroid disease is an important part of women's health practice.

Thyroid disease is three- to fourfold more common among women than men.[1] The reason is unknown, although most thyroid disorders are autoimmune in nature, and autoimmune diseases in general are more common in women.

Physiologically, thyroid activity is governed by thyroid-stimulating hormone (TSH) from the pituitary under the permissive control of the hypothalamus through thyrotropin-releasing hormone (TRH). TSH stimulates the thyroid to produce thyroxine (T4), which is relatively inactive. T4 is peripherally metabolized to triiodothyronine (T3), the active form. T4 provides negative feedback control of TSH.

Hypothyroidism

The prevalence of hypothyroidism in women is approximately 1%–2%, with about 0.3% being overt. Up to 4.6% of women have been found to have biochemical or subclinical disease.[2, 3] The high proportion of subclinical disease and the variation in symptoms requires a high degree of awareness and willingness to test among women's health providers.

Hypothyroidism has several important clinical associations. These include use of amiodorone, lithium, or interferon and age greater than 65, at which point prevalence rises to 10%. It is also more common in the postpartum period. Women over 65 with loss of appetite, weight changes, or other changes suggestive of physical deterioration or mental status changes should be screened for hypothyroidism.

Most hypothyroidism is autoimmune in origin. Hypothyroidism associated with goiter is Hashimoto's disease.[4] Iatrogenic hypothyroidism, caused by use of radioactive iodine or surgery for hyperthyroidism, must also be considered.

Presentation can be quite variable (see Table 32-1). In addition to specific gynecologic problems, symptoms also include many common complaints for women, such as constipation, weight gain, and fatigue. Myalgias should also prompt evaluation. Physical examination findings are typically nonspecific. Dry, dull hair and skin and decreased deep tendon reflexes may be seen. Table 32-1 lists several common presenting complaints.

Initial screening with TSH alone is adequate, since subclinical hypothyroidism is defined as an elevated TSH with normal thyroid function. Adding free T4 allows definitive diagnosis of the degree of thyroid dysfunction without additional visits or lab draws for the patient and with little added cost. When TSH alone

Table 32-1 Presenting symptoms of hypothyroidism

Common	Less common	Uncommon	Ob/gyn specific
Fatigue	Myalgias	Edema	Amenorrhea
Weakness	Dry skin	Bradycardia	Menorrhagia
Somnolence	Brittle hair	Hypertension	Premenstrual symptoms
Cold intolerance	Constipation	Hyperlipidemia	Galactorrhea
Memory changes		Myxedema	Recurrent pregnancy loss
		Coma	

Office Care of Women, ed. Martin E. Olsen and Botros Rizk. Published by Cambridge University Press.

Table 32-2 Conditions causing transient TSH elevation

Steroid usage
Recent inflammatory illness
Thyroiditis, recent and resolved

is abnormal it should be repeated in two to three weeks, since various conditions may cause transient TSH elevation (see Table 32-2). Other evaluation may include prolactin screening, EKG, and lipids when indicated.

Management is with T4 (levothyroxine) replacement. The required dose is approximately 1.6 mcg/Kg, with the typical range being 75 mcg–150 mcg daily. Obesity, medication usage, and age all can have a substantial effect, and dosing is always individualized. Requirements are reduced by about 30% in elderly women. Dosing should be started at 50 mcg daily and then raised in two weeks, especially in the elderly, to avoid cardiovascular complications.[5] Patients with a complex, multisystem presentation, or those who respond inappropriately to replacement management, should be referred to a medical endocrinologist.

Empiric treatment with T4 in the absence of an elevated TSH is not indicated. Weight gain is not a prominent symptom of hypothyroidism, and empiric treatment is especially not indicated for either weight loss or infertility management. Conversely, evaluation of all women with recurrent pregnancy loss should include TSH elevation.

TSH falls only slowly, and should be checked in 8–12 weeks but not sooner. Treatment is most effective when TSH is in the lower range of normal (<2.0 mIU/L).[4] Once a stable dose is established, monitoring can be done with TSH alone every 3–12 months. Return of function of the pituitary-thyroid axis can occur as the degree of inflammatory thyroid damage may change. Variation in thyroid function is not uncommon given the autoimmune nature of most hypothyroidism. Replacement may be discontinued after a prolonged period of treatment to evaluate this possibility.

Pregnancy presents minor variations in management of hypothyroidism. Thyroid replacement doses rise about 20%, the consequence of increased body water and serum protein binding capacity as well as a decrease in iodine availability. TSH should be measured upon presentation, and again at the end of the first trimester. It should be measured monthly for the remainder of the pregnancy. A new diagnosis of hypothyroidism is rare in pregnancy; hypothyroidism is associated with anovulatory infertility. Women's health providers should be alert for postpartum changes in thyroid function, especially new onset symptoms. Liberal use of screening is appropriate.[6, 7]

Table 32-3 Causes of hyperthyroidism

Graves' disease
Toxic goiter (multinodular or simple)
Solitary nodule
Thyroid cancer
Iodine excess
Gestational trophoblastic disease

Hyperthyroidism

Hyperthyroidism is less common than hypothyroidism. In addition, gynecologists and other women's health providers are typically less involved in its management because its manifestations are primarily cardiac, in contrast to the multiple gynecologic symptoms of hypothyroidism.

Hyperthyroidism can be both overt and subclinical, as in hypothyroidism. Family history, especially of Graves' disease, is an important association. Amiodorone can also be associated with hyperthyroidism.

The two most common causes of hyperthyroidism are Graves' disease and toxic multinodular goiter. Graves' disease is a specific clinical syndrome; the eponym is not a synonym for hyperthyroidism. Toxic goiter may be simple or multinodular. Hyperthyroidism may also arise from a solitary nodule or, rarely, from iodine excess. Gestational trophoblastic disease must be considered in the pregnant patient. (See Table 32-3 for a list of causes of hyperthyroidism.)

Symptoms, although variable, are more common and more consistent than in hypothyroidism. Graves' disease has a specific symptom triad of exophthalmos, pretibial edema, and hyperthyroidism. Other symptoms are listed in Table 32-4. Common symptoms include tachycardia, tremor, sweating, and heat intolerance. Marked hyperthyroidism can lead to cardiac failure and thyroid storm. Thyroid storm is a marked exacerbation of hyperthyroidism, usually the result

Table 32-4 Symptoms of hyperthyroidism

Common	Uncommon	Thyroid storm	Ob/gyn specific
Tachycardia	Diarrhea	Fever (>101°F)	Hyperemesis gravidarum
Palpitations	Dyspnea	Vomiting	Hydatidiform mole
Tremor	Oligomenorrhea	Diarrhea	
Sweating	Hair loss	Agitation	
Goiter	Emotional lability	Heart failure	
Nervousness		Marked arrhythmia	
Weight loss			

of nontreatment or occasionally by exacerbation secondary to an acute illness. Thyroid storm is an acute medical emergency requiring hospitalization. Symptoms include high fever, marked tachycardia or cardiac arrhythmias, vomiting, diarrhea, and agitation. Symptoms have been scored using a scale developed by Burch and Wartofsky.[8] The use of this scale and management of patients with advanced degrees of hypothyroidism are generally outside the scope of general gynecology practice.

Unlike hypothyroidism, which is associated with amenorrhea and anovulation, patients with hyperthyroidism typically ovulate. Such women are thus capable of becoming pregnant, and therefore become at risk for hyperemesis gravidarum. Gynecologic manifestations of hyperthyroidism are less common, but gynecologic care providers need to be aware of the symptoms of hyperthyroidism and to investigate and test liberally, given the higher incidence of thyroid disease in women. Table 32-4 lists symptoms associated with hyperthyroidism.

Diagnosis is made by hormonal testing. Like hypothyroidism, subclinical disease can occur. These patients have a TSH <0.4 but normal T4. No treatment for asymptomatic patients with a normal T4 is necessary; however, most of these women will progress to overt hyperthyroidism, and close serologic monitoring is essential.[9] Further, subclinical hyperthyroidism is a significant risk factor for atrial fibrillation, and all women's health providers should be aware of this association.[10] TSH below 0.4 mIU/L and elevated T4 or T3 establish the diagnosis of hyperthyroidism. In overt disease, evaluation of the thyroid gland itself is necessary, utilizing radioactive iodine. Management from this point is based on results of the iodine uptake. The fundamental choice is between medical suppression, radioactive thyroid ablation and surgery.

Toxic goiter with diffuse uptake can be managed with medication or radioactive ablation. A solitary nodule may be managed with radioactive iodine, but surgery is often preferred as nodules may recur, leading to high doses of radiation exposure. Both radioactive iodine and surgery have a risk of secondary, iatrogenic hypothyroidism.

Methimazole and propylthiouracil (PTU) are both used for the medical management of hyperthyroidism. They are equivalent in effectiveness, but methimazole is the drug of choice because it has fewer side effects. Typical initial oral dose is 10 mg–20 mg daily, falling to 5 mg–10 mg daily. PTU dosing is typically 50 mg–100 mg TID. The half-life of T4 is one week; thus TSH rises and T4 falls relatively slowly. Maximum effect of medication on thyroid function tests is at eight weeks.[9]

Thyroid storm is a life-threatening medical emergency. Hospitalization and often intensive care are necessary. Management includes Tylenol and cooling blankets for fever, beta blockers for arrhythmias and tachycardia, and inorganic iodine (Lugol's iodine) and methimnazole to reduce thyroid hormone production.[11]

Gynecologic surgeons and other women's health providers should be aware of Struma Ovarii as a cause for hyperthyroidism. A struma is a benign cystic teratoma composed completely or nearly completely of thyroid tissue. Patients typically present with hyperthyroidism without other cause or association. A pelvic ultrasound can rapidly direct management appropriately. Thyroid carcinoma can arise rarely within a struma, and even more rarely can metastasize out of the dermoid into the pelvis. Should this be found, oncologic management is indicated.

The management of established hyperthyroidism in pregnancy is well within the scope of general ob/gyn care providers. Methimazole should not be used in the first trimester. It is discontinued in women using it, and PTU substituted. Once out of the first trimester, patients should be converted back to methimazole. TSH and T4 should be measured monthly, and care taken to avoid iatrogenic hypothyroidism.[12]

Hyperthyroidism and thyroid storm may be caused by gestational trophoblastic disease. Patients presenting with new onset hyperthyroidism in pregnancy should be evaluated for hydatidiform mole, and patients with a partial molar pregnancy and a viable fetus are at risk for hyperthyroidism and thyroid storm. Such patients require a multidisciplinary team, including perinatology and internal medicine. Unless the labor floor has the capability of providing intensive treatment including hemodynamic monitoring, these patients typically require management off the labor floor in an intensive care unit. Thyroid storm in pregnancy has in particular increased risks of cardiac failure, pulmonary edema, and fetal death.

Hyperthyroidism may also present in pregnancy as hyperemesis. All patients with hyperemesis should be screened with a TSH.[13, 14]

Aside from established disease in pregnancy, the choices and managements for hyperthyroidism are generally outside the purview of general ob/gyn providers. Patients newly diagnosed with hyperthyroidism by an ob/gyn provider should be referred promptly to a medical endocrinologist.

Sheehan's syndrome

Sheehan's syndrome is a distinct form of pituitary failure characterized by hypoperfusional necrosis. This is distinct from other cases of panhypopituitarism, which are usually the result of pressure necrosis from a space-occupying lesion in the sella turcica. Its incidence has fallen with modern obstetrical care. In one review the incidence was 5.1/100,000 women.[15] In developing countries the incidence is substantially higher.[16] The large majority of patients in all reviews have had antecedent obstetric hemorrhage. Home birth is also associated with this disorder due to difficulties in estimating total blood loss and delays in management.[17, 18]

The pathophysiology is distinct, as described by Sheehan in his own monograph.[19] The anterior hypophysis receives its blood supply via the pituitary portal venous circulation from the hypothalamus. Pressure in this circulation is approximately 10 mmHg. Decreases in maternal blood pressure associated with hemorrhage lead to decreased pituitary perfusion and necrosis. The necrosis is often patchy, leading to a range of complaints, in contrast to the predictable pattern of pituitary failure associated with pressure infarction.

Table 32-5 Symptoms of Sheehan's syndrome and associated hormonal deficiencies

Symptom	Hormone
Agalactia	Prolactin
Amenorrhea	FSH, LH
Asthenia, fatigue	TSH, ACTH
Pubic and axillary hair loss/thinning	FSH, LH
Circulatory collapse, hypotension	ACTH

FSH – follicle-stimulating hormone, LH – luteinizing hormone, TSH – thyroid-stimulating hormone, ACTH – adrenocorticotropic hormone

Presentation is based on the extent of necrotic destruction and is quite variable. The most common ones are agalactia and amenorrhea, but more than 90% of patients also have hypothyroidism and adrenal insufficiency of varying degrees.[18] Symptoms can range from near immediate postpartum circulatory collapse from adrenal insufficiency to longstanding subclinical hypothyroidism. Table 32-5 lists symptoms of Sheehan's syndrome and their associated hormonal deficiencies.

An unfortunate phenomenon for patients with Sheehan's is the delay in diagnosis. In developing countries this can be as long as 20 years, although the average delay is 13 years. In developed countries a delay of 3.6 years has been reported.[15, 18] Because many patients with a postpartum hemorrhage have a curettage under difficult conditions, amenorrhea may be passed off as secondary to synechiae, and bottle feeding can obscure agalactia. Physicians who care for postpartum women need to be alert and sensitive to the possibility of Sheehan's syndrome. Patients with amenorrhea, especially those with agalactia or "failure" of breastfeeding, should be carefully examined and questioned about other symptoms.

Diagnosis is made by serologic testing. This should include follicle-stimulating hormone (FSH) and luteinizing hormone (LH), but also fasting prolactin, cortisol, and TSH. More definitive elucidation of the degree of endocrine dysfunction requires differential stimulatory testing done by endocrinologists. Awareness of and sensitivity to the diagnosis can shorten the interval between pituitary necrosis and diagnosis. The most important role of general obstetric providers in Sheehan's syndrome, however, is prevention through aggressive obstetrical management of massive hemorrhage.

Central hypogonadism

Amenorrhea is a common presenting complaint for patients with central hypogonadism. Evaluation of patients with primary amenorrhea includes examination, FSH, and LH. Other evaluation, as appropriate, may include bone age, 17-hydroxy progesterone, cortisol, and androgens. Information about the presence and patency of the vagina can be readily obtained with a gentle and simple examination. More invasive examination is not necessary, as ultrasound can and should take its place in establishing the presence or absence of the mullerian duct structures. Once the diagnosis is established, all subsequent evaluation and management of patients with congenital hypogonadotropic hypogonadism is performed by endocrinologists.

The terminology for hypogonadism is often confusing or off-putting when in fact it is completely straightforward, if polysyllabic. A woman with gonadal (ovarian) failure has hypogonadism. The failure may be primary (i.e., the woman never had functioning ovaries) or secondary (meaning the woman has ovaries that no longer function). The gonads are stimulated by the gonadotropic hormones FSH and LH. Women with hypogonadism will have either elevated or low/normal FSH and LH. Those with elevated FSH and LH are hypergonadotropic – their gonadotropic hormones are elevated. Women with low or normal FSH and LH are hypogonadotropic. Thus a woman may have **hypo**gonadotropic **hypo**gonadism or **hyper**gonadotropic **hypo**gonadism. Either situation may be primary or secondary. A brief classification of the causes of each is listed in Table 32-6.

Hypogonadotropic hypogonadism represents a pituitary failure whose origin depends on the age and presentation of the patient. The consideration of hypogonadotropic hypogonadism arises in almost all cases from evaluation of amenorrhea. In hypogonadotropic hypogonadism, FSH and LH are often quite low, but they may also be normal. In the typical negative feedback loop, an end-organ hormone such as estrogen provides negative feedback control on the production of the tropic hormone, such as FSH. If the end organ stops making its hormone, then the tropic hormone level should be unsuppressed and become elevated. Thus normal tropic hormone levels in the presence of end-organ failure represent a central failure. The tropic hormones are all produced in the pituitary, which in turn is regulated by the hypothalamus. The term "central failure" thus refers to a failure of the pituitary and/or hypothalamus to produce sufficient tropic hormone. Normal values are also seen in other causes of amenorrhea, such as müllerian agenesis.[20, 21]

Congenital hypogonadotrophic hypogonadism

Patients with congenital hypogonadotropic hypogonadism present as teens with amenorrhea. They have Tanner 1 breast and genital development. Stature is typically normal if karyotype is normal. The most common congenital presentation is Kallmann's syndrome, the combination of hypogonadism and anosmia (loss or absence of sense of smell). Kallmann's syndrome accounts for 50% of hypogonadotropic hypogonadism in females, but the incidence is quite low, about 1/10,000. Although stature is normal there may be numerous other abnormalities, including cleft palate, craniofacial defects, and neural hearing loss.

The specific defect in Kallmann's syndrome is unknown; however, gonadotropin-releasing hormone (GnRH) is not produced, indicating the fundamental failure is actually hypothalamic rather than pituitary. The combination of anosmia, hypothalamic dysfunction, neural hearing loss, and central facial defects all suggest a failure of organization and development at the base of the brain and basal central cranium. Isolated genetic defects have not been associated. Given the complexity and variation of the presentation, and its rarity, it is likely a multifactorial problem.

Genetic abnormalities of the FSH gene, abnormalities of its receptor, and abnormalities of GnRH receptors constitute identified but rare causes of hypogonadotropic hypogonadism. Tumors, notably craniopharyngioma, are another rare cause.

One cause of hypothalamic amenorrhea is anorexia nervosa, which generally presents with secondary amenorrhea; however, it is a potential consideration in congenital hypogonadotropic hypogonadism,

Table 32-6 Schematic for evaluation of hypogonadism/amenorrhea

FSH low or normal: hypogonadotropic hypogonadism		FSH high: hypergonadotropic hypogonadism	
Primary	**Secondary**	**Primary**	**Secondary**
Kallmann's syndrome	Anorexia	Turner's syndrome	Premature ovarian failure
Craniopharyngioma	Exercise induced	Swyer's syndrome	Menopause
Receptor abnormalities	Chronic illness		
Constitutional delay	Pituitary tumor		
Other causes		**Other causes**	
Rokitansky syndrome		Testicular feminization	
Adrenal hyperplasia		5-alpha reductase deficiency	

especially in those who are markedly underweight. Constitutional delay of puberty accounts for 25% or so of cases of delayed puberty. It is thus extremely important that the generalist ob/gyn provider aggressively seek other causes before assigning the diagnosis of constitutional delay.

Modern solid organ transplant and management of childhood tumors may also produce pubertal delays and hypogonadotropic hypogonadism. Organ failure can produce pubertal delays, with marked and rapid development after transplantation. Conversely, steroid immunosuppression can produce pubertal delays and a clinical picture suggestive of central gonadal failure. Gynecologic providers who care for teens treated for malignancies and transplant patients must be alert for effects on their pubertal development.[22, 23] Marked and rapid developments in transplant immunosuppression regimens require that gynecologic providers for transplanted teens coordinate their care closely with the transplant team.

Acquired hypogonadotropic hypogonadism

Patients with acquired hypogonadotropic hypogonadism have a history of normal menses and secondary sexual development but then present with secondary amenorrhea. The reader should note the distinction is between conditions such as menopause and premature ovarian failure (both are **hyper**gonadotropic hypogonadism) from hypogonadotropic hypogonadism.

Acquired hypogonadotropic hypogonadism is relatively uncommon. The two most common causes, excluding hyperprolactinemia, are anorexia nervosa and exercise induced amenorrhea (see Chapter 38). As in the congenital presentation, acquired symptoms can be the result of chronic illnesses such as renal failure or tumors, notably lymphomas and leukemias. Pituitary and cerebral tumors should be excluded with MRI before settling on a diagnosis.

Unlike congenital hypogonadotropic hypogonadism, acquired disease can be managed by the appropriately trained and experienced women's health physician. The fundamental goal of treatment is preservation of bone mass and vulvovaginal tissues. Monthly menstruation is not essential; four menses yearly is adequate. Oral contraceptives can be used for hormone replacement, with supplemental estrogen cream for the vulva and vagina added as necessary. Micronized estradiol can also be used, and withdrawal bleeds then produced by periodic use of a progestational agent. If micronized estradiol is used, dose requirements are more variable than with equine estrogens as it is metabolized much more easily. Dose requirements are also higher in young women than for menopausal replacement. A daily dose of 3–4 mg is not unreasonable, with adjustment based on symptoms and serum estradiol and FSH. Ultimately, resolution depends on the management of the underlying problem. If fertility is desired, ovulation induction with menotropins is necessary.

Diabetes insipidus

Diabetes insipidus (DI) is a rare disorder characterized by marked polyuria and polydipsia as a result of an inability to concentrate urine. There are two forms: central and nephrogenic.

In the normal patient 90% of glomerular filtrate is reabsorbed in the proximal and distal tubules. The remaining 10% is presented to the collecting tubules, which are the site of action of antidiuretic hormone (ADH). About 90% of the tubular fluid is resorbed under the influence of ADH, subject to the person's degree of hydration. Thus in a person with a filtration rate of 125 cc/min about 12.5 cc is presented to the collecting tubule. Of this about 1.25 cc/min of urine is formed. In the patient with DI the entire 12.5 cc/min of tubular fluid may be excreted as urine, or about 750 cc/hour, up to 18,000 cc daily although patients typically have urine volumes in the range of 5–6 liters daily.

Patients present with marked thirst and polyuria. There is typically a predilection for cold drinks. Thirst may be so intense that patients will drink toilet water and other sources of "gray" water. Patients also complain of nocturia, fatigue, and weakness. If water is not available or there are other fluid losses from gastroenteritis or exercise, the patient can become rapidly dehydrated, with serum sodium elevations, delirium, coma, and death.[24]

Urine shows a specific gravity of less than 1.005, but serum electrolytes are typically normal or show only mild elevations of sodium as long as dehydration does not occur. There are no other physical examination findings. Urine osmolality is low, between 50 and 200 mOsms/L, and does not rise in response to dehydration.

Approximately 50% of cases presenting to a primary care physician are idiopathic. Major causes are outlined in Table 32-7. Sheehan's syndrome, while described for the anterior pituitary hypophysis, can also affect the posterior hypophysis, producing DI.

Nephrogenic DI is more uncommon than central DI. There are two congenital forms: an autosomal recessive receptor defect and an X-linked recessive form.

The latter has been demonstrated in specific populations, notably those of Scottish descent. Advanced renal disease destroys the kidney's ability to respond to ADH, producing isosthenuria and polyuria. Lithium is well known to produce nephrogenic DI, but there are other drugs that may produce DI as a side effect.

The differential is between psychogenic polydipsia and DI. Psychogenic polydipsia patients typically have little or no nocturia, in contrast to patients with DI.

Table 32-7 Causes of diabetes insipidus

Central DI	Idiopathic
	Traumatic
	Pituitary surgery Basilar skull fracture Head injury Cranial surgery Sheehan's syndrome
	Congenital
	Genetic defect Neurofibromatosis
	Infiltrative disease
	Histiocytosis X Sarcoidosis
	Neoplasms
	Pituitary tumor Craniopharyngioma Lymphoma Hypothalamic tumors Metastases
Nephrogenic	Congenital
	Receptor defect Absent receptor
	Acquired
	Lithium Hypercalcemia

Diagnosis is established by the water deprivation test. Patients are prevented from drinking for six hours, and their serum and urine osmolality are calculated. Urinary osmolality should rise in response to water deprivation, excluding DI as a cause of symptoms. If it does not rise, then vasopressin is administered. If this raises osmolality, then a diagnosis of central DI is established. If it does not, then the patient has nephrogenic DI. This testing is done only by endocrinologists in a highly controlled hospital setting, as the patients can become quite ill during evaluation, and may also frantically seek any source of water if not monitored closely.

Management of central DI is administration of the vasopressin analog 1-desamino-8-D-arginine vasopressin. The generic name is desmopressin; the common trade name is DDAVP. This may be administered as a nasal spray or in tablets. Management is typically highly successful, although patients must remain cautious about sodium and water intake.

Management of nephrogenic DI depends on the cause. Drug-induced nephrogenic DI is initially managed by withdrawal of the drug. On occasion this is impossible or inadvisable. For these patients and those with congenital forms of nephrogenic DI, management is with thiazide diuretics, amiloride, and/or indomethacin. The basis of management is to reduce glomerular filtration, thus reducing total fluid presented to the collecting tubule. In addition, thiazides reduce free water excretion and increase sodium resorption, further reducing urine volume in this pathologic state.[25, 26]

Pregnancy has two potential effects on diabetes insipidus. Gestational diabetes insipidus can occur, in which do novo symptoms of polyuria and thirst arise. This is caused by the production of vasopressinase by the placenta. In patients with preexisting central diabetes insipidus, symptoms are typically improved as a result of diffusion of fetal ADH across the placenta. This must be considered in management, as DDAVP requirements may change substantially. Patients with nephrogenic DI will worsen in pregnancy as a result of increased glomerular filtration in pregnancy.[27]

All patients with DI of any type require management by an endocrinologist. Management of pregnancy complicated by DI requires close coordination of care with the endocrinologist, but does not a priori require perinatal care, as other aspects of the pregnancy are normal.

Women with complete failure of the posterior pituitary do not make oxytocin. This has no effect on the onset or progress of labor, as maternal oxytocin is not produced in significant amounts until after delivery of the placenta. It can have a marked effect on lactation, however, as the primary role of maternal oxytocin is milk letdown. Current research also describes substantial roles for oxytocin in socialization, contentment, and infant bonding.[28, 29]

Cushing's disease and Addison's disease

It is sufficient for most gynecologists to be familiar with the presentation and screening of Cushing's and Addison's disease in order to make appropriate and timely referrals.

Cushing's disease is the result of oversecretion of cortisol. It may arise centrally from pituitary overactivity (the eponymous Cushing's disease), or peripherally from the adrenal gland or elsewhere. Peripheral causes are much less common, and include paraneoplastic secretion of adrenocorticotropic hormone (ACTH) and autonomous secretion of cortisol by the pituitary.

Presentation is variable, but classically includes moon facies and a "buffalo hump" of fat between the shoulders. Patients have truncal obesity with leg muscle atrophy. Women commonly have hirsutism. Other findings include fatigue, irritability, elevated serum glucose, and depression.[30, 31]

Screening is done with serum cortisol. An overnight, 1 mg dexamethasone suppression test can be done, with an 0800 fasting cortisol drawn. Values less than 5 mcg/dL exclude Cushing's disease of any source. Confirmation of disease is done with 24-hour urinary cortisol testing. Differentiation of peripheral and central disease is done with two- to six-day dexamethasone suppression testing. It is important to remember that although Cushing's disease is a common reason for referral to an endocrinologist, it is one of the least common of diagnoses. It is thus important to be familiar not only with its presentation but with the evaluation of hirsutism, to avoid unnecessary tests and referrals.

Addison's disease is the result of adrenal insufficiency. Cushing's disease has substantial implications for long-term health, but Addison's disease can lead to death abruptly from Addisonian crisis unless appropriately diagnosed and treated. Of note, autoimmune disease can be a cause of Addison's disease as well as of premature ovarian failure and thyroid disease. Consideration should be given to multiple endocrine failures when one such failure is found.[32]

Presentation is usually insidious. Common symptoms include orthostatic hypotension, hypoglycemia, fatigue, and muscle weakness. In an Addisonian crisis, patients present acutely ill, with nausea, vomiting, confusion to the point of psychotic symptoms, syncope, and multiple electrolyte disturbances.[33]

Addison's disease is not in the purview of any gynecology provider. If the diagnosis is suspected, patients should be sent to an endocrinologist or for emergency care, as appropriate.

Table 32-8 Tumors associated with MEN

Tumor	Incidence in MEN		
	MEN 1	MEN 2a	MEN 2b
Pituitary adenoma	66%	–	–
Pancreatic tumors	20%–50%	–	–
Parathyroid hyperplasia	90%	50%	–
Medullary thyroid CA	–	100%	85%
Pheochromocytoma	–	50%	–
Neuroma	–	–	100%
Lipoma	17%	–	–

Multiple endocrine neoplasia

Multiple endocrine neoplasia (MEN) is syndrome of tumors arising in various endocrine organs. It is divided into MEN 1 and 2, and MEN 2 is further divided into 2a and 2b. Prevalence is extremely low, between 1/40,000 and approximately 1/1,000,000 people. MEN has significant genetic associations. The genetic focus for MEN 1 is found on chromosome 11, whereas ongene associations are known for MEN 2.[34]

The importance of MEN to the gynecology provider is to be aware of it and its common associations. Medullary thyroid carcinoma is seen in 85%–100% of patients with MEN 2a and 2b; 90% of patients with MEN 1 have parathyroid tumors. Any patient with medullary thyroid carcinoma or a parathyroid tumor should at least be investigated for MEN. Other tumors seen in MEN include multiple endocrine active pancreatic tumors, pituitary adenomas, lipomas, and neuromas. Table 32-8 lists the tumors seen in MEN.

The evaluation and management of MEN is done by oncologists and surgeons. The women's health provider's role is to suspect in appropriate conditions, ask, and refer as appropriate.

Adult onset congenital adrenal hyperplasia

Virilization at puberty

A variety of disorders can produce virilization at puberty. The most common is adult onset congenital adrenal hyperplasia (CAH). Most cases of CAH are diagnosed at or shortly after birth, or upon failure of pubertal development. All the adrenal enzymatic defects are autosomal recessives but have marked variation in phenotypic expression based on zygosity and penetrance.

The most common adrenal enzymatic disorder is 21-hydroxylase deficiency. This is also the most common one to have pubertal expression. At adrenarche, adrenal production of dehydroepiandrosterone sulfate (DHEAS) and androstenedione increases markedly. A mild, partial 21-hydroxylase block that produces no symptoms during childhood may manifest upon pubertal increases in ACTH. Since ACTH acts to stimulate the conversion of cholesterol to pregnenolone but is regulated by cortisol, any block between pregnenolone and cortisol leads to hyperstimulation and overproduction of intermediate compounds. The result is massive overproduction of DHEAS and androstenedione, leading to hirsutism. Girls who present with sudden excess hair growth at or near puberty should be evaluated for partial 21-hydroxylase deficiency. Although less common, 11 hydroxylase deficiency may present in this manner as well.

Delta 4–5 isomerase and 3 beta-ol dehydrogenase are responsible for production of more clinically active steroid hormones. Complete deficiency of these enzymes is incompatible with life, as the individual cannot make aldosterone or cortisol. Mild partial deficiencies, however, occur in both adrenal and gonad. The interference in estradiol and testosterone production leads to anovulation and oligoamenorrhea without hirsutism. These girls are typically diagnosed as having polycystic ovary syndrome (PCOS). Although their management is usually not affected, as the partial defect can be overcome with ovarian stimulation, on occasion it is important to know the actual source of the patient's problems. Appropriate differential testing will demonstrate this. Up to 10% of PCOS patients are thought to have partial deficiency syndromes of 3 beta-ol dehydrogenase or delta 4–5 isomerase. Testing, evaluation and management is outside the scope of generalist ob/gyn providers.[35]

Androgen receptor defects can also present as virilization at puberty. Complete androgen receptor deficiency is testicular feminization. Incomplete deficiency is Reifenstein syndrome. Complete forms of the disorder present as amenorrheic teens lacking a vagina, elevated FSH and LH, and a male karyotype. Incomplete syndromes can lead to massive virilization at puberty, as pubertal androgen secretion overcomes what is only a relative degree of receptor absence.

A 5-alpha reductase deficiency may also present as pubertal virilization. Like adrenal enzymatic blocks, this is an autosomal recessive disorder with variable penetrance. The virilization can be so complete as to cause sex role reversal and induction of a small but functional phallus in a previously female phenotypic individual. This is the basis of the guevedoces syndrome in the Dominican Republic.[36]

Any girl who presents with marked hirsutism or overt virilization should be referred promptly for gynecologic endocrine evaluation.

Concluding remarks

With the exception of thyroid disease, the endocrine disorders discussed in this chapter are not common. Some of their nomenclature is confusing. Yet it is for these very reasons that understanding them is so important. Endocrine disorders have multiorgan effects, and knowledge of them greatly increases the diagnostic abilities of any practitioner.

References

1. Vanderpump MP, Tunbridge WM, French JM, et al. The incidence of thyroid disorders in the community: a twenty-year follow-up of the Whickham Survey. *Clin Endocrinol (Oxf)* 1995 Jul; **43**(1): 55–68.
2. Hollowell JG, Staehling NW, Flanders WD, et al. Serum TSH, T4, and thyroid antibodies in the United States population (1988 to 1994): National Health and Nutrition Examination Survey (NHANES III). *J Clin Endocrinol Metab* 2002; **87**: 489–499.
3. Canaris GJ, Manowitz NR, Mayor G, Ridgway EC. The Colorado thyroid disease prevalence study. *Arch Intern Med* 2000; **160**: 526–534.
4. Roberts CGP, Ladenson PW. Hypothyroidism. *Lancet* 2004; **363**:793–803.
5. Baskin HJ, Cobin RH, Duick DS, et al. for the American Association of Clinical Endocrinologists. American Association of Clinical Endocrinologists medical guidelines for clinical practice for the evaluation and treatment of hyperthyroidism and hypothyroidism. *Endocr Pract* 2002; **8**: 457–469.
6. Glinoer D, de Nayer P, Bourdoux P, et al. Regulation of maternal thyroid during pregnancy. *J Clin Endocrinol Metab* 1990; **71**: 276–287.
7. ACOG. Subclinical hypothyroidism in pregnancy. Committee Opinion 381. October 2007, (reaffirmed 2012).
8. Burch, HB, Wartofsky, L. Life-threatening thyrotoxicosis – thyroid storm. *Endocrinol Metab Clin North Am* June 1993; **22** (2): 263–277.
9. Franklyn, JA. The management of hyperthyroidism. *New Engl J Med* 1994; **330**: 1731–1738.
10. Sawin CT, Geller A, Wolf PA, et al. Low serum thyrotropin concentrations as a risk factor for atrial fibrillation in older persons. *New Engl J Med* 1994; **331**: 1249–1252.
11. Klubo-Gwiezdzinska J, Wartofsky L. Thyroid emergencies. *Med Clin North Am* 2012 March; **96**(2): 385–403.
12. Hackmon R, Blichowski M, Koren G. The safety of methimazole and propylthiouracil in pregnancy: a systematic review. *J Obstet Gynaecol Can* 2012; **34** (11): 1077–1086.
13. Tan JY, Loh KC, Yeo GS, Chee YC. Transient hyperthyroidism of hyperemesis gravidarum. *BJOG*. 2002 Jun; **109**(6): 683–688.
14. Dozeman R, Kaiser FE, Cass O, Pries J. Hyperthyroidism appearing as hyperemesis gravidarum. *Arch Intern Med* 1983; **143**(11): 2202–2203.
15. Kristjansdottir HL, Bodvarsdottir SP, Sigurjonsdottir HA. Sheehan's syndrome in modern times: a nationwide retrospective study in Iceland. *Eur J Endocrinol* 2011 Mar; **164**(3): 349–354.
16. Zargar AH, Singh B, Laway BA, et al. Epidemiologic aspects of postpartum pituitary hypofunction (Sheehan's syndrome). *Fertil Steril* 2005; **84**: 523–528.
17. Gei-Guardia O, Soto-Herrera E, Gei-Brealey A, Chen-Ku CH. Sheehan syndrome in Costa Rica: clinical experience with 60 cases. *Endocr Pract* 2011 May–Jun; **17**(3): 337–344.

18. Tessnow AH, Wilson JD. The changing face of Sheehan's syndrome. *Am J Med Sci* 2010 Nov; **340**(5): 402–406.
19. Sheehan HL, Davis JC. *Post-partum Hypopituitarism.* Springfield, IL: Charles C. Thomas, 1982.
20. Skałba P1, Guz M. Hypogonadotropic hypogonadism in women. *Endokrynol Pol.* 2011; **62**(6): 560–567.
21. Silveira LF, Latronico AC. Approach to the patient with hypogonadotropic hypogonadism. *J Clin Endocrinol Metab* 2013; **98**(5): 1781–1788.
22. Burdelski M, Nolkemper D, Ganschow R, et al. Liver transplantation in children: long-term outcome and quality of life. *Eur J Pediatr* Dec 1999; **158**(Suppl 2): S34–S42.
23. Bartosh SM, Thomas SE, Sutton MM, et al. Linear growth after pediatric liver transplantation. *J Pediatr* Nov 1999; **135**(5): 624–631.
24. Wong, H. Management of diabetes insipidus. *J Mich Pharmacist* 1985 Feb; **23**: 4–5, 25–27.
25. Ziai, F. Walter, R. Rosenthal, IM. Treatment of central diabetes insipidus in adults and children with desmopressin: synthetic analog of vasopressin. *Arch Int Med* 1978 Sept; **138**: 1382–1385.
26. Zaben M. El Ghoul W. Belli A. Post-traumatic head injury pituitary dysfunction. *[Review] Disabil Rehabil* 2013; **35**(6): 522–525.
27. Gabbe SG, Niebyl JR, Simpson JL. Obstetrics. In: *Normal and Problem Pregnancies.* Philadelphia: Elsevier, 2007: **1039.**
28. Takayanagi Y, Yoshida M, Bielsky IF, et al. Pervasive social deficits, but normal parturition, in oxytocin receptor-deficient mice. *P Natl Acad Sci USA* 2005; **102** (44): 16096–16101.
29. Young WS 3rd, Shepard E, Amico J, et al. Deficiency in mouse oxytocin prevents milk ejection, but not fertility or parturition. *J Neuroendocrinol* 1996; **8**(11): 847–853.
30. Newell-Price J, Bertagna X, Grossman AB, Nieman LK. Cushing's syndrome. *Lancet* 2006; **367**(9522): 1605–1617.
31. Newell-Price J, Grossman A. Diagnosis and management of Cushing's syndrome. *Lancet* 1999 Jun 19; **353**: 2087–2088.
32. Eisenbarth GS, Gottlieb PA. Medical progress – autoimmune polyendocrine syndromes. *New Engl J Med* 2004; **350**(20): 2068–2079.
33. Baker SJ, Wass JA. Addison's disease. *BMJ* 2009 July 2; **339**: NIL_0007–NIL_0010.
34. Callender GG, Rich TA, Perrier ND. Multiple endocrine neoplasia syndromes. *Surg Clin North Am.* 2008 Aug; **88**(4): 863–895.
35. New MI. Extensive clinical experience: nonclassical 21-hydroxylase deficiency. *J Clin Endocrinol Metab* 2006; **91**(11): 4205–4214.
36. Imperato-Mcginley J, Peterson RE, Gautier T, Sturla E. Androgens and the evolution of male-gender identity among male pseudohermaphrodites with 5α-reductase deficiency. *New Engl J Med* 1979; **300**(22): 1233–1237.

Chapter 33

Office management of female reproductive tract anomalies

Brigid Hayden

Introduction

Congenital anomalies of the female genital tract are uncommon. As a consequence, office-based physicians rarely encounter a patient with such a condition. It is, however, important for all generalists, pediatricians, and gynecologists to be aware of the presenting features. Familiarity with the conditions described in this chapter will allow health-care providers to make a preliminary assessment, to communicate appropriately with the patient and her family, and to refer appropriately. A definitive diagnosis would consequently be made, and a proposed plan of management would be devised. Should surgery be required, patients with all but the most straightforward conditions (such as imperforate hymen) would be referred to a specialist. Subsequent care may also include important psychological support.

The British Society for Paediatric and Adolescent Gynaecology (BritSPAG) has devised a "UK Map of Services," which is freely available on its website (www.BritSPAG.org).[1] As a complement to the Map of Services, BritSPAG has produced a document entitled "Clinical Standards for Service Users in Paediatric & Adolescent Gynaecology," which is also freely available on the same website.

The UK government Department of Health has recently acknowledged the need for a network of specific centers to deal with the most specialized PAG cases, including disorders of sexual development (DSD; previously referred to as "intersex") and other rare and complex conditions.[2] BritSPAG's Clinical Standards document specifies that there should be PAG service provision in all acute hospitals providing gynecological services, with a designated lead clinician for PAG. It goes on to state that care needs to be in a setting appropriate for children, adolescents, and their families, including a child-friendly outpatient facility, supported by suitably qualified nursing staff.[3, 4]

The document further specifies that specialist centers are expected to maintain links with patient peer support groups, and it is noted that adolescents require information and advice on sexual health, contraception, and fertility. Close links are required between pediatric and adolescent services, ideally with joint transition clinics, to avoid the often haphazard transfer of care as adolescents become adults.

Embryology

A basic grasp of embryology is crucial in order to appreciate the various anomalies of the reproductive tract.

When discussing the gestation at which developments occur, it is important to remember that embryologists refer to the number of weeks post-fertilization. This contrasts with the system used in clinical practice, whereby the gestation is calculated as the number of weeks after the onset of the last menstrual period. The latter calculation will generally be two weeks longer than the former.[5]

Genital development is the same for both sexes up to week seven of in-utero life – that is, nine weeks after the mother's last menstrual period. This is known as the "indifferent stage." The urinary and reproductive systems of both sexes develop from the intermediate mesoderm of the developing embryo. This forms the urogenital ridge, located on either side of the aorta. This ridge is composed of the nephrogenic cord and the gonadal ridge.[6, 7]

The mesonephric ducts (alias wolffian ducts) are part of the developing urinary system. Lying lateral to these ducts are the paramesonephric ducts (also called müllerian ducts). The SRY gene (the sex-determining region of the Y chromosome) triggers male development. Testosterone from the fetal testis, along with the anti-müllerian hormone, determines

Office Care of Women, ed. Martin E. Olsen and Botros Rizk. Published by Cambridge University Press.

male sexual differentiation. In the absence of the SRY gene, female development occurs, whether or not there are ovaries present.[6]

Two X chromosomes are needed to bring about normal ovarian development. A greater number of X chromosomes than usual (e.g., XXX or XXY) has no effect on sexual organ development.

In the male fetus, the mesonephric (wolffian) ducts contribute to the reproductive system, whereas in the female fetus they regress. It is the paramesonephric (müllerian) ducts that play the greater role in female development. These ducts descend, meet in the midline, and fuse in the pelvic region to form the uterovaginal primordium, from which the uterus develops.[7]

The external genitalia appear similar in both sexes up to the ninth week of embryological development (i.e., the eleventh week after the mother's last menstrual period). The upper two-thirds of the vagina originates from the uterovaginal primordium, whereas the lower third arises from the vaginal plate, which becomes canalized during its development. In the female, the genital tubercle develops into the clitoris, and the urogenital groove develops into the vestibule, which contains the openings of the vagina and the urethra. The labia minora are formed from the urogenital folds, and the labioscrotal swellings become the labia majora.[6, 7]

Gonad formation comes about as a result of the migration of germ cells to the gonadal ridge at the beginning of week five (seven weeks from the mother's last menstrual period). The ovaries descend into the pelvis, and the gubernaculum, a peritoneal attachment to the gonads, goes on to form the round and ovarian ligaments.[5]

Specific congenital anomalies

Mullerian anomalies

Anomalies of development of the müllerian system range from very minor findings, requiring no intervention (such as arcuate uterus), through the minor condition known as imperforate hymen, to the most severe form, namely Mayer-Rokitansky-Kuster-Hauser syndrome, where the uterus and upper vagina completely fail to develop. See Figure 33-1 for diagrams of representative congenital anomalies of the uterus. These conditions may frequently be identified on ultrasound, but magnetic resonance imaging (MRI) may be indicated to more exactly define the nature of a specific anomaly.

Arcuate uterus and heart-shaped uterine fundus lie at the most minor end of the spectrum of müllerian fusion anomalies of the uterus, manifesting as incidental findings on ultrasound scan or at cesarean section. The arcuate uterus is noted to have a top that is flat rather than convex, and the heart-shaped uterus has an indentation at the fundus. Neither of these conditions generally requires any intervention, although they may occasionally be associated with abnormal fetal lie in late pregnancy.

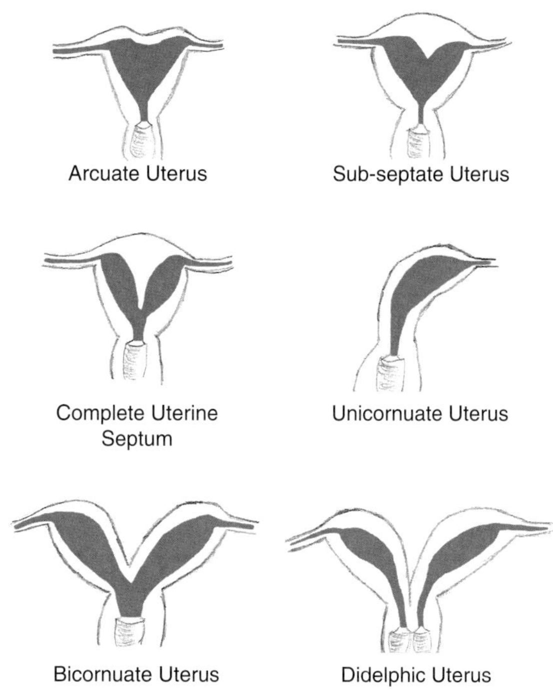

Figure 33-1 Representative congenital anomalies of the uterus.

A more significant anomaly on the müllerian fusion spectrum is the bicornuate uterus, which has two independent uterine canals. There may be a common vagina, or two distinct vaginas. Patients may present with difficulty inserting tampons, or with dyspareunia. This may confuse the unwary healthcare provider when performing vaginal examination. The condition may also be associated with abnormal fetal lie in pregnancy, and/or premature labor.

One variant is the uterine anomaly known as communicating uteri, where an isthmic communication connects two separate uterocervical cavities.[8, 9]

In situations where one vagina is blind ending, the young woman will present with severe dysmenorrhea. As she will be menstruating via the unaffected vagina, it may be many months, or even years, before the condition is recognized. Treatment consists of surgical removal of the septum. This creates a single vagina,

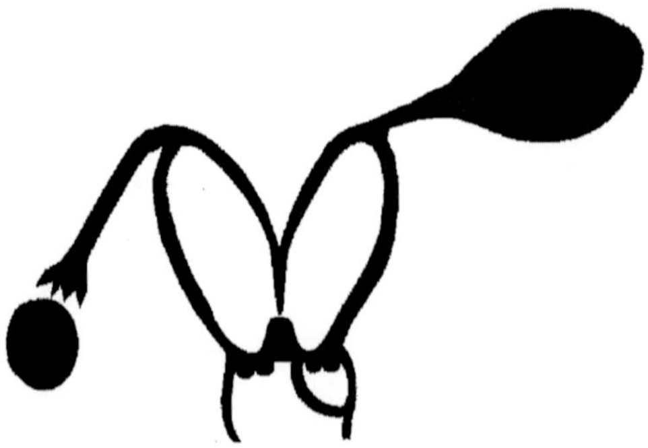

Figure 33-2 Toaff type 5A communicating uterine anomaly, one of several forms of the communicating uterine malformation. The patient in this example also had an endometrioma on the side of the obstructed hemivagina. *(Reprinted with permission, Olsen M, Thatcher SS, Breuel KF. Communicating Double Uterus with Obstructed Hemivagina and Subsequent Abscess Formation: A Case Report,* Adolesc Pediatr Gynecol. *1995;8:35–38.)*

which naturally contracts to a normal vaginal caliber. Nine different forms of this uterine anomaly (with variations) have been described by Toaff et al.[8] A representative example is seen in Figure 33-2.

A unicornuate uterus occurs through normal development of only one müllerian duct. It may be associated with abnormal fetal lie and premature labor. Occasionally, a rudimentary uterine horn may coexist with a unicornuate uterus. If the canal of the horn is blind ending (not communicating with the main uterine body), then severe dysmenorrhea will occur as the horn fills cyclically with menstrual fluid. The modern treatment is excision of the rudimentary horn, which is generally carried out laparoscopically. In years gone by, attempts were made to join the two horns together surgically, but the outcomes were not as good as with resection.[10] If pregnancy occurs in a rudimentary uterine horn, uterine rupture may occur, with potentially catastrophic results.

The most severe of the müllerian anomalies is Mayer-Rokitansky-Kuster-Hauser syndrome (MRKH), where the uterus and the upper vagina fail to develop as a consequence of failure of migration of both the wolffian and müllerian ducts.[11, 12] Development of secondary sexual characteristics takes place, as the ovaries are present, and there is characteristically no suspicion of a problem until primary amenorrhea is experienced. The incidence is approximately 1 in 5,000 female births.

Ultrasound evaluation of these patients will reveal an absent uterus with ovaries, which may be more difficult to see than usual, as they may be situated laterally, on the pelvic sidewall. MRI will be required to more accurately define the findings, and to delineate the amount of vagina present.

Three main areas of concern for patients with MRKH are psychological, sexual, and reproductive.

The diagnosis is potentially devastating for the patient and her family. Discussion must be handled very sensitively, with input from a clinical psychologist. For most patients, puberty will have progressed normally prior to the recognition of primary amenorrhea; the diagnosis is thus likely to be sudden and completely unexpected for the patient and her family. This generates serious concerns and anxieties in relation to body image as well as to sexual function and future reproductive potential.

The first-line treatment for creating a neo-vagina is the use of vaginal dilators. The success of this treatment is dependent on compliance, as 30 minutes of treatment daily on a regular basis is required. Once the girl engages in sexual activity, further natural dilation of the vagina will be achieved.

Surgical alternatives to dilation exist, including the Vechietti procedure. The procedure utilizes traction to create a vagina over the space of a week during inpatient hospitalization. Ongoing dilation is subsequently necessary, either by dilators or by sexual intercourse. Occasionally, a prolapse of the neo-vagina occurs, as the tissues are unsupported. This can be treated surgically with a sacrocolpopexy, attaching the vault of the neo-vagina to the anterior aspect of the sacrum.

Adoption and surrogacy (potentially with donor ovum) are currently the standard methods available to address fertility. Great progress is being made in the field of uterine transplantation. The first baby was born after this procedure in 2014.[13]

As has been discussed, the embryological development of the mesonephric and para-mesonephric ducts occur concurrently; therefore, uterine anomalies commonly coexist with abnormalities of development of the urinary tract. Renal tract anomalies are even more frequently seen in patients with the didelphic uterus congenital anomaly.

The renal anomaly may be a single kidney, or a horseshoe kidney, and the ureters may be duplicated or ectopic, or sometimes blind-ended. Consequently, it is imperative to carry out imaging of the urinary tract when müllerian abnormalities are diagnosed.[14] Figure 33-3 shows an intravenous pyelogram (IVP) of a patient with a single kidney and a müllerian anomaly.

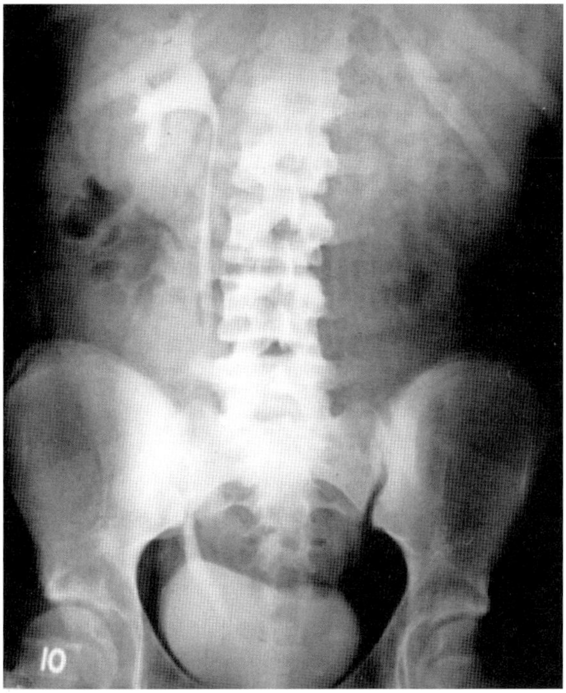

Figure 33-3 Intravenous pyelogram of the patient with the uterine anomaly seen in Figure 33-2. Note that the absent kidney is on the same side as the obstructed hemivagina.

The hymen is a thin membrane that lies at the embryological junction of the sinovaginal bulb and the urogenital sinus. It usually becomes perforated during fetal life, but may remain imperforate. Although obstruction to menstrual flow has been referred to previously in relation to a blind-ending duplicated vagina, and a noncommunicating uterine horn, an imperforate hymen is the most commonly encountered cause of obstruction to menstrual flow. The incidence of imperforate hymen is 1/1,000 female births.[15] See Figure 33-4 for an image of imperforate hymen/hematocolpos.

Girls with imperforate hymen usually present with primary amenorrhea, with a history of pelvic pain, which may or may not be cyclical. A palpable pelvic mass due to hematometra may be present.

The patient may present with such severe abdominal pain for which a diagnosis of appendicitis may be considered. When the labia are parted during examination, a bulging bluish membrane is seen. This is sufficient evidence to make the diagnosis. Confirmation is often sought by ultrasound scan.

Treatment is by resection of the hymen under anesthesia, via a cruciate incision, with excision of

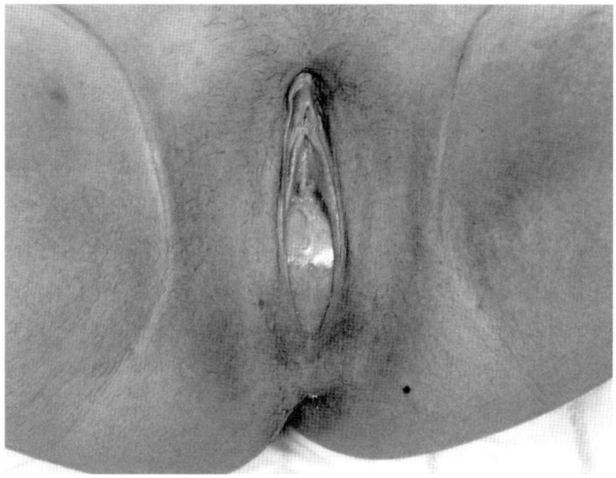

Figure 33-4 Image of imperforate hymen/hematocolpos.

the hymeneal remnants. Up to two liters of old blood may be released by this procedure. Full recovery without sequelae usually occurs after this procedure. An association between imperforate hymen and endometriosis exists, presumably due to backflow of menstrual fluid through the fallopian tubes.

Far less common than imperforate hymen is transverse vaginal septum, which occurs due to embryological failure of canalization of the müllerian ducts.[16] It presents with the same symptoms, but the characteristic bulging membrane is not seen on inspection. It is of crucial importance to refer the patient to a specialist for appropriate assessment and surgical management. An MRI is required to delineate the septum and to plan the surgical intervention. Induction of amenorrhea should take place with gonadotropin-releasing (GnRH) analogues while investigations are underway.

Transverse vaginal septa may occur anywhere along the length of the vagina; they are classified as upper, mid, and lower. The position will determine the surgical approach, which will be either vaginal or combined abdomino-vaginal. Vaginal dilators will be required to maintain patency of the vagina postoperatively.

Cervical agenesis is even more rare. In the past, hysterectomy was the standard treatment, but recently uterovaginal anastomosis has been performed successfully.

Disorders of sexual development

Disorders of sexual development (DSDs, formerly known as intersex disorders) include complete androgen insensitivity syndrome (CAIS). In this rare X-linked recessive condition, formerly known as testicular feminization, the karyotype is 46XY, but the phenotype is female. The gonads are testes, located in the abdomen or inguinal canals. Testosterone is produced, but the androgen receptors in the end-organ tissues are unresponsive.

In CAIS, during in-utero development, the müllerian structures regress due to normal secretion of the testicular müllerian inhibitory factor. Normal breast development occurs due to peripheral conversion of testosterone to estrogen, and the pubic and axillary hair are generally sparse or absent. CAIS commonly presents with primary amenorrhea, and the vagina is generally found to be short and blind ending.

Partial androgen insensitivity (PAIS) may exist to varying degrees, often presenting at birth as ambiguous genitalia.

In both CAIS and PAIS, sensitive disclosure of the diagnosis to the patient and her family is essential, with the ongoing support of a clinical psychologist. The issue of timing of removal of the gonads must be addressed due to the risk of malignant transformation of the internal testicles.[17]

Congenital adrenal hyperplasia (CAH) is the most common cause of ambiguous genitalia at birth. The majority of cases are due to an enzyme defect known as 21-hydroxylase deficiency. In its most severe form, this can lead to a salt-wasting crisis which is life threatening; therefore, it is imperative to diagnose or exclude this condition as soon as possible after birth.

CAH may occur in either boys or girls. When it affects girls, it brings about masculinization of the external genitalia. Surgical correction entails a vaginal and a clitoral component, and may be carried out in stages, prior to puberty and/or thereafter. A specialist will require careful consideration to determine the type and timing of surgery.

When evaluating the genitalia of a newborn, it is crucial to remember that it is not possible to assign a sex at the time of birth to babies with ambiguous genitalia. A large clitoris and a small penis, with or without hypospadias, may be indistinguishable; genital folds may be either scrotal or labial; and there may be only a single opening on the perineum, which is not clearly urethral or vaginal. Clinical inspection cannot provide a diagnosis, so the clinician must explain the situation to the parents and avoid the temptation to hazard a guess.

Other forms of DSD include Turner syndrome and mixed gonadal dysgenesis.

Turner syndrome has an incidence of 1 in 2,000–3,000 live female births.[16] The classical karyotype is 45X, but many affected girls have mosaic forms such as 45X/46XX or 45X/46XY. The phenotype can vary greatly, and the diagnosis is commonly not made until the girl is in her teens.

Patients with mixed gonadal dysgenesis, which is very rare, generally have female internal genitalia, but with a testis on one side (often in the inguinal ring) and an undifferentiated gonad on the other side.

Communication

The care of a female patient with reproductive tract anomaly is multifaceted. This poses diagnostic and management challenges. One important aspect which the physician must never overlook is communication, thereby practicing the art of medicine in addition to fulfilling its scientific roles.[17–19] Withholding information is not an option. In the past, a paternalistic approach of information restriction was often taken. This would lead to a situation where the patient had no knowledge or understanding of the condition that was central to her health and well-being.

Because of the potentially serious consequences of these congenital anomalies, recognizable similarities exist to breaking bad news in the context of malignant disease and life-changing injuries. Multidisciplinary input is crucial in the context of these complex discussions. A clinical psychologist, preferably with background experience in this area of practice, is an essential member of the team.[19]

The office environment lends itself well to the pre-consultation preparation required to facilitate a satisfactory meeting. Such a meeting will address the needs of the patient and of her accompanying parent or guardian. All available information about the patient's condition and her background health must be reviewed in advance; any investigation results must be scrutinized. The layout of the room may be adjusted, such as arranging a semicircle of chairs rather than a desk-and-chairs format.

The patient and her accompanying adult(s) should be greeted and made welcome to contribute to the discussion. The age and emotional maturity of the patient should be taken into consideration, along with the apparent educational level of her accompanying adult(s). Where English is not the first language spoken, consideration should be given to arranging the services of an interpreter. Many aspects of the condition will need to be addressed, including concerns about body image, sexual functioning, and future reproductive potential.

Opportunities for a one-on-one discussion with the patient alone should be built into the consultation in order to allow an exchange of more sensitive information. The input of experienced nursing colleagues is invaluable in such situations, and it is mandatory if an examination is required on that occasion. It may, of course, be appropriate to defer the examination to a later consultation, to allow time to build up confidence and rapport with the patient and her family.

The terminology used in the course of any consultation is important, but it is particularly so in this context. For example, the physician should avoid outdated terms such as "intersex" and "hermaphrodite," which have negative connotations, and use the acronym DSD, which stands for "disorders of sexual development" or "diverse sexual development."[19]

Explanations of complex concepts in layman's language should be well considered in advance, with avoidance of clumsy explanations such as "a girl in a boy's body" for androgen insensitivity syndrome. Such a mistake may cause misunderstanding and psychological harm. With this particular diagnosis, basic background information should be provided regarding chromosome numbers, for example, explaining that only one X is necessary to create a female, and that while most females are XX, some are XY.

It can be very difficult to manage the balance between effective information gathering and intrusiveness. Having a patient or her relative feel offended, patronized, or excluded will create a barrier to effective communication, understanding, and compliance with treatment. To paraphrase the great American author Maya Angelou, people may forget what a provider says and does, but they will not forget the way the provider made them feel. Once rapport has been achieved, the scene is set for explanation of the condition, any investigations required, and the likely treatment options. It is important to state clearly and compassionately that the sexual organs have not developed normally and, depending on the condition, whether or not the patient has a womb and whether or not she can produce eggs. In the case of androgen insensitivity syndrome, the need for hormonal treatment up to the usual age of menopause will need to be explained, as well as the need for the "abnormal ovaries" to be removed in order to prevent harm.

One important area, which is being increasingly explored, is the degree of control that a patient has during the consultation, and during the totality of the management of her illness or condition. One end of the spectrum of control would be a physician stating, "We are planning X intervention." The other end would be a physician stating, "These are the management options," and then following the patient's lead in providing more information by asking questions such as "How do you feel about this?" and "What's on your mind?" The concept of care-orientated and cure-orientated interventions is intrinsic to this notion.

The patient and her family must have the opportunity to gather the information they require; this is fundamental to obtaining informed consent. This entails outlining the risks and benefits of any investigation modalities and treatment options, taking into account the patient's age and maturity as well as the legal age of consent in the jurisdiction of residence.

It may take many consultations, sometimes over several years, for the patient and her family to come to terms with her condition. The presence of parents or guardians is invaluable during the consultation for the reasons already outlined, but also because they have a legitimate stake in the patient's future, which may potentially include issues relating to reproductive capability. For example, a post-menopausal woman has recently become the donor for a successful uterine transplantation in a young woman with MRKH in Gothenberg, Sweden; patients' parents are increasingly likely to seek information about such developments.[13]

Shame-free discussion about atypical sexual anatomy is to be encouraged during the consultation and thereafter within the patient's family and social circle. It should be clear that the aim is to enable rather than curtail sexual diversity; a vagina is not essential for satisfactory sexual activity.

Many websites and online support groups exist, which may be greatly helpful to girls and their relatives and close friends, providing information and psychological support.[20–23]

Physicians potentially harbor the same inhibitions and prejudices as their societies of origin; some may not find it easy to engage in these dialogues within an office environment. Role-play sessions, either face-to-face with an experienced facilitator or in a "serious gaming" online simulation set-up, may be invaluable in acquiring skills in this area.[20–24]

Concluding remarks

Congenital anomalies of the female genital tract are relatively uncommon and vary greatly in severity. It is important for the office physician, whether generalist, gynecologist, or pediatrician, to be aware of such conditions in order to make an initial assessment and to refer appropriately as needed. Communication with patients and their families is a more challenging process than with many diagnoses, but an effective discussion is critical to patient satisfaction.

References

1. British Society for Paediatric & Adolescent Gynaecology. Available at: www.BritSPAG.org. Accessed 25 Feb 2015.
2. MacDougall J, Creighton SM, Wood PL. Clinical networks in paediatric and adolescent gynaecology. *BJOG* 2010;**117**:131–133.
3. Department of Health. Transition: getting it right for young people. 2006. Available at: webarchive .nationalarchives.gov.uk. Accessed 25 Feb 2015.
4. Department of Health. You're welcome – quality criteria for young people friendly health services. 15 April 2011. Available at: www.gov.uk. Accessed 25 Feb 2015.
5. Fitzgerald MJT, Fitzgerald M. *Human Embryology*. London: Bailliere Tindall, 1994: 142–150.
6. Moore KL, Persaud TVN. *The Developing Human*, 8th Edition. Philadelphia: Elsevier, 2008: 243–284.
7. Webster S, de Wreede R. *Embryology at a Glance*, 1st Edition. Oxford: Wiley-Blackwell, 2012: 78–81. Companion website: www.wiley.com/go/embryology.
8. Toaff ME, Lev-Toaff AS, Toaff R. Communicating uterine anomalies. *Fertil Steril* 1984;**44**:661–679.
9. Toaff ME, Lev-Toaff AS, Toaff R. Communicating uteri: review and classification with introduction of two previously unreported types: *Fertil Steril* 1984;**41** (5):661–679.
10. Pandis GK, Michala L, Creighton SM, Cutner AS. Minimal access surgery in adolescent gynaecology. *BJOG* 2009;**116**:214–219.
11. Griffin JE, Edwards C, Madden JD, et al. Congenital absence of the vagina: the Mayer Rokitansky Kuster Hauser syndrome. *Ann Intern Med* 1976;**85**:224–236.
12. Valappil S, Chetan U, Wood N, Garden A. Mayer-Rokitansky-Kuster-Hauser syndrome: diagnosis and management. *Obstetrician & Gynaecologist.* 2012;**14**:93–98.
13. Brannstrom M, Johannesson L, Bokstrom H, et al. Livebirth after uterus transplantation. *Lancet* 2015 Feb 12;**385**(9968):607–616. Published online October 6, 2014.
14. Hall-Craggs MA, Kirkham A, Creighton SM. Renal and urological abnormalities occurring with Mullerian anomalies. *J Pediatr Urol* 2013;**9**:27–32.
15. Tseng JJ, Ho JY, Chen WH, Chou MM. Prenatal diagnosis of isolated fetal hydrocolpos secondary to imperforate hymen. *J Chinese Med Assoc* 2008 June;**71** (6):325.
16. Edmonds DK, Rose GL. Outflow tract disorders of the female genital tract. *Obstetrician & Gynaecologist* 2013 Jan;**15**(1):11–17.
17. Berra M, Liao LM, Creighton SM, Conway GS. Long-term health issues of women with XY karyotype. *Maturitas* 2010;**65**:172–178.
18. Garden AS, Topping J. *Paediatric & Adolescent Gynaecology for the MRCOG and Beyond*. London: RCOG Press, 2001.
19. Creighton SM, Liao LM. Changing attitudes to sex assignment in intersex. *BJU* 2004;**93**:659–640.
20. MRKH Foundation. Available at: http://mrkh.org. Accessed 25 Feb 2015.
21. Intersex Society of North America. Available at: www .isna.org. Accessed 25 Feb 2015.
22. DSD Families. Available at: dsdfamilies.org. Accessed 25 Feb 2015.
23. Androgen Insensitivity Syndrome Support Group. Available at: aissg.org. Accessed 25 Feb 2015.
24. Congenital Adrenal Hyperplasia Support Group. Available at: livingwithcah.com. Accessed 25 Feb 2015.

Chapter 34

Office care of breast disorders

Manjusha Sahni and Patrice M. Weiss

Evaluating patients with breast complaints

History

Evaluation of breast complaints begins with obtaining a detailed history of the patient. The goal is to aid the diagnosis and management of benign breast disorders and to identify women who are at higher risk for developing breast cancer in their lifetimes. The initial history should include the following:

- **Age** is the strongest risk factor for breast cancer. A woman's risk of developing breast cancer increases with age. The risk at age 40 is 1.47% and progressively increases to 3.56% at age 60.[1]
- **Commonly reported symptoms** of the breast are the presence of a lump, cyclic or noncyclic pain, nipple discharge, and skin changes or inflammation.
- **Duration** of breast symptoms and any changes over time should be noted. Slowly or rapidly growing masses are more concerning than those that stay stable in size.
- **Laterality** of the symptoms to one or both breasts.
- **Associated findings** such as tenderness, skin changes, nipple discharge, and history of trauma or radiation to the chest.
- **Systemic symptoms** such as weight loss or gain. Menstrual cycle or bowel habit changes suggest thyroid disorders. Headaches or changes in peripheral vision suggest a pituitary tumor compressing on the optic chiasm.
- **Possibility of pregnancy** or continued lactation should be considered especially in women with nipple discharge.
- **Previous history of breast cancer or benign breast diseases** and/or breast biopsies. Women diagnosed with breast cancer at age <40 have a 4.5 times increased risk of developing subsequent breast cancer.[2] Benign breast disorders such as atypical hyperplasia, lobular carcinoma in situ, and certain variants of fibroadenomas carry an increased risk of breast cancer and need to be surgically removed.
- **Breast implants**, although not associated with an increased risk for cancer, can make the evaluation technically challenging.
- **Family history** of breast or ovarian cancer in first-degree relatives is associated with significant increased risk of breast cancer in a woman. The risk is four times higher for women with two or more first-degree relatives.[2]
- **Genetic predisposition** because 5%–10% of breast cancers are a result of inherited genetic mutations such as *BRCA1* and *BRCA2*.[3] Inheritance pattern is autosomal dominant. In the general population, the carrier rate for such mutations is less than 1%, although in certain populations it is much higher. An estimated 1 in 40 Ashkenazi Jews carries a *BRCA1* or *BRCA2* founder gene mutation.[3] The estimated lifetime risk of breast cancer for a woman with *BRCA1* or *BRCA2* mutation is 65%–74%, and the risk for ovarian cancer is 20%–46%.[3] Patients, who are at a higher risk of being carriers of inherited gene mutations should be identified and offered genetic consultation.[2, 3]
- **Age of menarche or menopause.** Women with early menarche (before age 12) and late menopause (after age 55) have a slightly higher risk of breast cancer due to longer exposure to reproductive hormones. Conversely, earlier pregnancy (before age 30) and breastfeeding for over a year is protective against breast cancer.[2]
- **High breast tissue density** usually indicated by a previous mammography is an independent risk factor for developing breast cancer.

Office Care of Women, ed. Martin E. Olsen and Botros Rizk. Published by Cambridge University Press.

- **Postmenopausal use of combined estrogen and progesterone hormones** has shown to increase the risk of developing breast cancer in the Women's Health Initiative randomized trial. Updated results from this study failed to show an increased risk when estrogen alone was used in women without a uterus.[4]
- **Obesity and weight gain.** The risk of breast cancer is two times higher in postmenopausal women who are obese, likely due to high estrogen levels.[2]
- **Lifestyle and social history.** Current use of alcohol and tobacco can increase the risk of breast cancer in women by 12%. Conversely, regular physical activity has been shown to decrease risk of breast cancer in postmenopausal women by 10%–20%.[2]
- **Environmental risks.** Exposure to radiation between 10 and 30 years of age, exposure to diethylstilbestrol directly or in-utero (used until the 1960s), and high levels of ethylene oxide in commercial sterilization facilities have been shown to have strong association with development of breast cancer.[2]

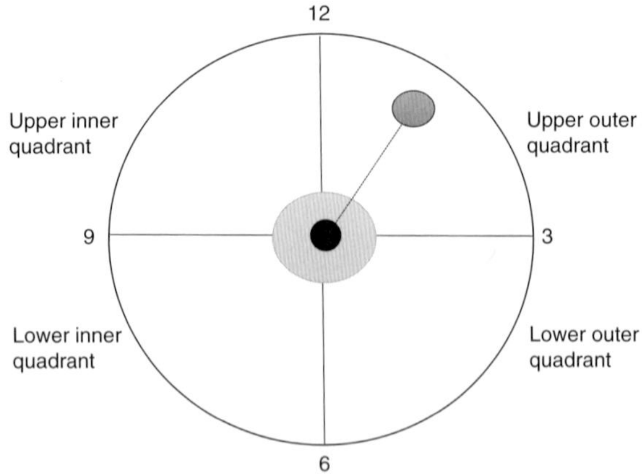

Figure 34-1 Representation of the left breast with a 2 cm palpable mass in the upper outer quadrant at 1'o clock position, 6 cm from the nipple.

Physical examination

General examination should be guided by history and review of systems and may include examination of visual fields, thyroid gland, chest wall, and lungs. The hallmark for evaluating any breast-related complaint is the ability to perform a thorough breast examination. The sensitivity and specificity of the clinical breast examination are estimated to be 54% and 94%, respectively, depending on the thoroughness of the examiner.[5]

Clinical breast exam

The clinical breast examination is performed with the patient in a sitting and then supine position. A breast is visualized as a face of a clock with vertical and horizontal lines intersecting at the nipple dividing the breast into four quadrants; upper inner and outer and lower inner and outer (Figure 34-1). The breast tail extends from the upper outer quadrant into the axillary region. The description of any abnormal finding should include the laterality of the breast, location of the abnormality in a quadrant, at o'clock position and its distance from the nipple in inches or cm (as shown in Figure 34-1).

Inspection of the breasts should be performed with the patient in sitting up and leaning forward positions, first hands on her sides and then on her hips. The breasts should be inspected for size, symmetry, skin changes, dimpling or retraction, edema or ulcerations, and scars from previous biopsies. The nipples are inspected for any asymmetry, inversion, eczema-like skin changes, and nipple discharge. Erythema of the breast can be a sign of an infection or inflammatory carcinoma of the breast. An eczematous appearing skin rash represent Paget's disease, which is a surface manifestation of an underlying malignancy. Any piercings and discharge or changes around the piercings should be noted.

Palpation of the breast tissue should be performed while the patient is supine with her arms behind her head. The examiner should use both the flat surface of the palm and pads of the fingers to palpate the breast tissue against the chest wall in a systematic fashion, either concentric circles from the nipple or vertical grids, so as to cover the entire breast.[6] Any abnormal finding should be noted as demonstrated in Figure 34-1. A mass should be noted for its location, size, mobility or fixity from the surrounding tissue, consistency (whether fluctuant, firm, or hard), smooth or irregular borders, and any associated retraction or edema of the overlying skin. The subareolar nipple complex should be examined in a similar manner and gently compressed to elicit discharge. Nipple discharge should be described for its laterality, color, involvement of single or multiple ducts, spontaneity versus expressed, and volume.

Palpation of the axillary, supraclavicular, and subclavian nodes in a sitting position completes the breast examination.

Diagnostic modalities

Mammography

Mammography is currently the best available imaging tool for detecting breast cancer. The procedure utilizes application of low dose radiation through compressed breast tissue to obtain multiple images of the inner structure of the breast. Full-field digital mammography has mostly replaced screen film mammography because of the use of a lower dose of radiation, the ability to manipulate images to obtain an optimal view, electronic storage, and easy accessibility. Digital mammography has been reported to be more accurate in premenopausal women younger than 50 years of age with dense breasts on mammography.[7]

Mammographic screening has the potential to detect a nonpalpable mass as small as 1 mm, at least three years or more before it increases to a palpable size of about 2 cm.[8] Tumors detected at an early stage are more likely to be optimally treated with lesser interventions, resulting in better quality of life and improved five-year survival rate. The sensitivity of screening mammography ranges from 83% to 95% and specificity rates between 90% and 95%.[9]

A 2011 Cochrane review assessed the effect of screening for breast cancer with mammography on mortality and morbidity; seven randomized trials were found to be eligible. Only three of these seven trials were noted to have adequate randomization and failed to show a significant reduction in breast cancer mortality after 10 years. When all seven trials were combined, the mortality rate was significantly lower.[10] However, another analysis suggests a decrease in the mortality rate in women older than 40 by 28% since screening mammography was introduced; several observational studies make a similar claim.[9]

Limitations of screening mammography include:

- False positive results. An almost 10% recall rate requires further testing; only 5% of these women have cancer.
- Overdiagnosis or finding of clinically insignificant cancers which may not have progressed. Rates are variable, ranging from 0% to more than 30%.[2]
- Decreased sensitivity in dense breasts leads to confusion and patient anxiety. A possible need for additional studies using ultrasonography or magnetic resonance imaging (MRI) then exists.
- Decreased sensitivity in younger women (under 30–35 years of age) exists due to higher breast density.

Breast cancers screening recommendations are highly controversial for women who are at average risk of breast cancer. The American Congress of Obstetricians and Gynecologists (ACOG) recommends initiating mammography annually at the age of 40 and clinical breast examination along with self-breast awareness starting at age 20. Updated 2015 guidelines from the American Cancer society, recommended initiating breast cancer screening at age 45.

Risks, benefits, and possible outcomes of screening mammography should be discussed with eligible patients, and screening recommendations individualized based on a woman's risk of breast cancer.

Indications for diagnostic mammography include the following:

- to evaluate breast masses and suspicious breast changes reported clinically
- to evaluate patients with pathological nipple discharge or eczematous skin changes for underlying malignancy
- to search for occult breast cancer in patients suspected of having a primary cancer of unknown location and metastasis to axillary lymph nodes[11]
- to obtain stereotactic breast biopsies in patients who have suspicious micro calcifications on a screening mammography

Ultrasonography

Breast ultrasonography is used as an adjunct to mammography to characterize breast findings or to screen dense breasts. It is the preferred modality to differentiate a solid from a cystic mass. Ultrasonography is the test of choice when evaluating younger patients (less than 30 years of age) with breast complaints or those who are pregnant or lactating. It can be used as an adjunct for screening with MRI in women who are at high risk for breast cancer. It is an excellent tool for guiding interventional procedures such as core needle biopsies, cyst aspiration, or drainage of breast abscess. The accuracy of the findings is highly dependent on operator technique and availability of high-resolution, real-time, linear array scanners.

The use of combined ultrasonography and mammography has been advocated to improve the detection of benign etiologies for palpable findings, thus, reducing the need for unnecessary biopsies. The addition of ultrasonography can increase the ability to detect cancers that are occult on mammography by 93%–100%. The negative predictive value can be more than 97% when mammography and ultrasonography findings are negative in the setting of a benign palpable mass.[12]

Magnetic resonance imaging

Contrast-enhanced breast MRI is currently being used as an adjunct for screening high-risk patients for breast cancer, especially those who are younger and have dense breast tissue. It is best used as part of a multimodality approach (along with mammography and ultrasonography) in detecting disease in high-risk women with dense breasts. The sensitivity reaches almost 100% with a specificity of 65%.[9]

Fine needle aspiration cytology

Fine needle aspiration cytology (FNAC) is an office-based procedure that involves collection of cellular material or cyst aspirate with a 23-gauge needle and preparation of direct smears for submission for cytological analysis. The procedure is operator dependent and can result in high inadequate rates, sampling errors, and false positive or false negative diagnosis.[4] Even in experienced hands, aspiration cytology can yield a false negative rate of up to 15% for breast cancer in patients with a palpable mass.[13] FNAC is an excellent, cost-effective tool where resources are limited; however, it should be performed by an experienced cytopathologist for optimum results.

Core needle biopsy

Tissue biopsy obtained by image-guided core needle biopsy (CNB) or excisional biopsy remains the gold standard for evaluation of suspicious or equivocal breast findings. Core biopsy of a palpable mass has been shown to be more sensitive, specific, and accurate in histological grading than FNAC.[12]

Evaluation of the breast mass

Introduction

A palpable breast mass is the most reliable clinical indicator of breast cancer. Breast cancer is the most common female cancer and the second leading cause of cancer-related death for women in the United States. About 1 in 8 women (12%) in the United States develop invasive breast cancer during their lifetime. It is estimated that in the year 2015, more than 2 million new cases of invasive breast cancer will be diagonised and 40,000 women will die of breast cancer in United States.[2] Age is the strongest risk factor for breast cancer, but 70% of women diagnosed with breast cancer have an additional identifiable risk factor. There are several models to help stratify breast cancer risk for any individual woman. The most widely used is the Gail model, which estimates five-year and lifetime breast cancer risk (see www.cancer.gov/bcrisktool).

Scope of the problem

In women presenting with breast masses, age plays the most important role. In a study of 542 women younger than age 30 and with palpable breast masses, only 2% were found to have invasive breast cancer; 72% of the masses were fibroadenomas, 8% fibrocystic changes (a term no longer used), 6% phyllodes tumor, 5% other, 4% breast cysts, and 3% breast abscess or mastitis.

Although a majority of the palpable masses in younger women are benign, a low index of suspicion for cancer can harmfully delay diagnosis and treatment in this age group.[15] A validated approach is needed to identify those who can be conservatively managed versus those who need surgical intervention. In contrast, older women with a palpable mass would need a more aggressive approach, including tissue diagnosis to rule out cancer and high-risk lesions.

Evaluating patients with a palpable breast mass

Evaluation of a woman with a palpable breast mass should always begin with a complete history, cancer risk assessment, and thorough breast examination as detailed earlier in this chapter. An attempt should be made to classify the findings as clinically benign, clinically suspicious, or indeterminate to guide further management.

- A **clinically benign** mass is generally smooth, firm or soft, freely mobile, with distinct smooth margins, and absent of nodularity. There is an absence of breast tissue retraction, overlying skin or nipple changes, or palpable axillary lymph nodes. Age-based diagnostic imaging is recommended, and a percutaneous needle biopsy is preferable for patients who prefer conservative management (see Table 34-1). Patients with higher risk for cancer based on family or personal history or known *BRCA* mutation or other inherited syndromes should be referred to a breast surgeon.

Table 34-1 Recommended management of clinically benign palpable breast masses

Patient age (in years)	Diagnostic imaging	Result (in relationship with clinical findings)	Management
<30	Targeted breast ultrasonography	Concordant	Repeat ultrasonography every 6 months for 2 years to determine stability, with or without; percutaneous needle biopsy; (biopsy recommended in high-risk patients)
		Discordant	CNB or referral to breast surgeon for excisional biopsy
>30	Diagnostic mammography +/– targeted breast ultrasonography	Concordant	Image-guided CNB or excisional biopsy recommended; or repeat breast imaging and CBE every 6 months for 2 years acceptable (if risk of malignancy is less than 2%)
		Discordant	Biopsy recommended; urgent referral to breast surgeon
All ages	Breast ultrasonography +/– diagnostic mammography	Simple cyst	Repeat ultrasonography and CBE every 6 months for 2 years; routine screening mammography >40 years of age; needle aspiration if enlarging, painful cysts; biopsy or surgical excision if aspirate is dry or bloody
		Complex cyst	Referral to breast surgeon; excision of cyst or CNB recommended

CNB – core needle biopsy, CBE – clinical breast exam
Source: References 4, 12, 15.

- A **clinically suspicious** mass is generally firm to hard, immobile, and fixed to surrounding parenchyma with poorly defined margins. Associated changes of overlying skin or nipple-areolar complex (edema, puckering, retraction, ulceration, rashlike lesion), or axillary lymphadenopathy may be present. Women who have findings suspicious for malignancy should be referred to a breast surgeon for tissue diagnosis.
- **Indeterminate** findings are those of a clinically undetected mass or presence of multiple glandular lumps, focal thickening, or asymmetric nodularity. Such patients should have a repeat breast examination after one or two months in the early phase of the menstrual cycle. In case of focal thickening, a diagnostic mammography and/or ultrasonography are recommended. If symptoms are persistent and findings unclear on breast examination, the patient should be referred to a breast specialist and diagnostic imaging obtained.

Common benign breast masses

Fibroadenomas are the most common benign breast masses in younger women and adolescents.[16] They present as well circumscribed, nontender, smooth, mobile, firm, and rubbery lesions measuring 2 cm–3 cm in diameter. They are usually single and unilateral. Approximately 10%–20% of fibroadenomas can be multiple and 10% are bilateral.[17] Giant fibroadenomas exceed 6 cm in size and can enlarge to 10 cm–15 cm. A giant fibroadenoma can mimic Phyllodes tumor, which has a malignant potential and needs to be surgically excised.

Sonographically, a fibroadenoma appears well encapsulated and uniformly hypo echoic. Diagnosis is based on ultrasonography and/or diagnostic mammography. Tissue biopsy is recommended for mass size greater than 2 cm, or unclear radiological findings.

Natural history of fibroadenomas is that of regression in up to 50% of patients, growth in 25%, and no change in 25% after five year of surveillance.[18]

A conservative approach involving percutaneous biopsy and long-term surveillance is cost-effective and associated with less morbidity compared to excisional biopsies in younger women.[15] Surgical excision is recommended in older women and in those with giant fibroadenomas or proliferative atypical lesions on histopathology. Cosmetic and less invasive procedures such as vacuum assisted removal or cryoablation performed in the office is suggested by some experts for smaller fibroadenomas.[19]

Phyllodes tumors are rare and account for <1% of breast tumors in all age groups.[20] These are fibroepithelial tumors with malignant potential which are difficult to distinguish from a fibroadenoma clinically or radiologically.[11] Diagnosis is established by core needle biopsy. Referral to a breast surgeon is recommended; treatment is wide local excision.

Breast cysts are most commonly seen between 35 and 55 years of age. Breast cysts can be multiple and bilateral. Palpable cysts can enlarge and may become painful in the premenstrual phase of the cycle. Cyst recurrence is seen in 30% of patients.

Diagnosis is established by breast sonography. *Simple cysts* appear smooth with thin walls and an absence of internal echoes. They are benign. A needle aspiration of the cyst fluid can be performed for painful cysts. The aspirate is usually straw to green colored. Tissue biopsy or excision of the cyst is recommended when the needle aspirate is dry, bloody, or thick or when ultrasonography features suggest an intracystic mass, internal echoes, or complex cyst.[11] Simple cysts are managed by close surveillance.

Hamartomas are rare benign breast tumors most commonly seen among women aged 30–50 years.[20] They account for 0.7%–4.8% of benign breast tumors and are characterized by disorganized overgrowth of mature breast tissue elements.[21] Hamartomas are palpable, painless, well-circumscribed, and mobile masses that are often misdiagnosed as fibroadenomas clinically and radiologically. A tissue biopsy is often necessary to confirm the diagnosis and also to identify any atypical features. In the absence atypical features, hamartomas can be managed by observation alone. Breast hamartomas have been reported in association with Cowden syndrome, which is characterized by the presence of multiple hamartomas in the breasts as well as the skin and mucus membranes of other anatomical locations. Patients with Cowden syndrome are at an increased risk of developing breast, thyroid, endometrial, and other cancers.

Lactating adenomas are the most common cause of palpable breast masses during pregnancy and lactation period. They present as well circumscribed masses, measuring up to 4 cm, which usually involute after completion of lactation. They can be complicated by infarction or hemorrhage in 5% of cases. A tissue biopsy is usually needed to confirm diagnosis. Surgical excision is recommended if the mass persists or grows.[20]

Nipple discharge

Introduction

Nipple discharge (ND) is a common breast complaint reported by up to 10% of women presenting for routine examination.[22] Incidence of breast carcinoma in patients with nipple discharge, who undergo operative excision, is reported to be 9.3%–21.3%.[23] Most women who present with ND have benign disease, but up to 15% of patients have an underlying malignancy and 7%–10% have an underlying high-risk lesion (HRL), such as atypical ductal hyperplasia or lobular carcinoma in situ.[22]

Scope of the problem

In a retrospective study of 416 patients, 129 patients (31%) were diagnosed to have physiological ND and were managed expectantly.[22] At a median follow-up of 18 months, 128 of 129 patients (99%) remained with no evidence of disease. The remaining patient (<1%) presented with an invasive ductal carcinoma at an interval of eight years or more. Her cancer was unrelated to the nipple-areolar complex and was not associated with persistent ND.[22]

Subsequently, 287 of the 416 (69%) patients were diagnosed to have pathological discharge and underwent image-guided diagnostic biopsies and/or surgical duct excision. A causative lesion was identified in 90% of these patients, of which 37% were either malignant or HRL. The authors of the study concluded that neither the clinical characteristics nor preoperative studies such as cytology, diagnostic imaging, or ductography could reliably distinguish between benign and malignant pathology. Surgical duct excision, therefore, was found to be the gold standard to exclude underlying malignancy in patients with pathological nipple discharge.[22]

Table 34-2 Stratification of nipple discharge based on clinical evaluation

ND characteristics	Clinically benign	Clinically suspicious
Duration	Self-limited	Persistent
Laterality	Bilateral	Unilateral
Color	Variable (milky, white, green, brown, black)	Bloody, clear, serosanguinous
Occurrence	Provoked	Spontaneous
Ductal involvement	Multiple ducts	Single duct
Clinical reproducibility	Usually absent	Usually present
Clinical breast exam	Normal	Normal/abnormal
Palpable mass	Absent	Sometimes present

Evaluating patients with nipple discharge

A clinical stratification can reliably distinguish patients with physiological nipple discharge who can be managed expectantly from those with pathological ND who need referral to a breast surgeon (see Table 34-2).

History

The history should include the age of the patient, number of pregnancies and lactation, duration of symptoms, color and laterality of discharge, whether the discharge is spontaneous or provoked, and sexual activity. Associated symptoms, such as palpable breast mass, weight gain or loss, staining of the brassiere (which could indicate an overlying skin infection or Paget's disease), recurrent headaches, visual field (pituitary involvement), and/or menstrual cycle irregularities (thyroid, pituitary disorders), should be noted. A high index of suspicion for cancer should be entertained in patients who are smokers or postmenopausal, or those who have persistent ND, a personal history of benign breast disease, or a strong family history of breast or ovarian cancer.

Physical examination

A clinical breast examination includes a careful palpation of the nipple-areolar complex. Special attention should be paid to any underlying masses, nipple retractions or overlying skin changes. An attempt should be made to express the discharge by applying pressure around the areola in a clockwise manner. The color of the discharge and whether it is expressed form a single or multiple ducts and one or both breasts should be noted. A Hemoccult card has a sensitivity for blood of about 50%). A bloody, serous or serosanguinous discharge originating spontaneously from a single duct is considered pathologic and should warrant a referral to the breast surgeon.

Based on the history and physical examination, the ND can be characterized as clinically benign (physiologic, pregnancy or lactation related, nonpuerperal galactorrhea, mammary duct ectasia) or clinically suspicious (pathologic) and subsequent management can be based on this stratification (see Table 34-2).

In cases where the differentiation is unclear, the patient need to be evaluated for a possible underlying malignancy. A diagnostic mammography and a subareolar ultrasonography should be obtained and the patient referred to a breast surgeon.

Cytology of ND has been shown to have a wide range of sensitivity (from 11% to 50%) and specificity ranging from 76% to 95%.[24] Use of duct cytology for the assessment of nipple discharge has been found to be of limited diagnostic value and is no longer advocated for initial evaluation of spontaneous nipple discharge.[25]

Ductography has been used as a diagnostic test in patients with single duct pathologic discharge. A filling defect usually indicates the presence of a tumor but does not help with differentiation of a benign from malignant lesion. Its use is therefore limited to identifying the precise location of intraductal lesions to aid with surgery.[26, 27]

The use of breast MRI for evaluation of ND is controversial and carries a high false positive rate. It is shown to be useful in evaluating patients with pathological ND who have equivocal mammographic or ultrasonographic findings.[28]

Although clinical stratification reliably identifies patients at risk for underlying pathology, nearly half of the patients diagnosed with cancer or HRL have a normal clinical breast exam and/or mammographic findings.[22] Bloody ND does not reliably predict the presence of an underlying malignancy; almost 55% of patients with malignant/HRL pathology have non-bloody ND by color alone.

Evaluation and management of clinically benign discharge

Once the ND is characterized as clinically benign, further investigation is based on patient and ND characteristics.

Physiologic discharge is usually patient reported, intermittent, nonmilky in color, scant in amount, and often not reproducible in the clinic. It is associated with excessive nipple stimulation or breast manipulation. If age- or risk-based screening mammography is up to date, no further investigation is indicated. The patient should be reassured and asked to avoid repeated nipple stimulation (including frequent checking for nipple discharge) and wear a supportive brassiere. A three- to six-month follow-up is recommended.

Nonpuerperal galactorrhea indicates a bilateral, milky white discharge seen in women who are not pregnant or lactating. Initial evaluation should include a pregnancy test. Once pregnancy is ruled out, the underlying cause for galactorrhea should be investigated. Common causes include use of medications that inhibit dopamine such as methyldopa, reserpine, verapamil, metoclopramide, oral contraceptives, and certain antipsychotics especially haloperidol. Other causes are thyroid disorders or hyperprolactinemia due to pituitary adenomas. Prolactin and thyroid-stimulating hormone levels should be obtained to screen for these disorders. A head MRI may be warranted in patients with unexplained significantly elevated prolactin levels to evaluate for pituitary tumors. Correction of underlying causes is usually adequate to treat galactorrhea.

Mammary duct ectasia (MDE) is a benign abnormality characterized by chronic inflammation and dilatation of the mammary duct.[29] It is usually seen in perimenopausal and menopausal women. The most common clinical presentation is a bilateral, multicolored nipple discharge. Colors range from yellow, green to brown, and black. The diagnosis is usually clinical if age-based screening mammography is up to date. Additional diagnostic imaging studies such as mammography and ultrasonography are reserved for patients who have additional findings such as alterations in the nipple-areolar complex (nipple retraction or distortion), palpable mass, or associated skin changes. Mammary duct ectasia usually resolves spontaneously after six to nine months and can be managed with close surveillance. In a validation study of 192 patients with pathologic nipple discharges who underwent further investigation and were diagnosed with MDE, the risk of carcinoma was 0%.[23] If the clinical presentation suggests pathological ND and/or mammographic findings are suggestive of malignancy, a duct excision is recommended.[20]

Any persistent or unresolved nipple discharge should be considered suspicious and further evaluation undertaken.

Evaluation of clinically suspicious or pathologic discharge

The initial evaluation of patients with pathologic ND should include a thorough clinical breast exam, diagnostic mammography, along with targeted ultrasonography of the nipple subareolar complex. Most of these patients will eventually need excisional biopsies.

Intraductal papilloma is the most common cause of pathological nipple discharge. It is a benign tumor of the major lactiferous ducts and is commonly observed in women 30–50 years of age. A solitary intraductal papilloma has not been shown to have a malignant potential. Intraductal papillomas can be multiple in approximately 10% of cases and are susceptible for malignant transformation. Initial evaluation is the same as for pathological ND and may include a ductography for appropriate visualization of the affected duct system. Diagnosis is based on biopsies, and treatment is surgical excision of the involved duct.[30]

High-risk lesions demonstrate proliferative change with atypical hyperplastic cells; they carry a 7- to 12-fold increased risk for developing breast cancer.[2] They are usually classified as atypical ductal hyperplasia or atypical lobular hyperplasia and usually present as palpable breast masses or pathological nipple discharge or are found incidentally on routine mammographic screening. Diagnosis is established by core needle biopsy, and treatment is surgical excision.

Other high-risk lesions that carry an increased risk for associated cancer are lobular carcinoma in situ, papillomatosis; and atypical papillomas; diagnosis and treatment as described earlier in the chapter.

Inflammatory disorders of the breast

Introduction

Mastitis is defined as an inflammatory condition of the breast that may or may not be associated with systemic signs of infection. It is usually unilateral and has the potential to develop into an abscess and rarely sepsis. Mastitis is typically seen in lactating women, but it can be a part of other processes such as skin-associated infections, chronic disease (e.g., diabetes, tuberculosis), autoimmune disorders (e.g., lupus), trauma, and rarely malignancy. Inflammatory carcinomatosis is an extremely aggressive form of breast cancer with poor prognosis and requires a high index of suspicion, early diagnosis, and treatment. A thorough history (including medical, surgical, family history) and review of systems for any systemic signs such as fever, chills, malaise, weight loss, nausea, or vomiting should be obtained by the clinician. Risk factors include cracked nipples, lactation, smoking, previous infections, nipple piercings, breast surgery, or trauma.[20] Any erythema, induration, fluctuancy, masses, drainage, and lymphadenopathy should be noted on CBE.

Lactational mastitis is discussed in Chapter 3.

Nonlactational mastitis

Breast infections in nonlactating women are commonly associated with superficial or deep parenchymal infections, and rarely associated with an underlying cancer, infectious disease, autoimmune vasculitis, or breast implants.

Infections of the nonlactating breasts can be categorized into central or subareolar infections and peripheral infections.[31] Infections are more commonly seen in women who smoke or have diabetes. These women are also more likely to experience recurrences and treatment failures.

Initial evaluation and management of nonlactational mastitis or abscess is similar to lactation-related breast infections. After an initial history and breast examination, a diagnostic ultrasonography and/or mammography or biopsy is obtained as indicated. The infection is treated with an antibiotic course for 10–14 days. In cases of recurrent fever or unresolved symptoms, an abscess should be suspected and treated with ultrasound-guided aspiration or surgical incision and drainage.[20] For unresolved inflammation, an evaluation for breast cancer is strongly recommended. Recurrences are common and require surgical excision of the involved duct or mass.

Granulomatous mastitis (GM) is a rare, benign inflammatory condition of the breast usually affecting women of childbearing age in the third or fourth decades.[32] GM can clinically mimic breast cancer and usually has an unclear pathogenesis and etiology. It has been associated with oral contraceptive use, immune mediated disorders, vasculitis such as polyarteritis nodusa, wegener's granulomatosis, systemic lupus erythematosus, and chronic granulomatous diseases such as tuberculosis.[32]

Clinical presentation can include presence of a breast mass with fixation to the underlying muscles or to the overlying skin, skin ulcerations, sinus tracts, and axillary lymphadenopathy.[38] It is usually unilateral and idiopathic.

Granulomatous mastitis can be mistaken for breast cancer. Radiologic findings on mammography can mimic malignancy, but ultrasonography can be useful to detect abscess. A combined modality is usually recommended. A breast biopsy is diagnostic.

Treatment is controversial and commonly involves wide local excision of the mass, antibiotic coverage for both aerobic and anaerobic bacteria, and a steroid course when infection has been ruled out.

Inflammatory carcinoma of the breast represents 1%– 5% of breast cancers.[33] It can clinically mimic an infectious process. It is an aggressive breast cancer with poor prognosis.

Inflammatory breast cancer should be considered in all women with unresolved inflammation or infection despite appropriate course of treatment. Initial evaluation with a diagnostic mammography and ultrasonography is recommended with breast biopsies based on clinical or radiological findings of suspicious lesions.

Mastalgia

Introduction

Mastalgia or breast pain is one of the most common breast symptoms reported by women.[20] It accounts for up to 66% of office visits for breast-related problems.[34, 35] Mastalgia is believed to be related to luteal phase hormonal variations of the menstrual cycle leading to an increase in the stromal water content.[35] Other more recent studies suggest that an increased sensitivity to hormones play a major role.[20] It is usually self-limited and benign. Approximately 10%–22% of patients have persistent pain that requires treatment.[36] Mastalgia can be confused with infection, malignancy, or other mammary conditions such as costochondritis, myocardial infarction or angina, pneumonia, pleuritis, esophageal spasm, rib fracture, shingles, and cervical radiculopathy. Figure 34-1 shows a flowchart demonstrating etiologies of breast pain.

Evaluating a patient with breast pain

History

A detailed history should elicit the duration, nature (cyclic versus noncyclic), location (focal or diffuse), radiation (to the axilla, shoulders, or dermatomes), aggravating or alleviating factors, lifestyle and diet (use of caffeine, fatty foods), exercise and any recent weight changes. Typically patients complain of breast pain that is cyclic, bilateral, and diffuse, occurring in the luteal phase only. Noncyclic pain is unrelated to the menstrual cycle and may be due to pregnancy, lactation, trauma, and medication or hormonal use (see Figure 34-2). A list of medications used by the patient including any nonprescription drugs should be documented. A history of trauma or surgery to the chest may be associated with fat necrosis.

Physical examination

The patient's posture, breast support, and bra marks on the skin should be carefully noted to evaluate for any musculoskeletal issues. The breasts should be examined for the presence of erythema or abscess (indicating an underlying infection, trauma, or malignancy) or a vesicular rash in a specific

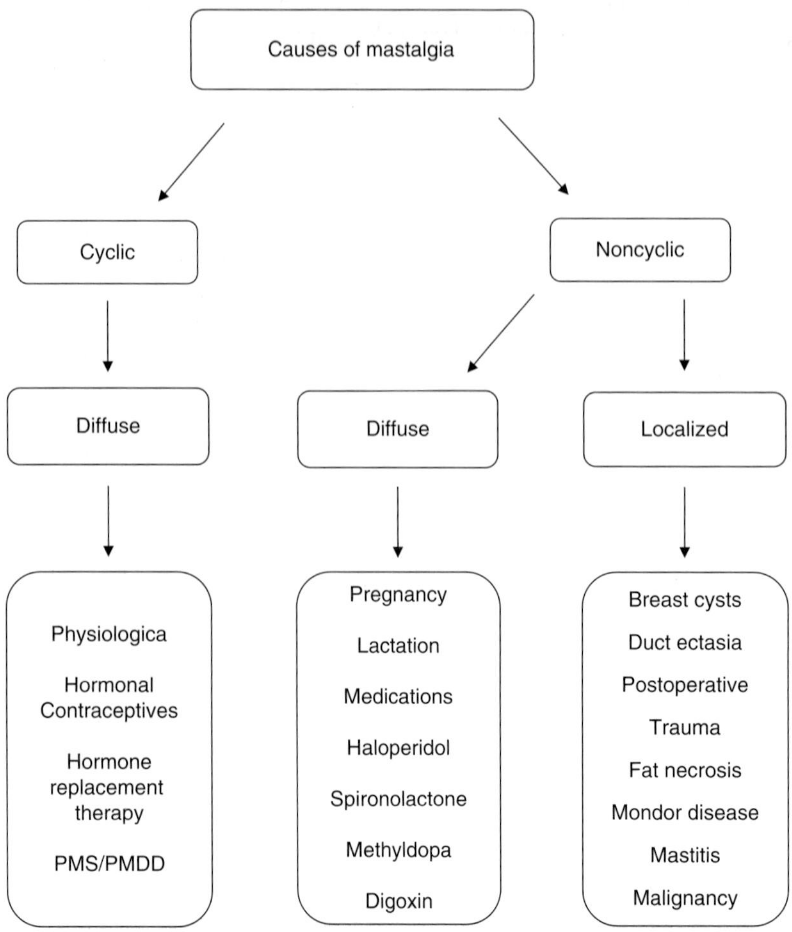

Figure 34-2 Flowchart demonstrating the possible etiologies of breast pain.

distribution (suggesting shingles). To evaluate the chest wall, the patient should be turned to her right or left side to displace her breast. The chest wall is then palpated by finger pads along the ribs and intercostal spaces going from the midaxillary line toward the midsternum.

Diagnostic test

Pregnancy, thyroid disorders, and prolactin disorders should be ruled out. Malignancy is an unlikely cause of mastalgia. If the clinical examination is normal and pain is cyclic and diffuse, no further testing is needed in low-risk women who are less than 30 years of age. Diagnostic mammography can be obtained in older women for reassurance and would be indicated in women older than 40.[20]

If the clinical examination is abnormal or if the pain is localized, an age-based diagnostic mammogram and/or targeted breast ultrasonography can be useful.[37] A breast biopsy is needed when diagnostic studies are insufficient, such as in fat necrosis. A core needle or excisional biopsy is indicated to rule out inflammatory breast carcinomatosis.

Treatment

Breast pain is persistent in 15% of patients and requires medical intervention (see Table 34-3). Most of the patients can be initially treated with reassurance, lifestyle modification, supportive measures, and analgesics. However, for patient with persistent breast pain, medications such as tamoxifen, bromocriptine, or danazol can provide much needed relief. These medications are associated with significant side effects that can be unacceptable to some patients. Pregnancy must be avoided with these medications. Low-dose tamoxifen has the least distressing effects and may be a first-line therapy.[38]

Evening primrose oil has been shown to be beneficial in some studies; however, a meta-analysis of randomized controlled trials comparing this with placebo failed to show a better outcome.[38]

Noncyclic breast pain is treated based on the underlying cause; most of these etiologies have been discussed in separate sections of this chapter. Pain associated with breast trauma or fat necrosis usually resolves without treatment and with

Table 34-3 Treatment measures for cyclic breast pain

First-line therapy, follow-up in 3–6 months
Reassurance
Lifestyle modifications: supportive underwire-free bra, exercise, low-fat intake, caffeine restriction, smoking cessation, vitamin E or multivitamin supplementation, daily pain score diary, heat or cold packs, cessation of exogenous hormones.
Nonsteroidal anti-inflammatory medications: Consider SSRI (luteal phase or continuous) in patients with symptoms of PMS or PMDD. Progesterone-only hormones may be effective in some premenopausal women.[39]
Second-line therapy, if pain persistent and debilitating
Tamoxifen[40] Dose: initiate at 10 mg daily for 3 months; if symptoms relapse continue for a total of 6 months Side effects: hot flashes, vaginal dryness, joint pain, leg cramps. Also increases risk for thromboembolic events, uterine cancer, and cataracts.
Danazol[38, 41] Dose: 200 mg once daily during luteal phase, only for 3 months Side effects: androgenic (nonreversible), lipid changes, hepatic impairment, intracranial hypertension, thromboembolic events
Bromocriptine[42] Dose: 2.5 mg twice daily for 3–6 months Side effects: significant cardiovascular and neurological effects limit use; high dropout rate in trials.
Goserelin (zoladex) has been shown to be effective in some trials[43].

supportive measures alone. *Mondor disease* is usually a result of trauma or surgery and is described as superficial thrombophlebitis of the anterior thoracoabdominal wall. It presents as tender, cordlike indurations palpated between the epigastric and axillary lesions. Diagnosis is confirmed by ultrasonography, and treatment is with anti-inflammatory medications.[20]

Concluding remarks

Physicians who care for women commonly see breast disorders. Although most complaints result from benign conditions, practitioners may miss serious health conditions if they fail to adequately evaluate breast concerns.

References

1. National Cancer Institute. Breast cancer risk in American women. Available at: www.cancer.gov/cancertopics/factsheet/detection/probability-breast-cancer. Accessed April 2014.
2. American Cancer Society. Breast cancer fact and figures 2013–2014. Available at: www.cancer.org/acs/groups/content/@research/documents/document/acspc-042725.pdf. Accessed April 2014.
3. ACOG. Hereditary breast and ovarian cancer syndrome. Practice Bulletin 103. Reaffirmed 2013.
4. Women's health initiative. Available at: www.nhlbi.nih.gov/whi. Accessed August 2014.
5. Santen RJ, Mansel R. Benign breast disorders. *N Engl J Med* 2005;**353**:275–285.
6. Swartz MH. The breast. In: *Textbook of Physical Diagnosis*, 7th edition. Philadelphia: Saunders, 2014: 409–438.
7. Gadd MA. Screening for breast cancer. In: Cameron JL, Cameron AM (eds). *Current Surgical Therapy: Expert Consult*, 11th edition. Philadelphia: Saunders, 2014: 568–571.
8. ACOG. Breast cancer screening. Practice Bulletin 122. August 2011.
9. Nelson AL. Controversies regarding mammography, breast self-examination and clinical breast examination. *Obstet Gynecol Clin N Am* 2013; **40**(3):413–427.
10. Gotzsche PC, Jorgensen KJ. Screening for breast cancer with mammography. *Cochrane Database Syst Rev* 2013 Jun 4;**6**:CD001877.
11. Grube BJ, Giuliano AE. Benign breast disease. In: Berek JS (ed). *Berek and Novak's Gynecology*, 14th edition. Philadelphia: Lippincott Williams & Wilkins, 2007: 637–668.
12. American College of Radiology. ACR Appropriateness Criteria. Clinical condition: palpable breast masses. Last review date: 2012. Available at: www.acr.org/~/media/ACR/Documents/AppCriteria/Diagnostic/PalpableBreastMasses.pdf. Accessed April 2014.
13. Winchester DP, Sener S, Immerman S, Blum M. A systematic approach to the evaluation and management of breast masses. *Cancer* 1983 June 15; **51**:2535–2539.
14. Green VL. Breast cancer risk assessment, prevention, and the future. *Obstet Gynecol Clin N Am* 2013; **40**:525–529.
15. Vargas HI, Vargas MP, Eldrageely K, et al. Outcomes of surgical and sonographic assessment of breast masses in women younger than 30. *Am Surg* 2005 Sep;**71**(9):716–719.
16. Fallat ME, Ignacio RC. Breast disorders in children and adolescents. *J Pediatr Adolesc Gynecol* 2008;**21**:311–316.
17. Bassett LW, Jackson VP, Fu KL, Fu YS. *Diagnosis of Diseases of the Breast*, 2nd edition. St. Louis: WB Saunders, 1997: 424.
18. Smallwood JA, Roberts A, Guyer PD, Taylor I. The natural history of fibroadenoma. *Br J Clinic Prac* 1988;**56**(Suppl):86–87.
19. Kaufman. CS, Littrup PJ, Freeman-Gibb LA, et al. Office-based cryoablation of breast fibroadenomas with long-term follow-up. *Breast Journal* 2005;**11** (5):344–350.
20. Onstad M, Stuckey A. Benign breast disorders. *Obstet Gynecol Clin N Am* 2013 Sep;**40**(3):459–473.
21. Chang HL, Lerwill MF, Goldstein AM. Breast hamartomas in adolescent females. *Breast Journal* 2009;**15**(5):515–520.
22. Morrogh M, Park A, Elkin EB, King TA. Lessons learned from 416 cases of nipple discharge of the breast. *Am Journ of Surg* 2010;**200**:73–80.
23. Ashfaq A, Senior D, Pockaj BA, et al. Validation study of a modern treatment algorithm for nipple discharge. *Am Journ of Surg*. Published online April 3, 2014. DOI: http://dx.doi.org/10.1016/j.amsurg.2013.12.035.
24. Moriarity AT, Schwartz MR, Laucirica R, et al. Cytology of spontaneous nipple discharge: Is it worth it? *Arch Pathol Lab Med* 2013 Aug;**137**(8):1039–1042.
25. Dolan RT, Butler JS, Kell MR, et al. Nipple discharge and the efficacy of duct cytology in evaluating breast cancer risk. *The Surgeon* 2010;**8**(5):252–258.
26. Sickles EA. Galactography and other imaging investigations of nipple discharge. *Lancet* 2000;**356**:1622–1623.
27. Paterok EM, Rosenthal H, Sabel M. Nipple discharge and abnormal galactogram: results of a long-term study (1964–1990). *European Jour of Obstet & Gynecol & Reproduce boil* 1993;**50**:227–234.

28. Orel SG, Dougherty CS, Reynolds C, et al. MRI imaging in patients with nipple discharge: initial experience. *Radiology* 2000;**216**(1):248–254.
29. Rahal RM, de Freitas-Júnior R, Carlos da Cunha L, et al. Mammary duct ectasia: an overview. *Breast J* 2011 Nov–Dec;**17**(6):694–695.
30. Al Sarakbi W, Worku D, Escobar PF, Mokbel K. Breast papillomas: current management with a focus on a new diagnostic and therapeutic modality. *Int Semin Surg Oncol* 2006;**3**(1):1.
31. Dixon JM, Khan LR. Treatment of breast infections. *BMJ* 2011;**342**:d396.
32. Ocal K, Dag A, Turkmenoglu O, et al. Granulomatous mastitis: clinical, pathological features and management. *Breast J* 2010 Mar–Apr;**16**(2):176–182.
33. Boutet G. Breast inflammation: clinical examination, aetiological pointer. *Diagnostic and Interventional Imaging* 2012;**93**:78–84.
34. National Program of Cancer Registries. US cancer stats; 1999–2007. Cancer incidence and mortality data. www.nccd.cdc.gov. Accessed April 2014.
35. Euhus DM. Breast disease, In: Hoffman BL, Schorge JO, Schaffer JI, et al. (eds). *Williams Gynecology*, 2nd edition. New York: McGraw-Hill, 2012:333–355.
36. Salzman B, Fleegle S, Tully A. Common breast problems. *Am Fam Physicians* 2012;**86**(4):343–349.
37. Leung JW, Kornguth PJ, Gollway MB. Utility of targeted sonography in the evaluation of focal breast pain. *J Ultrasound Med* 2002;**21**(5):521–526.
38. Srivastava A, Mansel RE, Arvind N, et al. Evidence-based management of mastalgia: a metaanalysis of RCTs. *Breast* 2007;**16**:503–512.
39. Euhus DM, Uyehara C. Influence of parenteral progesterones on the prevalence and severity of mastalgia in premenopausal women; a multi-institutional cross-sectional study. *J AM Coll Surg* 1997;**184**(6):596.
40. Fentiman IS, Caleffi M, Hamed H, Chaudary MA. Dosage and duration of tamoxifen treatment for mastalgia: a controlled trial. *Br J Surg* 1988;**75**(9):845–846.
41. O'Brien PM, Abukhalil IE. RCT of the management of PMS and premenstrual mastalgia using luteal phase only danazol. *Am J Obstet Gynecol* 1999;**180**:18–23.
42. Mansel RE, Preece PE, Hughes LE. A double blind trial of the prolactin inhibitor bromocriptine in painful benign breast. *Br J Surg* 1978;**65**(10):724–727.
43. Mansel RE, Goyal A, Preece P, et al. European randomized, multicentre study of goesrelin (zoladex) in the management of mastalgia. *Am J Obstet Gynecol* 2004;**191**(6):1942–1949.

Chapter 35

Urinary tract infections

Jeffrey D. Quinlan

Introduction

Urinary tract infection (UTI) is the most common type of infection in women. Recent estimates indicate that evaluation and treatment of urinary tract infections result in $1.6 billion in direct costs annually in the United States. The most common infectious agent associated with UTIs is *Escherichia coli*. Risk factors include sexual activity, spermicide use, prior UTI, urinary obstruction, and congenital anomalies of the urinary tract. In women with typical symptoms, empiric treatment may be initiated without the need for an office visit or laboratory evaluation. Nitrofurantoin, trimethoprim-sulfamethoxazole, fluoroquinolones, and β-lactams have been shown to be effective in the treatment of UTIs. Prophylaxis should be considered in women with recurrent infections. Special considerations should be given to pregnant women, postmenopausal women, and women with diabetes mellitus or indwelling catheters who develop UTIs.

Scope of the problem

Urinary tract infections are important in women's health because they are the most common bacterial infection.[1] Review of the 2009–2010 combined data of the National Ambulatory Medical Care Survey (NAMCS) and the National Hospital Ambulatory Medical Care Survey (NHAMCS) estimates that UTIs account for an estimated 5.4 million primary care office visits annually and another 2.3 million emergency room visits annually.[2] Although most patients with UTIs are treated as outpatients, 16.7%, or approximately 110,000 annually, require hospitalization.[3] Recent estimates are that evaluation and treatment of UTIs result in $1.6 billion in direct costs annually in the United States.[3]

Definitions

"Bacteriuria" is defined as the presence of 10^5 colony-forming units of bacteria per milliliter of urine collected from midstream urine on two consecutive urinations.[4] When a patient has bacteriuria but no associated symptoms, she is diagnosed with asymptomatic bacteriuria. This is particularly important in pregnant patients and will be discussed in detail later in the chapter.

Symptomatic infection of the urinary tract is a UTI and may involve the urethra, bladder, ureters, and/or kidneys.[5] Infections of the lower tract (bladder and urethra) are commonly referred to as cystitis; whereas, infections of the upper tract (kidney and ureters) are referred to as pyelonephritis.

The vast majority of UTIs are uncomplicated and do not progress to more serious infections; these are referred to as uncomplicated UTIs. On the other hand, patients who are pregnant, have chronic medical conditions (e.g., diabetes, neurogenic bladder, immunosuppression, or renal insufficiency), urinary obstruction, or calculi and who present with UTIs are considered to have complicated UTIs.[6] As seen later in the chapter, UTIs in these patients have implications for both length of treatment and empirical antibiotic treatment choice.

A final important differentiation is between recurrent and resistant UTIs. Resistant UTIs are those that fail to demonstrate resolution of bacteriuria following 7–14 days of appropriate antibiotic treatment.[7] Recurrent UTIs are defined as a subsequent UTI following successful treatment of an initial UTI in a six-month period of time or at least three UTIs within a year.[5]

Pathophysiology

Urinary tract pathogens reside as normal flora in the bowel. Prior to the development of a UTI, these

Office Care of Women, ed. Martin E. Olsen and Botros Rizk. Published by Cambridge University Press.

bacteria colonize the vagina and/or urethra. The bacteria may subsequently spread to the urethra and then ascend to the bladder. Men are thus less likely than women to develop UTIs. The distance between the anus and the opening of the urethra is significantly greater in men. The tissue surrounding the opening of the urethra is dry in men; the moist environment in women facilitates both bacterial migration and growth. Moreover, the urethra is longer in men than in women.[8]

Vaginal colonization appears to be an important step in the development of UTI in most women. Colonization is more likely in women with changes in the normal vaginal flora and specifically lactobacilli.[9] Additionally, in some women pathologic bacteria are able to adhere more readily to the vaginal mucosa. Research has demonstrated that these women are more likely to develop recurrent UTIs.[10]

Once bacteria have entered the bladder, the organisms must adhere to the epithelium of the bladder. In pathogenic bacteria, particularly *E. coli*, adhesive organelles called Type 1 pili have a terminal molecule, FimH, which binds to the uroepithelium.[11] The bacteria can then invade the epithelial cells and begin to replicate, ultimately forming biofilms.[12] These biofilms are able to resist the host defenses of white blood cell influx and shedding of the bladder epithelium.[12]

The virulence of the uropathogenic bacteria is enhanced by the presence of a variety of structural components that assist in decreasing the effectiveness of the body's immune and inflammatory responses. These include the presence of fimbria, flagella, a polysaccharide coating, adhesins such as FimH, and siderophores.[13]

Proteus mirabilis produces a urease that converts urea to ammonia and leads to precipitation of struvite and apatite crystals around the bacteria. These crystals provide a defense for *P. mirabilis* against antibiotics and can serve as a nidus for growth of other bacteria as well. Therefore, in patients with known calculi and symptoms of UTI, *P. mirabilis* infection should be strongly considered even if the culture does not grow out the species. Likewise, when urinary cultures grow *Proteus*, the patient should be evaluated for the presence of urinary calculi.[14]

Epidemiology/risk factors

Urinary tract infections are more common in women than men, with NAMCS and NHAMCS data demonstrating that 84% occur in women.[3] Furthermore, the infections occur with increased frequency in sexually active women.[15] In women over the age of 18, 10.8% report at least one UTI annually, and it is estimated that by age 24, one in three women will have at least one UTI requiring treatment.[16] Over the course of their lifetimes, women have an approximately 60% risk of having at least one UTI.[16]

Both modifiable and nonmodifiable factors have been associated with an increased risk of recurrent UTI. Several studies have demonstrated that specific blood group phenotypes (Lewis nonsecretors in particular) have higher rates of UTI secondary to increased adherence of bacteria to the epithelial cells.[17] Additionally, other nonmodifiable risk factors include a prior history of UTI, urinary obstruction, and congenital anomalies of the urinary tract.[15, 18] Furthermore, at least one study identified an increased risk of UTI in women whose mother had a history of UTI.[19]

Modifiable risk factors include those related to contraceptive use (spermicides, spermicide-coated condoms, and oral contraceptives) and those related to frequency of intercourse (≥4 times/month).[19] Spermicides increase the risk for UTI by allowing increased growth of *E. coli* following alteration of normal vaginal flora.[20] A study of sexually active college women demonstrated that compared to women who had not had intercourse during the week, women who had had intercourse three times had a 2.6-fold increase in relative risk whereas women who had daily intercourse had a ninefold increase in relative risk of UTI development.[21] Data suggests that this increase in risk is related to both trauma to the urethra and the mechanical introduction of bacteria into the urethra.[22, 23]

Research has failed to show a relationship between voiding habits, personal hygiene practices, and beverage consumption and recurrent UTIs.[19]

History

Patients with uncomplicated lower tract UTIs will frequently describe dysuria (difficulty and/or pain with urination), frequency (decreased latency between episodes of urination often associated with small volumes of urination), and/or urgency (sensation that one has to urinate immediately). They may also report hematuria, pyuria, and suprapubic discomfort or pain. Patients with upper tract infections, in addition to the symptoms just mentioned, may report nausea, vomiting, fevers, chills, and flank pain.

Although dysuria is common in women with UTIs, it can also be seen in women with urethritis and vaginitis. Differentiation of the three potential etiologies may be possible based on concomitant symptoms and timeline of symptom development. UTIs are commonly associated with pyuria and hematuria, but only pyuria is seen in urethritis, and neither is typically seen in vaginitis. Symptoms in UTI are typically acute in onset and severe in nature, whereas symptoms in urethritis and vaginitis tend to be more gradual in onset and milder in nature. Furthermore, vaginitis is often associated with vaginal discharge, odor, and pruritus not seen in UTI or urethritis.[24]

History of previous UTI is important to assess, as is a history of any complicated UTI.

Medical and surgical history should focus on factors that would increase the risk of UTI in general and also complicated UTI. Such factors include pregnancy, diabetes, neurogenic bladder, immunosuppression, renal insufficiency, urinary obstruction, or history of calculi. A history of urogenital surgeries should be obtained.

Physical exam

In general, physical examination is not diagnostic in the evaluation of UTI. It may be useful in differentiating lower tract infections from upper tract infections as both fever and costovertebral angle tenderness are more consistent with upper tract infections.[25] Additionally, in patients with vague or unclear symptoms, pelvic examination may reveal a vaginal source of symptoms instead of a urinary source.

Laboratory

Urinalysis and urine culture are the gold standards of UTI diagnosis. Typically, women are instructed to provide a midstream urine sample for evaluation after cleansing the perineum with a bacterial wash and while spreading the labia to prevent contamination. The use of these three techniques in the collection of the urine is designed to minimize the risk of contamination of the sample with skin flora. One randomized controlled trial (RCT) has called these techniques into question demonstrating similar contamination rates (29% and 32%, respectively) in women who provided a nonmidstream urine sample without cleansing versus women who provided properly collected midstream urine.[26]

Urinalysis can confirm the presence of bacteriuria and pyuria in patients with UTI symptoms. Pyuria is commonly defined as the presence of 10 or more leukocytes per high-powered field when examining an unspun urine.[27] As noted earlier, bacteriuria is the presence of $>10^5$ colony-forming units of bacteria per milliliter of urine.[4]

Urinalysis is frequently carried out with a dipstick instead of a microscope. Urine dipsticks evaluate for a combination of factors present in the urine including nitrite, leukocyte esterase, protein, glucose, ketones, hemoglobin, bilirubin, urobilinogen, acetone, pH, and specific gravity. A meta-analysis of studies looking at the sensitivity and specificity of the components of a urine dipstick used to diagnose UTI found that either a positive nitrite or leukocyte esterase are associated with a sensitivity of 75% and a specificity of 82%.[28] Individual studies have demonstrated sensitivities of 75%–96% and specificities of 94%–98% with a positive leukocyte esterase.[29]

Urine culture should be considered in all women who have symptoms consistent with pyelonephritis, women with both UTI symptoms and vaginal discharge, women with recurrent UTIs, and women with a history of resistant UTIs.[6, 30, 31]

Additionally, in patients with symptoms consistent with pyelonephritis or with comorbid conditions which increase the risk of sepsis (e.g., diabetes mellitus), blood cultures should be obtained.[32]

Microbiology

Between 70% and 95% of uncomplicated UTIs are a result of *Escherichia coli* infection and 5%–20% as a result of *Staphylococcus saprophyticus*. Small numbers have been associated with *Klebsiella*, *Enterococcus faecalis*, and *Proteus mirabilis*.[29] The organisms associated with complicated UTIs are similar to *E. coli*, continuing to account for the vast majority of infections. Additionally, *Enterococci*, coagulase negative staphylococci, *Serratia* and *Providencia stuartii* have been associated with complicated UTIs.[33] Table 35-1 summarizes bacteria commonly associated with UTIs.

Radiology

The vast majority of UTIs do not require any form of radiologic imaging. If there is a concern about possible urocalculi, obstruction, or anatomic anomaly, imaging may be helpful. Although plain films can be useful in identifying a radiopaque stone, ultrasound, computerized tomography (CT), and magnetic resonance imaging (MRI) offer the ability to identify anatomic anomaly, hydronephrosis, abscess, and stones.

Table 35-1 Common bacterial pathogens in UTIs

Uncomplicated UTI	Percentage	Complicated UTI	Percentage
Escherichia coli	70–90	*Escherichia coli*	21–54
Staphylococcus saprophyticus	5–20	*Proteus mirabilis*	1–10
Klebsiella	1–2	*Enterococci*	1–23
Proteus mirabilis	1–2	*Klebsiella*	2–17
Enterococcus faecalis	1–2	*Pseudomonas aeruginosa*	2–19
Citrobacter		*Enterobacter*	2–10
Group B *Streptococcus*		*Staphylococcus aureus*	1–2
Staphylococcus aureus		Coagulase-negative staphylococci	1–4
		Providencia stuartii	
		Serratia	

Source: Adapted from references 29, 33, 38.

Table 35-2 Indications for radiologic evaluation in UTIs

On initial presentation:

- Recurrent infections
- Severe symptoms/concern for pyonephrosis
- Unclear diagnosis
- Concern for other diseases (stone, infarct, etc.)
- Immunocompromised
- Diabetes mellitus

After initial treatment:

- Failure of standard treatment (no clinical improvement in >72 hours)

Source: Adapted from reference 34.

[34] Indications for imaging our summarized in Table 35-2.

Treatment

Strategy

Recently, clinical practice guidelines have evaluated the need for physical and laboratory evaluation in the treatment of uncomplicated UTIs. These guidelines are based on evidence that history alone can be highly sensitive in the diagnosis of UTI, a low threshold for treating UTIs, and a desire to introduce cost-effective evaluation and treatment. Studies have demonstrated 67%–77% of women with dysuria and frequency and without vaginal discharge had cystitis compared to 4%–14% of women who had vaginal discharge without dysuria and frequency.[35] As a result, in patients with typical symptoms and without comorbid conditions (e.g., diabetes mellitus) or risk for complicated UTI, empiric treatment with antibiotics is appropriate.[36] In these patients, cost savings can be realized by avoiding both an office visit and associated laboratory evaluation.[36]

A recent systematic review, however, has noted the increasing rate of antibiotic resistance in typical infecting organisms, and called this approach into question. It recommended that all women with UTIs should have urine cultures performed prior to initiation of antibiotics. Antibiotic regimens would then be based on the results of the urine culture to ensure sensitivity to treatment.[37] In many cases, this would necessitate an office visit as well.

Providers should be aware of local antibiotic resistance patterns and base their strategy for the evaluation and management of UTIs on resistance rates in their community. In communities with low rates of resistance, the former strategy may remain appropriate; however, in communities with higher rates of resistance, the latter should be considered.

Cystitis

The 2010 Infectious Diseases Society of America (IDSA) and European Society of Microbiology and Infectious Diseases (ESMID) jointly developed

Table 35-3 Antibiotics for the treatment of uncomplicated UTIs

Antibiotic	Dosage	Duration	Notes
Nitrofurantoin	100 mg twice daily	5 days	
Trimethoprim-sulfamethoxazole	160/800 mg twice daily	3 days	Not recommended as first-line treatment if local resistence if ≥20%
Fosfomycin trometamol	3 gm as single dose	1 day	
Pivmecillinam	400 mg twice daily	3–7 days	Not available in the United States
Fluoroquinolones Ofloxacin Ciprofloxacin Levofloxacin	200 mg–400 mg twice daily 250 mg twice daily 250 mg daily	3 days	Should be used as an alternative
β-lactams Amoxicillin-clavulanate Cefdinir Cefaclor Cefpodoxime-proxetil	500/125 mg twice daily 300 mg twice daily 250 mg three times daily 100 mg twice daily	3–7 days	Tend to have more side effects and be less efficacious than other β-lactams.

Source: Adapted from reference 31.

clinical practice guidelines for the treatment of acute uncomplicated cystitis, summarized in Table 35-3.[31] As a result of both increased bacterial resistance and poor clinical efficacy, neither amoxicillin nor ampicillin is recommended as first-line or alternative antibiotics in the treatment of uncomplicated UTI.[31] Additionally, given the increasing rate of resistance to trimethoprim-sulfamethoxazole, it should not be used as first-line therapy if local rates of resistance are greater than 20%.[31]

In patients with complicated cystitis, a seven-day course of antibiotics is typically recommended; a 10–14 day course of treatment is recommended for patients with upper tract disease or more severe symptoms.[33]

Pyelonephritis

Table 35-4 summarizes the 2010 IDSA and ESMID jointly developed clinical practice guidelines for the treatment of acute uncomplicated pyelonephritis.[31] In women who can tolerate oral antibiotics and do not require hospitalization for other reasons, oral fluoroquinolones may be used empirically while urine culture results are pending.[31] Initial one-time intravenous antibiotic treatment with ciprofloxacin 400 mg, ceftriazone 1 gm, or a consolidated 24-hour dose of an aminoglycoside antibiotic may precede oral dosing if local rates of antibiotic resistance exceed 10%.[31]

In women who require hospitalization, intravenous antibiotics should be initiated. Appropriate options include fluoroquinolones, aminoglycosides (with or without ampicillin), extended-spectrum cephalosporins, extended-spectrum penicillins, and carbapenem. Local antibiotic resistance rates and susceptibility as determined by urine culture should be utilized to determine which antibiotic to choose.[31] Patients may be transitioned to oral antibiotics once they are tolerating oral fluids.

Prevention

Antibiotic prophylaxis has been demonstrated to decrease the rate of recurrent UTI by 95%.[38] It has been recommended for women who have had two or more UTIs in the past six months or three or more UTIs in the past year.[38, 39] Both low-dose continuous antibiotic prophylaxis and postcoital antibiotic prophylaxis have been demonstrated to be effective strategies for the prevention of recurrent UTI.

Low-dose antibiotic prophylaxis can be initiated after demonstration of resolution of the most recent UTI via a negative urine culture obtained one to two weeks following treatment. The choice of antibiotic should be based on both the patient's allergies and previous culture results. Typical antibiotics include trimethoprim, trimethoprim-sulfamethoxazole, or nitrofurantoin.[40] A Cochrane review failed to

Table 35-4 Antibiotics for the treatment of uncomplicated pyelonephritis

Antibiotic	Dosage	Duration	Notes
Ciprofloxacin	500 mg twice daily orally 1,000 mg extended release once daily	7 days	Initial one-time intravenous antibiotic may precede oral dosing.* Recommended if rates of resistance exceed 10%.
Levofloxacin	750 mg once daily	5 days	Initial one-time intravenous antibiotic may precede oral dosing.* Recommended if rates of resistance exceed 10%.
Trimethoprim-sulfamethoxazole	160/800 mg twice daily	14 days	Only if susceptibility to agent is known. Initial one-time intravenous antibiotic should precede oral dosing if susceptibility is unknown.*

* Ciprofloxacin 400 mg, ceftriazone 1 gm, or consolidated 24-hour dose of an aminoglycoside antibiotic.
Source: Adapted from reference 31.

demonstrate a best antibiotic or an optimal duration of treatment;[41] however 6–24 months of treatment is typically recommended.[38]

In women whose UTIs are related to sexual activity, a single postcoital dose of antibiotics may be as effective as daily low-dose antibiotic prophylaxis.[42] Studies have demonstrated that single doses of trimethoprim-sulfamethoxazole, nitrofurantoin, cephalexin, and fluoroquinolones are comparable in their ability to decrease rate of recurrence.[43, 44]

Several nonpharmacologic prophylaxis strategies have been suggested including the use of cranberry and probiotics such as lactobacillis. A Cochrane review found some evidence for cranberry's effectiveness in young women with recurrent UTIs.[45] Studies examining the use of lactobacilli to colonize the vaginal flora have found mixed results.[46]

Special considerations

Pregnancy

Approximately 10% of women are diagnosed with asymptomatic bacteriuria during pregnancy.[47] Asymptomatic bacteriuria can have serious health effects for both the mother and the fetus. Women with asymptomatic bacteriuria are 15 to 20 times more likely to develop pyelonephritis during pregnancy than pregnant women without asymptomatic bacteriuria.[48] Additionally, their babies are more likely to be born prematurely and have low birth weights.[48] Women who receive antibiotic treatment for their asymptomatic bacteriuria during pregnancy significantly reduce their rate of developing pyelonephritis (20%–35% incidence without treatment and 1%–4% incidence with treatment).[49] Likewise, studies have shown that treatment with antibiotics in these patients decreases the rate of both preterm birth and low birth weight infants.[50]

Special caution should be used to avoid use of teratogenic antibiotics during pregnancy. Penicillins, cephalosporins, and nitrofurantoin are safe throughout pregnancy. Fluoroquinolones are known to affect cartilage development and trimethoprim-sulfamethoxazole may reduce folate levels in the developing fetus and lead to birth defects if used in the first trimester. Additionally, it has been associated with neonatal hyperbilirubinemia when used in the third trimester.

Postmenopausal women

Risk factors for UTIs in postmenopausal women include catheterization, declining functional status, atrophic vaginitis, incontinence, incomplete voiding, cystocele, and history of UTI prior to menopause.[8] Additionally, decreased estrogen and resulting vaginal atrophy appear to be associated with increased rates of UTI in these women. There is some evidence that intravaginal estrogen replacement can decrease the rate of UTI in postmenopausal women.[8] Treatment for UTI in postmenopausal women is similar to that of premenopausal women. Short duration treatment (two or three days) has been demonstrated to be as effective as longer duration treatment (seven days) and is better tolerated.[51]

Diabetes mellitus

The incidence of both asymptomatic bacteriuria and UTI in women with diabetes mellitus is higher than in women without diabetes.[33] Additionally, women with diabetes are more likely to have UTIs complicated by bacteremia, abscess, papillary necrosis, and emphysematous or xanthogranulomatous pyelonephritis.[8, 33] As with all patients with complicated UTIs, cystitis should be treated for seven days, and pyelonephritis or severe symptoms should be treated for 10–14 days.[33]

Women with indwelling catheters

The most common nosocomial infection is catheter-acquired UTI. In patients with long-term catheters (>30 days), the prevalence of UTI is 100%. In addition to a seven-day course of antibiotics, catheter change is recommended for these patients when they have a UTI. Prophylaxis is not recommended in patients with indwelling catheters as it promotes antibiotic resistance and subsequent infection with resistant bacteria.[33]

Concluding remarks

Urinary tract infections are a common problem in women resulting in significant morbidity for women and financial burden on the health-care system. Appropriate use of office visits and laboratory evaluation, as well as antibiotic prophylaxis in women with recurrent UTIs as described in this chapter may decrease that burden. Providers must understand local antibiotic resistance patterns in order to select appropriate therapy. Special caution should be used in the treatment of pregnant and postmenopausal women as well as those with diabetes or indwelling catheters.

References

1. Nicolle LE. Epidemiology of urinary tract infections. *Infect Med* 2001; **18**:153–62.
2. http://www.cdc.gov/nchs/data/ahcd/combined_tables/192009-2010_combined_web_table01.pdf. Accessed December 12, 2014.
3. Sammon JD, Sharma P, Rahbar H, et al. Predictors of admission in patients presenting to the emergency department with urinary tract infection. *World J Urol* 2014; **32**:813–9.
4. Nicolle LE, Bradley S, Colgan R, et al. Infectious Diseases Society of America guidelines for the diagnosis and treatment of asymptomatic bacteriuria in adults. *Clin Infect Dis* 2005; **40**(5):643–54.
5. Barber AE, Norton JP, Spivak AM, et al. Urinary tract infections: current and emerging management strategies. *Clin Infect Dis* 2013; **57**(5):719–24.
6. Hooton TM. Clinical practice. Uncomplicated urinary tract infection. *N Engl J Med* 2012; **366**(11):1028–37.
7. Nossier SB, Lind LR, Winkler HA. Recurrent uncomplicated urinary tract infections in women: a review. *J Womens Health* 2012; **21**(3):347–54.
8. Hooton TM. Pathogenesis of urinary tract infections: an update. *J Antimicrob Chemother* 2000; **46**:1–7.
9. Hooton TM, Stamm WE. The vaginal flora and UTIs. In: Mobley HLT & Warren JW, eds. *Urinary Tract Infections: Molecular Pathogenesis and Clinical Management.* Washington, DC: ASM Press; 1996: 67–94.
10. Fowler JE, Stamey TA. Studies of introital colonization in women with recurrent urinary infections. VII. The role of bacterial adherence. *J Urol* 1977; **117**:472–6.
11. Mulvey MA, Lopez-Boado YS, Wilson CL, et al. Induction and evasion of host defences by type 1-piliated uropathogenic Escherichia coli. *Science* 1998; **282**:1494–7.
12. Anderson GG, Palermo JJ, Schilling JD, et al. Intracellular bacterial biofilm-like pods in urinary tract infections. *Science* 2003; **301**:105–7.
13. Johnson JR. Microbial virulence determinants and the pathogenesis of urinary tract infection. *Infect Dis Clin North Am* 2003; **17**:261–78.
14. Holmgren K. Urinary calculi and urinary tract infection: a clinical and microbiological study. *Scand J Urol Nephrol Suppl* 1986; **98**:1–71.
15. Foxman B, Gillespie B, Koopman J, et al. Risk factors for second urinary tract infection among college women. *Am J Epidemiol* 2000; **151**:1194–1205.
16. Foxman B, Barlow R, d'Arcy H, et al. Urinary tract infection: self-reported incidence and associated costs. *Ann Epidemiol* 2000; **10**:509–15.
17. Sheinfeld J, Schaeffer AJ, Cordon-Cardo C, et al. Association of the Lewis blood group phenotype with recurrent urinary tract infections in women. *N Engl J Med* 1989; **320**:773–7.
18. Twaij M. Urinary tract infection in children: a review of its pathogenesis and risk factors. *J R Soc Health* 2000; **120**:220–6.
19. Scholes D, Hooton TM, Roberts DL, et al. Risk factors for recurrent urinary tract infection in young women. *J Infect Dis* 2000; **182**:1177–82.
20. Hooton TM, Fennell CL, Clark AM, Stamm WE. Nonoxynol-9: differential antibacterial activity and enhancement of bacterial adherence to vaginal epithelial cells. *J Infect Dis* 1991; **164**(6):1216–19.
21. Hooton TM, Scholes D, Hughes JP, et al. A prospective study of risk factors for symptomatic urinary tract infection in young women. *New Eng J Med* 1996; **335**:468–74.

22. Hooton TM, Hillier S, Johnson C, et al. *Escherichia coli* bacteriuria and contraceptive method. *JAMA* 1991; **265**:64–9.
23. Foxman B, Marsh J, Gillespie B, et al. Condom use and first-time urinary tract infection. *Epidemiology* 1997; **8**:637–41.
24. Stamm WE, Hooton TM. Management of urinary tract infections in adults. *N Engl J Med* 1993; **329**:1328–34.
25. Bent S, Saint S. The optimal use of diagnostic testing in women with acute uncomplicated cystitis. *Dis Mon* 2003; **49**:83–98.
26. Lifshitz E, Kramer L. Outpatient urine collection: does collection technique matter? *Arch Intern Med* 2000; **160**:2537–40.
27. Stamm WE. Measurement of pyuria and its relation to bacteriuria. *Am J Med* 1983; **75**:53–8.
28. Hurlbut TA III, Littenberg B. The diagnostic accuracy of rapid dipstick tests to predict urinary tract infection. *Am J Clin Pathol* 1991; **96**:582–8.
29. Hooton TM, Stamm WE. Diagnosis and treatment of uncomplicated urinary tract infection. *Infect Dis Clin North Am* 1997; **11**:551–81.
30. Nosseir SB, Lind LR, Winkler HA. Recurrent uncomplicated urinary tract infections in women: a review. *J Womens Health* 2012; **21**(3):347–54.
31. Gupta K, Hooton TM, Naber KG, et al. International clinical practice guidelines for the treatment of acute uncomplicated cystitis and pyelonephritis in women: a 2010 update by the Infectious Diseases Society of America and the European Society of Microbiology and Infectious Diseases. *Clin Infect Dis* 2011; **52**:e103–20.
32. Franco AV. Recurrent urinary tract infections. *Best Pract Res Clin Obstet Gynaecol* 2005; **19**(6):861–73.
33. Nicolle LE. A practical guide to antimicrobial management of complicated urinary tract infection. *Drugs & Aging* 2001; **18**(4):243–54.
34. Browne RFJ, Zwirewich C, Torreggiani WC. Imaging of urinary tract infection in the adult. *Eur Radiol* 2004; **14**:E168–83.
35. Berg AO, Heidrich FE, Fihn SD, et al. Establishing the cause of genitourinary symptoms in women in a family practice: comparison of clinical examination and comprehensive microbiology. *JAMA* 1984; **251**:620–5.
36. Bent S, Saint S. The optimal use of diagnostic testing in women with acute uncomplicated cystitis. *Am J Med* 2002; **113**(1A):20S–28S.
37. Schmiemann G, Kniehl E, Gebhardt K, et al. The diagnosis of urinary tract infection, a systematic review. *Dtsch Arztebl Int* 2010; **107**(21):361–7.
38. Nicolle LE, Ronald AR. Recurrent urinary tract infection in adult women: diagnosis and treatment. *Infect Dis Clin North Am* 1987; **1**:793–806.
39. Ronald AR, Conway B. An approach to urinary tract infections in ambulatory women. *Curr Clin Top Infect Dis* 1988; **9**:76–125.
40. McLaughlin SP, Carson CC. Urinary tract infections in women. *Med Clin North Am* 2004; **88**:417–429.
41. Albert X, Huertas I, Pereiro II, et al. Antibiotics for preventing recurrent urinary tract infection in non-pregnant women. *Cochrane Database Syst Rev* 2004; **3**:CD001209.
42. Melekos MD, Asbach HW, Gerharz E, et al. Post-intercourse versus daily ciprofloxacin prophylaxis for recurrent urinary tract infections in premenopausal women. *J Urol* 1997; **157**:935–9.
43. Chew LD, Fihn SD. Recurrent cystitis in nonpregnant women. *West J Med* 1999; **170**:274–7.
44. Stapleton A, Latham RH, Johnson C, Stamm WE. Postcoital antimicrobial prophylaxis for recurrent urinary tract infection: a randomized, double-blind, placebo-controlled trail. *JAMA* 1990; **264**:703–6.
45. Jepson RG, Williams G, Craig JC. Cranberries for preventing urinary tract infections. *Cochrane Database Syst Rev* 2012; **10**:CD001321.
46. Stapleton A. Novel approaches to prevention of urinary tract infections. *Infect Dis Clin North Am* 2003; **17**:457–71.
47. Gratacos E, Torres PJ, Vila J, et al. Screening and treatment of asymptomatic bacteriuria in pregnancy prevent pyelonephritis. *J Infect Dis* 1994; **169**:1390–2.
48. Kincaid-Smith P, Bullen M. Bacteriuria in pregnancy. *Lancet* 1965; **191**:395–9.
49. Smaill F. Antibiotics for asymptomatic bacteriuria in pregnancy. *Cochrane Database Syst Rev* 2001; **2**: CD000490.
50. Mittendorf R., Williams MA, Kass EH. Prevention of preterm delivery and low birth weight associated with asymptomatic bacteriuria. *Clin Infect Dis* 1992; **14**:927–32.
51. Vogel T, Verreault R, Gourdeau M, et al. Optimal duration of antibiotic therapy for uncomplicated urinary tract infection in older women: a double-blind randomized controlled trial. *CMAJ* 2004; **170**(4): 469–73.

Chapter 36

Office care of premenstrual syndrome and premenstrual dysphoric disorder

Hal Elliott

Introduction

Premenstrual dysphoric disorder (PMDD) and premenstrual syndrome (PMS) are distinct cyclical disorders in which women experience distressing mood and behavioral symptoms in the late luteal or premenstrual phase of their menstrual cycle. PMDD is the most extreme or severe form of PMS. Women with PMDD experience marked dysphoria, irritability, mood lability, anxiety, fatigue, change in appetite, and the subjective sense of feeling overwhelmed. The most common complaint is irritability.

It is common for women to experience changes in mood and to have physical symptoms such as pain and bloating in the one to two weeks leading to their menstrual period. However, although up to 75% of women will experience physical and emotional symptoms before their menses and 12.6%–31% will experience symptoms significant enough to describe as moderate to severe PMS, only 3%–8% will experience symptoms severe enough to qualify for a diagnosis of PMDD.[1]

Scope of the problem

Although there had been some debate as to the unique nature of PMDD, there now appears to be a consensus that PMDD is a separate and distinct psychiatric disorder.[2] PMS/PMDD is more likely to occur in women who have histories of abuse, who have histories of mood disorders, or who have a histories of anxiety disorders. The biological basis of PMDD, however, is supported by twin studies indicating that PMDD is inherited[3] and by studies indicating that medical or surgical suppression of ovulation will eliminate premenstrual symptoms.[4, 5] Menstrual mood disorders are associated with blunted sympathetic reactivity to stress but to a heightened autonomic reactivity to auditory stimuli. In addition, the predictable cyclical recurrence in relation to the menstrual cycle and the remission of symptoms during that cycle is further evidence of PMDD as a distinct and biologically driven syndrome.[6]

Diagnosis

The diagnosis of PMS/PMDD is based on the presence of at least five of the following symptoms during the postovulatory period prior to menses: depressed mood, anxiety, affective lability, irritability, decreased interest in usual activities, decreased concentration, lack of energy, change in appetite (increased or decreased), change in sleep pattern (increased or decreased), sense of feeling overwhelmed, and physical symptoms (breast tenderness, bloating, headache, joint or muscle pain). Essential to diagnosis is the presence or absence of symptoms in different phases of the menstrual cycle and that the symptoms are severe enough to interfere with social or occupational functioning. Women with PMS/PMDD typically will have onset of their symptoms in the last one to two weeks of their menstrual cycle with remission of their symptoms by the end of the menstrual flow. Occasionally, there will be an increase in PMS/PMDD symptoms at ovulation; however, symptoms generally will begin in a fairly predictable pattern linked to the luteal, or postovulatory, phase of the cycle and remit after menses begins or ends.

Because patients can misinterpret, underemphasize, or overemphasize symptoms as relating to their menstrual cycles, it can be quite useful to have them chart their symptoms throughout the month. Multiple instruments can be used to chart symptoms including the Daily Rating Form, the Menstrual Distress Questionnaire, the Premenstrual Assessment Form, the Calendar of Premenstrual Experiences, the Premenstrual Symptoms Screening Tool, and the Prospective Record of the Impact and Severity of Menstrual Symptoms calendar. All of these instruments aid in

Office Care of Women, ed. Martin E. Olsen and Botros Rizk. Published by Cambridge University Press.

identifying and quantifying the timing and impact of symptoms during the menstrual cycle. Charting allows the clinician to differentiate PMDD from other psychiatric or medical disorders and establish a cyclical basis for symptoms. Alternatively, the clinician can direct patients to rate their symptoms on a simple scale of one to five or one to ten in terms of pain or mood symptoms. The key is to have a scale of symptoms related to a patient's menstrual cycle in order to correlate symptoms with that cycle.

In addition to PMS/PMDD, many women report an exacerbation of other psychiatric disorders in the late luteal phase of their menstrual cycle. Depression, bipolar disorder, panic disorder, generalized anxiety disorder, and attention deficit disorder symptoms all can worsen in the premenstrual period. The difference is that patients with a pure PMDD diagnosis generally will have a full remission or nearly full remission of their symptoms when not in the postovulatory period of their cycle. In addition to exacerbation of psychiatric disorders, premenstrual changes in hormone levels can exacerbate underlying medical conditions such as migraine headache, irritable bowel syndrome, asthma, seizure disorders, and various endocrine disorders such as diabetes.[7, 8]

Other medical causes of dysphoria or PMS/PMDD symptoms should not be overlooked. A complete history and physical should be performed and routine laboratory tests obtained to rule out other etiologies of premenstrual complaints, depressive or anxiety symptoms, and premenstrual or menstrual pain and bloating. The differential diagnosis could include hypothyroidism, autoimmune disorders, diabetes, anemia, parathyroid disorders, and endometriosis.

Etiology

PMS and PMDD are closely linked to the hypothalamic-pituitary-gonadal (HPG) axis. Although women might ask for their "hormone levels" to be checked, there is no demonstrable gonadal hormone level abnormality in women with PMS and PMDD.[9] Rather, it is more likely that women with PMS and PMDD have heightened central nervous system (CNS) sensitivity to normal ovarian cycling of gonadal steroids. Sensitivity exists to the change in hormone levels throughout the menstrual cycle as opposed to any measurable ongoing abnormality in any specific gonadal hormone.

Serotonin (5-HT) functions in a reciprocal relationship with the HPG axis. As women with PMS and PMDD cycle through the late luteal phase of their menstrual cycle and progesterone levels drop, availability of 5-HT is reduced. This abrupt reduction in serotonin could trigger symptoms known to be associated with 5-HT depletion. Symptoms of serotonin depletion include irritability, dysphoria, impulsivity, and carbohydrate craving.[10]

Several studies have implicated altered 5-HT function in women with PMDD. Blood 5-HT levels and platelet uptake of 5-HT are reduced in patients with PMDD.[9, 11] In addition, acute depletion of tryptophan, a precursor of serotonin, aggravates and precipitates symptoms of PMS/PMDD in women who have had PMS/PMDD symptoms in the late luteal phase.[12]

Although dysregulation of serotonin mediated through the HPG axis could be one cause of PMS and PMDD symptoms, there also is evidence that other neurotransmitters could play a significant role. Reduced gamma-aminobutyric acid (GABA) levels have been noted in patients with PMDD and PMS.[13] Studies using naltrexone and naloxone have suggested a possible acute endogenous opioid withdrawal in the late luteal phase of the menstrual cycle, thus causing irritability and mood lability characteristic of such withdrawal.[14, 15] Women with PMDD given the opiate antagonists naltrexone and naloxone during the non-luteal phase of their cycle experience irritability and mood lability similar to premenstrual symptoms experienced in the late luteal phase.

Finally, the unusually rapid action of the selective serotonin reuptake inhibitors (SSRIs) in PMS/PMDD has led to the theory that these agents perhaps work by a different mechanism in patients with PMS/PMDD than in patients with symptoms of depression or anxiety. Typically, SSRIs take two to four weeks to begin working in depressed patients and up to four to six weeks to show full effect. Patients with PMS/PMDD can see improvement in symptoms within days of beginning or increasing their prescribed SSRI.

Allopregnenolone, a metabolite of progesterone, decreases anxiety by binding to central GABA receptors. Women with PMDD have lower levels of progesterone and alloprognenolone in the luteal phase of their menstrual cycle. In PMDD patients, SSRIs might work by indirectly increasing allopregnenolone synthesis from progesterone. This may account for the rapid onset of action of the SSRIs in patients with PMS/PMDD.[16, 17]

Regardless, it appears that most likely PMDD is mediated by a complex interplay within the HPG axis and that the cause of symptoms is a central sensitivity to normal fluctuations of gonadal steroids as opposed to any peripheral gonadal hormonal level abnormality. Decreased availability of serotonin and allopregnenolone centrally may cause heightened symptoms of dysphoria, irritability, and anxiety.

Therefore, treatment should focus on the correction or compensation for central sensitivity or on stopping the fluctuations in gonadal hormones altogether instead of just modifying the existing monthly hormonal cycle.

Treatment

Currently, the SSRIs have the best evidence of efficacy and appear to be effective in up to 70% of patients with PMDD. Sertraline, fluoxetine, paroxetine, citalopram, and escitalopram all have controlled trial evidence of efficacy in and are approved by the FDA for the treatment of PMS and PMDD symptoms.

As noted earlier, SSRIs work rapidly in the treatment of PMS/PMDD symptoms and much more quickly than for treatment of depression, panic disorder, or obsessive-compulsive disorder. Because women often see improvement in the first day or two after initiating therapy with an SSRI, several studies have investigated whether SSRIs work for PMDD when taken only in the late luteal phase. Indeed, it appears that SSRIs are effective for PMDD when taken only in the one to two weeks before menses. In fact, a 1998 study by Wikander and colleagues suggested that intermittent dosing of citalopram might be better than continuous dosing for PMDD symptoms.[18]

Side effects for the SSRIs include weight gain and sexual dysfunction. Intermittent/postovulatory dosing can decrease the intensity and frequency of these side effects.

Other antidepressant medications that also have serotonin reuptake effects, such as venlafaxine and duloxetine and clomipramine, might be useful in treating PMS and PMDD symptoms. Note that non-serotonin enhancing antidepressants, such as bupropion or the standard tricyclics, do not appear to have efficacy in the treatment of PMS/PMDD symptoms. Lithium also is ineffective.

In May of 2007, the FDA proposed that all antidepressants carry a warning for a possible increase in suicidal thinking and behavior in patients between 18 and 24 years of age. The risk of suicidality is most likely greatest in the first several months of treatment, but clinicians should be aware of this risk and screen patients, especially in the 18–24 age range, while treating them for PMS/PMDD with antidepressant medication.

Although SSRIs target central sensitivity to menstrual cycling, ovulation suppression strategies focus on halting the menstrual cycling. Gonadotropin-releasing hormone (GnRH) agonists act centrally on the hypothalamus, causing anovulation by decreasing follicle-stimulating (FSH) and luteinizing hormone (LH) levels, which, in turn, decreases estrogen and progesterone synthesis. Despite there being evidence of some efficacy in women with PMDD, GnRH agonists do not work as well in women with severe dysphoria in the late luteal phase or who have exacerbation of preexisting major depression in the late luteal phase.[19]

Danazol has also been studied in the treatment of PMDD/PMS. Results for use of danazol have been mixed, but a positive response appears to be linked to suppression of ovulation.[20] However, use of danazol has been linked to acne, facial hair, weight gain, and depression. In addition, long-term reduction of estrogen is linked to decreased bone density.

Other proposed treatments for PMS/PMDD have included oral contraceptives and luteal phase addition of progesterone. Despite widespread use of standard 21–28-day oral contraceptives as treatment of PMS/PMDD symptoms, there is no real evidence of efficacy. In fact, there is at least one study indicating a worsening of PMDD symptoms with the continuous use of 21–28-day oral contraceptives.[21] Because of the anxiolytic properties of allopregnenolone, there has been interest in the addition of its precursor progesterone in the luteal phase; however, several controlled trials have not shown the addition of progesterone in the postovulatory phase to be more effective than placebo.[22]

The addition of androgen hormones has been associated with worsening of PMS/PMDD symptoms.

A relatively new oral contraceptive containing low-dose estrogen and drospirenone apparently reduces water retention and some symptoms of PMDD.[23] In addition, newer, longer duration oral contraceptive pills (levonorgestrel/ethinol) can decrease the number of menstrual periods to between one and four times per year by continuing the hormone medication pills and decreasing the intervals of placebo pills. These newer preparations of oral contraceptives will deliver low-dose oral contraceptives more continuously and thereby suppress menstruation and late luteal phase symptoms. Although there might not be a decrease in intensity of symptoms when the late luteal phase does occur, a decrease in frequency might be a useful option and a welcome relief for patients suffering from significant PMS or PMDD.

Because of their action on GABA, benzodiazepines have been studied in the treatment of PMS/PMDD symptoms. The results have been mixed, with some studies showing mild efficacy and other studies failing to show any superiority of alprazolam over placebo. Several studies showed mild improvement in severe PMS symptoms with the addition of low-dose alprazolam, but the improvement rate appears significantly less than the improvement rate for SSRIs. Furthermore, alprazolam should be used with caution in patients with a history of substance abuse. Because benzodiazepines may cause disinhibition in some patients, they should be used with caution in patients with a history of impulse control difficulties.

Buspirone, a novel anxiolytic with serotonergic properties, has shown some efficacy in decreasing or mitigating PMS-associated irritability and anxiety. Buspirone has the advantage of not causing disinhibition or dependency. However, it should be taken ongoing and not on an as needed basis.

Results of studies with vitamin and mineral supplements have also been mixed with the best evidence of efficacy having been demonstrated with calcium supplementation. A large 1998 study using calcium carbonate with vitamin D showed a 48% improvement rate compared with 30% placebo.[24] The rate of response is less than that for SSRIs, but calcium carbonate with vitamin D is an inexpensive and nonintrusive option for treatment of PMS/PMDD symptoms.

Vitamin B_6 has received attention for treatment of PMS. Again, the results of controlled trials have been mixed, showing perhaps a very mild benefit at doses of 50 mg–100 mg daily. Doses of B_6 should be kept in the 50 mg–100 mg range to minimize the risk for the neurotoxicity that can occur at higher doses. There has been at least one study indicating improvement in PMDD symptoms with magnesium supplementation,

BOX 36-1 Key points in the diagnosis and management of severe PMS or PMDD

- The diagnosis should be established with patient charting of symptoms throughout the course of her menstrual cycle.
- A medical cause or an exacerbation of an underlying psychiatric disorder must be excluded from the differential diagnosis. A thorough history, performance of a medical/gynecologic examination, and assessment of appropriate baseline laboratory tests should be undertaken. Particular care should be given to ruling out endocrine abnormalities.
- Depending on severity, consider nonintrusive interventions such as calcium supplementation and a multivitamin with magnesium and B_6, an increase in complex carbohydrates and exercise, and a decrease in caffeine and tobacco. Also consider herbal treatments such as chaste tree depending on patient's level of interest.
- Consider referral for cognitive behavioral therapy/interpersonal therapy and/or referral for relaxation therapy, especially if there are external stressors that exacerbate symptoms.
- If residual symptoms are present or minimal improvement occurs, consider adding an SSRI in the late luteal phase; if intermittent dosing is ineffective or if there are ongoing depressive or anxiety symptoms throughout the cycle, begin an SSRI on a continuous schedule and, if needed, consider an increase in dosage in the 10–14 days before menses.
- Monitor all patients for increased suicidality while on antidepressant medications. Particular caution should be exercised in patients between the ages of 18 and 24.
- Benzodiazepines can be useful as an adjunctive treatment of PMDD, especially if anxiety is a significant factor; however, they should be used with some caution in patients with a history of substance abuse or with a history of impulse control problems.
- Depending on the severity of symptoms, another option would be to suggest ongoing fixed dose oral contraceptive without allowing for onset of menses; this strategy may decrease PMDD symptoms to one to four times a year.
- If the patient continues to be refractory to interventions and/or the PMDD is of significant severity, the clinician should consider a referral for medical or surgical suppression of the ovulatory cycle and referral to a psychiatrist for consultation.

but a more recent study indicated only improvement in fluid retention.[25]

Significant interest has been found with herbal treatments of PMDD, such as oil of primrose or St. John's wort. Despite this interest, no significant proof of efficacy for herbal treatments in randomized clinical trials has been documented.[26] However, the results of a prospective randomized placebo-controlled study of 17 women indicated some efficacy for treating PMDD with *Vites agnus castus* (chaste tree).[27]

Nonmedication interventions, including dietary recommendations, exercise, and cognitive and relaxation therapy, can also be of significant benefit. An increase in complex carbohydrates, a decrease in caffeine and tobacco, and more frequent meals in the premenstrual phase can be helpful. Carbohydrate craving in the premenstrual period may be an attempt to increase tryptophan, a precursor of serotonin. Exercise may also increase endogenous endorphin levels, alleviating anxiety and dysphoria. Finally, both relaxation techniques and cognitive behavioral therapy have been reported as effective in relieving PMS/PMDD and in improving coping mechanisms for the core symptoms.[28]

Concluding remarks

Premenstrual dysphoric disorder (PMDD) and premenstrual syndrome (PMS) are significant cyclical disorders in which patients experience distressing mood and behavioral symptoms in the late luteal or premenstrual phase of their menstrual cycle. Patients should chart their symptoms to confirm that these correlate with the menstrual cycle. The clinician should rule out a medical cause or exacerbation of an underlying psychiatric disorder by obtaining a thorough history, performing a medical/gynecologic examination, and by ordering appropriate laboratory tests. Nonintrusive treatments include calcium supplementation, an increase in complex carbohydrates and exercise, a decrease in caffeine and tobacco, and referral for relaxation/ CBT therapy. If there are residual symptoms, consider adding an SSRI in the late luteal phase or on a continuous basis. With excellent treatment, these patients can experience significant symptom improvement.

Box 36-1 highlights steps for a reasonable approach to a patient who is reporting severe PMS or PMDD.

References

1. Steiner M, McDougall M, Brown E. The premenstrual symptoms screening tool for clinicians. *Arch Womens Mental Health*. 2003; **6**:203–209.
2. Endicott J, Amsterdam J, Eriksson E, et al. Is premenstrual dysphoric disorder a distinct clinical entity? *J Womens Health Gender-Based Med*. 1999; **8**:663–679.
3. Condone JT. The premenstrual syndrome: a twin study. *Br J Psychiatry*. 1993; **162**:481–486.
4. Schmidt PJ, Nieman LK, Danaceau MA, et al. Differential behavioral effects of gonadal steroids in women with and in those without premenstrual syndrome. *Am J Obstet Gynecol*. 1990; **162**:99–105.
5. Casson P, Hahn PM, Van Vugt DA. Lasting response to ovariectomy in severe intractable premenstrual syndrome. *Am J Obstet Gynecol*. 1991; **162**:99–105.
6. Klatzkin R, Bunevicius A, Fomeris C, Girdler S. Menstrual mood disorders are associated with blunted sympathetic reactivity to stress. *J Psychosom Res*. 2014 Jan; **76**(1):46–55.
7. Case AM, Reid RL. Menstrual cycle effects on common medical conditions. *Compr Ther*. 2001; **27**:65.
8. Altman G, Cain KC, Motzer S, et al. Increased symptoms in female IBS patients with dysmennorhea and PMS. *Gastroenterol Nurs*. 2006; **29**:4.
9. Roca CA, Schmidt PJ, Bloch M, et al. Implications of endocrine studies of premenstrual syndrome. *Psychiatr Ann*. 1996; **26**:576–580.
10. Rapkin AJ, Edelmuth E, Chang LC, et al. Whole blood serotonin in premenstrual syndrome. *Obstet Gynecol*. 1987; **70**:533–537.
11. Taylor DL, Mathew RJ, Ho BT, et al. Serotonin levels and platelet uptake during premenstrual tension. *Neuropsychobiology*. 1984; **12**:16–18.
12. Menkes DB, Coates DC, Fawcett JP. Acute tryptophan depletion aggravates premenstrual syndrome. *J Affect Disord*. 1994; **32**:37–44.
13. Albreich U, Petty F, Yonkers K, et al. Low plasma gamma-aminobutyric acid levels during the late luteal phase of women with premenstrual dysphoric disorder. *Am J Psychiatry*. 1996; **153**:718–720.
14. Rapkin AJ, Shouple D, Reading A, et al. Decreased central opioid activity in premenstrual syndrome: leutenizing hormone response to naloxone. *J Soc Gynecol Investig*. 1996; **3**:93–96.
15. Chuong CJ, Coulam CB, Bergstralh EJ, et al. Clinical trial of naltrexone in premenstrual syndrome. *Obstet Gynecol*. 1988; **72**:332–336.
16. Rapkin AJ, Morgan M, Goldman L, et al. Progesterone metabolite allopregnanolone in women with premenstrual syndrome. *Obstet Gynecol*. 1997; **90**:709.

17. Guidotti A, Costa E. Can the antidysphoric and anxiolytic profiles of selective serotonin reuptake inhibitors be related to their ability to increase brain 3 alpha, 5 alpha-tetrahydroprogesterone (allpregnenolone) availability? *Biol Psych.* 1998; **44**:865–873.
18. Wikander I, Sundblad C, Andersch B, et al. Citalopram in premenstrual dysporia: is intermittent treatment during luteal phases more effective than continuous medication throughout the menstrual cycle? *J Clin Psychopharmacol.* 1998; **18S**:390–398.
19. Freeman EW, Sonheimer SJ, Rickels K. Gonadotropin-releasing hormone agonist in treatment of premenstrual symptoms with and without ongoing dysphoria: a controlled study. *Psychopharmacol Bull.* 1997; **33**:303–309.
20. Halbreich U, Rojansky N, Palter S. Elimination of ovulation and menstrual cyclicity (with Danazol) improves dysphoric menstrual syndromes. *Fert Steril.* 1991; **56**:1066–1069.
21. Bancroft J, Rennie D. The impact of oral contraceptives on the experience of perimenstrual mood, clumsiness, food craving and other symptoms. *J Psychosom Res.* 1993; **37**:195–202.
22. Wyatt K, Dimmock P, Jones P, et al. Efficacy of progesterone and progestogens in management of premenstrual syndrome: a systematic review. *BMJ.* 2001; **323**:134.
23. Yonkers KA, Brown C, Pearlstein TB, et al. Efficacy of a new low dose oral contraceptive with drospirenone in premenstrual dysphoric disorder. *Obstet Gynecol.* 2005; **106**:492.
24. Thys-Jacobs S, Starkey P, Bernstein D, et al. Calcium carbonate and the premenstrual syndrome: effects on premenstrual and menstrual symptoms. *Am J Obstet Gynecol.* 1998; **179**:444–452.
25. Walker AF, De Souza MC, Vicker MF, et al. Magnesium supplementation alleviates premenstrual symptoms of fluid retention. *J Womens Health.* 1998; **7**:1157–1165.
26. Stevenson C, Ernest E. Complementary/alternative therapies for premenstrual syndrome: asystematic review of randomized controlled trials. *Am J Obstet Gynecol.* 2001; **185**:227.
27. Schellenberg R. Treatment for premenstrual syndrome with angus castus fruit extract: prospective randomized placebo-controlled study. *BMJ.* 2001; **322**:134.
28. Blake F, Salkovskis P, Gath D, et al. Cognitive therapy for premenstrual syndrome: a controlled trial. *J Psychosom Res.* 1998; **45**:307.

Evidence-based references

Douglas S. Premenstrual syndrome: evidence-based treatment in family practice. *Can Fam Physician.* 2002; **48**:1789.

Rapkin AJ. A review of treatment of premenstrual syndrome and premenstrual dysphoric disorder. *Psychoneuroendocrinology.* 2003 Aug; **28**(Suppl 3):39–53.

Cunningham J, Yonkers K, O'Brien S, Eriksson E. Update on research and treatment of premenstrual dysphoric disorder; *Harv Rev Psychiatry.* 2009; **17**(2):120–137.

Chapter 37

Office management of depression

Sarah M. Appleton

Introduction

Approximately 21% of women suffer from depression during their lifetimes.[1, 2] The rate of depression in women is twice that of men.[1] Depression often affects women during key transitional phases of their lives: adolescence, early adulthood, postpartum,[3] and during the menopausal transition.[4]

Depression can also be associated with or a manifestation of other mood or psychiatric disorders including anxiety, bipolar disorder, eating disorders, or premenstrual dysphoric disorder (PMDD). This chapter will specifically focus on the diagnosis and initial treatments of depression in the outpatient setting.

Scope of the problem

The rates of depression in women greatly impact the outpatient obstetrician-gynecologist (ob-gyn). Nearly one-third of women consider their ob-gyn as their primary care physician,[5] and one-third of outpatient visits for women less than 65 years old are provided by an ob-gyn.[6] Moreover, women with a lower socioeconomic status or those in minority groups are more likely to seek care from their gynecologist than from a primary care provider.[6] Despite the high prevalence of depression, only 20%–33% of women are accurately diagnosed by their ob-gyn.[7, 8] Patients with undiagnosed, and thus, untreated, depression are at highest risk for suicidal ideation. Suicide attempts have been reported to be as high as 15% in those with affective disorders, with an increase in this risk as severity or agitation increases.[9]

The financial impact of depression in the United States is staggering. Depression alone accounts for over $43 billion in health-care costs and an additional $17 billion in lost productivity annually.[10] By 2020, depression is projected to become the second leading cause of disability.[11]

As such, ob-gyns are needed to be the first line in the recognition, diagnosis, and facilitation of treatment for depression.

Screening

Given the prevalence of depression, much discussion has occurred regarding the utility of universal screening in the primary care setting as well as the in nonobstetrical population of the ob-gyn practice. Although screening has been shown to increase recognition rates of depression, the data is mixed regarding the impact of such screening on outcomes.[12, 13] Studies demonstrate that screening improves outcomes only if partnered with treatment opportunities.[14, 15] The United States Preventive Services Task Force (USPSTF), therefore, recommends screening only in a setting that can ensure accurate diagnosis, effective treatment, and appropriate follow-up.[15]

Many validated instruments exist for depression screening, and none are superior.[15] If the screening instrument is positive, a full diagnostic interview should be arranged to assess for depression and other mood disorders using standard diagnostic criteria (see also "Diagnosis"). Two commonly used screening instruments are the patient health questionnaire: the PHQ-2 and the PHQ-9.

The PHQ-2 is a validated, ultrashort screen that may rule out, but not definitively diagnose, depression.[17] It is as effective as longer screening instruments including the widely used Zung depression scale and the Beck depression inventory.[18, 19] In adults, the PHQ-2 has been reported to be 97% sensitive and 67% specific[19]; in adolescents it is 74% sensitive and 75% specific.[20] See Table 37-1.

The PHQ-9 is a slighter longer validated instrument commonly used for both depression screening as well as treatment monitoring. It takes, on average, two to

Office Care of Women, ed. Martin E. Olsen and Botros Rizk. Published by Cambridge University Press.

Table 37-1 Patient Health Questionnaire-2

	Not at all	Several days	More than one-half the days	Nearly every day
Over the past two weeks, how often have you been bothered by any of the following problems?				
Little interest or pleasure in doing things	0	1	2	3
Feeling down, depressed, or hopeless	0	1	2	3

Note: If the patient has a positive response to either question, consider administering the PHQ-9 or asking the patient more questions about possible depression.

five minutes to complete. It has demonstrated 61% sensitivity and 94% specificity for mood disorders in adults and 89% sensitivity and 77% specificity in adolescents.[21] See Table 37-2.

History

The initial and most impactful tool for the diagnosis of depression is a well-taken history. In addition, a thorough history and physical exam should be performed to rule out organic causes for depression and to delineate a diagnosis of depression from other mood disorders. Rarely will a patient present with a directed chief complaint of depression. The majority of patients seeking care will complain of vague somatic symptoms such as fatigue, headache, abdominal distress, or weight changes or numerous complaints without a clear clinical pattern.[22]

In obtaining a review of symptoms, the practitioner must evaluate for neurovegetative symptoms. A common pneumonic for this is "SIGECAPS" – "a prescription for energy capsules." Inquiring about changes in sleep habits, appetite, and energy patterns can determine if further investigation is needed. See Table 37-3.

It is important to evaluate a patient's past medical history as patients with a history of a prior depressive episode have up to a 75% risk of suffering a subsequent episode; 10%–30% will continue to demonstrate residual symptoms from a previous episode.[23, 24] Those patients with chronic medical problems including coronary artery disease, diabetes mellitus, and stroke are also at higher risk of depression.[25–28]

A careful review of medications should be conducted as many medications can contribute to depressive symptoms. Some contributing prescription medications include reserpine, beta blockers, alpha-methyldopa, levodopa, calcium channel blockers, hormone replacement therapies, statins, barbiturates, and benzodiazepienes.

The review of a patient's social history should include any instances of abuse of prescription medication, illicit drugs, or alcohol, which can lead to development of depression or reflect an attempt at self-treatment by the depressed patient. Moreover, the patient's social history should also be reviewed for social support structures to assess a patient's prognosis or risk of suicide or self-harm.

An inquiry regarding suicide ideation is warranted in those patients with depression or depressive symptoms. Major depressive episode is the most common psychiatric diagnosis among suicide victims and attempters (56%–87%).[29] Further, more than half of suicide victims contact their primary care provider within four weeks of their suicidal act.[29] Patients will have an increase in their energy level in response to therapy; therefore, their risk of acting on suicidal thoughts increases.

Physical exam

Depression is not based primarily on physical findings, but rather a combination of a well-gathered history as well as a mental status exam (MSE). The physical exam can assist in exclusion of common

Table 37-2 Patient Health Questionnaire-9

	Not at all	Several days	More than one-half the days	Nearly every day
Over the past two weeks, how often have you been bothered by any of the following problems?				
Little interest or pleasure in doing things	0	1	2	3
Feeling down, depressed, or hopeless	0	1	2	3
Trouble falling or staying asleep, or sleeping too much	0	1	2	3
Feeling tired or having little energy	0	1	2	3
Poor appetite or overeating	0	1	2	3
Feeling bad about yourself – or that you are a failure or have let yourself or your family down	0	1	2	3
Trouble concentrating on things, such as reading the newspaper or watching television	0	1	2	3
Moving or speaking so slowly that other people could have noticed. Or the opposite – being so fidgety or restless that you have been moving around a lot more than usual	0	1	2	3
Thoughts that you would be better off dead, or of hurting yourself in some way	0	1	2	3
Totals				

Total score:	Depression severity:
1 to 4	Minimal
5 to 9	Mild
10 to 14	Moderate
15 to 19	Moderately severe
20 to 27	Severe

organic causes for depressive symptoms. These etiologies fall into categories including:

1. Medications: medication side effects, abuse of prescriptive or illicit drugs
2. Endocrine disorders: thyroid disease (both hypo- and hyper-), electrolyte imbalances, diabetes mellitus
3. Neurologic disorders: stroke, subdural hematoma, multiple sclerosis, Parkinson's, Huntington's, epilepsy (uncontrolled), dementias, vitamin B12 deficiency, pellagra
4. Infections: syphilis, viral infections
5. Tumors or carcinomas: brain tumors (especially those in the frontal lobe), other carcinomas

The MSE should be a part of the clinical assessment if a provider is concerned about depression or another psychiatric illness. It is a structured means of describing a patient's state of mind under the domains of appearance, attitude, behavior, mood and affect, speech, thought process, thought content, insight, and judgment. See Table 37-4.

Laboratory assessment

As with the physical exam, utilizing a targeted laboratory assessment can help to rule out organic causes for depressive symptoms. A detailed history can guide the

Table 37-3 SIGECAPS

	Symptoms	Question examples
S	Sleep disruptions	Do you struggle to fall or stay asleep? Do you sleep too much?
I	Interest or pleasure has decreased	Do you have less interest or pleasure in activities that were previously enjoyable?
G	Guilt feelings or feelings of worthlessness	Do you feel guilty or worthless frequently?
E	Energy changes or fatigue	Is your energy lower than usual? Do you feel tired even with a full night's sleep?
C	Concentration impairment	Do you have difficulty concentrating?
A	Appetite changes	Are you eating more or less than you typically do?
P	Psychomotor disturbances	Do people close to you feel your speech or movement is slower or faster than previously?
S	Suicidal thoughts	Do you have thoughts of hurting yourself? Do you ever think you would be better off dead?

practitioner regarding which labs are indicated. See Table 37-5.

Diagnosis

The diagnosis of a major depressive episode should be made using the fifth edition of the *Diagnostic and Statistical Manual of Mental Disorders* (DSM-5), which was updated by the American Psychiatric Association.[30] The diagnostic criteria are similar to previously used DSM-IV criteria. The most significant change that occurred is removal of the exclusion criterion for times of bereavement.

The criteria for a major depressive episode include:[30]

- Five (or more) of the following symptoms have been present during the same two-week period and represent a change from previous functioning; at least one of the symptoms is either (a) depressed mood or (b) loss of interest or pleasure.

  Note: Do not include symptoms that are clearly due to a general medical condition, or mood-incongruent delusions or hallucinations.

  1. Depressed mood most of the day, nearly every day, as indicated by either subjective report (e.g., feels sad or empty) or observation made by others (e.g., appears tearful). Note: In children and adolescents, can be irritable mood.
  2. Markedly diminished interest or pleasure in all, or almost all, activities most of the day, nearly every day (as indicated by either subjective account or observation made by others).
  3. Significant weight loss when not dieting or weight gain (e.g., a change of more than 5% of body weight in a month), or decrease or increase in appetite nearly every day. Note: In children, consider failure to make expected weight gains.
  4. Insomnia or hypersomnia nearly every day.
  5. Psychomotor agitation or retardation nearly every day (observable by others, not merely subjective feelings of restlessness or being slowed down).
  6. Fatigue or loss of energy nearly every day.
  7. Feelings of worthlessness or excessive or inappropriate guilt (which may be delusional) nearly every day (not merely self-reproach or guilt about being sick).
  8. Diminished ability to think or concentrate, or indecisiveness, nearly every day (either by subjective account or as observed by others).
  9. Recurrent thoughts of death (not just fear of dying), recurrent suicidal ideation without a specific plan, or a suicide attempt or a specific plan for committing suicide.

- The symptoms cause clinically significant distress or impairment in social, occupational, or other important areas of functioning.
- The symptoms are not due to the direct physiological effects of a substance (e.g., a drug of abuse, a medication) or a general medical condition (e.g., hypothyroidism).

Before making the diagnosis of major depression, the possibility of other mood disorders should be evaluated. Anxiety can coincide with depression. Further, providers should assess for bipolar disorder by inquiring about any previous episodes of mania or

Table 37-4 Mental status exam

Domain	Definition	Observations or questions for patient
Appearance	Patient's appearance and change in appearance over time	Observe patient's grooming and hygiene
Attitude	Patient's approach to the interview process	Observe patient's facial expressions and behavior toward the examiner
Behavior	Patient's level of activity during the interview	Observe specific abnormal movements, eye contact, and gait
Speech	Concerned with the production of speech, not the content	Observe the patient's spontaneous speech including volume, rate, and quantity
Mood	Sustained emotion that the patient is experiencing	How do you feel most days?
Affect	The apparent emotion conveyed by the patient's nonverbal behaviors	Observe the patient's generalized emotion based on nonverbal cues
Thought process	The quantity and form (logical coherence) of thought	Infer from the patient's speech and connection of thought
Thought content	A description of what the patient is thinking about regularly	Explore a patient's thoughts with open-ended questions
Insight	Patient's ability to understand her own circumstances	What do you think is causing your problems?
Judgment	Ability for the patient to make appropriate decisions in appropriate situations	If you found a letter on the ground in front of a mailbox, what would you do with it?

Table 37-5 Laboratory assessment for depression

Lab test	Diagnosis to exclude
Complete blood count	Anemia
Electrolytes	Electrolyte abnormalities
Liver function evaluation	Drug effects, liver dysfunction
Renal function evaluation	Drug effects, renal dysfunction
Thyroid function tests	Thyroid disease
EEG	If seizure disorder is suspected

hypomania. In selecting treatment, ruling out bipolar disorder is critical to avoid inducing a manic episode with many common antidepressants.

Once a diagnosis of major depressive episode is made, the patient should be assessed for any risk of suicide ideation. The patient should then be offered initiation of treatment.

Treatment

Although ob-gyns recognize the importance of depression treatment and management, many cite barriers to doing so, including lack of training and inadequate resources for appropriate follow-up.[31] Evidence supports that there exist larger gaps in diagnosis and treatment of depression in the ob-gyn office than in primary care.[32]

The goals of therapy for depression include relieving acute symptoms, returning patient to normal functioning level, preventing relapse, and decreasing the risk of self-harm. Choosing initial treatment should be based on the severity of disease. Patients with mild to moderate disease do not exhibit severe features, which include suicidal or homicidal ideation, no psychotic features, and intact judgment. As such, treatment can occur in an outpatient setting. Any person with one or more of the severe features should be referred to a psychiatrist and/or require inpatient management.

For mild to moderate depression, randomized trials support initiating pharmacotherapy and psychotherapy simultaneously as combination treatment has been found to be more effective.[33] However, it is reasonable to offer pharmacotherapy or psychotherapy alone as either may be more acceptable or available to the patient.

Pharmacologic treatment

The choice of initial medical treatment should be based on safety, anticipated side effects, and cost. Approximately one-third of patients with depression achieve complete resolution of symptoms after three months of therapy, and about half of depressed patients will have at least a partial response to pharmacotherapy with some residual symptoms.[34, 35] Treatment monitoring should include efficacy, side effects, and suicidality. Dose changes should occur if a patient has not achieved improvement after 4–12 weeks of treatment.[36]

Selective serotonin reuptake inhibitors and serotonin norepinephrine reuptake inhibitors

Selective serotonin reuptake inhibitors (SSRIs) have become the most widely prescribed treatment for depression in the United States as a result of their efficacy, acceptable side effect profile, and ability to treat concurrent anxiety. SSRIs treat depression by increasing the serotonergic activity in the brain. Because this class of medications has little affinity for other receptors, the medications typically have few adrenergic, histaminic, or cholinergic side effects. SSRIs are metabolized by hepatic cytochrome P450, and, thus, there exists a wide array of potential drug–drug interactions.

Prior to starting a patient on an SSRI, the practitioner should review the risks and potential side effects. Expectations for the treatment effect should be made clear; while initial clinical response may occur within two weeks, the mean time to substantial improvement or remission is 8–12 weeks.[37, 38] Further, patients should be counseled that abrupt discontinuation of the medication can lead to "discontinuation syndrome," with symptoms of dizziness, sadness, fatigue, chills, and myalgias.

Common side effects of SSRIs include sexual dysfunction (17%), dowsiness (17%), weight gain (12%), insomnia (11%), anxiety (11%), dizziness (11%), and headache (10%).[39] SSRIs can also prolong the QT interval, most significantly with citalopram. Serotonin syndrome can potentially occur with SSRIs as a result of overstimulation of serotonin receptors.

Serotonin norepinephrine reuptake inhibitors (SNRIs) are typically second-line therapy. They are trialed when patients have a poor response or are intolerant of the side effects of SSRIs. They function by blocking the reuptake of both serotonin and norepinephrine in the brain.

As they do with SSRIs, clinicians should discuss risks, side effects, and treatment expectations with a patient before starting an SNRI. A full clinical response may take 8–14 weeks, and a similar "discontinuation syndrome" can occur if these medications are stopped abruptly.[40] The most common side effects with this class of medication include nausea, dizziness, and diaphoresis.

For dosing of both SSRIs and SNRIs, see Table 37-6.

Tricyclic antidepressants

Tricyclic antidepressants (TCAs) block norepinephrine reuptake receptors, and partially block serotonin reuptake receptors. With TCAs, the number needed to treat to achieve one responder is four patients.[34] Because of their actions on cholinergic, adrenergic, and histaminic receptors, TCAs frequently cause undesirable side effects including sedation, constipation, dry mouth, weight gain, and orthostatic hypertension. The number needed to harm (side effects bothersome enough to stop treatment) is 5–11 patients.[34] Given their narrow therapeutic index, these medications are used less frequently than SSRIs or SNRIs.

TCAs also have pharmacologic interactions and risks that should be reviewed with the patient prior to starting. First, TCAs have been associated with increasing risk of cardiovascular events in patients with pre-existing ischemic heart disease. Second, they are metabolized by hepatic cytochrome P450 and thus

Table 37-6 SSRI, SNRI, and atypical antidepressant dosing

	Generic name	Trade name	Starting dose/day	Dosing range/day
SSRIs	Citalopram	Celexa	20 mg	20 mg–40 mg
	Escitalopram	Lexapro	10 mg	10 mg–20 mg
	Fluoxetine	Prozac	20 mg	20 mg–60 mg
	Fluvoxamine	Luvox	50 mg	50 mg–200 mg
	Paroxetine	Paxil	20 mg	20 mg–40 mg
	Sertraline	Zoloft	50 mg	50 mg–200 mg
SNRIs	Desvenlafaxine	Pristiq	50 mg	50 mg–400 mg
	Duloxetine	Cymbalta	30 mg	30 mg–120 mg
	Milnacipran	Savella	12.5 mg	100 mg–200 mg
	Venlafaxine	Effexor	37.5 mg	75 mg–375 mg
Atypical	Buproprion	Wellbutrin	200 mg	150 mg–450 mg
	Mirtazapine	Remeron	15 mg	15 mg–45 mg

can have varying blood levels and interactions with various other medications metabolized by this pathway. Lastly, an overdose of TCAs can be lethal due to their cardiac, pulmonary, and neurologic impact.

Atypical antidepressants

Atypical antidepressants are pharmacologically distinct from other antidepressants and are often initiated in patients who do not respond to first-line therapies or have significant side effects to those modalities. In the United States, the two atypical antidepressants available are bupropion and mirtazapine.

Bupropion is a dopamine norepinephrine reuptake inhibitor with little effect on other neurotransmitters. It is often used in patients with sexual side effects with other antidepressants either as an adjunct therapy or in replacement of the previous medication. It is metabolized by hepatic cytochrome P450 causing potential interactions with other medications. A dose dependent risk of seizures is associated with the use of bupropion. This is especially problematic in those patients with eating disorders. Other side effects included dry mouth (21%), nausea (13%), insomnia (12%), and dizziness (10%).[41]

Mirtazapine is not a reuptake inhibitor; rather, it contributes to a blockade of the adrenergic receptors causing an increased release of norepinephrine and serotonin. It does have a high affinity for histamine H1 receptors, which likely contributes to its sedating effects. However, the sedation has an inverse relationship to the dose – seen more predominantly at 15 mg daily than doses greater than 30 mg daily. It is not metabolized by hepatic cytochrome P450, and thus, it is often used in patients taking other medications metabolized by this route. Reported side effects include dry mouth (25%), drowsiness (23%), sedation (19%), increased appetite (11%), and increased weight (10%).[42] Mirtazapine has also been associated with QT prolongation, especially in those patients at increased for QT prolongation or in cases of mirtazapine overdose.

Psychotherapy

There are a variety of psychotherapies which have been demonstrated to be effective in treating depression.[36, 43, 44] There is, however, little compelling data that support one modality over the others. A therapy choice should therefore be tailored to the needs and personality of the patient. The most common, and thus most widely available, are cognitive behavioral therapy (CBT) and interpersonal therapy (IPT). Other forms of therapies can include individual, family, motivational interviewing, or group therapy.

CBT is a combination program of cognitive therapy, in which the therapist guides the patient in identifying and correcting maladaptive beliefs, and behavioral therapy, which uses mental exercises or activities to help facilitate symptom reduction. It often includes coping skill development, stress reduction, relaxation techniques, and education. The patient best suited for success with CBT is the highly motivated patient who desires a problem-solving approach to therapy.

IPT is a therapy which focuses on the patient's interpersonal relationships that may be problematic and related to the patient's depressive episode. Depressive symptoms and interpersonal relationships have a reciprocal relationship and as one improves, as does the other leading to lessening of symptoms and improved interpersonal functioning.[45]

Other therapies

Electroconvulsive therapy

Electroconvulsive therapy (ECT) has been demonstrated to be more effective in treatment of severe depression than other therapy modalities. Its impact on symptoms is rapid; however, it has many drawbacks including safety concerns and adverse effects on memory and cognitive function.

Exercise

Exercise has been used as monotherapy or as a treatment adjunct depending on the severity of a patient's depression. Although exercise has been supported in practice guidelines,[36] it has not been shown to be effective for treatment of depressive disorders.[46, 47]

Behavioral activation

Behavioral activation (BA) incorporates relaxation techniques as well as reintroducing positive activities into a patient's life. Rather than waiting until the patient feels better, it is encouraged for patients to re-engage in enjoyable activities to help relieve depressive symptoms. Relaxation techniques include progressive muscle relaxation, diaphragmatic breathing, and relaxation imagery. A meta-analysis did not show this to be superior to psychotherapy, but it can be used as an adjunct therapy.[48]

Depression and the reproductive life cycle

There are key phases in a woman's life that are associated with change in mood and, thus, with higher risk for depressive symptoms. These have been hypothesized to be associated with hormonal changes as well as concurrent role transitions.

Premenstrual dysphoric disorder

Premenstrual dysphoric disorder (PMDD) and premenstrual syndrome (PMS) are characterized by both physical and emotional symptoms which occur consistently during the end of the luteal phase and which interfere with the patient's life. As these symptoms can be quite distressing, it is important to accurately diagnose these syndromes and treat them appropriately. In addition, it is important to rule out these conditions before diagnosing major depressive episode.

The American Congress of Obstetricians and Gynecologists (ACOG) defines PMS as the presence of at least one symptom (physical or psychological) which occurs during the luteal phase of the cycle and leads to significant impairment in daily functioning. PMDD is defined by DSM-5 criteria:[30]

One or more of the following symptoms must be present:

1. mood swings, sudden sadness, increased sensitivity to rejection
2. anger, irritability
3. sense of hopelessness, depressed mood, self-critical thoughts
4. tension, anxiety, feeling on edge

and one or more of the following symptoms must be present to reach a total of five symptoms overall:

1. difficulty concentrating
2. change in appetite, food cravings, overeating
3. diminished interest in usual activities
4. easy fatigability, decreased energy
5. feeling overwhelmed, or out of control
6. breast tenderness, bloating, weight gain, or joint/muscles aches
7. sleeping too much or not sleeping enough

The treatments for PMS and PMDD consist of both pharmacologic and nonpharmacologic options. For patients with mild symptoms, nonpharmacologic treatments can be advised, although it is still unclear if the benefit of most of these is due to placebo effect. Limited evidence suggests that exercise [49, 50] as well as relaxation techniques [51] may help patients with mild symptoms.

For those with more significant symptoms, medication therapy is recommended. First-line therapy is typically an SSRI which has been shown to be effective.[52, 53] Medications approved by the US Food and Drug Administration (FDA) include sertraline, fluoxetine, and paroxetine-controlled release. SSRI therapy can be administered daily or only during the luteal phase (beginning on day 14 and continuing until menses begins). Although luteal phase treatment can decrease side effects, it has been reported to be less effective than daily therapy.[54]

Pregnancy and postpartum

Although the focus of this chapter is not obstetrical care, it is important to recognize the risks of preexisting depression on future pregnancies and the postpartum period as well as the risk of a subsequent major depressive episode after diagnosis of postpartum depression.

About 9%–16% of women will develop postpartum depression. Those who have previously suffered from postpartum depression have a 40% risk of developing postpartum depression with a subsequent pregnancy. There are numerous risk factors for prenatal and postpartum depression, but in a variety of studies, the most significant risk is a past history of depression.[55, 56] In addition, those with a history of postpartum depression have an increased risk of developing depression over her lifetime.

Perimenopause

It is common to see increased depressive symptoms at times of transition, and depression associated with menopause is typically linked to vasomotor symptoms. Depression in the perimenopausal period is diagnosed and treated in a similar manner to depression in premenopausal patients. Women can be treated with estrogen replacement as appropriate to improve vasomotor symptoms. However, major depression is still optimally treated with antidepressants and/or psychotherapy.

Physician and legal responsibility

It is well understood by providers that patient confidentiality can be violated if there are concerns that the patient is a threat to herself or to others. However, many practitioners are still concerned about their ability to accurately interpret a suicide threat. The law recognizes that suicide is the result of a complicated intersection of factors, and, as such, there are no criteria for prediction.[57] In evaluating a patient for suicidality, the expected standard of care is based on the concept of "foreseeability." This includes whether the provider took a thorough history, identified applicable risk factors, and offered a treatment plan to prevent a completed suicide.[58]

Concluding remarks

Depression is common and treatable. With such a large percentage of women affected by depression, it is paramount that ob-gyn providers play an active role in identifying patients at risk, diagnosis, and initiation of treatment. Patients with depression should be assessed for suicide risk and offered treatment or referral to a specialist as needed.

References

1. Kessler RC. Epidemiology of women and depression. *J Affect Disord.* 2003 Mar;**74**(1):5–13.
2. Kessler RC, McGonagle KA, Zhao S, et al. Lifetime and 12-month prevalence of DSM-III-R psychiatric disorders in the United States: results from the National Comorbidity Survey. *Arch Gen Psychiatry.* 1994 Jan;**51** (1):8–19.
3. Gavin NI, Gaynes BN, Lohr KN, et al. Perinatal depression: a systematic review of prevalence and incidence. *Obstet Gynecol.* 2005 Nov;**106**(5 Pt 1):1071–83.
4. Cohen LS, Soares CN, Vitonis AF, et al. Risk for new onset of depression during the menopausal transition: the Harvard study of moods and cycles. *Arch Gen Psychiatry.* 2006 Apr;**63**(4):385–90.
5. Scholle SH, Kelleher K. Assessing primary care performance in an obstetrics/gynecology clinic. *Women Health.* 2003;**37**(1):15–30.
6. Scholle SH, Chang JC, Harman J, McNeil M. Trends in women's health services by type of physician seen: data from the 1985 and 1997–98 NAMCS. *Womens Health Issues.* 2002 Aug;**12**(4):165–77.
7. Spitzer RL, Williams JB, Kroenke K, et al. Validity and utility of the PRIME-MD patient health questionnaire in assessment of 3000 obstetric-gynecologic patients: the PRIME-MD Patient Health Questionnaire Obstetrics-Gynecology Study. *Am J Obstet Gynecol.* 2000 Sep;**183**(3):759–69.
8. Smith MV, Rosenheck RA, Cavaleri MA, et al. Screening for and detection of depression, panic disorder, and PTSD in public-sector obstetric clinics. *Psychiatr Serv.* 2004 Apr;**55**(4):407–14.
9. Blumenthal SJ, Kupfer DJ, eds. *Suicide over the Life Cycle: Risk Factors, Assessment, and Treatment of*

Suicidal Patients. Washington, DC: American Psychiatric Association; 1990.

10. Chisholm D. The economic costs of depression. In: Dawson A, Tylee A, eds. *Depression: Social and Economic Timebomb*. London: BMJ Books; 2001.
11. Murray CJ, Lopez AD. Evidence-based health policy – lessons from the Global Burden of Disease Study. *Science*. 1996;**274**(5288):740–3.
12. Rucker L, Frye EB, Cygan RW. Feasibility and usefulness of depression screening in medical outpatients. *Arch Intern Med*. 1986 Apr;**146**(4):729–31.
13. Zung WW. The role of rating scales in the identification and management of the depressed patient in the primary care setting. *J Clin Psychiatry*. 1990 Jun;**51**(Suppl):72–6.
14. Schade CP, Jones ER, Wittlin BJ. A ten-year review of the validity and clinical utility of depression screening. *Psychiatr Serv*. 1998 Jan;**49**(1):55–61.
15. O'Connor EA, Whitlock EP, Gaynes B, Beil TL. Screening for Depression in Adults and Older Adults in Primary Care: An Updated Systematic Review [Internet]. Rockville, MD: Agency for Healthcare Research and Quality (US); 2009 [cited 2014 Aug 29]. Available from: www.ncbi.nlm.nih.gov/books/NBK36403. Accessed 12 Dec 2015.
16. US Preventive Services Task Force. Screening for depression in adults: summary of the evidence. *Ann Intern Med*. 2002;**136**:765–76.
17. Mitchell AJ, Coyne JC. Do ultra-short screening instruments accurately detect depression in primary care? A pooled analysis and meta-analysis of 22 studies. *Br J Gen Pract*. 2007 Feb;**57**(535):144–51.
18. Arroll B, Khin N, Kerse N. Screening for depression in primary care with two verbally asked questions: cross sectional study. *BMJ*. 2003 Nov 15;**327**(7424):1144–6.
19. Whooley MA, Avins AL, Miranda J, Browner WS. Case-finding instruments for depression: two questions are as good as many. *J Gen Intern Med*. 1997 Jul;**12**(7):439–45.
20. Richardson LP, Rockhill C, Russo JE, et al. Evaluation of the PHQ-2 as a brief screen for detecting major depression among adolescents. *Pediatrics*. 2010 May;**125**(5):e1097–1103.
21. Nease DE Jr, Maloin JM. Depression screening: a practical strategy. *J Fam Pract*. 2003;**52**(2):118–24.
22. Kirmayer LJ, Robbins JM, Dworkind M, Yaffe MJ. Somatization and the recognition of depression and anxiety in primary care. *Am J Psychiatry*. 1993 May;**150**(5):734–41.
23. Mueller TI, Leon AC, Keller MB, et al. Recurrence after recovery from major depressive disorder during 15 years of observational follow-up. *Am J Psychiatry*. 1999 Jul;**156**(7):1000–6.
24. Keller MB, Lavori PW, Rice J, et al. The persistent risk of chronicity in recurrent episodes of nonbipolar major depressive disorder: a prospective follow-up. *Am J Psychiatry*. 1986 Jan;**143**(1):24–8.
25. Ford DE, Mead LA, Chang PP, et al. Depression is a risk factor for coronary artery disease in men: the precursors study. *Arch Intern Med*. 1998 Jul 13;**158**(13):1422–6.
26. Ciechanowski PS, Katon WJ, Russo JE. Depression and diabetes: impact of depressive symptoms on adherence, function, and costs. *Arch Intern Med*. 2000;**160**(21):3278–85.
27. Robinson RG, Bolduc PL, Price TR. Two-year longitudinal study of poststroke mood disorders: diagnosis and outcome at one and two years. *Stroke*. 1987;**18**(5):837–43.
28. Taylor CB, Youngblood ME, Catellier D, et al.; ENRICHD Investigators. Effects of antidepressant medication on morbidity and mortality in depressed patients after myocardial infarction. *Arch Gen Psychiatry*. 2005;**62**(7):792–8.
29. Rihmer Z, Dome P, Gonda X. The role of general practitioners in prevention of depression-related suicides. *Neuropsychopharmacol Hung*. 2012 Dec;**14**(4):245–51.
30. American Psychiatric Association. *Diagnostic and Statistical Manual of Mental Disorders*. 5th ed., text revision. Washington, DC: American Psychiatric Association; 2013.
31. LaRocco-Cockburn A, Melville J, Bell M, Katon W. Depression screening attitudes and practices among obstetrician-gynecologists. *Obstet Gynecol*. 2003 May;**101**(5 Pt 1):892–8.
32. Kelly R, Zatzick D, Anders T. The detection and treatment of psychiatric disorders and substance use among pregnant women cared for in obstetrics. *Am J Psychiatry*. 2001 Feb;**158**(2):213–19.
33. Cuijpers P, Dekker J, Hollon SD, Andersson G. Adding psychotherapy to pharmacotherapy in the treatment of depressive disorders in adults: a meta-analysis. *J Clin Psychiatry*. 2009 Sep;**70**(9):1219–29.
34. Arroll B, Macgillivray S, Ogston S, et al. Efficacy and tolerability of tricyclic antidepressants and SSRIs compared with placebo for treatment of depression in primary care: a meta-analysis. *Ann Fam Med*. 2005;**3**(5):449–56.
35. Trivedi MH, Rush AJ, Wisniewski SR, et al.; STAR*D Study Team. Evaluation of outcomes with citalopram for depression using measurement-based care in STAR*D: implications for clinical practice. *Am J Psychiatry*. 2006;**163**(1):28–40.
36. American Psychiatric Association: *Practice Guideline for the Treatment of Patients with Major Depressive Disorder*, 3rd ed. Washington, DC: American Psychiatric Association; 2010.

37. Quitkin FM, Petkova E, McGrath PJ, et al. When should a trial of fluoxetine for major depression be declared failed? *Am J Psychiatry*. 2003 Apr;**160**(4): 734–40.

38. Posternak MA, Baer L, Nierenberg AA, Fava M. Response rates to fluoxetine in subjects who initially show no improvement. *J Clin Psychiatry*. 2011 Jul;**72** (7):949–54.

39. Hu XH, Bull SA, Hunkeler EM, et al. Incidence and duration of side effects and those rated as bothersome with selective serotonin reuptake inhibitor treatment for depression: patient report versus physician estimate. *J Clin Psychiatry*. 2004 Jul;**65**(7):959–65.

40. Nierenberg AA, Fava M, Trivedi MH, et al. A comparison of lithium and T(3) augmentation following two failed medication treatments for depression: a STAR*D report. *Am J Psychiatry*. 2006 Sep;**163**(9):1519–30; quiz 1665.

41. Clayton AH, Gillespie EH. Bupropion. In: Schatzberg AF, Nemeroff CB, eds. *The American Psychiatric Publishing Textbook of Psychopharmacology*, 4th ed. Washington, DC: American Psychiatric Publishing, Inc.; 2009.

42. Montgomery SA. Safety of mirtazapine: a review. *Int Clin Psychopharmacol*. 1995 Dec;**10**(Suppl 4):37–45.

43. Parikh SV, Segal ZV, Grigoriadis S, et al. Canadian Network for Mood and Anxiety Treatments (CANMAT) clinical guidelines for the management of major depressive disorder in adults. II. Psychotherapy alone or in combination with antidepressant medication. *J Affect Disord*. 2009 Oct;**117**(Suppl 1):S15–25.

44. Churchill R, Moore THM, Furukawa TA, et al. "Third wave" cognitive and behavioural therapies versus treatment as usual for depression. *Cochrane Database Syst Rev*. 2013;**10**:CD008705.

45. Cuijpers P, Geraedts AS, van Oppen P, et al. Interpersonal psychotherapy for depression: a meta-analysis. *Am J Psychiatry*. 2011 Jun;**168**(6):581–92.

46. Cooney GM, Dwan K, Greig CA, et al. Exercise for depression. *Cochrane Database Syst Rev*. 2013;**9**: CD004366.

47. Chalder M, Wiles NJ, Campbell J, et al. Facilitated physical activity as a treatment for depressed adults: randomised controlled trial. *BMJ*. 2012;**344**:e2758.

48. Jorm AF, Morgan AJ, Hetrick SE. Relaxation for depression. *Cochrane Database Syst Rev*. 2008;**4**: CD007142.

49. Steege JF, Blumenthal JA. The effects of aerobic exercise on premenstrual symptoms in middle-aged women: a preliminary study. *J Psychosom Res*. 1993;**37** (2):127–33.

50. Aganoff JA, Boyle GJ. Aerobic exercise, mood states and menstrual cycle symptoms. *J Psychosom Res*. 1994 Apr;**38**(3):183–92.

51. Goodale IL, Domar AD, Benson H. Alleviation of premenstrual syndrome symptoms with the relaxation response. *Obstet Gynecol*. 1990 Apr;**75**(4):649–55.

52. Stone AB, Pearlstein TB, Brown WA. Fluoxetine in the treatment of late luteal phase dysphoric disorder. *J Clin Psychiatry*. 1991 Jul;**52**(7):290–3.

53. Wood SH, Mortola JF, Chan YF, et al. Treatment of premenstrual syndrome with fluoxetine: a double-blind, placebo-controlled, crossover study. *Obstet Gynecol*. 1992 Sep;**80**(3 Pt 1):339–44.

54. Shah NR, Jones JB, Aperi J, et al. Selective serotonin reuptake inhibitors for premenstrual syndrome and premenstrual dysphoric disorder: a meta-analysis. *Obstet Gynecol*. 2008 May;**111**(5):1175–82.

55. Beck CT. Predictors of postpartum depression: an update. *Nurs Res*. 2001 Oct;**50**(5):275–85.

56. Nonacs R, Cohen LS. Postpartum mood disorders: diagnosis and treatment guidelines. *J Clin Psychiatry*. 1998;**59**(Suppl 2):34–40.

57. Simon RI. *Psychiatry and Law for Clinicians*. Washington, DC: American Psychiatric Press; 1992.

58. Swartz M. Malpractice liability for suicide. Clinical, legal, and rhetorical dimensions. *Psychiatric Forum*. 1988;**14**(1):45–53.

Chapter

38

Eating disorders

Mark Schnee

Introduction

Eating disorders are among the most common psychiatric disorders affecting young women.[1] Most notably, anorexia nervosa and bulimia nervosa are significant causes of morbidity and mortality among adolescent and adult females. Because many of these women suffer in silence, the diagnosis of eating disorders can be elusive, and more than half of all cases go undetected.[2] These conditions are associated with serious medical and psychological consequences, including death, depression, osteoporosis, developmental and growth delay, and family disruption. A Finnish study determined that reproductive outcomes are adversely compromised with lower pregnancy and childbirth rates noted in women with eating disorders compared to controls.[3] Early detection and prompt treatment are essential for improving outcomes in what can become a chronic and debilitating condition.[4] Simple screening questions and key physical findings such as low body mass index (BMI), amenorrhea, bradycardia, gastrointestinal disturbances, changes in skin and dentition can lead to the detection of eating disorders.

Gynecologists and other women's health providers are in ideal positions to screen for these problems and be part of a multidisciplinary team; menstrual cycle irregularities, osteoporosis, infertility, and pregnancy related risk factors are all affected by eating disorders.

The *American Psychiatric Association's Diagnostic and Statistical Manual*, Fifth Edition (DSM-5), identifies the feeding and eating disorders listed in Table 38-1.[5]

The principal eating disorders that will be discussed in this chapter are anorexia nervosa, bulimia nervosa, and binge-eating disorder. The core features of both anorexia nervosa and bulimia nervosa are preoccupation with weight gain and excessive self-evaluation of body weight and shape. These disorders occur 10–20 times more often in females than males, especially females aged 15 to 24.[6] It is estimated that 4% of adolescent girls have an eating disorder of which 0.3% have anorexia nervosa. Anorexia nervosa peaks at age 17 to 18 years old. Bulimia nervosa typically has a later onset but is more prevalent than anorexia nervosa.[7] The lifetime prevalence rate of anorexia nervosa has been estimated to be between 0.5% and 3.7%.[8] These entities are psychiatric disorders that have physical complications. Anorexia nervosa has the highest mortality rate of any of the psychiatric diagnoses; the patients die from suicide or a complication of the eating disorder such as an arrhythmia.[9] Therefore, initiation of therapy is essential to facilitate a reduction in associated health risks to the gynecologic patient.

Table 38-1 List of eating disorders

- Pica
- Rumination disorder
- Avoidant/restrictive food intake disorder
- Anorexia nervosa
- Bulimia nervosa
- Binge-eating disorder
- Other specified feeding or eating disorder
- Unspecified feeding or eating disorder

Anorexia nervosa

The three core essential features of anorexia nervosa are:

- persistent food restriction that leads to an abnormally low body weight
- intense fear of gaining weight and becoming fat or persistent behavior that interferes with weight gain
- disturbance in self-perceived weight or shape

Anorexia nervosa characteristics are described in Table 38-2. Psychological and behavioral signs and

Office Care of Women, ed. Martin E. Olsen and Botros Rizk. Published by Cambridge University Press.

Table 38-2 Anorexia nervosa characteristics

- Body weight significantly lower than what is expected for age, sex, and height
- Intense fear of gaining weight
- Body image distortion
- Amenorrhea no longer included in DSM-5
- Subtypes: restrictive and binge/purge

symptoms that are associated with anorexia nervosa are listed in Table 38-3.

The individual with anorexia nervosa maintains a significantly low body weight defined as a weight that is less than that set at a minimally normal level for age, sex, developmental trajectory, and physical health. For adults, the Centers for Disease Control and Prevention (CDC) and the World Health Organization (WHO) have set the lower limit of normal body weight as a BMI of 18.5 kg/m^2.

The BMI percentiles used to determine level of current severity are as follows:

Mild: BMI 17 kg/m^2 –18.49 kg/m^2

Moderate: BMI 16 kg/m^2–16.99 kg/m^2

Severe: BMI 15 kg/m^2–15.99 kg/m^2

Extreme: BMI <15 kg/m^2

Anorexia nervosa has two subtypes: restricting type and binge-eating/purging type. Individuals with the restricting type have not engaged in recurrent binge or purging behavior for the past three months with weight loss accomplished primarily through fasting, dieting, and/or excessive exercise. On the other hand, the binge-eating/purging subtype has engaged in recurrent episodes binge-eating or purging (i.e., self-induced vomiting or the misuse of laxatives, diuretics, or enemas) during the past three months.

Table 38-3 Anorexia nervosa signs and symptoms

- Preoccupation with thoughts of food
- Avoidance of fatty foods
- Overusing artificial sweeteners
- Overestimating caloric content consumed
- Avoidance of social eating (prefer eating in their room)
- Hiding dishes, food wrappers, or containers (closet, car trunk, backpack)
- Secret eating (eat late at night)
- Compulsive exercise patterns (e.g., set daily running distance or swimming specific number of lapses in the pool)
- Insomnia
- Reduced libido
- Always feeling cold
- Limited social spontaneity (e.g., resists changes in schedule or environment)
- Body checking: repeated weighing, mirror gazing, measuring the size of body parts
- Wear lose fitting clothing (e.g., sweat shirts, sweaters, and baggy pants)
- Minimize or deny symptom severity
- Inhibited expression of emotions (e.g., becomes sad if feels happy)
- Misuse of laxatives, diuretics, or diet pills
- Preoccupation with insatiable desire to be thin

Bulimia nervosa

Core essential features of bulimia nervosa are:

- recurrent episodes of binge eating
- recurrent inappropriate compensatory behaviors to prevent weight gain
- binge eating and inappropriate compensatory behaviors must occur, on average, at least once per week for three months
- self-evaluation that is unduly influenced by body shape and weight

Inappropriate compensatory behaviors to prevent weight gain include self-induced vomiting; misuse of laxatives, diuretics, or other medications; fasting; or an excessive amount of exercise.

As defined in the DSM-5, an episode of binge eating is characterized by both of the following: (1) the individual eats in a discrete period of time, usually less than two hours, an amount of food that is definitely larger than what most individuals would consume in a similar period of time under similar circumstance; (2) the individual senses a lack of control over eating during the episode. An indicator of loss of control is characterized by the inability to refrain from eating or to stop once the binge has started. A single episode of binge eating is not restricted to one setting. For example, it can begin in one location and continue to another.

The minimum level of severity is based on the frequency of inappropriate compensatory behaviors per week.

Mild: an average of 1–3 episodes of inappropriate compensatory behaviors per week

Moderate: an average of 4–7 episodes of inappropriate compensatory behaviors per week

Table 38-4 Bulimia nervosa characteristics

- Recurrent episodes of binge eating (eating more food than normal in a two-hour period with lack of control)
- Recurrent inappropriate compensatory behaviors to prevent weight gain such as vomiting, laxative abuse, diuretics, enemas, or excessive exercise
- Binge and purge behaviors occur at least once a week for three months
- Self-evaluation is influenced by body shape and weight
- Can be purging or nonpurging type (fasting, exercise)

Severe: an average of 8–13 episodes of inappropriate compensatory behaviors per week

Extreme: 14 or more episodes of inappropriate compensatory behaviors per week

Individuals with bulimia nervosa place undue importance on body shape or weight in their self-evaluation. Individuals with this disorder share some resemblance to anorexia nervosa by their fear of gaining weight, a desire to lose weight, or in their level of dissatisfaction with their appearance. However, adult individuals with bulimia nervosa typically are within the range with a BMI $\geq$18.5 kg/m^2–30 kg/m^2. Bulimia nervosa can occur, although uncommon, in obese individuals. Bulimic individuals typically restrict their diet to low-calorie foods and avoid foods that they perceive as fattening or that trigger a binge.

Bulimia nervosa characteristics are described in Table 38-4.

Binge-eating disorder

The essential feature of a binge-eating disorder is recurrent episodes of binge eating. Each episode is characterized by consuming an amount of food within two hours that exceeds a normal amount that is usually consumed in a similar time period under similar circumstances. A binge-eating episode is associated with at least three of the following:

- eating more rapidly than a normal rate
- eating until uncomfortably full
- consuming large amount of food when not actually physically hungry
- eating alone due to an embarrassed feeling about the quantity of food being eaten
- feelings of disgust, depression, or guilt after the binge episode

Additionally, the affected individual demonstrates marked distress regarding the presence of binge eating. The binge eating occurs on average at least once a week for three months. As opposed to bulimia nervosa, the binge eating is not associated with a recurrent use of an inappropriate compensatory behavior. The frequency of binge eating episodes determines the level of security.

Mild: 1–3 binge eating episodes per week

Moderate: 4–7 binge episodes per week

Severe: 8–13 binge episodes per week

Extreme: 14 or more binge episodes per week

Binge-eating disorder occurs in normal-weight, overweight, and obese individuals. The disorder is characterized by individuals consuming more calories and has greater functional impairment, more subjective distress, and psychiatric comorbidity than obese individuals who do not engage in recurrent binge eating.

Common comorbid disorders include depression, anxiety, and bipolar disorders and to a lesser extent substance abuse. Overvaluation of body weight and shape are higher in obese individuals with the disorder than those without the disorder. The psychiatric component is linked to the severity of binge eating and not the degree of obesity. Remission rates and successful treatment outcomes are higher for individuals with the binge-eating disorder. Crossover from binge-eating disorder to other eating disorders is generally not felt to be common,[5] but in one study, crossover from binge eating to bulimia nervosa was high.[10]

Epidemiology

The estimated lifetime prevalence of anorexia nervosa in women is 0.4%, whereas bulimia nervosa is nearly 1.5% and binge eating is estimated to be 1.6%.[5]

Data from the National Comorbidity Replication Survey indicated the median age of onset is 12–13 years old. Teenagers reported significant rates of comorbidity, as well as mental impairment and suicidal ideation.[11]

Predisposed individuals may initially engage in eating disorder behaviors at times of profound body changes, such as those associated with puberty and pregnancy, or of significant life change, such as moving away or starting college. Subtle criticism of weight by parents, peers, boyfriends, coaches, or teachers also can trigger the onset of an eating disorder in a susceptible individual.

Although many are initiated by dieting behavior, eating disorders become self-sustained because they are related to a desperate need for control when life is out of harmony.

Pathogenesis

The most potent risk factor for developing an eating disorder is female gender. The degree of association that is attributed to biological versus social factors is not clear. Twin and family studies indicate that anorexia nervosa, bulimia nervosa, and binge-eating disorder are complex genetic diseases, and each disorder has an estimated heritability range between 50% and 83%.[12–14] A study of 133 families with at least one bulimia nervosa proband provided evidence of significant linkage on chromosome 10p.[15] Additionally, a linkage analysis study of 192 families with anorexia nervosa suggested evidence for the presence of an anorexia nervosa susceptibility locus on chromosome 1p.[16]

Recent MRI studies demonstrated an increased gray matter volume of the medial orbitofrontal cortex (gyrus rectus) in women with restrictive-type anorexia nervosa and those with bulimia nervosa.[17] Orbitofrontal cortex function is associated with a value attributed to food stimuli and to food avoidance.[18, 19] It has been postulated that a larger gyrus rectus in eating disorders is associated with stronger sensory experience of food stimuli, which may be experienced as overwhelming; this then triggers food avoidance.[18, 20] The underlying cause for an increased gyrus rectus volume is unclear. Analyses also indicated other morphologic differences.

The antero-ventral insula gray matter volume was increased on the right side in anorexia nervosa and on the left side in the bulimia nervosa group compared to the control group. The right anterior insula has been recognized in being associated with self -recognition and interoceptive awareness.[21, 22] The fixed perception of being fat while severely underweight in anorexia nervosa could theoretically be related to the right-sided increased anterior ventral insula volume and dysfunction.[23] But, activation of the left anterior ventral insula is related to gastric distention and self-reported fullness.[24] Therefore, an altered anterior insula interferes with the normal interoception in bulimia nervosa, which contributes to a reduced ability to sense satiation and trigger the urge to purge after excessive food intake and the guilt experienced over eating. To summarize, both anorexia nervosa and bulimia nervosa have altered gray matter volume in the gyrus rectus that may be a trait – related structural abnormality.

Another biologic risk factor that has been shown to put female offspring at a higher risk for bulimia nervosa is that of in utero exposure to excessive androgen. Fetal exposure to androgen excess has been attributed to the subsequent development of polycystic ovarian syndrome which is a highly comorbid condition with binge eating and bulimia nervosa.[25] Eating disorders are not of the individual's own free will, although dieting often precedes it. For some vulnerable individuals, the weight loss originated in an attempt to improve performance or at the suggestion of a coach, but unfortunately, the behaviors became compulsive or excessive. That individual is then caught up in this dilemma and spirals out of control.

Medical complications

Eating disorders have been shown to adversely affect every organ system of the human body. The numerous medical complications of anorexia nervosa are a direct result of caloric restriction and weight loss. Starvation causes protein and fat catabolism that leads to decreased cellular volume and atrophic changes of the heart, brain, liver, intestines, kidneys, and muscles. Some of these complications are reversible with weight gain, but bone mineral density loss is not totally reversed.[26]

Purging leads to most medical complications identified in the patient with bulimia nervosa.

Dermatologic

Dermatologic changes in patients with severe anorexia nervosa include the development of xerosis (dry scaly skin) on the back and arms due to reduced sebaceous gland secretion. It has been found in 97% of patients with anorexia nervosa.[27] Lanugo hair is frequently seen on the back, abdomen, and forearms. This is fine hair growth that serves to conserve heat. Carotenoderma or a yellowish-orange skin discoloration develops as a result of elevated serum carotene levels from increased carotenoid-rich vegetable consumption. Other skin changes of eating disorders include acne, telogen effluvium (hair loss), hyperpigmentation, seborrheic dermatitis, acrocyanosis, paronychia, pruritus, abdominal striae distensae, poor skin turgor, and slow wound healing. Patients with bulimia nervosa frequently develop the Russell's sign or a callus on the dorsum of the knuckles from the pressure of the teeth pressing against the skin due to the self-induced vomiting. They may also demonstrate scars from self-injurious behavior such as cutting or burning.[28]

Neurologic

Neurological issues can manifest as seizure activity triggered by electrolyte abnormalities in patients who purge. Cerebellar atrophy, enlarged cortical sulci, and ventriculomegaly are evident on neuroimaging in patients with anorexia nervosa compared to controls.[29]

Cardiovascular

Cardiovascular complications of eating disorders, especially anorexia nervosa, are related to changes in the heart itself. Structural changes manifest as decreased cardiac mass, decreased cardiac chamber volume, and the development of mitral valve prolapse in 20% of anorexic patients. These changes lead to decreased cardiac output, reduced exercise capacity, fatigue, and orthostatic hypotension. There are no known cases of mitral regurgitation that have required mitral valve surgery. With refeeding and weight gain in the patient, the compromised heart regains mass and its cardiac volume normalizes over months.[30, 31] Pericardial effusion has been reported in 22% of adolescent patients with anorexia nervosa. Likewise, within three months of refeeding, the pericardial effusions disappeared in 62% of patients.

Bradycardia with heart rates between 25 and 60 beats per minute (bpm) have been found in anorexia nervosa. The bradycardia is an adaptive compensatory response to conserve energy.[32] Hospitalization is recommended for heart rates less than 40 bpm. Similarly, bradycardia and orthostatic pulse changes generally resolve once body weight is restored to an amount greater than 80% of ideal body weight.[33]

Gastrointestinal

Gastroparesis and constipation are common complications of anorexia nervosa. Other gastrointestinal complications include elevated liver functions (aspartate aminotransferase and alanine aminotransferase alkaline phosphatase and bilirubin), superior mesenteric artery syndrome, and pancreatitis. Patients often have dental caries and decalcification of the teeth caused by exposure to gastric acid in patients with chronic vomiting (perimylolysis), parotitis (sialadenosis), pancreatitis, and gastroesophageal reflux disease or Mallory-Weiss tears. Severe constipation or laxative dependence syndrome is caused by damage to the myenteric plexus by stimulant laxative abuse.[34]

Endocrine

Anorectics have abnormal levels of multiple hormones including low levels of gonadotropin-releasing hormone (GnRH), luteinizing hormone (LH), follicle-stimulating hormone (FSH), insulin-like growth factor 1 (IGF-1), free testosterone, triiodothyroxine (T3), and thyroxine (T4). Growth hormone and cortisol are increased in anorectic patients. The hypothalamus is essentially in starvation mode; reduced secretion of GnRH leads to anovulation and a functional hypothalamic amenorrhea. Two hormones that have a major role in the regulation of food intake and body weight are leptin and ghrelin. Leptin, which is the product of the ob gene (located at 7q31.3) and is produced mainly in adipose tissue, is a mediator for long-term regulation of energy balance by suppressing food intake and by stimulation of the metabolic rate. Ghrelin is secreted from the stomach and functions as an appetite-stimulator. Serum leptin levels are reduced in association with low body weight and percent body fat in subjects with anorexia nervosa compared to normal controls. Leptin levels were determined to correlate highly with weight, percent body fat, and IGF-I in subjects with anorexia nervosa,[35] suggesting that the physiological regulation of leptin is maintained in relation to nutritional status even at an extreme of low weight and body fat.[36]

Thyroid abnormalities such as euthyroid hypothroxinemia may develop. It is characterized by normal thyroid-stimulating hormone (TSH) level and normal to decreased serum levels of thyroxine (T4) and triiodothyronine (T3). Thyroid replacement is not indicated.

Reproductive cycle

Eating disorders are associated with fertility issues, unplanned pregnancies, and increased risk of induced and spontaneous abortions.

Bulimia nervosa was shown to be associated with an increased risk for induced abortion compared to controls, but higher rates of spontaneous abortion were noted in patients with binge-eating disorders.[3]

In anorexia nervosa, the pulsatile secretion of GnRH is reduced, which frequently leads to secondary amenorrhea and infertility. It has been determined that a weight loss of approximately 15% of normal body weight disrupts the menstrual cycle in many women. This may be compounded by the weight loss from excessive exercise commonly seen in anorectic patients. Fortunately, the menstrual cycle resumes functioning when the patient has attained 90% her ideal body weight. But, amenorrhea can persist in 10%–30% of patients despite gaining weight due to ongoing abnormal eating behaviors such as purging or excessive exercise.[37] Female athletes with eating disorders who also have amenorrhea and low bone mineral density are commonly long distant runners, gymnasts, figure skaters, or ballet dancers. They are at a high risk for stress fractures secondary to the hypoestrogenemia and intense physical activity.

Osteoporosis

Studies in anorexia nervosa subjects have demonstrated that osteoporosis develops in nearly 34% and places the patient at a higher fracture risk.[38] The decreased bone mineral density is primarily identified in trabecular bone and the lumbar spine, proximal femur, and distal radius.[39] The severity of the osteoporosis correlates with the lean body mass and the duration of amenorrhea. Studies have shown that a BMI of 15 kg/m^2 and amenorrhea for at least six months leads to bone loss.[40] Bone mineral density should be measured in anorectic patients with amenorrhea for six months or more and then every two years. The findings may have the benefit of promoting a positive behavioral change and seek treatment for anorexia nervosa. Weight gain and the restoration of menstrual function are the current best treatment options for the development of decreased bone mineral density.[41]

Renal

Electrolyte abnormalities are complications secondary to purging induced by vomiting, laxatives, and diuretics. Through vomiting, a metabolic alkalosis results from hydrogen, chloride, and potassium loss. Laxative abuse leads to losses of potassium and bicarbonate ions in the stool, resulting in hypokalemic, nonanion gap metabolic acidosis. Diuretic abuse can result in hypokalemic metabolic alkalosis through renal losses of potassium and hydrogen ions. Severe hypokalemia can lead to cardiac arrhythmias, muscle weakness, memory impairment, and confusion.[42] Low creatinine, secondary to muscle wasting, is associated with restrictive anorexia nervosa.[43] Electrolyte abnormalities typically correct after discontinuing purging behaviors.

Screening tool

Of the eating disorders, anorexia nervosa has the highest mortality rate as compared to other mental illnesses. The mortality rate attributed to anorexia nervosa is 12 times higher than the death rate associated with all other causes of death for females 15–24 years old. Nearly 50% of those suffering from it meet the criteria for depression.[44] Female athletes in weight-dependent sports such as gymnastics, ballet, and figure skating are at a higher risk.[45] Patients in high-risk categories for eating disorders should be screened during routine gynecological office visits.

A screening tool that has been developed to identify patients with an eating disorder is the SCOFF questionnaire. It consists of five questions (see Box 38-1). It has a sensitivity of 84.6% and a specificity of 89.6%.[46]

Management and prognosis

When a patient with an eating disorder is identified, the physician must then assemble a team to care for the patient. The team should include a psychotherapist, nutritionist, internist, and psychiatrist. A gynecologist should not manage all areas of the patient's condition. Because stable remission in eating disorders is often low and treatment is time consuming, the physician often feels excessively concerned,

BOX 38-1 SCOFF questionnaire

- Do you make yourself Sick because you feel uncomfortably full?
- Do you worry you have lost Control over how much you eat?
- Have you recently lost more than One stone (14 lb or 6.35 kg) in a three-month period?
- Do you believe yourself to be Fat when others say you are too thin?
- Would you say that Food dominates your life?
Scoring: Each "yes" = 1 point. A score of 2 points indicates a likely diagnosis of anorexia nervosa.

exhausted, and frustrated. The women's health provider must remember to remain firm yet compassionate and encourage the patient to become an active participant in her own recovery effort. Furthermore, the physician must be aware of the pro-eating disorder websites and communities that have emerged, wherein users can find material to support the progression of eating disorders. The patient should be counseled to avoid these websites at all costs. These groups are known as Pro-Ana (pro-anorexia), Pro-Mia (pro-bulimia), and Pro-ED (pro-eating disorder).[47] These are dangerous websites that serve only to reinforce an eating disorder by demonstrating explicit methods on how to avoid hunger pangs, to misled health-care providers, and suggest new methods of purging.

Main general treatment goals are to restore and maintain a healthy nutritional status and formulate coping skills that deal with the underlying psychosocial issues that may have given rise to the eating disorder. Unfortunately, treatment resistance is an omnipresent frustration for many individuals with an eating disorder. In anorexia nervosa, the severity of the core features of the preoccupations with body image, weight gain, eating, and exercise predicts a greater resistance for seeking treatment. Furthermore, an anxiety disorder coupled with perfectionism may confer greater treatment resistance for anorexics. With bulimia nervosa, individuals are less resistant to treatment, but treatment failures are related to body image concerns, depression, impulsivity, and severe diet restriction. For individuals afflicted with binge-eating disorders, childhood obesity often confers treatment failure.[48]

Current evidence for an effective pharmacologic or psychosocial treatment of anorexia nervosa is lacking based on a recent Cochrane review.[49] Prescribing selective serotonin reuptake inhibitors (SSRIs) such as fluoxetine to anorexic individuals immediately upon restoration of normal weight did not provide any substantial benefit in maintaining weight.[50]

Additionally, combined family-based therapy for those with anorexia nervosa was found to equally effective as compared to other forms of psychotherapy interventions,[51] but families with extreme overprotection or criticism have better outcomes with separated family therapy. Parents often become overly burdened by the behaviors and symptoms of a child with an eating disorder, and they should seek group educational interventions to help them cope.[52]

In contrast to anorexia nervosa, a 2009 Cochrane review provided evidence supporting cognitive behavioral therapy (CBT) in the treatment of bulimia nervosa and binging. CBT achieved an outcome of 37% cumulative binge-eating abstinence as compared to no treatment.[53] Additionally, SSRIs have been shown to reduce binge eating and vomiting and also to improve mood and anxiety symptoms in individuals with bulimia nervosa. Specific SSRIs evaluated included fluoxetine, citalopram, sertraline, and fluvoxamine.[54]

Concluding remarks

Eating disorders develop in susceptible individuals due to a combination of certain personality traits, environmental factors, and a genetic predisposition. These illnesses are associated with a high rate of morbidity and mortality. The deleterious medical consequences of eating disorders can be irreversible or have later repercussions on health. Eating disorders adversely affect all human systems. Malnutrition is the primary cause for complications in patients with anorexia nervosa, whereas purging leads to most of the complications in bulimia nervosa. It is crucial for ob/gyn physicians and other women's health providers to help align these patients with appropriate additional health providers to combat this appalling disease process. Recovery is always possible; however, the patient ultimately has to attain a stable sense of self-control that is not manifested as weight control.

References

1. Kreipe RE, Birndorf SA. Eating disorders in adolescents and young adults. *Med Clin North Am* 2000; **84**:1027–49.
2. Becker AE, Grinspoon SK, Klibanski A, Herzog DB. Eating disorders. *N Engl J Med* 1999; **340**:1092–8.
3. Linna MS, Raevuori A, Haukka J, et al. Reproductive health outcomes in eating disorders. *Int J Eat Disord* 2013; **46**(8):826–33.
4. Herzog DB, Nussbaum KM, Marmor AK. Comorbidity and outcome in eating disorders. *Psychiatr Clin North Am* 1996; **19**:843–59.
5. American Psychiatric Association. Diagnostic and Statistical Manual of Mental Disorders, *5th edition.* Washington, DC: American Psychiatric Association; 2013: 329–54.
6. Mitchell AM, Bulik CM. Eating disorders and women's health: an update. *J Midwifery Women's Health* 2006; **51**(3):193.

7. Hoek HW. Incidence, prevalence and mortality of anorexia nervosa and other eating disorders. *Curr Opin Psychiatry* 2006; **19**(4):389.
8. Pearlstein T. Eating disorders and comorbidity. *Arch Womens Ment Health* 2002; **4**:67–78.
9. Fisher M. The course and outcome of eating disorders in adults and adolescents: a review. *Adolesc Med* 2003; **14**(1):149–58.
10. Allen KL, Bryne SM, Oddy WH, et al. DSM-IV-TR and DSM-5 eating disorders in adolescents: prevalence, stability, and psychological correlates in a population-based sample of male and female adolescents. *J Abnorm Psychol* 2013; **122**(3):720–32.
11. Swanson SA, Crow, SJ, Le Grange DL, et al. Prevalence and Correlates of Eating Disorders in Adolescents. *Arch Gen Psychiatry* 2011 July; **68**(7):714–23. doi:10.1001/archgenpsychiatry.2011.22. Epub 2011 Mar 7.
12. Javaras KN, Laird NM, Reichborn-Kjennerud T, et al. Familiality and heritability of binge eating disorder: results of a case–control family study and a twin study. *Int J Eat Disord* 2008; **41**:174–9.
13. Bulik CM, Slof-Op't Landt MC, van Furth EF. The genetics of anorexia nervosa. *Ann Rev Nutr* 2007; **27**:263–75.
14. Bulik CM, Tozzi F. The genetics of bulimia nervosa. *Drugs Today* 2004; **40**:741–9.
15. Bulik CM, Devlin B, Bacanu SA, et al. Significant linkage on chromosome 10p in families with bulimia nervosa. *Am J Hum Genet* 2003; **72**(1):200–7.
16. Grice DE, Halmi KA, Fichter MM, et al. Evidence for a susceptibility gene for anorexia nervosa on chromosome 1. *Am J Hum Genet* 2002; **70**(3):787–92.
17. Frank GK, Shott ME, Hagman JO, et al. Alterations in brain structures related to taste reward circuitry in ill and recovered anorexia nervosa and in bulimia nervosa. *Am J Pschiatry* 2013; **170**:1152–60.
18. Plassmann H, O'Douherty JP, Rangel A. Appetitive and aversive goal values are encoded in the medical orbitofrontal cortex at the time of decision making. *J Neurosci* 2010; **30**:10799–808.
19. Uher R, Murphy T, Brammer MJ, et al. Medial prefrontal cortex activity associated with symptom provocation in eating disorders. *Am J Psychiatry* 2004; **161**:1238–46.
20. Frank, GK, Reynolds JR, Shott ME, et al. Altered temporal difference learning in bulimia nervosa. *Biol Psychiatry* 2011; **37**: 2031–46.
21. Devue C, Collette F, Balteau E, et al. Here I am: the cortical correlates of visual self-regulation. *Brain Res* 2007 Apr 27; **1143**:169–82. Epub 2007 Jan 25.
22. Critchley HD, Wiens S, Rotshtein P, et al. Neural systems supporting interoceptive awareness. *Nat Neurosci* 2004; **7**:189–95.
23. Konstantakopoulos G, Varsou E, Dileos D, et al. Delusionality of body image beliefs in eating disorders. *Psychiatry Res* 2012; **200**:482–8.
24. Craig AD. How do you feel-now? The anterior insula and human awareness. *Nat Rev Neurosci* 2009; **10**:59–70.
25. Kothari R, Gafton J, Treasure J, et al. 2D:4D ratio in children at familial high-risk for eating disorders: The role of prenatal testosterone exposure. *Am J Hum Biol* 2014 Mar–Apr; **26**(2):176–82. doi:10.1002/ajhb.22495. Epub 2013 Dec 10.
26. Powers PS, Santana CA. Eating disorders: a guide for the primary care physician. *Primary Care* 2002; **29**: 81–98.
27. Glorio R, Allevato M, Pablo A, et al. Prevalence of cutaneous manifestations of eating disorders in 200 patients with eating disorders. *Int J Dermatol* 2000; **39**:348.
28. Strumia R. Skin signs in anorexia nervosa. *Dermatoendocrinol* 2009; **1**:268.
29. Titova OE, Hjorth OC,Schioth HB, et al. Anorexia nervosa is linked to reduced brain structure in reward and somatosensory regions: a meta-analysis of VBM studies. *BMC Psychiatry* 2013; **13**:110.
30. Goldberg SJ, Comerci GD, Feldman L. Cardiac output and regional myocardial contraction in anorexia nervosa. *J Adolesc Health Care* 1988; **9**:15.
31. Mehler PS, Winkelman AB, Andefrson DM, et al. Nutritional rehabilitation: practical guidelines for refeeding the anorectic patient. *J Nutr Metab* 2010; 2010. pii: 625782. doi: 10.1155/2010/625782. Epub 2010 Feb 7.
32. Miller KK, Grinspoon SK, Ciampa J, et al. Medical findings in outpatients with anorexia nervosa. *Arch Intern Med* 2005; **165**:561.
33. Shamim T, Golden NH, Arden M, et al. Resolution of vital sign instability: an objective measure of stability in anorexia nervosa. *J Adolesc Health* 2003; **32**:73.
34. Mehler PS. Clinical practice: bulimia nervosa. *N Eng J Med* 2003; **349**:875–81.
35. Misra M, Miller KK, Almazan C, et al. Hormonal and body composition predictors of soluble leptin receptor, leptin and free leptin index in adolescent girls with anorexia nervosa and controls and relation to insulin sensitivity. *J Clin Endocrinol Metab* 2004 Jul; **89**(7): 3486–95.
36. Grinspoon S, Gulick T, Askari H, et al. Serum leptin levels in women with anorexia nervosa. *J Clin Endocrinol Metab* 1996; **81**: 3861–3.
37. Katz MG, Vollenhoven B. The reproductive endocrine consequences of anorexia nervosa. *BJOG* 2000; **107**:707.
38. Miller KK, Grinspoon SK, Ciampa J, et al. Medical findings in outpatients with anorexia nervosa. *Arch Intern Med* 2005; **165**:561.

39. Grinspoon S, Thomas E, pitts S, et al. Prevalence and predictive factors for regional osteopenia in women with anorexia nervosa. *Ann Intern Med* 2000; **133**:790.

40. Mehler PS, Mackenzie TD. Treatment of osteopenia and osteoporosis in anorexia nervosa: a systematic review of the literature. *Int J Eat Disord* 2009; **42**:195.

41. Mirsa M, Prabhakaran R, Miller KK, et al. Weight gain and restoration of menses as predictors of bone mineral density change in adolescent girls with anorexia nervosa-1. *J Clin Endocrinol Metab* 2008; **93**(4):1231–7.

42. Birmingham CL, Alothman AF, Goldner EM. Anorexia nervosa: refeeding and hypophosphatemia. *Int J Eat Disord* 1996; **20**:211–13.

43. American Psychiatric Association. Treatment of patients with eating disorders, third edition. American Psychiatric Association. *Am J Psychiatry* 2006; **163**(7 Suppl):4–54.

44. Sullivan PF. Mortality in anorexia nervosa. *Am J Psychiatry* 1995; **152**:1073–4.

45. Sundgot-Borgen J, Torstveit MK. Prevalence of eating disorders in elite athletes is higher than in the general population. *Clin J Sport Med* 2004; **14**:25–32.

46. Morgan JF, Reid F, Lacey JH. The SCOFF questionnaire: assessment of a new screening tool for eating disorders. *BMJ* 1999; **319**:639–55.

47. Borzekowski DL, Schenk S, Wilson J, et al. e-Ana and e-Mia: a content analysis of pro-eating disorder web sites. *Am J Public Health* 2010; **100**: 1526–34.

48. Halmi KA. Perplexities of treatment resistance in eating disorders. *BMC Psychiatry* 2013; **13**:292.

49. Claudino AM, Silva de Lima M, Hay PPJ, et al. Antidepressants for anorexia nervosa. *Cochrane Database Syst Rev* 2006; **1**:CD004365.

50. Walsh BT, Kaplan AS, Attia E, et al. Fluoxetine after weight restoration in anorexia nervosa: a randomized controlled trial. *JAMA* 2006; **295**: 2605–12.

51. Fisher CA, Hetrick SE, Rushford N. Family therapy for anorexia nervosa. *Cochrane Database Syst Rev* 2010; **4**: CD004780.

52. Zucker NL, Marcus M, Bulik C. A group parent-training program: a novel approach for eating disorder management. *Eat Weight Disord* 2006;**11**:327–30.

53. Hay PPJ, Bacaltchuk J, Kashyap P. Psychological treatments for bulimia nervosa and binging. *Cochrane Database Syst Rev* 2009; **4**:CD000562.

54. Bacaltchuk J, Hay P. Antidepressants vs. placebo for people with bulimia nervosa. *Cochrane Database Syst Rev* 2003; **4**:CD003391.

Chapter 39

Office care of obese patients

Sharon Luent Seidel and Jessica R. Jackson

Introduction

The past 25 years have shown an ongoing epidemic of obesity. Despite increasing public awareness of the consequential health risks of obesity, the number of American adults who are obese continues to increase. In 2000, the release of the *Healthy People 2010* report set national objectives for the reduction in the prevalence of obesity in the United States. The goal was to reduce the obesity prevalence to 15%.[1] In the 2001 *Surgeon General's Call to Action to Prevent and Decrease Overweight and Obesity*, an attempt was made to warn the public of the detrimental effects of obesity on health and promote the recognition of overweight and obesity as a major public health problem.[2] Despite this initiative, the trend did not reverse. *The Surgeon General's Vision for a Healthy and Fit Nation 2010* was launched in response to the ongoing obesity epidemic. The goal is to achieve optimal health for all at every stage of life.[3]

The health detriments of obesity impact women during the reproductive years and continue through menopause. Many women utilize their ob-gyn for both preventive and problem-focused health-care needs. Therefore it is imperative that ob-gyns appreciate the risks of obesity and associated diseases. Each patient encounter is an opportunity to address obesity and lifestyle behavior, as proactive management and treatment are necessary to achieve and maintain weight loss. Prevention is also important to achieve optimal health and minimize a woman's likelihood of developing obesity with associated comorbidities. This chapter serves to aid women's health providers with the diagnosis, management, treatment, and prevention of obesity as it relates to the overall health of a woman in addition to entities that are specific to obstetrics and gynecology.

Scope of the problem

More than two-thirds of American adults are overweight (69%) and just over one-third (35.1%) are obese.[4] The prevalence of obesity in the United States has risen dramatically from 13.4% in 1980 to 35.1% in 2011.[3] In 2011–2012, the prevalence of obesity was higher among middle-aged adults (39.5% aged 40–59) than among younger adults (30.3% aged 20–39) or older adults (35.4% aged 60 and older). There also exists a slight difference between the prevalence of obesity among men (33.5%) and women (36.1%).[5] In fact, women are at even greater risk of more severe obesity, with 18.1% being Class II obese (BMI ≥35 kg/m^2) and 8.1% being Class III obese (BMI ≥40 kg/m^2) compared with 12.5% and 4.4% of men being Class II and Class III obese, respectively.[6]

The prevalence of obesity also differs with race and ethnicity. In 2011–2012, the prevalence of obesity was higher in non-Hispanic black women (56.6%) than Hispanic (44.4%), non-Hispanic white (32.8%), and non-Hispanic Asian (11.4%) women.[5] Disparities are also noted among the prevalence of obesity in regard to socioeconomic status. Among women, obesity prevalence increases as income decreases. Of women who live in households with income at or above 350% of the poverty level, 29% are obese compared to 42% of women with income below 130% of the poverty level. The prevalence of obesity also increases in women as the education level decreases. Of women with a college degree, 23.4% are obese compared to 42.1% of women with less than a high school education. Interestingly, this disparity between education level and obesity does not exist among men.[7]

Obesity prevalence in the United States also varies across states and regions. According to the 2012 Centers for Disease Control and Prevention (CDC) report, obesity prevalence ranged from 20.5% in

Office Care of Women, ed. Martin E. Olsen and Botros Rizk. Published by Cambridge University Press.

Table 39-1 Prevalence* of self-reported obesity among US adults (2012)

State	Rate (%)	State	Rate (%)
Alabama	33	Montana	24.3
Alaska	25.7	Nebraska	28.6
Arizona	26	Nevada	26.2
Arkansas	34.5	New Hampshire	27.3
California	25	New Jersey	24.6
Colorado	20.5	New Mexico	27.1
Connecticut	25.6	New York	23.6
Delaware	26.9	North Carolina	29.6
District of Columbia	21.9	North Dakota	29.7
Florida	25.2	Ohio	30.1
Georgia	29.1	Oklahoma	32.2
Hawaii	23.6	Oregon	27.3
Idaho	26.8	Pennsylvania	29.1
Illinois	28.1	Rhode Island	25.7
Indiana	31.4	South Carolina	31.6
Iowa	30.4	South Dakota	28.1
Kansas	29.9	Tennessee	31.1
Kentucky	31.3	Texas	29.2
Louisiana	34.7	Utah	24.3
Maine	28.4	Vermont	23.7
Maryland	27.6	Virginia	27.4
Massachusetts	22.9	Washington	26.8
Michigan	31.1	West Virginia	33.8
Minnesota	25.7	Wisconsin	29.7
Mississippi	34.6	Wyoming	24.6
Missouri	29.6		

* Prevalence reflects methodological changes in 2011, and these estimates should not be compared to those before 2011.
Source: Adapted from Centers for Disease Control and Prevention. Adult obesity facts. Available at: www.cdc.gov/obesity/data/adult.html. Retrieved July 5, 2014.

Colorado to 34.7% in Louisiana. No state had an obesity prevalence less than 20% (Table 39-1). Higher prevalence of obesity was found in the Midwest (29.5%) and the South (29.4%) compared to the Northeast (25.3%) and the West (25.1%). No state met the *Healthy People 2010* goal to reduce the prevalence of obesity to 15%. In fact, in 2010 there were 12 states with an obesity prevalence of 30%, in comparison to no state with an obesity prevalence greater than 30% in 2000.[8] If the obesity prevalence would have remained at 15%, medical savings would have totaled $1.9 trillion.[9]

Just as obesity is common, it is serious and costly. Approximately 300,000 obesity-related deaths occur each year in the United States.[2] Obesity is a risk factor for numerous medical conditions including hypertension, dyslipidemia, type 2 diabetes, coronary heart disease, stroke, gallbladder disease, osteoarthritis, sleep apnea and respiratory problems, gynecological problems including abnormal menses and infertility, along with endometrial, breast, and colon cancers.[10] Obesity is also associated with an increase in all-cause mortality. Depending on age and race, obesity has been shown to be associated with a 6- to 20-year decrease in life expectancy.[11] In addition to the physical morbidities associated with obesity, emotional hardships can also develop in obese individuals in the form of social stigmatization and discrimination.[12]

Furthermore, obesity significantly impacts the economy. It is estimated that the annual medical cost of obesity in the United States was $147 billion in 2008. Medical costs for obese people were reported to be $1,429 higher than those of normal weight.[9]

Evaluation and diagnosis of the obese patient

Every patient encounter is an opportunity to address prevention and management of obesity in order to optimize the patient's health. Evaluation and diagnosis for overweight status or obesity is the first step. The National Heart, Lung, and Blood Institute classify overweight and obesity based on body mass index (BMI), which correlates with total body fat content. BMI is calculated as weight (kg)/height (m^2). Obesity is classified as a BMI ≥30 (Table 39-2).[12] Waist circumference, which is measured just above the anterior superior iliac spines at the end of expiration, can be used as in independent predictor of morbidity associated with obesity. Abdominal fat distribution positively correlates with a greater risk of heart disease and type 2 diabetes in comparison to fat deposits elsewhere. This is true for women with a waist circumference >88 cm (>35 inches). By adding waist circumference to BMI, the prediction of obesity-related morbidity is enhanced. This holds true as long as the BMI is ≤35, as patients with a higher BMI likely exceed the cutoff value.[12, 13]

Table 39-2 Classification of overweight and obesity by BMI

	Obesity class	BMI (kg/m2)
Underweight		<18.5
Normal		18.5–24.9
Overweight		25.0–29.9
Obesity	I	30.0–34.9
	II	35.0–39.9
Extreme obesity	III	≥40

Source: Adapted from Clinical Guidelines on the Identification, Evaluation, and Treatment of Overweight and Obesity in Adults – the Evidence Report. National Institutes of Health. Available at: www.nhlbi.nih.gov/guidelines/obesity/ob_galns.htm. Retrieved July 5, 2014.

In addition to stratifying the degree of overweight/obesity, the National Heart, Lung, and Blood Institute recommends conducting a risk assessment to determine the patient's overall risk of morbidity related to obesity. Disease conditions that are classified as very high risk for complications include coronary artery disease, other atherosclerotic diseases, type 2 diabetes, and sleep apnea. Other obesity-related diseases include osteoarthritis, gallstones, gynecological abnormalities, and stress incontinence. Cardiovascular risk factors to screen include cigarette smoking, hypertension or utilization of antihypertensive agents, high-risk LDL cholesterol ≥160 mg/dL, low HDL cholesterol <35 mg/dL, impaired fasting glucose 110 mg/dL–125 mg/dL, family history of premature coronary heart disease, and age ≥55 years or postmenopausal for female patients. The patient is classified as having high absolute risk for obesity-related morbidity if she screens positive for three of the preceding risk factors. Clinical management is usually required to reduce these risk factors. In the presence of physical inactivity and elevated serum triglycerides >200 mg/dL, the risk of obesity-related morbidity is markedly higher and weight loss is paramount for optimal health.[12]

Screening for overweight and obesity

The US Preventive Services Task Force (USPSTF) recommends screening all adults for overweight and obesity.[11] Although there is no established frequency interval, screening for overweight status and obesity should be part of a woman's annual well check.[13] Discussing healthy lifestyle behaviors at each visit could facilitate open dialogue with the patient and optimize weight loss goals and strategies.[14] Many factors must be considered when determining the cause of obesity. Anything that promotes an imbalance of caloric intake and energy consumption will play a role in developing obesity. As a result, body weight is the end product of a person's makeup of genetics, metabolism, behavior, environment, culture, socioeconomic status, diseases, and drugs. When screening for overweight and obesity, all of these factors must be considered (Box 39-1).

BOX 39-1 Risk factors for obesity

Dietary factors

- High fat diet
- Overeating
- Frequency of eating
- Infant feeding practices

Social and behavioral factors

- Socioeconomic status
- Ethnicity
- Binge eating
- Night eating
- Psychologic conditions (depression, stress)
- Sedentary lifestyle

Genetic factors

- Prader-Willi syndrome
- Angelman syndrome
- Possible other genetic factors

Neuroendocrine factors

- Polycystic ovary syndrome
- Cushing syndrome
- Seasonal affective disorder
- Hypogonadism

Iatrogenic causes

- Drugs that cause weight gain (antidepressants, steroids)

Other factors

- Low birth weight

Source: Adapted from Steele, KE, Burke, AE. Obesity. In: Stenchever M, Artal R, eds. *Clinical Updates in Women's Health Care.* Vol XII, 2013.

Treatment for obesity

According to the National Heart, Lung, and Blood Institute, three main goals exist for weight loss and management: prevent further weight gain, reduce body weight, and maintain long-term lower body weight. The initial goal of weight loss treatment is to reduce body weight by 10%, which can reasonably be accomplished in six months. Randomized trials suggest that weight loss at a rate of one to two pounds per week usually occurs for up to six months, and further loss and maintenance thereafter depends on implementation of a weight maintenance program.[12]

Three main options exist for weight loss management: lifestyle modification (including dietary changes, physical activity, and behavioral therapy), pharmacotherapy, and weight loss surgery. Initial weight loss is usually achieved with caloric reduction. Dietary changes require a consumed calorie reduction of approximately 500–1,000 kcal/day in order to achieve a weight loss of one to two pounds per week. Caution should be exercised with patients utilizing a very low calorie diet (800 kcal/day or less), due to the intensive monitoring and compliance needed. Reducing dietary fat and carbohydrates has proven to be more successful than reducing dietary fat alone for weight loss.[12]

Increased physical activity is most helpful in maintaining weight loss and preventing regain. It also decreases abdominal fat and increases cardiopulmonary fitness, which can reduce risks associated with cardiovascular disease and diabetes. Ideally, long-term goals should include at least 30 minutes of moderate physical activity five to seven days a week. However, patients should set exercise goals that are realistic and manageable.[12]

Behavioral therapy has also proven beneficial when incorporated into lifestyle modifications. These strategies serve to overcome barriers to compliance with dietary modifications and increased physical activity. These therapies target self-monitoring of dietary and physical activity, stress management, problem solving, stimulus control, contingency management, cognitive restructuring, and social support.[12] Several studies have examined the efficacy of self-monitoring for weight loss. One study of 220 obese women found an association between long-term weight loss success and a combination of high frequency plus high consistency of dietary information recorded.[15]

Lifestyle modifications are usually most successful at achieving weight loss, maintenance, and prevention of regain. Only when six months of lifestyle modification fails to achieve weight loss should pharmacotherapy be considered. Weight loss drugs should always be used in conjunction with lifestyle modification and never alone. The drug should be continued as long as it is deemed efficacious and there are no serious adverse effects.[12] Pharmacologic treatment for obesity is limited. To date, orlistat is the only FDA-approved drug for chronic weight loss management. Other drugs have been FDA approved for short-term use, but they have come under scrutiny due to adverse side effects. Orlistat reduces fat absorption by inhibiting gastrointestinal lipases. Although the most common side effect is steatorrhea, there are additional complications such as hepatotoxicity, nephrotoxicity, pancreatitis, and kidney stones. In combination with a controlled diet, orlistat can help induce weight loss, prevent weight regain, and improve fasting low-density lipoprotein and insulin levels.[16] One randomized controlled trial found that caraway extract showed a significant reduction of weight, body mass index, body fat percentage, and waist-to-hip ratio when compared to placebo. However, there were no changes in lipid profile, urine-specific gravity, or blood pressure.[17]

The first-line treatments already discussed have been associated with somewhat poor results and high relapse rates. Those patients with a BMI ≥40 or ≥35 with comorbidities who have failed first-line therapies, and who have an increased risk for obesity-related morbidity and mortality are candidates for bariatric surgery.[12] This is the most effective and lasting long-term weight loss management. It is promoted by the National Institutes of Health (NIH) as an effective method for long-term weight control. Selection criteria are stringent, and the patient must agree to reliable, strict follow-up.[13]

Providers are encouraged to approach obesity treatment from a multifactorial standpoint. Issues to be considered include emotional health, history of weight struggles and previous attempts at weight loss, eating patterns, social support, environmental triggers, psychiatric well-being, and obesity-related comorbidities. The patient's readiness and motivation to start and maintain lifestyle modifications should be addressed prior to implementation, as the likelihood of success is low if she is not committed.[13]

Physicians are encouraged to initiate a conversation with patients regarding lifestyle modification at each encounter. Motivational interview techniques can aide in developing a long-term commitment to weight loss. Discussions regarding a healthy lifestyle, including exercise and food choices, should be addressed. Educational material with recommendations for dietary intake, including preparation of low-calorie meals, and physical activity should be provided. Physicians can help overcome barriers to healthy living by advocating for free exercise and wellness programs as well as safe outdoor recreational facilities. Support of data collections for tracking obesity and chronic diseases is also important to optimize patient health.[14]

Obesity and pregnancy

Overweight and obesity is a common problem in pregnancy, affecting more than one-half of pregnant women in the United States.[6] Both maternal and fetal complications occur due to obesity. Maternal complications include increased risk of gestational diabetes, hypertension, preeclampsia, cesarean delivery, and postpartum weight retention. Fetal complications include macrosomia, prematurity, stillbirth, congenital anomalies such as neural tube defects, large-for-gestational-age infants, and obesity later in life. Potential intrapartum complications in the obese patient are also of concern. Anesthesia management can be challenging and an antepartum consultation should be arranged. Estimating fetal weight can be difficult as well as monitoring and interpreting external fetal heart rate and contraction patterns. There is also an increased risk of complicated and emergent cesarean delivery.[18] Obese women are more likely to be admitted earlier in labor requiring induction with oxytocin and have longer labor. They are also less likely to have a successful vaginal birth after cesarean delivery.[19]

In 2009 the Institute of Medicine revised the pregnancy weight gain guidelines based on pre-pregnancy BMI recommended by the WHO. These new guidelines recommend a total pregnancy weight gain of 15–25 pounds for overweight women, and 11–20 pounds for obese women. These goals differ from the 25–35 pounds recommended for a woman of normal weight.[20] These goals should be addressed, preferably before conception, but definitely during the first prenatal visit. Providers should assist their patients in setting realistic diet and exercise plans to help during pregnancy as well as postpartum. A multidisciplinary approach using a nutritionist may be helpful.

A meta-analysis conducted in 2014 assessed effects of behavioral interventions in pregnancy versus standard maternity care. Behavioral interventions were statistically associated with reducing gestational weight gain in obese women without comorbid conditions. However, behavioral interventions were not associated with reduced pregnancy weight gain in overweight or morbidly obese women. Behavioral interventions also had no effect on postpartum weight loss or infant birth weight.[21]

One question to consider with obesity in pregnancy is mode of delivery. The rate of cesarean delivery is higher among obese women, with a cesarean rate of 33% for BMI of 30–34.9 and 43% for BMI ≥35. This compares to a cesarean rate of 21% for BMI <30.[22] Cesarean delivery in obese women poses increased complications, including excessive blood loss, prolonged operative time, wound infection and breakdown, endometritis, and venous thromboembolism.[18] Interestingly, a retrospective cohort study performed at the University of Alabama, Birmingham, evaluated mode of delivery in women with class III obesity, comparing planned cesarean with induction of labor. In the study 661 women with a BMI >40 were evaluated. There were no significant differences in maternal morbidity or neonatal morbidity between the two groups. Maternal morbidity included operative complications, infections, wound morbidity, venous thromboembolism, and maternal death. Fetal complications included stillbirth, hypoxic ischemic encephalopathy, neonatal intensive care unit admission for more than 72 hours, mechanical ventilation for more than 24 hours, grade III or IV intraventricular hemorrhage, respiratory distress syndrome, necrotizing enterocolitis, suspected sepsis, culture-proven sepsis, or neonatal death.[23]

Women who have undergone bariatric surgery constitute a unique population of pregnant women. Bariatric surgery presents a set of specific considerations for pregnancy. It is recommended to delay childbearing for 12–24 months after bariatric surgery to allow time for rapid weight loss.[18, 24] Nutritional and microelemental deficiencies are common, particularly vitamin B12, folic acid, calcium, vitamin D, and iron. The American Association of Clinical Endocrinologists, the Obesity Society, and the American Society for Metabolic and Bariatric Surgery (ASMBS) formulated guidelines for patients after bariatric surgery, including women who become pregnant. Recommended micronutrient supplementation for pregnant women after bariatric surgery include one prenatal vitamin daily (prenatal vitamins containing 400 mcg of folic acid are generally sufficient to prevent neural tube defects), calcium citrate 1,200 mg daily with 400–800 IU of vitamin D), elemental iron 40 mg–65 mg daily (in addition to prenatal vitamin), and at least 350 mcg of vitamin B12 orally daily.[25] Vitamin A deficiencies affect 10% of patients after gastric bypass. Vitamin A is essential, especially in the second and third trimesters, for normal fetal lung development. Excessive vitamin A is teratogenic to the fetus. It is recommended that vitamin A levels should be monitored periodically, and supplementation started if needed, but not to exceed the dose of 5,000 IU/day.[19, 24]

A study published in the *European Journal of Obstetrics & Gynecology and Reproductive Health* found that, when compared with controls, obese pregnant women who had undergone bariatric surgery preconceptually had lower rates of preeclampsia, gestational diabetes, and large neonates. However, they did have higher rates of small neonates, preterm birth, admission to neonatal intensive care unit, and maternal anemia. Interestingly, laparoscopic adjustable banding did not appear to increase the risk of small-for-gestational-age infants found with other forms of gastric surgery.[26]

Obesity and contraception

For obese women who desire contraception, the ob-gyn must be familiar with the current safety and efficacy profiles for all forms of contraception. Providers should not deny obese women contraception, as the risks of pregnancy far outweigh the risks associated with contraception and obesity. According to the CDC's US Medical Eligibility Criteria for Contraceptive Use, 2010, all contraceptive methods are safe and appropriate for use in obese women (Table 39-3).[27]

Unfortunately, evidence is lacking regarding the efficacy of hormonal contraception in obese women. Most efficacy trials to date have excluded obesity from the study population. Research is ongoing to determine the effects on pharmacokinetics of contraceptive hormones in obese women. A Cochrane review of 11 studies examined the effectiveness of hormonal

Table 39-3 Medical eligibility criteria for selected contraceptive methods in obese women

Contraceptive method	MEC category
Intrauterine contraception	1
Progestin implant	1
DMPA	1
Progestin only pills	1
Emergency contraceptive pills	1
Combined contraceptive pill, patch, ring	2

Source: Adapted from US Medical Eligibility Criteria for Contraceptive Use, 2010. Centers for Disease Control and Prevention. MMWR Recomm Rep 2010; 59: 1–86. Category 1: no restriction for use of the contraceptive method; Category 2: advantages of using the method generally outweigh the theoretical or proven risks; Category 3: risks generally outweigh advantages; Category 4: method should not be used. DMPA: Depot medroxyprogesterone acetate.

contraceptives in preventing unplanned pregnancies among overweight and obese women in comparison to women of lower weight or BMI. It concluded that unintended pregnancy was almost twice as likely in overweight and obese women on combination oral contraceptives than women of normal weight.[28] By contrast, an analysis of data from the Contraceptive CHOICE Project found no increase in contraceptive failure rate by BMI for combination oral contraceptives, transdermal patch, or vaginal ring.[29] Although there is limited data, long-acting reversible contraceptives have been shown to maintain excellent efficacy in obese women and may be an excellent option for this patient population.[30] Injectable contraception (depot medroxyprogesterone acetate) is another effective option, as obesity does not reduce its efficacy; however weight gain is a possible side effect that must be addressed with the patient.[13, 30]

Although obesity alone is not a contraindication to any contraceptive method, obesity and combination oral contraceptives are independent risk factors for venous thromboembolism (VTE). Obese women are twice as likely to experience VTE as normal weight women, and if on combination oral contraceptives, the VTE risk is tenfold higher than for women of normal weight not on combination oral contraceptives.[31] However, the risk of VTE in pregnancy and postpartum are substantially higher than the risk of VTE from combination contraceptive use.[30] There are no safety concerns with the use of progestin-only contraceptive methods in obese women, including pills, injectables, intrauterine devices, and implants.[27]

The possibility of lower efficacy of combination oral contraceptives in obese women warrants consideration of utilizing long-acting contraceptives, as they provide the most reliable contraception for all women regardless of weight. However, if a woman makes an informed decision to use a combination oral contraceptive, she should not be denied based on weight or BMI alone.[30] Therefore, the patient's preference, expectations, and future fertility plans should be at the forefront when choosing the appropriate form of contraception.

Special consideration should be taken regarding women who undergo bariatric surgery. Patients are strongly advised to avoid pregnancy for two years after surgery.[19] It is very common that with the drastic weight loss experienced after surgery, resumption of normal menses and ovulation occurs.[32] Both malabsorptive and restrictive procedures could theoretically reduce the efficacy of oral contraceptives. It is for this reason that the US Medical Eligibility Criteria for Contraceptive Use, 2010, advises against the use of oral contraceptives after bariatric surgery. The efficacy of nonoral methods is not affected by bariatric surgery and are better suited for these patients (Table 39-4).[30, 33]

Obesity and menopause

The prevalence of obesity rises dramatically as a woman ages. In the United States in 2010, 66% of women aged 40–59 years and 73.5% of women aged 60 or greater were obese.[6] On average, a woman gains two to five pounds during the menopausal transition.[34] Consistent findings reveal that age is the main determinant of weight gain at midlife, but hormonal changes during the menopausal transition substantially contribute to obesity as well.[35] Hormonal changes promote adipose tissue expansion, especially in the central distribution. This increase in waist circumference is not only associated with an increase in cardiovascular disease, type 2 diabetes, and cancer, but it also has negative effects on sexual function and health-related quality of life. Slower metabolism and a decrease in physical activity also contributes to weight gain.[13]

Table 39-4 Medical eligibility criteria for selected contraceptive methods in women who have undergone bariatric weight-loss surgery

Contraceptive method	MEC category after restrictive surgery	MEC category after malabsorptive surgery
Intrauterine contraception	1	1
Progestin implant	1	1
Depot medroxyprogesterone acetate (DMPA)	1	1
Contraceptive patch, vaginal ring	1	1
Combined or progestin-only pill	1	3
Emergency contraceptive pill	1	3

Source: Adapted from US Medical Eligibility Criteria for Contraceptive Use, 2010. Centers for Disease Control and Prevention. MMWR Recomm Rep 2010; 59: 1–86. Category 1: no restriction for use of the contraceptive method; Category 2: advantages of using the method generally outweigh the theoretical or proven risks; Category 3: risks generally outweigh advantages; Category 4: method should not be used.

Weight gain during the menopausal transition can intensify menopausal symptoms, as obesity is an independent risk factor for more severe menopausal symptoms.[35] Weight reduction, lower BMI, and reduced abdominal circumference have been shown to decrease vasomotor symptoms in overweight and obese menopausal women.[36] Diet modification and exercise together have more positive effects on health-related quality of life and psychological health than either alone.[36, 37]

It has been questioned whether hormone therapy affects weight and body composition. According to a Cochrane review published in 2000, there is no evidence of adverse effects of estrogen-only or estrogen-progestin therapy on body weight or BMI.[38] In fact, studies have shown an overall reduction in abdominal fat with hormone therapy and improved insulin sensitivity with lower rates of type 2 diabetes.[35]

Older women should utilize the same strategies to maintain a healthy weight as younger women. The fundamental basis of weight control is lifestyle modification; however, this can be enhanced by pharmacotherapy and surgery. By encouraging physical activity, optimal weight may be achieved and maintained, which in turn can improve medical comorbidities for which overweight and obese women are at risk.

Challenges for the obstetrician-gynecologist

There are many barriers that make it challenging to care for overweight and obese patients. Society has created one of these barriers. There is a social stigma associated with obesity that must be eliminated. Society as a whole sees obesity as an abnormal state for which the individual is at fault. Obese women are blamed for overeating and not exercising. Their weight is seen as a product of their own bad choices. They face blame from their families, friends, peers, strangers, and even their physicians. A 2001 review revealed that health-care providers were more likely to have a negative attitude toward obese patients than those of normal weight.[39] Health-care providers need to create an environment in which obese patients feel safe and no judgments are cast. Physicians should care for obese patients in an unbiased manner, recognizing that the medical, social, cultural, and ethical implications need to be addressed in a manner that respects the patient's autonomy and dignity.[40]

Physicians need to dedicate more time to counseling obese patients regarding medical comorbidities and the appropriate management plans, and also follow their progress. Obese patients should be treated no differently than other patients with complex medical issues that require more time for appropriate care. If the physician feels that safe, effective care cannot be provided, then a referral or consultation is appropriate. Continuity of care should be maintained when possible. A multidisciplinary team approach including ob-gyns, nutritionists, dieticians, internal medicine specialists, bariatric surgeons, and mental health professionals, in conjunction with community programs, can help patients achieve weight loss and optimal health.[40]

Concluding remarks

Overweight status and obesity are epidemic in the United States, with the prevalence of obesity at 35% in adults. It is predicted that obesity prevalence will increase by 33% and severe obesity by 130% over the next two decades. If the obesity rate stays at that of 2010 instead of rising to 42% as predicted, then the United States could save more than $549.5 billion in weight-related medical expenditures from now until 2030.[9]

Given these statistics, ob-gyns will encounter more obese patients in their practice. Screening for obesity should take place at every patient encounter; physicians must be proficient in screening for, diagnosing, and evaluating obesity. Prevention and management plans should be formulated and executed with a multidisciplinary team when necessary. Patient progress should be followed with the appropriate counseling necessary to promote positive changes in patient behavior.

Treating obesity as a medical condition and a modifiable risk factor could help physicians provide unbiased care that promotes a positive patient-physician relationship. Improved understanding of social, cultural, and medical implications of obesity will allow physicians to realistically formulate management plans with obtainable goals. Physicians will then be more effective at caring for obese patients, resulting in successful outcomes and optimal patient health.

References

1. US Department of Health and Human Services. *Healthy People 2010: Understanding and Improving Health and Objectives for Improving Health*, 2nd ed. Washington, DC: US Government Printing Office; 2000.
2. US Department of Health and Human Services. *The Surgeon General's Call to Action to Prevent and Decrease Overweight and Obesity*. Rockville, MD: US Department of Health and Human Services, Public Health Service, Office of the Surgeon General; 2001.
3. US Department of Health and Human Services *The Surgeon General's Vision for a Healthy and Fit Nation*. Rockville, MD: US Department of Health and Human Services, Office of the Surgeon General; 2010.
4. Centers for Disease Control and Prevention. Obesity and Overweight (internet). Available at: www.cdc.gov/nchs/fastats/obesity-overweight.htm. Retrieved July 5, 2014.
5. Ogden CL, Carroll MD, Kit BK, Flegal KM. Prevalence of obesity among adults: United States, 2011–2012. NCHS Data Brief No. 131. Hyattsville, MD: National Center for Health Statistics; 2013. Available at: www.cdc.gov/nchs/data/databriefs/db131.pdf. Retrieved July 24, 2014.
6. Flegal KM, Carroll MD, Kit BK, Ogden, CL. Prevalence of obesity and trends in the distribution of body mass index among US adults, 1999–2010. *JAMA*. 2012; **307**: 491–7.
7. Ogden CL, Lamb MM, Carroll MD, Flegal KM. Obesity and socioecomonic status in adults: United States 2005–2008. NCHS Data Brief No. 50. Hyattsville, MD: National Center for Health Statistics; 2010. Available at: www.cdc.gov/nchs/data/databriefs/db50.pdf. Retrieved July 5, 2014.
8. Centers for Disease Control and Prevention. Adult obesity facts. Available at: www.cdc.gov/obesity/data/adult.html. Retrieved July 5, 2014.
9. Finkelstein EA, Khavjou OA, Thompson H, et al. Obesity and severe obesity forecasts through 2030. *Am J Prev Med*. 2012; **42**:563–70.
10. Centers for Disease Control and Prevention. Causes and consequences. Available at: www.cdc.gov/obesity/adult/causes/index.html. Retrieved July 5, 2014.
11. US Preventive Services Task Force. Screening for and management of obesity in adults. Available at: www.uspreventiveservicestaskforce.org/uspstf1/obeseadults/obesers.html. Retrieved August 5, 2014.
12. National Institutes of Health. Clinical guidelines on the identification, evaluation, and treatment of overweight and obesity in adults – the evidence report. Available at: www.nhlbi.nih.gov/guidelines/obesity/ob_galns.htm. Retrieved July 5, 2014.
13. Steele KE, Burke AE. Clinical updates in women's healthcare. *Obesity* 2013 Jan; **XII**:1.
14. American College of Obstetricians and Gynecologists. Challenges for overweight and obese women. Committee Opinion No. 591. *Obstet Gynecol* 2014; **123**:726–30.
15. Peterson ND, Middleton KR, Nackers LM, et al. Dietaryself-monitoring and long-term success with weight management. *Obesity (SilverSpring)* 2014 Jun 13. doi: 10.1002/oby.20807. [Epub ahead of print] PubMed PMID: 24931055.
16. Kim JW, Lin JE, Blomain ES, Waldman SA. Antiobesity pharmacotherapy: new drugs and emerging targets. *Clinical Pharmacology & Therapeutics*. 2014 Jan; **95**(1):53–66.
17. Kazemipoor M, Radzi C, Hajifaraji M, et al. Antiobesity effect of caraway extract on overweight and obese women: a randomized, triple-blind, placebo-controlled clinical trial. *Evidence-Base Complementary and Alternative Medicine* 2013; **2013**:1–8.

18. American College of Obstetricians and Gynecologists. Obesity and pregnancy. Committee Opinion No. 549. *Obstet Gynecol.* 2013 Jan; **121**(1):213–17.

19. American College of Obstetricians and Gynecologists. Bariatric surgery and pregnancy. Practice Bulletin No. 105. *Obstet Gyencol* 2009; **113**:1405–13.

20. Institute of Medicine of the National Acadamies. *Weight gain during pregnancy: reexamining the guidelines.* Washington, DC: National Academies Press; 2009.

21. Agha M, Agha R, Sandell J. Interventions to reduce and prevent obesity in pre-conceptual and pregnant women: a systematic review and meta-analysis. *PLOS one.* 2014 May; **9**(5):e95132.

22. Kominiarek, MA, Vanveldhuisen P, Hibbard J, et al. The maternal body mass index: a strong association with delivery route: Consortium of Safe Labor. *Am J Obstet Gynecol* 2010; **203**(264):E1–7.

23. Subramaniam A, Jauk VC, Goss AR, et al. Mode of delivery in women with class III obesity: planned cesarean compared to induction of labor. *American J of Obstet and Gynecol.* 2014; doi: 10.1016/j.ajog.2014.06.045.

24. Kaska L, Kobiela J, Abacjeq-Chmylko A, et al. Nutrition and pregnancy after bariatric surgery. *ISRN Obesity.* 2013 Jan 30; **2013**:492060. doi: 10.1155/2013/492060. eCollection 2013.

25. Mechanick JI, Kushner RF, Sugerman HJ, et al. American Association of Clinical Endocrinologists, The Obesity Society, and American Society for Metabolic & Bariatric Surgery medical guidelines for clinical practice for the perioperative nutritional, metabolic, and nonsurgical support of the bariatric surgery patient. *Surg Obes Relat Dis* 2008; **4**:S109–84.

26. Galazis N, Docheva N, Simillis C, Nicolaides K. Maternal and neonatal outcomes in women undergoing bariatric surgery: a systematic review and meta-analysis. *European Journal of Obstetrics & Gynecology and Reproductive Biology.* 2014 July; **181**:45–53.

27. Centers for Disease Control and Prevention. U.S. Medical Eligibility Criteria for Contraceptive Use, 2010. *MMWR Recomm Rep.* 2010; **59**:1–86.

28. Lopez LM, Grimes DA, Chen-Mok M, et al. Hormonal contraceptives for contraception in overweight or obese women. *Cochrane Database Syst Rev* 2010; **7**: CD008452.

29. McNicholas C, Zhao Q, Secura G, et al. Contraceptive failures in overweight and obese combined hormonal contraceptive users. *Obstet Gynecol* 2013; **121**:585–92.

30. Robinson JA, Burke AE. Obesity and hormonal contraceptive efficacy. *Women's Health.* 2013; **9**:453–66.

31. Abdollahi M, Cushman M, Rosendaal F. Obesity: risk of venous thrombosis and the interaction with coagulation factor levels and oral contraceptive use. *Thromb Haemost.* 2003; **89**:493–8.

32. Mehri ZO, Impact of bariatric surgery on female reproduction. *Fertil Steril.* 2009; **92**:1501–8.

33. Paulen ME, Zapata LB, Cansino C, et al. Contraceptive use among women with a history of bariatric surgery: a systematic review. *Contraception.* 2010; **82**:86–94.

34. Simkin-Silverman LR, Wing RR. Weight gain during menopause. Is it inevitable or can it be prevented? *Postgrad Med.* 2000; **108**:47–50, 53–56.

35. Davis SR, Castelo-Branco C, Chedraui P, et al. Understanding weight gain at menopause. *Climacteric.* 2012; **15**:419–29.

36. Huang AJ, Subak LL, Wing R, et al. An intensive behavioral weight loss intervention and hot flushes in women. *Arch Intern Med.* 2010; **170**:1161–7.

37. Imayama I, Alfano CM, Kong A, et al. Dietary weight loss and exercise interventions effects on quality of life in overweight/obese postmenopausal women: a randomized controlled trial. *Int J Behav Nutr Phys Act.* 2011; **8**:118.

38. Norman RJ, Flight IH, Rees MC. Oestrogen and progesterone hormone replacement therapy for peri-menopausal and postmenopausal women: weight and body fat distribution. *Cochrane Database Syst Rev.* 2000; **2**:CD001018.

39. Puhl R, Brownell KD. Bias, discrimination, and obesity. *Obes Res.* 2001; **9**:788–805.

40. American College of Obstetricians and Gynecologists. Ethical issues in the care of the obese woman. Committee Opinion No. 600. *Obstet Gynecol.* 2014; **123**:1388–93.

Chapter 40

Smoking cessation

David Gregory

Introduction

Tobacco use has contributed to more preventable deaths in the twentieth century than any other identified lifestyle choice, killing more than 100 million people worldwide,[1] and more than 480,000 people every year in the United States.[2] In addition, each year more than 41,000 nonsmoking US citizens die from diseases caused by second-hand exposure, with more than 34,000 dying from heart disease and 7,300 dying from lung cancer.[2] The health costs associated with tobacco use in the United States total more than $289 billion each year, with more than $133 billion from direct medical costs and $156 billion from lost work productivity.[2] Nearly all interventions that safely identify, educate, motivate, or empower smokers to quit are effective and cost efficient because of this enormous illness burden and societal cost.[3, 4]

Scope of the problem

According to the Centers for Disease Control and Prevention (CDC), tobacco smoke contains a mixture of more than 7,000 chemicals. In addition to nicotine, a neurostimulant with highly addictive qualities, cigarette smoke contains known carcinogens, toxic metals, and poisons. The carcinogens include formaldehyde, benzene, polonium, and vinyl chloride. Chromium, arsenic, lead, and cadmium are among the toxic chemicals found. Gaseous poisons in tobacco smoke include carbon monoxide, hydrogen cyanide, ammonia, butane, and toluene.

Contrary to the calming effect that many tobacco users report during smoking, nicotine found in tobacco stimulates human physiology, inducing elevated blood pressure and vascular constriction. Carbon monoxide and cyanide reduce the oxygen carrying capacity of hemoglobin to all organs of the body. The irritating effects of tobacco smoke and its many chemicals increases the risk of cancer in nearly all organs of the body. The result is an accumulating risk of morbidity and mortality from cardiovasular and pulmonary diseases, as well as cancers.

In 2010, 19.3% of adults in the United States admitted to smoking.[5] Between 2010 and 2011, more than half of surveyed smokers tried to quit, but only 6.3% were successful.[6] Outpatient medical practices in the United States, however, ask only 65.9% of patients about smoking status, resulting in missed opportunities for counseling. Even more concerning is the fact that, according to the CDC, when identified as smokers, less than 20% of these patients are counseled to quit.[6]

Smokers seeing a physician who asks about smoking and provides individual with counseling are more likely to be successful in quitting than those whose physician does not ask about their smoking habit.[7] Smokers who are advised and receive assistance to quit report greater satisfaction with their health care than those who do not.[8–10] Because so many smokers are in the process of quitting and a physician's individual counseling has such an effect, the singular physician behavior that has the most positive impact on the health of patients is simply to identify who smokes and ask if they are considering quitting.[3, 4] Unfortunately, less than 20% of physicians feel confident in their abilities to counsel smokers on cessation.[11] The remainder of this chapter will discuss the skills and tools needed by physicians to counsel smokers to quit.

Cessation strategies

Trans-theoretical model of change

Smoking cessation appears to be less of a "completed" or "not begun" task for smokers, and more of a process of quitting that progresses and regresses indefinitely. Even patients who have not smoked for

Office Care of Women, ed. Martin E. Olsen and Botros Rizk. Published by Cambridge University Press.

years may relapse into regular use. This acknowledged continuum of quitting has resulted in the "transtheoretical model of change" related to smoking cessation. This model suggests that smokers move through the following "stages of change" as they successfully change their smoking habit.[12]

- **Pre-contemplation** – Patients in this stage may have a neutral unawareness, psychological denial, or apparent disagreement with the effects of smoking on themselves, resulting in no apparent motivation to consider cessation.
- **Contemplation** – Patients in this stage are aware of the negative effects of smoking on themselves, are considering quitting, but may be overwhelmed or unaware of how cessation could be successful.
- **Preparation** – Patients in this stage have considered quitting and are aware of possible success if they could identify a plan that worked for them, but they may not be able yet to act upon a plan due to many barriers.
- **Action** – Patients in this stage have decided to do something because they perceive the benefits of quitting outweigh the amount of effort required, and they have been able to overcome enough barriers to enact their plan.
- **Maintenance** – Patients in this stage have been able to stop smoking but remain at risk for relapse and must be empowered with tools and strategies for avoidance of smoking.

When a physician asks a patient if she smokes, she may answer yes or no, but a follow-up question is needed to determine her stage of cessation. If the answer is no, it could be that the patient never smoked or is in the action or maintenance stages, where one can ask whether or not she is actively using cessation strategies and tools (which will be discussed shortly). If the answer is yes, the patient may be in any of the other stages; in this case, the physician can ask the patient if she has considered quitting. If she has not considered quitting, she is in the pre-contemplation stage, but if the patient has, she is in the contemplation or preparation stages.

A further follow-up question of smokers beyond the pre-contemplation stage – "Have you decided upon a date you would like no longer be smoking?" or asking about a quit date – can help discern the smoker in the contemplation stage from the preparation stage. Contemplation stage smokers have not yet made steps toward deciding on a definitive action, much less a quit date, whereas preparation stage smokers who may have decided on a potential quit date are more likely to be receptive to hearing further about the many tools available to them and gathering these in advance of the date.

Determining smoker's stage of change helps to find the tools she is in most need and accepting of for success. Trying to skip a stage is likely to result in poor progress. For example, a pre-contemplation smoker is not likely to be ready for the action stage until she has exceeded the contemplation stage, chosen a quit date, and id able to process the preparation needed for action. Progressing stage by stage has resulted in more success in moving smokers along all changes to cessation and can efficiently reserve cessation tools until a smoker is truly committed to quitting.[13, 14]

The 5 As

The Agency for Healthcare Research & Quality (AHRQ) has suggested there be "5 Major Steps to Intervention" for smoking cessation in the form of the 5 As, including:

- **Ask** routinely about tobacco use status and document this for every patient with every visit, providing opportunity to determine if there is smoking risk and opportunity for cessation.
- **Advise** to quit – clearly, firmly, and personally for every tobacco user, allowing pre-contemplation stage smokers to move into the contemplation stage through education and reaffirming for others that they are doing the right thing.
- **Assess** if the tobacco user is presently interested in quitting, allowing contemplation stage smokers to begin preparing to quit.
- **Assist** the tobacco user who is willing to quit by directing her to counseling and pharmacotherapy, allowing preparation stage smokers to begin acting and planning on a quit date.
- **Arrange** follow-up in person or by telephone, best within one week of the quit date, allowing all smokers, no matter their stage, accountability to progress to the next stage.[15]

Motivational interviewing

Regardless of the stage of change, several patients may remain unwilling to quit because of:

- a lack of understanding of tobacco's harmful effects

- a lack of resources to quit (financial, role models, etc.)
- concerns about quitting
- feelings of helpless because of previous relapse(s) [16–19]

These patients may respond to brief interventions based on the principles of motivational interviewing. Although there is evidence that motivational interviewing is effective in increasing future quit attempts,[20–25] it may or may not help to improve abstinence among individuals already motivated to quit smoking.[26, 27]

Motivational interviewing explores a tobacco user's psychosocial viewpoints toward her habit to facilitate the patient to develop her own "change talk" and "commitment language."[28–30] This outcome is highly desired because self-derived words are more transformative to patients than their clinician's recommendations, which in themselves can increase patients' resistance to change.[29]

There are four general principles of motivational interviewing:[31, 32]

1. **Show empathy** – Without feeling that you care, patients will not be open to the conversation.
2. **Make known to patients the inconsistencies between their reality and hopes** – Smokers have conflict with their habit, either known to themselves or not realized because of denial.
3. **Accept that there will be resistance to change** – Personal resistance is a normal reaction to required effort toward change, but some barriers to change may be very difficult to overcome by the patient.
4. **Build a patient's belief in her own ability to change** – Patients will not be successful if they cannot believe that change is possible and only they have the ability to make the change.

The kinds of things to discuss during motivational interviewing related to smoking can be summarized in the "5 Rs":

1. **Relevance** – Make quitting relevant to a patient's health concerns, social situation, age, gender, and barriers to quitting.
2. **Risks** – Emphasize the negative consequences that are most relevant to the patient.
3. **Rewards** – Reframe which of the positive benefits of quitting would be desired most by the patient.
4. **Roadblocks** – Have the patient self-identify the most significant barriers to success and potential solutions to overcome them.
5. **Repetition** – At each appointment revisit the discussion to remind the patient of relevant advantages.

Using the 5 Rs as a potential curriculum to motivate patients for change has been shown to increase the likelihood of patients trying to quit smoking.[33, 34]

Helping patients to quit smoking begins with asking if they smoke, and requires mindful consideration of a patient's commitment and barriers to change. These issues often require many visits and follow-up, but they have been performed effectively with only three minutes of added time.[35] Depending on your practice support and styles, clinicians for women may provide ongoing care and tools or refer a patient to ongoing primary care with goals of further smoking cessation care.

Cigarette smoking reduction

Many smokers, as a part of their cessation plan, will initiate a reduction in the number of cigarettes. It is important to note that although it may make sense that reducing cigarettes is generally better than smoking the same or more, cigarette smoking reduction is not associated with a decrease in mortality from tobacco-related diseases.[36] Therefore, the goal should still remain cessation for health benefit. Still, there is evidence that reduction of cigarette number prior to a smoker's quit eate can improve success in eventual cessation.[37]

Specific cessation tools

Many pharmacologic and nonpharmacologic tools have been used to help smokers quit. Most smokers who successfully quit do so without any of these tools, indirectly demonstrating that the most important ingredient for successful cessation is a patient's commitment to making it happen. The following tools are simply adjuncts to this commitment that will provide benefit to some patients if they decide to include the tools in their planning. Employing them in the care of a patient without her being ready to quit significantly reduces their efficacy. Only a few tools have strong evidence to support their widespread use among most smokers, although many have weak anecdotal evidence, which as long as they are not harmful and a patient is committed to their use, may support a specific patient's plan for cessation.

Nonpharmacologic tools

Brief advice from a doctor or nurse Patients visiting an outpatient clinic for a health concern, who are exposed simply to a statement from a nurse or doctor that quitting smoking is in the best interest of their health are up to two times as likely to successfully quit as those not receiving this simple message.[38, 39]

More intensive brief behavioral support A natural extension from the 5 As and motivational interviewing – that is, providing regular brief behavioral support (some may call it cheerleading) in person or by phone – can have a small but important impact on cessation progress, compliance, accountability, and prevention of relapses. Smokers are 10%–25% more likely to quit when they are provided active, positive behavioral support while they progress through the stages of quitting than those for whom the topic is not discussed. The effect is proportional to the amount of behavioral interventions that a patient receives.[40]

Self-help materials Support provided through generic self-help materials, such as written leaflets and manuals, audiotapes, videotapes, and computer programs, are often used as an adjunct to brief advice. Although they can reach many more people than interventions delivered by trained counselors, they have no additional benefit over brief personal advice.[41] These are most beneficial when a face-to-face contact is not available, and have only a small effect on cessation when compared with no intervention. Interestingly, however, when self-help materials are directed at a specific demographic, such as adolescent women or pregnant women, the effect is much stronger.[42] Going further, by adding a phone contact option to the self-help materials, results in even greater improved cessation success.[39]

Internet-based and mobile phone applications Neither internet sources of contact nor those found through mobile phone applications, such as social media contact, have been adequately evaluated to suggest a significant impact on long-term smoking cessation rates.[39, 43]

One-on-one versus group support Many smokers may prefer more support from one-on-one or group counseling. Although group therapy has been shown to be more effective than self-help materials,[44] there has been no significant difference in cessation between smokers seeking individual or group support – both increase the chances of quitting by 27% to 90% more than those not receiving counseling.[44, 45] Although group counseling is theoretically more cost-effective than individual, retention of a smoking cessation group's integrity limits this approach to settings where there may be many barriers to attendance.[39, 46]

Exercise Although clearly good for general health maintenance in women, exercise alone as a cessation intervention has limited evidence to conclude that it is an effective tool for smoking cessation.[47]

Acupuncture and related interventions Although short-term – under six months – positive effects on cessation have been shown with acupuncture, acupressure, and laser therapy, there has been significant bias to available studies and no long-term effects have been demonstrated. Electrostimulation appears ineffective in reducing smoking.[48]

Hypnotherapy Available randomized controlled trials show that hypnotherapy has little added benefit compared to other interventions.[49]

Pharmacologic tools

Nicotine replacement Smokers can reduce nicotine withdrawal symptoms that occur during smoking cessation by replacing nicotine in other forms, such as chewing gum, transdermal patch, nasal spray, inhaler, sublingual tablet, and lozenge (see Table 40-1). By doing so, smokers who have demonstrated withdrawal symptoms and who have been provided at least brief counseling, are 1.5 to 2 times more successful in quitting than those who do not.[50] All forms of replacement have similar effects and carry a risk of irritation in the site they are used; therefore, which form to use should be determined by patient preference. None has shown any significant benefit in use beyond eight weeks.[39, 51]

Varenicline (Chantix) A nicotine-receptor partial agonist, varenicline has demonstrated positive effects on smoking cessation (see Table 40-1). Used in standard doses, it has shown a two to three times increase in cessation success versus placebo. Lower doses can provide some benefit with fewer side effects. The most common adverse effect of varenicline is nausea, although mild and usually reducing with time. For varenicline to be effective and in full dosing, it must be started seven days prior to stopping smoking. Possible other serious adverse events, including worsening depression and cardiovascular events, cannot be ruled out. There is little evidence to support the use of this treatment beyond 12 weeks.[52]

Antidepressants and anxiolytics Only a few antidepressants have shown benefits to aid long-term smoking cessation. Bupropion (see Table 40-1) and

Table 40-1 Potential smoking cessation pharmacologic agents

Pharmacologic agent	Dosing	Cautions & contraindications
Nicotine replacement therapy	Start on or after "quit date" **Patches (Nicoderm CQ):** • 6–10 cigarettes/day: • 14 mg patch Qday × 6 weeks, then 7 mg patch Qday × 2 weeks, then stop • >10 cigarettes/day: • 21 mg patch Qday × 6 weeks, then 14 mg patch Qday × 2 weeks, then 7 mg patch Qday × 2 weeks, then stop **Gum/lozenges** • First cigarette >30 minutes after waking: • 2 mg Q1–2 hours × 6 weeks, then Q2–4 hours × 3 weeks, then Q4–8 hours × 3 weeks, then stop • First cigarette <30 minutes after waking • 4 mg Q1–2 hours × 6 weeks, then Q2–4 hours × 3 weeks, then Q4–8 hours × 3 weeks, then stop **Inhalers** • Start by replacing up to 16 cigarettes per day with up to 16 cartridges per day (no more); gradually taper dose over 6–12 weeks, then stop	**Caution:** • Do not smoke while using • May worsen high blood pressure • May worsen peptic ulcers • Use in pregnancy is not recommended • Treatment beyond 8 weeks has not been well studied **Contraindications:** • Allergic reaction • MI in last 2 weeks • Unstable angina • Arrhythmias
Varenicline (Chantix)	Start at least one week prior to "quit date": 0.5 mg po Qday × 3 days, then 0.5 mg po BID × 4 days, then 1.0 mg po BID × 12 weeks	**Caution:** • Requires renal dosing • Patients see worsening psychiatric disease • Cardiovascular disease patients may be at risk for cardiac side effects • Use during pregnancy is not recommended • Treatment beyond 12 weeks is not well studied **Contraindications:** • Allergic reaction • <18 years old
Bupropion ER (Zyban)	Start 5–7 days prior to "quit date": 150 mg Qday × 3 days, then 150 mg BID × 7–12 weeks (dosing >8 hours apart)	**Caution:** • Can cause increased suicidality and worsened psychiatric illness • Treatment beyond 12 weeks is not well studied **Contraindications:** • MAO inhibitor usage in last 14 days • Seizure disorder • Bulimia • Anorexia • Abrupt alcohol, benzodiazepine, sedative or antiepileptic discontinuation

nortriptyline appear to have benefits to quitting independent of their antidepressant effects, with rare serious adverse effects leading to stopping medication (though nortriptyline is not FDA approved for this purpose). They are about as effective as nicotine replacement therapy, with bupropion being less effective than varenicline. For bupropion to be effective and in full treatment dosing, it must be started five to seven days prior to tobacco cessation. Other antidepressants, such as selective serotonin reuptake inhibitors (SSRIs) and monoamine oxidase (MAO) inhibitors, do not appear to have benefits to smoking cessation.[53] Other anxiolytics have no evidence in helping smoking cessation.

Other pharmacologic agents Clonidine is FDA approved to treat hypertension, but it has not been FDA approved to treat tobacco abuse. It does have some of the same pharmacological effects as the antidepressants. It has been shown to be effective in helping patients quit smoking (30%–74% more effective than placebo), but its usefulness is reduced by common side effects of sedation and postural hypotension.[39, 54]

Aversion therapy By pairing the pleasurable stimulus of smoking with an unpleasant one, some have theorized that smoking cessation could be assisted. Aversive stimuli, such as silver acetate which causes an unpleasant taste while smoking, has had variable to no effect when studied.[39, 46]

Electronic cigarettes Many smokers have replaced cigarettes with E-cigarettes, with or without nicotine. When used with the intent of quitting cigarettes and then gradually reducing the nicotine content, they have demonstrated modest help in cessation rates, similar to other nicotine replacement forms, and few adverse effects. The overall risk and benefit of this tool compared to other forms of nicotine replacement has not yet been well evaluated.[55]

Barriers to success

Although women appear more likely to seek assistance to quit smoking than men, they generally benefit similarly to the same interventions offered to men.[56, 57] Women appear to face barriers to smoking cessation differently than men, such as having higher rates of depression, more concern for weight gain, and greater social motivations for smoking.[58] Very few studies have looked at gender-specific smoking cessation approaches addressing these barriers, but addressing them is important for patient-centered tobacco cessation planning in women. Overall, despite these unique barriers, similar smoking cessation rates are observed among men and women.[59, 60]

Finances

The Centers for Disease Control and Prevention (CDC) reports the average cost of a pack of cigarettes in the United States is $5.64, (costs vary from US state to US state) resulting in the average pack-per-day smoker spending more than $150 per month on cigarette purchases alone. The financial stress that this places on smokers can motivate them to begin a cessation plan, but most cessation tools may appear to add expense to smokers who are unaware that they are soon meant to replace the tobacco expense. In order to address this often perceived barrier to starting a plan, it is important to explicitly share when the costs of smoking can be removed in the plan. With those using nicotine replacement, emphasize that continued smoking is contraindicated, and will be much less expensive than continuing to smoke.

Weight gain

Weight gain is a common effect during smoking cessation. Women are especially concerned about this and often site this as a cause for not attempting or being successful in quitting. Bupropion or nicotine replacement therapy lessen the weight gain associated with cessation attempts. Dietary and exercise counseling have little effect on the weight gain from cessation and may actually reduce cessation success. Other pharmacologic agents, such as fluoxetine, naltrexone, and phenylpropanolamine, have also shown reduced weight gain, but more study comparing their effects to the more traditional agents already used for cessation is needed.[61] Women should be reminded that quitting smoking is more beneficial to their health, even if they gain weight, and that smoking is a more difficult thing to do for most women than losing weight.

Social

The social connections that exist with the smoking habit can be quite powerful for women, such as smoking while taking a work break, having coffee with friends, or while spending time in restaurants and bars. Women will not be as successful in quitting tobacco if a plan for dealing with these triggers is not prepared. Asking women what situations are the most significant triggers for them to have a cigarette, and identifying substituted behaviors during those social triggers or replacing these triggers, may allow women smokers to be more in control. Working with women to develop close friend and family support in quitting can have a positive impact on their success, especially if these friends are supportive of substituting social triggers.

Pregnancy

Cigarette smoking is one of the most modifiable risk factors for pregnancy-related morbidity and mortality in the United States.[62] Cigarette smoking causes stillbirths, spontaneous abortion, premature birth, low birth weight, placental abruption, and sudden infant death syndrome (SIDS).[63, 64] Preconception smoking cessation is best, but health benefits result from abstinence at any time of pregnancy.[65–67] Guidelines recommend that all pregnant smokers receive face-to-face psychosocial interventions, such as those discussed earlier in the chapter, to encourage smoking cessation as early as possible during gestation.[3] Use of other pharmacologic tools during pregnancy is not recommended, but requires further research.

Concluding remarks

Health-care workers have a significant impact on patients who smoke when the health workers ask if the patients smoke, advise them to quit, assess their stage of change, assist them in attaining the next stage, and arrange appropriate follow-up. Poorly motivated patients may benefit from motivational interviewing; making the discussion relevant; focusing on patient important risks, roadblocks, and rewards; and repeating the message as necessary. The most important characteristic of an effective strategy is one that a patient is committed to following. There are many effective tools from which patients can choose, such as nicotine replacement, varenicline, or bupropion. Women may have special stressors that impact their success which clinicians need to be able to discuss openly and encourage accommodation.

References

1. World Health Organization. Fresh and Alive: MPOWER. WHO Report on the Global Tobacco Epidemic Available at: www.who.int/tobacco/mpower/2008/en. Accessed Mar 30, 2015.
2. US Department of Health and Human Services. *The Health Consequences of Smoking – 50 Years of Progress: A Report of the Surgeon General.* Atlanta, GA: U.S. Department of Health and Human Services, Centers for Disease Control and Prevention, National Center for Chronic Disease Prevention and Health Promotion, Office on Smoking and Health, 2014.
3. Fiore MC, Jaen CR, Baker TB, et al. *Treating Tobacco Use and Dependence: 2008 Update. Clinical Practice Guideline.* Rockville, MD: US Department of Health and Human Services, Public Health Service; 2008. Available at: www.surgeongeneral.gov/tobacco/index.html. Accessed Sept 14, 2015.
4. Maciosek MV, Coffield AB, Edwards NM, et al. Priorities among effective clinical preventive services: results of a systematic review and analysis. *Am J Prev Med* 2006;**31**:52–61.
5. Vital signs: current cigarette smoking among adults aged ≥18 years – United States, 2005–2010. *MMWR Morb Mortal Wkly Rep.* 2011 Sep 9;**60**(35):1207–1212.
6. Centers for Disease Control and Prevention (CDC). Current cigarette smoking among adults-United States, 2011. *Morb Mortal Wkly Rep* 2012;**61**(44):889.
7. Lancaster T, Stead LF. Individual behavioural counselling for smoking cessation. *Cochrane Database Syst Rev* 2005;**2**:CD001292. doi: 10.1002/14651858.CD001292.pub2.
8. Quinn VP, Stevens VJ, Hollis JF, et al. Tobacco-cessation services and patient satisfaction in nine nonprofit HMOs. *Am J Prev Med* 2005;**29**:77–84.
9. Solberg LI, Boyle RG, Davidson G, et al. Patient satisfaction and discussion of smoking cessation during clinical visits. *Mayo Clin Proc* 2001;**76**: 138–143.
10. Barzilai DA, Goodwin MA, Zyzanski SJ, et al. Does health habit counseling affect patient satisfaction? *Prev Med* 2001;**33**:595–599.
11. Weaver KE, Danhauer SC, Tooze JA, et al. Smoking cessation counseling beliefs and behaviors of outpatient oncology providers. *Oncologist* 2012;**17**(3):455–462. doi: 10.1634/theoncologist.2011-0350. Epub 2012 Feb 14.
12. DiClemente CC, Prochaska JO, Fairhurst, SK, et al. The process of smoking cessation: an analysis of precontemplation, contemplation, and preparation stages of change. *Journal of Consulting and Clinical Psychology* 1991 Apr;**59**(2):295–304. http://dx.doi.org/10.1037/0022-006X.59.2.295.
13. Goldberg DN, Hoffman AM, Farinha MF, et al. Physician delivery of smoking-cessation advice based on the stages-of-change model. *American Journal of Preventive Medicine* 1994 Sep–Oct; **10**(5):267–274.
14. Norcross JC, Krebs PM, Prochaska JO. Stages of change. *Journal of Clinical Psychology*, Special Issue: Adapting psychotherapy to the individual patient. 2011 Feb;**67**(2):143–154.

15. Agency for Healthcare Research and Quality. Five Major Steps to Intervention (The "5 A's"). December 2012. Available at: www.ahrq.gov/professionals/clinicians-providers/guidelines-recommendations/tobacco/5steps.html. Accessed Mar 30, 2015.

16. Rundmo T, Smedslund G, Gotestam KG. Motivation for smoking cessation among the Norwegian public. *Addict Behav* 1997;**22**:377–386.

17. Alberg AJ, Carter CL, Carpenter MJ. Weight gain as an impediment to cigarette smoking cessation: a lingering problem in need of solutions. *Prev Med* 2007;**44**:296–297.

18. Donze J, Ruffieux C, Cornuz J. Determinants of smoking and cessation in older women. *Age Ageing* 2007;**36**:53–57.

19. Fagan P, Augustson E, Backinger CL, et al. Quit attempts and intention to quit cigarette smoking among young adults in the United States. *Am J Public Health* 2007;**97**:1412–1420.

20. Chan SS, Lam TH, Salili F, et al. A randomized controlled trial of an individualized motivational intervention on smoking cessation for parents of sick children: a pilot study. *Appl Nurs Res* 2005;**18**:178–181.

21. Butler CC, Rollnick S, Cohen D, et al. Motivational consulting versus brief advice for smokers in general practice: a randomized trial. *Br J Gen Pract* 1999;**49**:611–616.

22. Curry SJ, Ludman EJ, Graham E, et al. Pediatric-based smoking cessation intervention for low-income women: a randomized trial. *Arch Pediatr Adolesc Med* 2003;**157**:295–302.

23. Brown RA, Ramsey SE, Strong DR, et al. Effects of motivational interviewing on smoking cessation in adolescents with psychiatric disorders. *Tob Control* 2003;**12**(Suppl 4):IV3–10.

24. Steinberg ML, Ziedonis DM, Krejci JA, et al. Motivational interviewing with personalized feedback: a brief intervention for motivating smokers with schizophrenia to seek treatment for tobacco dependence. *J Consult Clin Psychol* 2004; **72**:723–728.

25. Lai DTC, Cahill K, Qin Y, Tang JL. Motivational interviewing for smoking cessation. *Cochrane Database Syst Revs* 2010;**1**:CD006936. doi: 10.1002/14651858.CD006936.pub2.

26. Hettema J, Steele J, Miller WR. Motivational interviewing. *Annu Rev Clin Psychol* 2005;**1**:91–111.

27. Ahluwalia JS, Okuyemi K, Nollen N, et al. The effects of nicotine gum and counseling among African American light smokers: a 2 × 2 factorial design. *Addiction* 2006;**101**:883–891.

28. Carpenter MJ, Hughes JR, Solomon LJ, et al. Both smoking reduction with nicotine replacement therapy and motivational advice increase future cessation among smokers unmotivated to quit. *J Consult Clin Psychol* 2004;**72**:371–381.

29. Amrhein PC, Miller WR, Yahne CE, et al. Client commitment language during motivational interviewing predicts drug use outcomes. *J Consult Clin Psychol* 2003;**71**:862–878.

30. Rollnick S, Miller WR, Butler CC. *Motivational Interviewing in Health Care: Helping Patients Change Behavior*. New York: The Guilford Press, 2008.

31. Miller WR, Rollnick S. *Motivational Interviewing: Preparing People for Change*, 2nd ed. New York: Guilford Press, 2002.

32. Rollnick S, Mason P, Butler C. *Health Behavior Change: A Guide for Practitioners*. Edinburgh: Churchill Livingstone, 1999.

33. Carpenter MJ, Hughes JR, Solomon LJ. et al. Both smoking reduction with nicotine replacement therapy and motivational advice increase future cessation among smokers unmotivated to quit. *J Consult Clin Psychol* 2004;**72**:371–381.

34. Carpenter MJ, Hughes JR, Keely JP. Effect of smoking reduction on later cessation: a pilot experimental study. *Nicotine Tob Res* 2003;**5**:155–162.

35. Atkinson AL, Sherlock D. Is smoking cessation counselling effective in the OB/GYN office? A prospective study. *International Journal of Medical Science and Public Health* 2013;**2**(3):558–561.

36. Godtfredsen NS, Hoist C, Prescott E, et al. Smoking reduction, smoking cessation, and mortality: a 16-year follow-up of 19,732 men and women from the Copenhagen Centre for Prospective Population Studies. *Am J Epidemiol* 2002 Dec 1;**156**(11):994–1001.

37. Bolliger CT, Zellweger JP, Danielsson T, et al. Smoking reduction with oral nicotine inhalers: double blind, randomised clinical trial of efficacy and safety. *BMJ* 2000 Aug 5;**321**(7257):329–333.

38. Rice VH, Stead LF, Cochrane Collaboration, editors. Nursing interventions for smoking cessation. *Cochrane Library*. Issue 3. Oxford: Update Software; 2000. Available at: www.cochranelibrary.com/enhanced/doi/10.1002/14651858.CD001188. Accessed Dec 21, 2015.

39. Lancaster T, Stead L, Silagy C, Sowden A. Effectiveness of interventions to help people stop smoking: findings from the *Cochrane Library*. *BMJ* 2000 Aug 5;**321** (7257):355–358.

40. Stead LF, Lancaster T. Behavioural interventions as adjuncts to pharmacotherapy for smoking cessation. *Cochrane Database Syst Rev* 2012;**12**:CD009670. doi: 10.1002/14651858.CD009670.pub2.

41. Lancaster T, Stead LF, Cochrane Collaboration, editors. Self-help interventions for smoking cessation. *Cochrane Library*. Issue 3. Oxford: Update Software; 2000. Available at: www.ncsct.co.uk/usr/pub/self-help-interventions.pdf. Accessed Dec 21, 2015.

42. Prochaska JO, Velicer WF. The transtheoretical model of health behavior change. *Am J Health Promot* 1997;**12**:38–48.
43. Whittaker R, Borland R, Bullen C, et al. Mobile phone-based interventions for smoking cessation. *Cochrane Database Syst Rev* 2009;**4**:CD006611. doi: 10.1002/14651858.CD006611.pub2.
44. Stead LF, Lancaster T, Cochrane Collaboration, editors. Group behaviour therapy programmes for smoking cessation. *Cochrane Library*. Issue 3. Oxford: Update Software; 2000.
45. Lancaster T, Stead LF, Cochrane Collaboration, editors. Individual behavioural counselling for smoking cessation. *Cochrane Library*. Issue 3. Oxford: Update Software; 2000.
46. Lancaster T, Stead LF. Cochrane Collaboration, editors. Silver acetate for smoking cessation. *Cochrane Library*. Issue 3. Oxford: Update Software; 2000.
47. Ussher MH, Taylor A, Faulkner G. Exercise interventions for smoking cessation. *Cochrane Database Syst Rev* 2012;**1**:CD002295. doi: 10.1002/14651858.CD002295.pub4.
48. White AR, Rampes H, Liu JP, et al. Acupuncture and related interventions for smoking cessation. *Cochrane Database Syst Rev* 2014;**1**:CD000009. doi: 10.1002/14651858.CD000009.pub4.
49. Barnes J, Dong CY, McRobbie H, et al. Hypnotherapy for smoking cessation. *Cochrane Database Syst Rev* 2010;**10**:CD001008. doi: 10.1002/14651858.CD001008.pub2.
50. Silagy C, Mant D, Fowler G, Lancaster T, Cochrane Collaboration, editors. Nicotine replacement therapy for smoking cessation. *Cochrane Library*. Issue 3. Oxford: Update Software; 2000.
51. Stead LF, Perera R, Bullen C, et al. Nicotine replacement therapy for smoking cessation. *Cochrane Database Syst Rev* 2012;**11**:CD000146. doi: 10.1002/14651858.CD000146.pub4.
52. Cahill K, Stead LF, Lancaster T. Nicotine receptor partial agonists for smoking cessation. *Cochrane Database Syst Rev* 2012;**4**:CD006103.
53. Hughes JR, Stead LF, Hartmann-Boyce J, et al. Antidepressants for smoking cessation. *Cochrane Database Syst Rev* 2014;**1**:CD000031. doi: 10.1002/14651858.CD000031.pub4.
54. Gourlay SG, Stead LF, Benowitz NL, Cochrane Collaboration, editors. Clonidine for smoking cessation. *Cochrane Library*. Issue 3. Oxford: Update Software; 2000.
55. Bullen, C, Howe C, Laugesen M, et al. Electronic cigarettes for smoking cessation: a randomised controlled trial. *Lancet* 2013;**382**(9905):1629–1637.
56. Zhu S, Melcer T, Sun J, et al. Smoking cessation with and without assistance: a population-based analysis. *Am J Prev Med* 2000;**18**:305–311.
57. Munafo M, Bradburn M, Bowes L, et al. Are there sex differences in transdermal nicotine replacement therapy patch efficacy? A meta-analysis. *Nicotine Tob Res* 2004;**6**:769–776.
58. Smith SS, Jorenby DE, Leischow SJ, et al. Targeting smokers at increased risk for relapse: treating women and those with a history of depression. *Nicotine Tob Res* 2003;**5**:99–109.
59. Jarvis MJ, Cohen JE, Delneo CD, Giovino GA. Dispelling myths about gender differences in smoking cessation: population data from the USA, Canada and Britain. *Tobacco Control* 2013 Sep; **22**(5):356–360.
60. Husky MM, Mazure CM, Paliwal P, McKee SA. Gender differences in the comorbidity of smoking behavior and major depression. *Drug and Alcohol Dependence* 2008 Jan 11;**93**(1–2):176–179.
61. Farley AC, Hajek P, Lycett D, Aveyard P. Interventions for preventing weight gain after smoking cessation. *Cochrane Database Syst Rev* 2012;**1**:CD006219. doi: 10.1002/14651858.CD006219.pub3.
62. Armour BS, Campbell VA, Crews JE, et al. Nicotine replacement and behavioral therapy for smoking cessation in pregnancy. *Am J Prev Med* 2007 Oct;**33** (4):297–305.
63. U.S. Department of Health and Human Services. *The health consequences of involuntary exposure to tobacco smoke: a report of the Surgeon General, U.S. Department of Health and Human Services, Centers for Disease Control and Prevention, National Center for Chronic Disease Prevention and Health Promotion, Office on Smoking and Health*. 2006. Available at: www.surgeongeneral.gov/library/reports/secondhandsmoke/fullreport.pdf. Accessed Dec 21, 2015.
64. American College of Obstetricians and Gynecologists. Smoking cessation during pregnancy. *Obstet Gynecol* 2005;**106**:883–888.
65. England LJ, Kendrick JS, Wilson HG, et al. Effects of smoking reduction during pregnancy on the birth weight of term infants. *Am J Epidemiol* 2001;**154**:694–701.
66. Lieberman E, Gremy I, Lang JM, et al. Low birthweight at term and the timing of fetal exposure to maternal smoking. *Am J Public Health* 1994 Jul;**84** (7):1127–1131.
67. DiClemente CC, Dolan-Mullen P, Windsor RA. The process of pregnancy smoking cessation: implications for interventions. *Tob Control* 2000;**9** (Suppl 3):III16–III21.

Chapter 41

Office evaluation and management of abdominal pain

Brett Worly

Introduction

Abdominal pain is a common presenting complaint in the outpatient office setting for primary health-care providers. This condition makes up to 50% of adult complaints and affects nearly every woman in her lifetime.[1] One-third of all patients have an underlying cause that cannot be specified; the most common etiologies are gastroenteritis (7.2%–18.7%), irritable bowel disease (2.6%–13.2%), urologic (5.3%), and gastritis (5.2%). Ten percent of abdominal pain patients have acute onset, such as appendicitis (1.9%), diverticulitis (3.0%), and biliary/pancreatic (4.0%), or neoplastic processes (1.0%); these require immediate therapy.[1] Abdominal pain has a rich, complex series of etiologies at the cellular and molecular level, with a complicated list of differential diagnoses. It is essential for the astute health-care provider to masterfully elicit appropriate history from the patient, quickly narrow the list of differential diagnoses with a skillful physical exam, then expertly order the appropriate tests. This chapter will evaluate abdominal pain from the cellular and molecular level, move to the clinical pearls for history taking and physical exam, then elucidate complex and more common etiologies and provide treatment options. This chapter thus provides a clear and concise perspective for a challenging topic.

Physiology of pain

Pain is often caused at the molecular level by various substances released by damaged cells, including substance P, cyclooxygenase-2, prostaglandin, aromatase, and interleukins.[2, 3] These substances lead to angiogenesis, fibrosis, adhesion formation, and altered immune function. Response to cell injury is modulated based on size and severity of injury, molecular release of the markers just noted, and serotonergic response with cortical processing. Free nerve endings of unmyelinated C fibers and Aδ fibers in the skin convey thermal, chemical, or mechanical stimuli as pain with moderate to extreme amounts of input. Inflammation makes sensory afferent neurons more sensitive through the release of bradykinin, prostaglandin, and leukotrienes. Cortical processing can be influenced by serotonin and norepinephrine.[2, 3]

Damage or overstimulation of these pathways can lead to dysesthesia, which are abnormal painful sensations usually found in an area of sensory loss. This pain is referred to as neuropathic pain and is usually described by the patient as burning, tingling, or shock-like. The causes of neuropathic pain include overly sensitive afferent nerves, a developed sensitivity to norepinephrine, and abnormal electrical current conduction or neuron recruitment. Synaptic reorganization can also occur at the level of the brain and spinal cord, amplifying signals differently in response to frequent pain. Neurotransmitters affecting pain interpretation include endorphins, serotonin, and norepinephrine; validating the biological plausibility of serotonin reuptake inhibitors, norepinephrine reuptake inhibitors, and opioids for pain control.[2, 3]

Types of pain

Many different types of pain exist. Historical assessment should identify the exact symptomatology. A discriminating question is, "What changed?" This question may help an interviewer better understand a potential inciting event, or a progressive process. Identification of new stresses or medical disorders may better direct questioning. Sharp pain is usually associated with a specific location and occurs from peritoneal irritation. Dull, aching, colicky pain can signify visceral pain, arising from distension or spasm of a hollow organ. Burning or shooting pain is usually associated with neuropathic pain. Cyclic pain may be related to hormonal fluctuations.[2, 3]

Office Care of Women, ed. Martin E. Olsen and Botros Rizk. Published by Cambridge University Press.

Other important symptoms

"PPQRST," a common mnemonic in evaluating pain, is used to narrow the differential diagnosis. "P" signifies provocation, identifying what was associated with the onset of pain, and what makes the pain worse. For example, mesenteric ischemia usually starts within one hour of eating, whereas peptic ulcers usually improve with eating. The next "P" helps identify the palliative factors and could include medicines taken and activities altered. Specific attention to bowel movements, menstrual cycles, and urination may be helpful, as pain relieved or worsened with bowel movements can suggest irritable bowel syndrome, whereas increased pain with a full bladder may be suggestive of painful bladder syndrome. Pain worse with menses may suggest endometriosis, adenomyosis, or uterine leiomyoma. "Q" helps identify the quality of the pain and can be especially helpful in distinguishing etiologies among visceral, neuropathic, and peritoneal pain etiologies. "R" is helpful for eliciting information about pain location and radiation. "S" enables the provider to identify the severity of the symptoms and how it affects the patient's life. The patient's psychological state in relation to the pain is important, so questions regarding psychotropic medications, opiate or illicit drug use, hospitalizations, psychiatric hospitalizations, and suicide attempts are essential to understanding the condition. A sexual history should be taken for all patients, with inquiries about pain during coitus, number of sexual partners, history of sexually transmitted infections, sexually transmitted infections or symptoms in partners, contraception use, and timing of pain in relation to menses. "T" is important to help understand the timing of the pain and identifying intermittent, constant, or cyclic pain.[4]

Acute versus chronic pain

One of the most important aspects of becoming a skilled care provider is being able to identify acute, severe, and life-threatening problems; separating them from those complaints that are not severe; and appropriately triaging resources, time, money, and energy. Symptoms of an acute emergency include pain severity, fever, vomiting, and signs of hypotension, severe hypertension, tachycardia, tachypnea, and an abdominal exam that includes rebound, guarding, or tenderness.[4]

Location

The location and radiation of pain are helpful for narrowing the many differential diagnoses to an appropriate and manageable number. This chapter will focus on pain in different locations, separating the abdomen into nine sections. Although some types of abdominal pain may cross these borders, many types of pain linger in one region.

The abdomen may be divided into four or nine sections, and the terminology for describing the location of the pain can be essential in communicating with other health-care providers (see Figure 41-1).[4] Table 41-1 gives common differential diagnoses based on the region of pain.

Migratory pain

Pain that migrates can be classified into several categories that usually pertain to the organ system in each anatomical location of the pain complaint. Bowel, musculoskeletal, endometriosis, and supratentorial pain etiologies can exist anywhere within the abdomen.

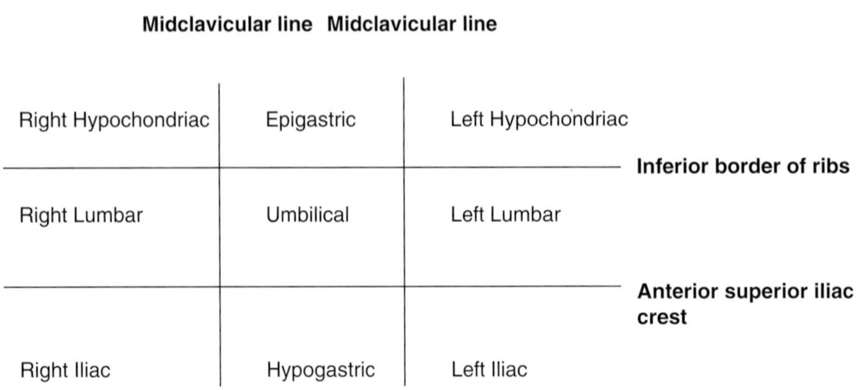

Figure 41-1 Abdominal regions.

Table 41-1 Causes of abdominal pain by geographic location

Right hypochondriac:	Epigastric:	Left hypochondriac:
Cholecystitis	Gastritis	Constipation
Cholelithiasis	Gastroesophageal reflux	Rib fracture
Gall bladder carcinoma	Myocardial infarction	
Liver abscess	Splenic infarct	
Cirrhosis	Aortic dissection	
Fitz-Hugh-Curtis syndrome	Gas pain	
Pneumonia	Stomach cancer	
Right lumbar	**Umbilical**	**Left lumbar**
Nephrolithiasis	Early appendicits	Nephrolithiasis
Pyelonephritis	Constipation/gas	Pyelonephritis
	Uterine leiomyoma	
	Sickle cell attack	
Right iliac	**Hypogastric**	**Left iliac**
Appendicitis	Pregnancy	Ovarian torsion
Ovarian torsion	Ectopic pregnancy	Adnexal mass
Adnexal mass	Uterine leiomyoma	Uterine leiomyoma
Uterine leiomyoma	Adnexal mass	Endometriosis
Endometriosis	IBS/IBD	Constipation/gas
Constipation/gas	Endometriosis	IBS/IBD
Irritable bowel syndrome (IBS)	Adenomyosis	Diverticulitis
Irritable bowel disease (IBD)	Painful bladder syndrome	Inguinal hernia
Inguinal hernia	Urinary tract infection	
	Pelvic inflammatory disease	
	Mittleschmerz	

Left iliac pain

Left iliac pain is usually associated with colon, small bowel, musculoskeletal, or urologic etiology. Sharp, colicky pain can indicate bowel or urologic etiology, and appropriate lab tests, imaging, and referral are essential to this evaluation. Pain caused by the female reproductive system can be identified in the iliac region, although other common causes of left lower quadrant pain include diverticulitis, inguinal hernia, and gas.

Hypogastric pain

Hypogastric pain can involve uterus, bladder, musculoskeletal systems, ovaries, and gastrointestinal systems. A patient history and physical exam, with diagnostic laboratory and imaging tests, are essential here. Urinary, gastrointestinal, and reproductive history should be areas of focus for the visit.

Right iliac pain

Reproductive, gastrointestinal, musculoskeletal, and urologic systems need to be evaluated in the history and physical exam portions of the visit with a complaint in this region. Appendicitis, ovarian cysts, and torsion are common etiologies. Appendicitis traditionally begins in the epigastric region with dull and aching visceral pain, and eventually evolves into sharp right lower quadrant pain at McBurney's point, two-thirds distance from the umbilicus on a spinoumbilical line, when parietal inflammation and irritation begin.[5]

Right hypochondriac pain

Right hypochondriac pain is commonly related to cholecystitis, cholelithiasis, and hepatomegaly. Older, overweight female patients with postprandial severe right hypochondriac pain nausea, vomiting, or fever should be evaluated for cholecystitis. Patients with chronic liver disease, a history of hepatitis, and alcoholism should undergo a thorough evaluation of the liver.

Organ system approach to abdominal pain

Several different organ systems can be responsible for abdominal pain. It is often important to think about the geographic location of the pain and then consider a differential diagnosis based on the organ systems potentially involved. Organ systems that could contribute to abdominal pain include the gastrointestinal tract, renal system, reproductive tract, musculoskeletal tract, immune system, cardiovascular system, the skin, and the nervous system including psychiatric causes.

Gastrointestinal tract

Gastrointestinal causes of pain could be indicated with many complaints, including abdominal pain of any location, and may present with sharp or dull pain, with associated symptoms of nausea and vomiting, constipation or diarrhea, fever, chills, sweats, and bloody or tarry stools.

Common causes of abdominal pain include inflammatory bowel disease (IBD) and irritable bowel syndrome (IBS). IBD consists of two separate entities: ulcerative colitis (UC) and Crohn's disease (CD).

IBS effects 15% of the US population and has three main subtypes: IBS-C for constipation dominant, IBS-D for diarrhea predominant, and IBS-M for mixed symptoms. IBS is thought to be an abdominal pain or discomfort associated with a change in consistency or frequency of stools, and relieved by defecation. Rome III criteria for diagnosis include 12 weeks in the past 12 months of abdominal pain or discomfort that has at least two of the following: symptoms improved with defecation, onset is associated with a change in the frequency of stool, or onset is associated with a change in the consistency of stool. Criteria that increase confidence of an IBS diagnosis include abnormal stool frequency noted to be greater than three episodes per day or less than three episodes per week; abnormal stool form described as lumpy, watery, or hard; abnormal stool passage with either straining, urgency, or incomplete evacuation; passage of mucous in stool; or bloating.

Treatment of IBS includes cessation of smoking and chewing gum and avoiding caffeine, carbonated beverages, lactose, sorbitol, and fructose. Anti-inflammatory medications such as sulfasalazine and glococorticoids; antispasmodics such as dicyclomine, peppermint oil, and hyoscyamine; selective serotonin reuptake inhibitors (SSRIs) such as citalopram, paroxetine, and fluoxetine; fiber with bran and psyllium; and tricyclic antidepressants such as amitriptylene, trimipramine, and desipramine have all been proven to be helpful in IBS patients. Constipation may be managed with adequate hydration, including 8–10 cups of water daily, and adequate fiber, as well as osmotic laxatives such as docusate. lactulose, polyethylene glycol, and magnesium citrate may also be used for constipation symptoms. Diarrhea may be managed with loperamide or cholestyramine.[6, 7]

UC is usually limited to the colonic mucosa and rectum, whereas CD is transmural and granulomatous. Although CD is most likely found in the distal ileum or colon, it can be found at any point in the gastrointestinal tract. Likely etiology of these conditions is an aberrant host immune response to gastrointestinal tract antigens. CD is characterized by inflammation and ulceration of the entire thickness of the bowel wall, potentially even involving mesentery and lymph nodes. The simultaneous deep mucosal inflammation with the submucosal thickening gives CD a "cobblestone" appearance. Further complications may result from this disease including abscess, perforation, fistula, and small bowel obstruction. Some patients with CD will also have inflammatory disorders of the skin, eye, mucous membranes, apthous ulcers, and migratory arthritis.

Both CD and UC present similarly, with complaints of bloody diarrhea leading to malabsorption and potentially to protein losing enteropathy and malnutrition. Because UC is usually limited to the mucosa, it is uncommon to see perforation, abscess formation, and small bowel obstruction. Unfortunately, UC is associated with carcinoma and toxic megacolon.

Further evaluation for these conditions would include complete blood count (CBC), electrolytes, liver function tests, amylase and lipase, stool hemoccult test, and colonoscopy. All tests except for colonoscopy should be normal in IBS patients. Celiac sprue antibody screening may also be performed to rule out this condition.

IBD flare is rare for some patients, but it can recur frequently for others. Sulfasalazine, or 5-amniosalicylic acid, is a common medication for IBD and is thought to have actions that modulate inflammatory response, with leukotriene and tumor necrosis factor (TNF) alpha effects. Other immune modulators may be used for IBD, including azathioprine, mercaptopurine, methotrexate, and infliximab. Treatment is aimed at symptoms and supportive care, and is not curative.[3]

Diverticular disease is another common etiology of abdominal pain in Caucasian populations, with increasing prevalence in those with advancing age, low fiber diet, and lack of physical exercise.[8] Diverticular disease is located more commonly in the left abdomen and occurs when the colonic mucosa and submucosa herniate through the underlying muscularis. This problem affects 10% of the US population; incidence increases with age. The most common presentation is intermittent left lower quadrant pain. Fevers and signs of acute abdomen may develop, including rebound, abdominal tenderness, and guarding. Bloody stools or positive hemoccult blood tests may also occur. Patients eating refined foods with decreased fiber are commonly associated with diverticular disease.

Most acquired diverticula occur in the colon, with 95% occurring in the sigmoid colon. Functional problems are usually associated with low fiber intake and chronic constipation, with increased transmural pressure from the lumen. Increased muscular contractions can cause abdominal pain lasting hours to days, with relief after passing flatus or feces. Constipation, diarrhea, and flatulence are common presenting symptoms.[3]

Diverticulitis is the most common complication of diverticulosis, and occurs when a focal diverticulosis inflammation occurs as a result of fecal material. Diverticulitis affects 25% of patients with left-sided colonic diverticulosis. Diverticulitis can produce fever, abdominal pain, abscess formation, and perforation. The three clinical criteria with the highest positive predictive value for diverticulitis include left lower quadrant abdominal pain, a C-reactive protein (CRP) value less than 50 mg/L, and the absence of vomiting. Additional imaging may be helpful. Perforation is usually self-contained, but it can lead to fistula formation and intestinal obstruction. Colonoscopy is recommended by many after the acute episode of diverticulitis to evaluate for carcinoma. Treatments for diverticular disease prevention include increased dietary fiber and rifaximin. Patients with acute diverticulitis may be followed as an outpatient if they are without fever, able to take oral liquids, have no excessive vomiting, have no marked peritonitis, and have a good support system with close follow-up available. Antibiotics are commonly recommended for patients with diverticulitis, particularly in patients with septicemia, poor general condition, pregnancy, or patients taking immunosuppressants. Surgery may be appropriate in select candidates.[8]

Renal system

Abdominal pain may also have a urologic etiology. These can include urinary tract infection, pyelonephritis, and nephrolithiasis. Nephrolithiasis can be caused by several different disorders; however, 75% of stones include calcium. Nephrolithiasis affects 1 in 11 people in the United States, with 50% of individuals having a recurrence within 10 years. The prevalence in women is 7.1%. Risk factors for stones include obesity/overweight, hypertension, and diabetes. Common presenting symptoms include severe, sharp, shooting pain from the flanks to the inguinal region, hematuria, and history of a stone. Clinical evaluation for patients with kidney stones includes dietary history, serum chemistries, urinalysis (microscopic and dipstick), urine culture, CBC, and renal ultrasound. Dietary history should include a focus on calcium intake, fluid intake, sodium intake, fruits and vegetables, and animal derived purines.[10] Increased oral hydration and avoidance of high-protein, high-sodium, and high-calcium diets may be helpful. Other protective factors include adjusting citrate and magnesium levels, avoiding sugar-sweetened beverages, and increasing dietary fiber.[10]

When nephrolithiasis occurs, renal stones commonly cause ureter, renal pelvis, or renal capsule distention. The severity of the pain is related to the degree of dilation. Rarely urinary tract obstruction can result, but this usually improves with expectant management, adequate oral hydration, pain control, and rest. Major concerns occur when this problem leads to hydronephrosis with possible permanent renal damage due to obstruction, infection, renal damage, and chronic hypertension.[3]

Painful bladder syndrome (PBS) occurs in 1%–11% of patients, and may be caused by disruption in the proteoglycan/glucosaminoglycan (GAG) layer, upregulated immune/inflammatory response, neural upregulation, and pelvic floor dysfunction.[11] This condition may present with hypogastric pain, particularly with a full bladder, urinary frequency, hematuria, pain after intercourse, and pain with menses or stress.[6] PBS is a disagreeable sensation (pain, pressure, or discomfort) perceived by the patient to be related to the urinary bladder; it is associated with lower urinary tract symptoms of more than 6 weeks duration, when infection or other causes are unidentifiable. On exam, these patients will frequently have suprapubic or bladder tenderness, with urinalysis showing sterile pyuria and Hunner's ulcerations seen on cystoscopy. Diet may play a part in worsening PBS pain; eliminating citrus fruits, tomato products, alcohol, cola, and spicy foods may be helpful. Pentosan sulfate may help replace the disrupted GAG layer. Amitriptyline may also be helpful by blocking serotonin and noradrenaline reuptake.[11] Oral cimetidine, hyaluronic acid, and dimethyl sulfoxide may be used as intravessical instillations. Immunotherapy agents may also be used.[6, 11]

Reproductive tract

The female reproductive tract is responsible for one-third of all complaints of pelvic pain, and may be a cause of abdominal pain as well.

The reproductive tract has many potential etiologies for pelvic pain. A thorough history taking, physical exam, and appropriate tests are essential at coming to a challenging diagnosis. Separating chronic pelvic pain, or pain that has lasted six months or longer, from acute pelvic pain may be instrumental to the diagnosis. Further understanding the timing of the pain quality, radiation, association with menstrual cycle timing, as well as bowel and bladder habits may also be important for determining the diagnosis. All patients of reproductive age should receive a pregnancy test as part of the evaluation. All patients with a positive pregnancy test will need to have their blood type and Rh factor identified.

Early pregnancy

If a current pregnancy is identified, miscarriage, normal pregnancy, and ectopic pregnancy need to be considered based on timing of pregnancy, obstetric and gynecologic history, smoking status, history of sexually transmitted disease, vaginal bleeding, pain, risk factors, physical exam, and ultrasound. Ectopic pregnancy is a life-threatening condition and occurs in 1.5%–2% of pregnancies. Ectopic pregnancy is a diagnosis that cannot be dismissed until a negative pregnancy test is found or an intrauterine pregnancy is clearly identified. For patients with a positive urine pregnancy test, a serum β-HCG quantitative test should be used to evaluate the pregnancy. For patients with an HCG above 1,500 mIU/mL–3,000 mIU/mL, initial signs of an intrauterine pregnancy should be identified on transvaginal ultrasound; otherwise an abnormal pregnancy should be declared. For patients who are below this discriminatory zone, transvaginal ultrasound may still be helpful in identifying the cause for pain, as evidence of an ectopic pregnancy may be seen, including free fluid in the posterior cul de sac, empty uterus, or adnexal mass. For patients with severe pain, vaginal bleeding, and a positive pregnancy test, evaluation needs to be prompt. Delays in evaluating and caring for a patient with an ectopic pregnancy can be disastrous. Pregnancies with an HCG value below the discriminatory zone in a stable patient with nondiagnostic ultrasound can be followed with serial HCG values every 48 hours. A minimum of a 53% rise for a normal pregnancy is expected, and repeat ultrasound is performed once the discriminatory zone is reached. Treatment for ectopic pregnancy includes methotrexate, a dihydrofolate antagonist, or surgery. Absolute contraindications to methotrexate include unstable patient, breastfeeding, immunodeficiency, blood dyscrasia, known sensitivity to methotrexate, active pulmonary disease, peptic ulcer disease, renal or hematologic dysfunction, alcoholism, or chronic liver disease. Relative contraindications include ectopic mass greater than 3.5 cm, embryonic cardiac motion, likely poor compliance, or HCG greater than 5,000 mIU/mL.[12]

For patients with a positive pregnancy test, vaginal bleeding, and an identifiable intrauterine pregnancy, threatened abortion can be a common diagnosis if the patient's cervix is closed. With an open cervix, an inevitable abortion is diagnosed. Expectant, medical, or surgical management may take place at this point. A positive pregnancy test with a transvaginal ultrasound showing a gestational sac greater than 25 mm, without a yolk sac or fetal pole should be identified as an anembryonic gestation; the patient should be informed of the pregnancy loss and offered appropriate management. For patients where a fetal pole is identified at greater than 7 mm, without fetal cardiac motion, embryonic demise should be identified, and the patient should be informed of the pregnancy loss with management options. Miscarriage is the most common complication of early pregnancy and occurs in 15%–20% of early clinical pregnancies.[12, 13] See Chapter 11 for additional discussion on ectopic pregnancy.

Pelvic inflammatory disease

Pelvic inflammatory disease (PID) is a common cause of acute pelvic pain with 1.2 million medical visits in the United States in 2000 alone, and estimated direct medical costs in 1998 were $1.88 billion. PID includes sequelae such as chronic pelvic pain, ectopic pregnancy, and infertility. Nongonoccal and nonchlamydial etiology are seen in 9%–23% of patients with PID. A diagnosis of PID should be considered for patients who have symptoms that include a history of pelvic inflammatory disease, risky sexual contacts, smoking, illicit drug use, and young age. Patient symptoms including vaginal discharge, fevers, and nausea or vomiting. Patients with a temperature greater than 100.4° Fahrenheit, abdominal tenderness, rebound, guarding, cervical motion tenderness, adnexal tenderness or mass, pus from the cervical os, leukorrhea [>10 white blood count (WBC)/high powered field on wet mount], erythrocyte sedimentation rate (ESR) greater than 15 mm/h, irregular vaginal bleeding, leukocytosis, and tubo-ovarian abscess on ultrasound need prompt treatment for PID. The examination should also include an abdominal exam with palpation of the right upper quadrant to consider Fitz-Hugh-Curtis syndrome, a vaginal speculum exam looking for friability of the cervix or mucopurulent discharge from the cervix, a bimanual exam, and a wet mount of vaginal discharge assessing for trichomonads, bacterial vaginosis, or leukorrhea. Thickened, fluid-filled tubes on transvaginal ultrasound have 85% sensitivity and 100% specificity for PID.[14]

Patients with PID who have surgical emergencies, are pregnant, lack clinical response after 72 hours of oral antibiotic therapy, are noncompliant, have signs or symptoms of sepsis, cannot tolerate medicines orally, or have tubo-ovarian abscess require inpatient therapy. Patients not fitting these criteria may be managed as an outpatient as long as they are given careful sepsis precautions and can be counted on to return to the outpatient office in 72 hours for further evaluation, while being compliant with their oral antibiotics.[14] Updated guidelines for antibiotics in patients with PID can be found at http://cdc.gov. Additional discussion on PID is undertaken in Chapter 17.

Endometriosis

Endometriosis is a common condition in women under 30 years of age, and usually presents with dysmenorrhea. Constant pelvic pain may be reported for severe cases. Whereas many patients with endometriosis report pain limited to their pelvis, endometriosis can be responsible for pain throughout the body, implanting in sites as far away as the diaphragm, brain, umbilicus, c-section scar, and fingers. Endometriosis is not identified readily on ultrasound, MRI, or with the serum Ca125 test, but it is often arrived upon as a diagnosis of exclusion, as it usually improves with hormonal contraceptive agents. In recalcitrant cases, diagnostic laparoscopy may be warranted. An official diagnosis of endometriosis can only be made with tissue biopsy.[2]

Hormonal contraception with a levonorgestrel-releasing intrauterine system has the most evidence of benefit in a Cochrane review, while gonadotropin-releasing hormone (GnRH) analogues and danazol may also be helpful. In patients where hormonal contraception fails, hypothalamic pituitary adnexal access inhibitors, such as leuprolide, may be used.[15]

A Cochrane review of surgical management of endometriosis through destruction of lesions may be helpful to patients, with laparoscopic surgery benefiting patients compared to diagnostic laparoscopy at 6 and 12 months postoperatively (odds ratios of 6.58 with 95% CI 3.31–13.10 and 10.00 with 95% CI 3.21–31.17, respectively).[16] A full discussion of endometriosis is undertaken in Chapter 25.

Uterine leiomyoma

Uterine leiomyoma (fibroids) affects 20%–80% of women of reproductive age and accounts for the most common cause of gynecologic emergency department visits in the UK. Fibroids are monoclonal tumors of uterine smooth muscle cells with collagen, fibronectin, and proteoglycan. Risk factors for fibroids include being of African descent, obese, and aged ≤35; increased alcohol and caffeine intake; decreased parity; and prolonged estrogen exposure with early menarche. Patients may share a history of severe menstrual cramping, pelvic pressure, dyspareunia, urinary incontinence or retention, and heavy menstrual bleeding. Pelvic exam and transvaginal ultrasound are helpful at evaluating this problem, while MRI shows increased sensitivity. Treatment needs to be tailored to the patient's wishes. Fibroid symptoms are commonly treated with hormonal contraceptives. Leuprolide with progestin add-back therapy may be helpful in shrinking fibroids by up to 30%–40%, increasing pre- and postoperative hemoglobin, and improving pelvic symptoms. Mifepristone, ulipristal acetate, anastrazole, and letrozole have also been shown to be effective in decreasing fibroid size and symptoms. Surgical management includes laparoscopic, hysteroscopic, and open myomectomy, with the understanding that excision of large fibroids could necessitate hysterectomy or c-section with each pregnancy, due to the uterine defect resulting from excision. Recurrence of fibroids is common in premenopausal patients who undergo myomectomy, and should be included in surgical counseling. Hysterectomy provides definitive treatment in patients who have completed their reproductive lives. Uterine fibroid or uterine artery embolization is a minimally invasive option for patients who desire treatment beyond what medication may allow, who are not good surgical candidates, and who have completed childbearing. Embolization can be highly effective in circumstances where there is a large intracavitary fibroid, where fibroids are few in number, and where patients fully understand the potential for fibroid necrosis. Uterine leiomyosarcoma occurs in 1 out of 500–1,000 women with fibroids, and most occur in those over 40 years of age with abnormal uterine bleeding, pelvic pain, and a growing palpable pelvic mass. Concerns about leiomyosarcoma have motivated the Food and Drug Administration (FDA) and many providers across the United States to discourage hand-held electric intraabdominal morcellation procedures, due to risk of malignant spread.[17] A full discussion of fibroids is undertaken in Chapter 23.

Adenomyosis

Adenomyosis is a common condition found in reproductive age women and is associated with heavy menstrual bleeding and cyclic dysmenorrhea. This common benign condition is defined by islands of ectopic endometrial tissue found in the myometrium. Definitive diagnosis is found on pathological analysis after hysterectomy, but indicators of adenomyosis include a globular, tender uterus on physical exam, thickened endometrial/myometrial junction, subendometrial hyperechoic striations, and asymmetric myometrial walls on ultrasound. Primary evaluation includes transvaginal ultrasound to rule out other etiologies, whereas MRI is better than ultrasound in terms of sensitivity and specificity. Treatment options include includes nonsteroidal anti-inflammatory agents (NSAIDs), hormonal contraceptives, oral progesterones, levonorgestrel-releasing intrauterine device, GnRH agonists, and uterine artery embolization, and hysterectomy.[18]

Ovarian torsion

Ovarian torsion may cause unilateral pelvic pain, which can be acute or intermittent. Torsion describes a condition where the ovarian and fallopian tube vasculature twists around the infundibulopelvic and broad ligaments, and the ovarian artery is intermittently or permanently occluded. Patients often note sudden, extreme sharp pelvic pain, with nausea, vomiting, abdominal tenderness, rebound, guarding, fever, and adnexal tenderness and mass on exam. Patients with torsion often have decreased Doppler blood flow to their ovary on pelvic ultrasound, although ultrasound is only 50% sensitive for torsion. Treatment is surgical, and the ovary must be untwisted as soon as possible, ideally less than 24 hours from the onset of severe pain, except in the poor surgical candidate where excision of the necrotic ovary or expectant management may be more appropriate.[19]

Adnexal masses

Adnexal masses are another gynecologic cause of pelvic pain. Patients who are premenopausal and have simple cystic masses without septations and less than

10 cm do not have cancer; however, these masses can cause substantial discomfort. Diagnosis is important in treatment planning, although the diagnosis can be very difficult despite imaging technologies. Multiple different types of cysts exist, including benign conditions – namely hemorrhagic, simple, theca lutein, endometrioma, cystadenoma, benign cystic teratoma, and corpus luteum cysts. Pelvic mass is discussed in Chapter 19.

Musculoskeletal and connective tissue etiology

The musculoskeletal and connective tissue etiologies for abdominal pain are frequently dismissed, but they deserve inclusion in an appropriate differential diagnosis.

Adhesive disease

Adhesive disease often occurs in patients with multiple abdominal surgeries, or who are four to six weeks out from abdominal surgery. Pain is usually focused in one particular location, with bowel-like complaints including nausea and vomiting, obstipation, diarrhea, sharp pain, or constipation. Adhesive tissue can form and cause intermittent strangulation or obstruction of bowel or other abdominal contents. Patients with severe pain and symptoms suggestive of ischemia will need emergency surgery to rectify the problem; however, patients with mild to moderate pain should be encouraged to consider expectant management, as surgery can resolve adhesions, but this often leads to more adhesions in the future, leaving most patients with no overall improvement at one year postoperatively.[6]

Musculoskeletal disease

Musculoskeletal etiology or trigger points can be described as intermittent or constant burning, shooting, or sharp abdominal pain, usually in one location. Diagnosis can be confirmed by Carnett's test, when the head is flexed from the supine position simultaneously with flexion of the abdominal muscles, and abdominal tenderness is palpated on exam. Trigger point injections into the location of pain may be curative immediately when using lidocaine 1% with bupivacaine 0.25%. Physical therapy may also be helpful for other musculoskeletal etiologies.[6]

Abdominal pain from etiologies outside of the abdomen

Psychogenic causes of abdominal pain are common. Depression; another psychiatric diagnosis; and a history of physical, sexual, or emotional abuse are frequently found in pain patients. These patients may have migratory intermittent pain that is sometimes associated with stressful life events or relationships. Psychological counseling or antidepressants may be helpful in this population, although many are reluctant to seek help due to social stigma about a psychologic diagnosis. Lab results, exam, and imaging in these patients will likely return with normal findings. It is essential that providers take seriously the complaints from patients diagnosed with psychogenic abdominal pain. Although their complaints typically remain psychogenic in origin, occasionally an additional new acute or emergent etiology may emerge. This cannot be missed.

Idiopathic pelvic pain

Idiopathic pelvic pain often responds to treatment with medroxyprogesterone acetate with a 50% reduction in visual analog scale pain rating, but patients do note side effects, including bloating and weight gain. Gosrelin, gabapentin, and amytriptylene have also been proven to be effective medications. Reassurance ultrasounds, psychologic counseling, distension of pelvic structures, and writing therapy are effective nonpharmacologic interventions.[20]

Concluding remarks

Abdominal pain is one of the more challenging symptoms in the outpatient setting. Evaluation may need to be immediate and emergent, or it may take months as various possible etiologies are eliminated. Although some cases of abdominal pain may be life threatening and need urgent care with prompt recognition, many cases require a broad differential diagnosis and thorough evaluation. Abdominal pain affects patients in all age ranges, and many patients with a chronic presentation are appreciative of the health-care provider who can effectively listen to the complaint, take a medical history with a focused history of present illness, perform a complete physical exam, evaluate appropriately, work toward identifying a diagnosis, and treat with success. Unfortunately, not all etiologies of abdominal pain are easily resolved, and many presentations of abdominal pain share multiple etiologies. Regrettably, some patients may live with chronic abdominal pain and need to learn healthful coping strategies while developing a strong relationship with their health-care provider.

References

1. Viniol A, Keunecke C, Biroga T, et al. Studies of the symptom abdominal pain – a systematic review and meta-analysis. *Family Practice* 2014; **0**: 1–13.
2. Worly B, Schlaff, W. Endometriosis and chronic pelvic pain. *Postgraduate Obstetrics & Gynecology* 2012; **18**: 1–7.
3. McPhee M, Lingappa V, Ganong W. *Pathophysiology of Disease: An Introduction to Clinical Medicine*, Fourth Edition. New York: Lange Medical Books/ McGraw-Hill Medical Publishing Division, 2003.
4. Bickley L, Szilagyi P. *Bates Guide to Physical Examination and History Taking*, Eleventh Edition. New York: Wolters Kluwer Health/Lippincott Williams & Wilkins, 2013.
5. Netter F. *Atlas of Human Anatomy*, Second Edition. Canada: Friesens Corporation, 1997.
6. Worly B, Schlaff W. Chronic pelvic pain unrelated to endometriosis. *Postgraduate Obstetrics & Gynecology* 2012; **19**: 1–7.
7. Trinkley K, Nahata M. Medication management of irritable bowel syndrome. *Digestion* 2014; **89**: 253–267.
8. Vennix S, Morton D, Hahnloser D, et al. Systematic review of evidence and consensus on diverticulitis: an analysis of national and international guidelines. *Colorectal Dis* 2014 Nov; **16**(11): 866–878.
9. Effective Health Care Program. Surgical management of inguinal hernia. *Agency for Healthcare Research and Quality* 2013; **12**: 1–3.
10. Pearle M, Goldfarb D, Assimos D, et al. Medical management of kidney stones: AUA guideline. *Journal of Urology* 2014; **192**: 316–324.
11. Dyer A, Twiss C. Painful bladder syndrome: an update and review of current management strategies. *Current Urology Reports* 2014; **384**: 1–10.
12. Barnhart K. Ectopic pregnancy. *New England Journal of Medicine* 2009; **361**: 379–387.
13. Doubilet P, Benson C, Bourne T, Blaivas M. Diagnostic criteria for nonviable pregnancy early in the first trimester. *New England Journal of Medicine* 2013; **369**: 1443–1451.
14. Mitchell C, Prabhu M. Pelvic inflammatory disease: current concepts in pathogenesis, diagnosis and treatment. *Infectious Disease Clinics of North America* 2013; **27**: 793–809.
15. Brown J, Farquhar C. Endometriosis: an overview of Cochrane Reviews. *Cochrane Collaboration* 2014; 3. Available at: www.cochrane.org/CD009590/MENSTR_endometriosis-an-overview-of-cochrane-reviews. Accessed Dec 21, 2015.
16. Duffy J, Arambage K, Correa F, Olive D, et al. Laparoscopic surgery for endometriosis. *Cochrane Collaboration* 2014; 4. Available at: www.update-software.com/BCP/WileyPDF/EN/CD011031.pdf. Accessed Dec 21, 2015.
17. Khan A, Shehmar M, Gupta J. Uterine fibroids: current perspectives. *International Journal of Women's Health* 2014; **6**: 95–114.
18. Levy G, Dehaene A, Laurent N, Lernout M. An update on adenomyosis. *Diagnostic and Interventional Imaging* 2013; **94**: 3–25.
19. Berman M, Randall-Whitis L. Management of adnexal masses. *ACOG Practice Bulletin* 2007; **83**: 1–14.
20. Cheong Y, Smotra G, Williams A. Non-surgical interventions for the management of chronic pelvic pain. *Cochrane Collaboration* 2014; 3. Available at: http://onlinelibrary.wiley.com/doi/10.1002/14651858.CD008797.pub2/full. Accessed Dec 21, 2015.

Chapter 42

Hypertension

Jennifer Frank

Scope of the problem

Hypertension is one of the most common chronic diseases in the United States, affecting approximately 30% of adults and uncontrolled in more than half of those with hypertension.[1] Rates are nearly equal between genders with 31.3% of men aged 20 and older affected compared with 29.6% of women. However, this is not the same across all age ranges. Men have higher rates of hypertension than age-matched premenopausal women. Between ages 45 and 64, the rates are similar in men and women. At 65 and older, women have higher rates of hypertension than men.[2] Up to 75% of American women older than 60 have hypertension.[3] For both genders, African-American people are affected more often than whites and prevalence increases with increasing age.

A National Health and Nutrition Examination Survey (NHANES) study of women aged 20–49 found that over a 10-year period, the proportion of women diagnosed with hypertension remained stable, although the proportion of women who were advised to start antihypertensive therapy and the number of women who reported compliance with an antihypertensive drug regimen showed a statistically significant increase, possibly reflecting increased attention to hypertension over time.[4]

Hypertension is associated with serious cardiovascular disease including stroke, myocardial infarction, and congestive heart failure as well as kidney disease and retinopathy.[5, 6] Although hypertension is often found in women with other risk factors (e.g., diabetes mellitus or dyslipidemia), elevated blood pressure is an independent risk factor for cardiovascular and renal disease, and the risk increases with rising blood pressure levels.[5] Cardiovascular disease is the leading cause of death among American women, and hypertension accounts for approximately 41% of the attributable risk, surpassing tobacco use and physical inactivity. The Women's Health Initiative study identified hypertension as a major independent risk factor for sudden cardiac death; sudden cardiac death is most common in postmenopausal women.[6]

Definition

Normal blood pressure is a systolic blood pressure (SBP) of <120 mmHg and a diastolic blood pressure (DBP) of <80 mmHg. Prehypertension is SBP 120 mm Hg–139 mmHg or DBP 80 mmHg–89 mmHg. Hypertension in adults (aged 18 and older) is defined as a systolic blood pressure equal to or greater than 140 mmHg or a diastolic blood pressure equal to or greater than 90 mmHg.[7, 8] It is further divided into stage 1 hypertension (SBP 140 mmHg–159 mmHg or DBP 90 mmHg–99 mmHg) and stage 2 hypertension (SBP ≥160 mmHg or DBP ≥100 mmHg).[5] Despite these definitions, it is important to remember that blood pressure and its association with cardiovascular risk is on a continuum. The definition of hypertension is based on the number at which treatment reduces risk.[8]

Hypertension can be primary (e.g., essential hypertension) or secondary (e.g., caused by other conditions). Although the majority of people have essential hypertension, the diagnosis of secondary hypertension is important for determining treatment and reducing future risk. Other types of hypertension include masked hypertension, pseudohypertension, resistant hypertension, and white-coat hypertension.

Masked hypertension

When a person has normal blood pressure measured in the clinic but elevated blood pressure readings outside of the clinic, it is termed isolated clinic hypertension or masked hypertension.[8] This condition has an overall prevalence of approximately 13% but may be higher in the subset of people with high normal blood pressure.[8] Elevated blood pressure outside of the clinic has

Office Care of Women, ed. Martin E. Olsen and Botros Rizk. Published by Cambridge University Press.

many potential causes including physical activity, anxiety, stress, and alcohol or tobacco use. It is both underdetected and undertreated and is associated with an increased risk of developing sustained hypertension, end-organ damage, and cardiovascular disease.[8]

Pseudohypertension

Pseudohypertension is found when the measured blood pressure by sphygmomanometer cuff is elevated compared with the intra-arterial pressure. It is caused by arterial stiffness and is more common in the elderly who also have atherosclerotic disease, renal insufficiency, and diabetes.[9] It can be a cause of treatment-resistant hypertension. Persistently elevated blood pressure without end-organ damage suggests the possibility of pseudohypertension.[10]

Resistant hypertension

Resistant hypertension is defined as failure to achieve blood pressure goal despite maximal therapy with three or more antihypertensive agents, one of which must be a diuretic.[5] The estimated prevalence is 10% of those with hypertension, although reported rates range from 5% to 30%.[8] Resistant hypertension significantly increases the risk of cardiovascular and renal disease.[8]

Establishing true resistant hypertension can be challenging. A common cause of apparent resistance to treatment is nondisclosed failure to adhere to the prescribed antihypertensive regimen. Causes of resistant hypertension include lifestyle factors that contribute to high blood pressure (e.g., obesity, alcohol use, excessive sodium intake), secondary causes of hypertension (e.g., pheochromocytoma, renovascular hypertension), obstructive sleep apnea, and advanced end-organ damage.[8]

Treatment of resistant hypertension includes a careful history and physical examination, appropriate laboratory and other diagnostic evaluation for suspected contributing or causative factors, and treatment intensification.[8] Referral to a specialist in hypertension management may be warranted.

White-coat hypertension

White-coat hypertension describes the finding of an elevated blood pressure in clinic despite a normal blood pressure reading on either ambulatory blood pressure monitoring or home blood pressure monitoring. The prevalence of white-coat hypertension across the population is approximately 13%, but it can affect up to one-third of patients with hypertension.[8] The diagnosis of white-coat hypertension should be confirmed in three to six months and then reassessed annually.[8, 11] White-coat hypertension is a risk factor for developing sustained hypertension and, in some studies, is associated with higher risk for cardiovascular disease compared with normotensive individuals (i.e., those with blood pressure <120/80 mmHg), although the risk for end-organ damage remains below that of individuals with hypertension.[8, 11] Current data is limited regarding the optimal treatment, although lifestyle modification is indicated.[11]

Risk factors

The etiology of essential hypertension is unknown, but many theories exist, including some specific to the development of hypertension in women. Independent risk factors for developing hypertension include obesity, age, ethnicity, diabetes mellitus, and chronic kidney disease.[12] Family history of hypertension, particularly early-onset is a risk factor for developing hypertension.[8] There are a number of established risk factors and conditions known to cause secondary hypertension. These include chronic kidney disease, coarctation of the aorta, Cushing's syndrome, obstructive sleep apnea, pheochromocytoma, primary aldosteronism, renovascular hypertension, and thyroid or parathyroid disease.[5]

Lifestyle factors that increase risk for developing hypertension include obesity, which may be the most significant modifiable risk factor.[12] Dietary factors linked to developing hypertension include total grain intake, salt consumption, ingestion of processed (compared to unprocessed) red meat, and low levels of fruit intake in nonobese women.[12–15] Recreational (as opposed to occupational) physical activity is inversely related to risk of hypertension.[16] Women getting five or fewer hours of sleep demonstrated increased risk of hypertension in the Nurses' Health Study.[17]

Vitamin D insufficiency may be a predictor of future risk of systolic hypertension.[18] Women with osteoporosis are significantly more likely to have hypertension; both diseases are associated with decreased dairy intake.[19]

Certain risk factors may be gender specific or influenced by gender. For example, women exposed to famine while in utero demonstrate an increased blood pressure measurement and were significantly more likely to have been diagnosed with and treated for hypertension than women who were not exposed to famine. The same relationship was not seen in male counterparts.[20] Although obesity significantly increases the risk of both hypertension and prehypertension in women and men, the magnitude of increased risk is greater in women.[21] Preeclampsia quadruples future risk of hypertension.[2, 8]

Diagnosis

In order to diagnose hypertension, the blood pressure must be obtained correctly. In the office, the sphygmomanometer is used; it should be calibrated periodically. Measurement is taken from the upper arm using an appropriately sized cuff, defined as the cuff bladder encircling at least 80% of the upper arm.[5] The patient should be seated for five minutes quietly prior to measurement. Measurement should be obtained while the patient is seated with the back supported and the feet on the floor while the arm is supported at heart level.[5] The blood pressure should be taken twice about one to two minutes apart and repeated if there is a significant difference. Since blood pressure may be significantly different between the left and right arm, on an initial visit, it is important to obtain both measurements, using the higher reading as the reference blood pressure. A difference in blood pressure between arms of more than 10 mmHg is associated with increased cardiovascular risk.[8] The first Korotkoff sound is the systolic blood pressure and the fifth (disappearance) sound is the diastolic.

There are common pitfalls to accurate measurement.[8] Clinicians may be susceptible to two types of error in recording the blood pressure measurement. The first is rounding bias in which the blood pressure is rounded up or down. The second is digit bias in which the number is recorded at a specific digit, for example at a number ending in a zero (e.g., 120, 130). The auscultatory gap, which is more common in elderly patients, refers to the disappearance of Korotkoff sounds as the cuff is being deflated, which then reappear at a lower pressure. The second set of sounds can be mistaken for the systolic blood pressure. Elderly patients are also at increased risk of manifesting pseudohypertension in which the pressure measured by the cuff exceeds the actual intra-arterial pressure because of vascular stiffness.[10]

History

Ask patients with hypertension about the length of diagnosis, previous blood pressure values (including home readings), and any history of antihypertensive therapy.[8] Many patients with hypertension have or are at risk for other cardiovascular disease, so a history of stroke or TIA, myocardial infarction, valvular heart disease, congestive heart failure, peripheral artery disease, kidney disease, and diabetes should be elicited. Specific to women, a history of gestational HTN, eclampsia or preeclampsia, and polycystic ovarian syndrome (PCOS) are associated with increased prevalence of hypertension.[8, 22]

It is important to carefully elicit any associated signs or symptoms that may be related to hypertension in order to identify comorbid conditions, causes of secondary hypertension, and presence of end-organ damage. Many patients with hypertension report no symptoms relatable to elevated blood pressure. Elevated blood pressure, however, can be associated with symptoms of end-organ damage or with symptoms that suggest a secondary cause of hypertension (i.e., hyperthyroidism, primary aldosteronism). Therefore, a complete review of systems should be elicited focusing on neurologic symptoms, symptoms of renal disease, cardiovascular symptoms, endocrinologic symptoms, any cognitive deficit, and history of snoring, apnea, or daytime somnolence that may suggest obstructive sleep apnea.[8]

Blood pressure is affected by a number of prescription and over-the-counter medications and supplements, so a careful history must elicit all substances that a woman is currently taking (Box 42-1). Oral contraceptive pills are a common medication taken by women and are associated with both elevated systolic and diastolic blood pressure as well as increased risk for prehypertension and hypertension when used for longer than 24 months.[23]

Women should be asked about tobacco, alcohol and illicit drug use as all three of these substances can result in elevated blood pressure. Furthermore, smoking cessation, reduction of alcohol intake, and avoidance of illicit substances are important components of hypertension treatment. Eliciting information about lifestyle including diet and physical activity may reveal opportunities for intervention.[8]

Understanding family history is important in the evaluation of a woman with hypertension. Patients should be asked about family history of hypertension and cardiovascular disease, especially an early onset of either condition. Additionally, it is important to elicit any history of diabetes, dyslipidemia, or chronic kidney disease (looking for polycystic kidney disease).[8]

BOX 42-1 Medications and substances that can raise blood pressure

Alcohol
Amphetamines
Antidepressants
Beta blockers (rebound hypertension when discontinued)
Bromocriptine
Cocaine
Clonidine
Combined oral contraceptives
Corticosteroid
Cyclosporine
Danazol
Desflurane
Erythropoietin
Ketamine
Ketoconazole
Methyldopa (may initially exacerbate hypertension)
Metoclopramide
NSAIDs
Natural licorice
Prochlorperazine
Sympathomimetics (oral decongestants, appetite suppressants, nasal sprays, eye drops containing epinephrine)

Source: Information from reference 29.

Physical examination

The physical examination of a patient with elevated blood pressure starts with the appropriate measurement of blood pressure. Height, weight, body mass index (BMI), and waist circumference should be measured. The examination should include auscultation of the heart; the presence of a heart murmur may warrant further investigation. The pulse at rest should be obtained; both tachycardia and arrhythmia should prompt additional testing. A careful examination should be made of the neck for thyroid disorders, the neurologic system, vascular system including auscultation of the carotid and renal arteries and palpation of peripheral pulses, and the abdomen for enlarged kidneys (associated with polycystic kidney disease). A fundoscopic examination can detect retinal hemorrhages and a skin examination may reveal sequelae of conditions associated with secondary hypertension (i.e., Cushing's syndrome or pheochromocytoma).[8]

It is important to consider potential causes of secondary hypertension, particularly in younger women. Women younger than age 40 with moderate to severe hypertension should be evaluated for renovascular hypertension related to fibromuscular dysplasia as this is significantly more common in women.[24] Pheochromocytoma should also be considered in younger women with characteristic symptoms. Both renovascular hypertension and pheochromocytoma are associated with pregnancy complications if untreated.[24]

Labs/diagnostic evaluation

The role of laboratory and other diagnostic testing has three goals: to identify causes of secondary hypertension, the presence of end-organ damage, and the presence of other cardiovascular disease.[8] Initial testing includes creatinine [and estimation of glomerular filtration rate (GFR)], fasting blood glucose, hemoglobin and hematocrit, lipids, potassium, sodium, uric acid, urinalysis, and a 12-lead electrocardiogram.[8] Additional testing, based on the history, physical examination, and results of initial testing may include abdominal ultrasound, ankle brachial index, carotid ultrasound, echocardiogram, hemoglobin A1c, Holter monitor, peripheral artery ultrasound, quantitative urine protein, and urine electrolytes.[8]

Ambulatory blood pressure monitoring

Ambulatory blood pressure monitoring (ABPM) provides additional information about blood pressure outside of the clinic, during normal activities, and while the patient is sleeping. To perform, a patient wears a portable blood pressure cuff for 24 hours and does her normal activity. Blood pressure measurement is done every 15 minutes while awake and every 30 minutes while asleep.[8] Normal blood pressures on ABPM are SBP of <135 mmHg while awake and <120 mmHg while asleep and DBP <85 mmHg while awake and <70 mmHg while asleep (ESC). ABPM is more sensitive and a better predictor than office blood pressure measurement of risk of end-organ damage and cardiovascular morbidity and mortality.[8]

Home blood pressure monitoring

Home blood pressure monitoring (HBPM) is performed by the patient or by a family member or support person in the patient's home over several days. The blood pressure is obtained by a cuff placed on the upper arm and in the same manner as in the office (e.g., after five minutes of rest, with arm at level of heart). Ideally, the blood pressure is monitored for three to seven consecutive days both morning and evening.[8] Similar to ABPM, it is a better predictor of end-organ damage (e.g., left ventricular hypertrophy) and cardiovascular morbidity and mortality than office blood pressure measurement. However, it is limited by a lack of data during the patient's normal activities as it is performed at rest and does not provide data on BP while the patient is sleeping.[8]

Table 42-1 Components of lifestyle modification for treatment of hypertension

Diet	Sodium intake ≤2.4 grams/day DASH diet (high intake of fruits, vegetables, and low-fat dairy, limit fat intake)
Exercise	30 minutes of physical activity most days of the week
Substance use	Limit alcohol intake to 1 drink/day for women Stop smoking
Weight	Maintain a BMI of 18.5 kg/m^2 –24.9 kg/m^2

Source: Information from references 5 and 8.

Treatment

Treating hypertension reduces a woman's risk of heart failure by approximately 50%, myocardial infarction by 20%–25%, and stroke by 35%–40% in trials of antihypertensive treatment.[5] Decisions about the treatment of hypertension must take into account several different factors including the blood pressure goal, comorbid conditions, age, and ethnicity. The Eighth Joint National Committee (JNC 8) released new guidelines in early 2014 that upheld the definition of hypertension but adjusted treatment recommendations from the previous guidelines.[7] Women aged 18–59 should initiate pharmacologic treatment starting at a SBP of 140 mmHg or higher or a DBP of 90 mmHg or higher and be treated to a goal of <140/90 mmHg. In women 60 years of age and older, a treatment goal of SBP of <150 mmHg and a DBP of <90 mmHg is recommended.[7] Women with chronic kidney disease or diabetes should be treated to a goal of <140/90 mmHg.[7] Elderly women 75 years of age and older demonstrate a survival benefit with systolic blood pressure in the range of 140 mmHg–145 mmHg.[10] Gender bias has been demonstrated in hypertension treatment, although women are more likely to have controlled hypertension than men, especially prior to age 65.[2]

Lifestyle modification

Lifestyle modification is recommended for all women with hypertension and should be continually emphasized even if pharmacologic therapy is initiated (Table 42-1).[5, 7, 8] The components of lifestyle modification advocated include physical activity, diet, weight reduction, moderation of alcohol intake, and smoking cessation.[5, 8] Ideal body weight (body BMI between 18.5 kg/m^2 and 24.9 kg/m^2)]can be associated with a lowering of SBP by 5 mmHg–20 mmHg for each 10 kg lost.[5] The Dietary Approaches to Stop Hypertension (DASH) diet emphasizes consumption of fruits, vegetables, and low-fat dairy with reduced intake of saturated and total fat and can be associated with a SBP reduction of 8 mmHg–14 mmHg. Limiting sodium intake to 2.4 grams per day may be particularly important for women and can lower SBP by 2 mmHg–8 mmHg. Physical activity is also recommended for 30 minutes most days of the week and has the potential to lower SBP by 4 mmHg–9 mmHg and reduce mortality by 20% or more.[8] However, women of all ages are less likely to engage in physical activity than men, and the amount of exercise decreases with increasing age.[2] Drinking more than two to three alcoholic beverages daily is associated with increased blood pressure, so women should be advised to limit alcohol consumption.[24] Limiting alcohol consumption to one drink per day in women is recommended and is associated with a reduction in SBP of 2 mmHg–4 mmHg. Counseling women to quit smoking is important as smoking is associated with an increased risk of cardiovascular disease and may acutely raise blood pressure.[8]

Reducing salt intake is a cornerstone of the DASH diet. Sodium restriction may be more effective in reducing blood pressure in women compared with men.[24] A Cochrane review found that, on average, modestly reducing dietary salt is associated with approximately 5 mmHg decrease in SBP and 3 mmHg decrease in DBP.[25] Further reducing salt intake is associated with further reductions in SBP. Hypertension in premenopausal women has been observed to be salt-resistant whereas it becomes salt-sensitive in postmenopausal women, likely related to the impact of sex hormones on the renin-angiotensin system.[2]

Although the importance of lifestyle in the management of hypertension is undisputed, women may not receive adequate education about dietary and exercise recommendations. Up to 10% of women reported having received no lifestyle education from their health-care providers, 25% reported having only been told to limit salt, and up to half of women reported not being told about the relationship between sugar consumption, diabetes, and hypertension.[26]

Choice of pharmacologic agents

Although blood pressure goals can be achieved in the majority of patients with hypertension, most will require at least two different medications (Table 42-2)[5]

Table 42-2 Selected antihypertensive agents

Drug	Class	Starting dose*	Maximum daily dose	
Benazepril	ACE inhibitor	10 mg/day	80 mg/day	
Captopril	ACE inhibitor	12.5–25 mg BID or TID	450 mg/day	Increase by 12.5–25 mg/dose every 1–2 weeks
Enalapril	ACE inhibitor	5 mg/day	40 mg/day	
Lisinopril	ACE inhibitor	10 mg/day	80 mg/day (doses >40 mg/day usually not more effective)	
Moexipril	ACE inhibitor	7.5 mg/day	30 mg/day	May divide BID
Quinapril	ACE inhibitor	10 mg/day	80 mg/day	May divide BID
Perindopril	ACE inhibitor	4 mg/day	16 mg/day	
Ramipril	ACE inhibitor	2.5 mg/day 1.25 mg/day if renal artery stenosis or hypovolemia	20 mg/day	May divide BID
Trandolapril	ACE inhibitor	1 mg/day 2 mg/day in black patients	8 mg/day	
Azilsartan	ARB	80 mg/day	80 mg/day	
Candesartan	ARB	16 mg/day	32 mg/day	
Eprosartan	ARB	600 mg/day	800 mg/day	Can be divided BID
Irbesartan	ARB	150 mg/day	300 mg/day	
Losartan	ARB	50 mg/day	100 mg/day	
Olmesartan	ARB	20 mg/day	40 mg/day	
Telmisartan	ARB	40 mg/day	160 mg/day	

Table 42-2 (cont.)

Drug	Class	Starting dose*	Maximum daily dose	
Valsartan	ARB	80 mg/day	320 mg/day	
Amlodipine	Dihydropyridine CCB	5 mg/day 2.5 mg/day if elderly or not monotherapy	10 mg/day	
Felodipine	Dihydropyridine CCB	5 mg/day 2.5 mg if elderly or hepatic impairment	10 mg/day	
Nifedipine	Dihydropyridine CCB	30 mg/day	120 mg/day	
Diltiazem	Non-dihydropyridine CCB	Depends on formulation 180 mg/day (long-acting form)	540 mg/day	
Verapamil	Non-dihydropyridine CCB	Depends on formulation 80–120 mg TID (immediate release)	480 mg/day	Start lower dose (40 mg tid for immediate release) in elderly or small stature
Chlorthalidone	Thiazide diuretic	12.5 mg/day	50 mg/day 25 mg/day in elderly	
Hydrochlorothiazide	Thiazide diuretic	25 mg/day 12.5 mg/day in elderly	50 mg/day	

* ACE inhibitors and ARBs: Consider a lower dose (50% of recommended) if on diuretic/has volume depletion
Source: Information from reference 30.

Multiple barriers to effective blood pressure lowering include failure to adopt lifestyle change, medication nonadherence, and failure to escalate drug therapy.[5] The majority of studies indicate that antihypertensive medications exert similar effects in both blood pressure lowering and cardiovascular risk reduction among men and women, therefore, treatment is not gender based.[2] However, differences in occurrence of side effects and frequency have been observed between men and women (Table 42-3 describes side effects in women). Women are more likely to develop hyponatremia or hypokalemia with diuretic therapy and to experience angiotensin-converting enzyme inhibitor-induced cough.[24] As with men, women can experience sexual dysfunction with antihypertensives especially with centrally acting agents, beta blockers, and diuretics.[6]

JNC 8 recommends that non-black women with or without diabetes receive a thiazide-diuretic, calcium

Table 42-3 Antihypertensive side effects in women

Antihypertensive	Effects seen in women
ACE inhibitors	Dry cough more common
Beta blockers	Sexual dysfunction more common
Calcium channel blockers	Edema more common
Diuretics	May reduce hip fractures Higher rates of hypokalemia and hyponatremia Lower rates of gout

Source: Information from reference 2.

channel blocker, angiotensin-converting enzyme inhibitor, or angiotensin receptor blocker as first-line therapy. Initial treatment of black women, including those with diabetes, includes a thiazide diuretic or calcium channel blocker. Women with chronic kidney disease should have an ACE-I or ARB as initial or add-on therapy regardless of race or presence of diabetes. For patients not able to achieve blood pressure goal or who have a contraindication to taking one of the three recommended agents (thiazide, CCB, or ACE-I/ARB), other antihypertensive agents can be used (e.g., beta blockers, alpha blockers).[7]

The efficacy of pharmacologic treatment should be reassessed one month after therapy is started, and if the patient is not at goal, it should be adjusted. There are three general strategies for advancing pharmacotherapy.[7] If the patient has failed to achieve her blood pressure goal, a single agent can be started and gradually titrated to a maximum dose before selecting a second agent, if needed. Alternatively, a second agent could be added before the first agent has been increased to the maximum dose. Finally, two agents can be started simultaneously as two separate pills or as a single-pill combination.[7] For patients with a SBP ≥160 mmHg or DBP ≥100 mmHg, it may be preferable to start two agents as it is unlikely that monotherapy will sufficiently lower the blood pressure to target.

Nonadherence to prescribed medications is a common and important problem in the treatment of hypertension. In one survey, 25% of women reported not taking their blood pressure medications continuously. Reasons for nonadherence included forgetfulness, cost, concern about side effects, and actual side effects.[26] Despite a lack of significant discrepancy in the number of antihypertensives prescribed for men and women, older women particularly are less likely to have adequate blood pressure control than their male counterparts.[6] The use of a fixed-dose, single-pill combination should be strongly considered as it improves adherence and is associated with improved rates of blood pressure control.[8] A number of single-pill combinations are available, including generic formulations.

Treatment in special populations

Elderly women

There is proven benefit to blood pressure control in women up to age 85, although the goal of blood pressure lowering may be less stringent as previously mentioned.[10] In addition to cardiovascular risk, hypertension in the elderly is associated with a cognitive decline, most clearly seen in executive function (e.g., remembering details, managing time, curbing inappropriate speech).[10] In approaching the treatment of the elderly, it is important to consider potential causes of secondary hypertension, including medications (e.g., nonsteroidal anti-inflammatory medications), sleep apnea, and hyperthyroidism.

The elderly may be particularly susceptible to wide fluctuations in blood pressure throughout the day, including a risk of orthostatic and postprandial hypertension. They, like other patients, may also experience a change in the normal circadian pattern of blood pressure. This may only be detectable with ambulatory blood pressure monitoring. However, the physiologic changes that may lead to hypotension after meals or with standing and which are more pronounced in the elderly may be improved with blood pressure regulation, leading to a lower risk of hypotension.[10]

As with women of other ages, treatment initially includes a focus on sodium restriction, physical activity, weight control, smoking cessation, and moderation of alcohol use. The choice of pharmacologic therapy mirrors that of younger women and is primarily based on comorbid conditions that may argue for one antihypertensive over another and cost. Additionally, thiazide diuretics are associated with decreased risk of hip fracture.[6]

Women of childbearing potential

Women with hypertension who may become pregnant are at increased risk of developing preeclampsia during pregnancy. Approximately one in five women with chronic hypertension will develop superimposed preeclampsia during pregnancy and it is more likely to be early-onset (i.e., before 34 weeks gestation).[27] The treatment goal for women of childbearing potential remains <140/90 mmHg. Pharmacologic treatment is likewise the same, although caution should be used with angiotensin-converting enzyme inhibitors and angiotensin receptor blockers as these are potentially teratogenic.[8] Caution should also be exercised with the use of mineralocorticoid receptor antagonists and direct renin inhibitors.[6]

Pregnant women

There are multiple hypertensive disorders of pregnancy. This chapter will focus on treatment of chronic hypertension during pregnancy, which is largely guided by expert opinion as randomized controlled trial data is lacking. Approximately 1%–5% of pregnancies are complicated by chronic hypertension with increasing prevalence seen with increased age.[27] Women with chronic hypertension are at increased risk for developing preeclampsia. Lifestyle modification remains an important component of treatment with emphasis on weight control and exercise.[6] Pharmacologic treatment is recommended for pregnant women with a systolic or diastolic blood pressure of 160 mmHg or 110 mmHg respectively and should be considered for women with persistent blood pressures ≤150/95 mmHg. In women with blood pressures of ≥140/90 who also have gestational hypertension, asymptomatic organ damage, or symptoms, pharmacologic treatment should be considered.[8]

Pharmacologic agents recommended in pregnant women include labetalol, methyldopa, or nifedipine. Pregnancy is a possible contraindication to the use of diuretics or beta blockers and an absolute contraindication to angiotensin-converting enzyme inhibitors or angiotensin receptor blockers.[8]

Prevention

In normotensive people, a modest reduction in dietary salt is associated with an average reduction in SBP and DBP of 2 mmHg and 1 mmHg, respectively.[25] A diet that is higher in nuts and dairy products and lower in meat has been associated with a reduced risk of developing hypertension.[28] Getting adequate sleep, at least seven hours per night may prevent hypertension, particularly in younger women.

Hormonal therapy and hypertension

Oral contraceptives (OC) are associated with elevations in blood pressure, raising SBP by 5 mmHg–6 mmHg and DBP by 1 mmHg–2 mmHg.[24] Hypertension is two to three times more common among users of OCs compared with age-matched peers, and occurs in approximately 5% of OC users.[8] The increased risk is seen even with use of contraceptives containing lower estrogen doses and increases with duration of use and potency of the progestin component.[24] Although the data is limited, the same effect has not been observed with the use of progestin-only pills. Women taking OCs should have their blood pressure monitored regularly. Women with hypertension who are smokers should generally not use OCs;[24] caution should be employed in women 35 years of age and older who smoke.[8] Women with hypertension who are using OCs may have improved blood pressure control with cessation of OCs.[8]

Hormone replacement therapy has also been associated with elevated blood pressure, although the relationship is not as clearly established as with OCs and the risk is generally low.[8] Hormone replacement therapy is not absolutely contraindicated in women with hypertension, but it is important to monitor such women closely and to remember that regardless of effects on blood pressure, hormone replacement therapy is associated with an increased risk of stroke.[24]

Concluding remarks

Hypertension affects approximately 30% of women and is a major risk factor for cardiovascular and renal disease. Women who are obese, have other cardiovascular disease, or have a history of hypertensive disorders of pregnancy are at increased risk for developing high blood pressure. Accurate diagnosis begins with correct measurement of blood pressure in the office. For younger women or for women who are treatment resistant, other contributing factors, including causes of secondary hypertension, must be considered. Treatment is not gender specific, but there are certain considerations, including childbearing potential, ethnicity, comorbid conditions, and potential for side effects.

References

1. National Center for Health Statistics. *Health, United States, 2012: With Special Feature on Emergency Care.* Hyattsville: US Government Printing Office; 2013.
2. Doumas M, Papademetriou V, Faselis C, Kokkinos P. Gender differences in hypertension: myths and reality. *Curr Hypertens Rep.* 2013;**15**(4):321–30.
3. Lima R, Wofford M, Reckelhoff JF. Hypertension in postmenopausal women. *Curr Hypertens Rep.* 2012;**14**(3):254–60.
4. Laz TH, Rahman M, Berenson AB. Trends in serum lipids and hypertension prevalence among non-pregnant reproductive-age women: United States National Health and Nutrition Examination Survey 1999–2008. *Matern Child Health J.* 2013;**17**:1424–31.
5. National Heart, Lung, and Blood Institute. *The Seventh Report of the Joint National Committee on Prevention, Detection, Evaluation, and Treatment of High Blood Pressure.* Bethesda: NHLBI Health Information Center; 2004.
6. Hage FG, Mansur SJ, Xing D, Oparil S. Hypertension in women. *Kidney Int Suppl (2011).* 2013;**3**(4):352–6.

7. James PA, Oparil S, Carter BL, Cushman WC, Dennison-Himmelfarb C, Handler J, et al. 2014 evidence-based guideline for the management of high blood pressure in adults: report from the panel members appointed to the Eighth Joint National Committee (JNC 8). *JAMA*. 2014;**311**(5):507–20.

8. Mancia G, Fagard R, Narkiewicz K, et al. 2013 ESH/ESC guidelines for the management of arterial hypertension. *J Hypertens*. 2013;**31**(7):1281–357.

9. Kleman M, Dhanyamraju S, DiFillipo W. Prevalence and characteristics of pseudohypertension in patients with "resistant hypertension." *J Am Soc Hypertens*. 2013;7(6):467–70.

10. Lipsitz LA. A 91 year-old woman with difficult-to-control hypertension. *JAMA*. 2013;**310**(12):1274–80.

11. Franklin SS, Thijs L, Hansen TW, et al. White-coat hypertension: new insights from recent studies. *Hypertension*. 2013;**62**(6):982–7.

12. Abramson BL, Melvin RG. Cardiovascular risk in women: focus on hypertension. *Can J Cardiol*. 2014;**30** (5):553–9.

13. Ha SK. Dietary salt intake and hypertension. *Electrolyte Blood Press*. 2014;**12**(1):7–18.

14. Song HJ, Paek YJ, Choi MK, Lee HJ. Gender differences in the relationship between risk of hypertension and fruit intake. *Prev Med*. 2014;**67**(C): 154–9.

15. Laouis M, Bijon A, Fagherazzi G, et al. Processed and unprocessed red meat consumption and hypertension in women. *Am J Clin Nutr*. 2014 Sep;**100**(3):948–52. doi: 10/3945/ajcn.113.080598. Epub 2014 Jul 30.

16. Huai P, Xun H, Reilly KH, et al. Physical activity and risk of hypertension: a meta-analysis of prospective cohort studies. *Hypertension*. 2013;**62**(6):1021–6.

17. Gangwisch JE, Feskanich D, Malaspina D, et al. Sleep duration and risk for hypertension in women: results from the Nurses' Health Study. *Am J Hypertens*. 2013;**26**(7):903–11.

18. Griffin FC, Gadegbeku CA, Sowers MS. Vitamin D and subsequent systolic hypertension among women. *Am J Hypertens*. 2011;**24**(3):316–21.

19. Varenna M, Manara M, Galli L, et al. The association between osteoporosis and hypertension: the role of a low dairy intake. *Calcif Tissue Int*. 2013;**93**(1):86–92.

20. Chen H, Nembhard WN, Stockwell HG. Sex-specific effects of fetal exposure to the 1959–61 Chinese famine on risk of adult hypertension. *Matern Child Health J*. 2014;**18**(3):527–33.

21. Wakabayashi I. Stronger associations of obesity with prehypertension and hypertension in young women than in young men. *J Hypertens*. 2012;**30**(7):1423–9.

22. Sirmans S, Pate K. Epidemiology, diagnosis, and management of polycystic ovarian syndrome. *Clin Epidemiol*. 2014;**6**:1–13.

23. Park H, Kim K. Associations between oral contraceptive use and risk of hypertension and prehypertension in a cross-sectional study of Korean women. *BMC Women's Health*. 2013;**13**:39.

24. August P. Hypertension in women. *Adv Chronic Kidney Dis*. 2013;**20**(5):396–401.

25. He FJ, Li J, MacGregor GA. Effect of longer-term modest salt reduction on blood pressure. *Cochrane Database Syst Rev*. 2013;**4**:CD004937.

26. Lotenberg LD, Clough LC, Mackey TA, et al. Lessons learned from a survey of the diagnosis and treatment of journeys of postmenopausal women with hypertension. *J Clin Hypertens*. 2013;**15**(8):532–41.

27. Chappell LC, Enye S, Seed P, et al. Adverse perinatal outcomes and risk factors for preeclampsia in women with chronic hypertension. *Hypertension*. 2008;**51**(4):1002–9.

28. Weng LC, Steffen LM, Szklo M, et al. A diet pattern with more dairy and nuts, but less meat is related to lower risk of developing hypertension in middle-aged adults: the Atherosclerosis Risk in Communities (ARIC) study. *Nutrients*. 2013;**5**(5):1719–33.

29. Frank JE, Sommerfeld D. Clinical approach in treatment of resistant hypertension. *Integrated Blood Pressure Control*. 2009;**2**:9–23.

30. Epocrates [Internet]. Drugs. Available at http://online.epocrates.com. Accessed August 20, 2014.

Chapter 43

Hyperlipidemia

Beth Anne Fox and Martin E. Olsen

Introduction

Cardiovascular disease (CVD) is the most common cause of death in both women and men in the developed world. The information that CVD is the number one killer of women is unfortunately unrecognized by many female patients and their physicians. This lack of recognition can sometimes promote a less aggressive management of cardiovascular risk because it is mistakenly believed that women are at lower risk for developing heart disease.[1, 2] A majority of women are unable to recall ever discussing heart disease risk with their physician.[1] Women receive fewer preventive recommendations such as lipid-lowering therapy than do men,[2, 3] and ob/gyns are less likely to recommend lipid lowering interventions than other specialties.[2] This chapter will promote CVD prevention in women by an appropriate diagnosis and management of lipid abnormalities.

Scope of the problem

Cardiovascular disease has been the leading cause of death for US women since 1919. More women than men die from CVD every year.[4] Although improvements have occurred, women remain underrepresented in biomedical research.[5] Evidence suggests that the majority of recommendations to prevent CVD are similar for women as those in men, but exceptions exist.[6] Women are at lower risk of CVD during the reproductive years, but the risk increases significantly at around 50 years of age. Patients seem to believe that their greatest risk of mortality is cancer; one of every 26 US women dies from breast cancer, but CVD kills one of every two women or 12 times as many women each year as breast cancer.[1] Women are less likely to be treated properly for CVD than men, and the survival rate of women is worse than for men.[7]

Screening

Cardiovascular disease is the leading cause of morbidity and mortality in women. Screening for lipid disorders is recommended as a means to identify those individuals who can benefit from targeted therapy to reduce cardiovascular (CV) risk. Lipid testing is only one component of the overall assessment of CV risk in women. Studies have consistently found a relationship between elevated levels of low-density lipoprotein cholesterol (LDL-C) and total cholesterol (TC) and CVD.[8] Women characterized as high risk include those with manifestations of CVD such as coronary heart disease, cerebrovascular disease, peripheral arterial disease, diabetes, chronic kidney disease, and abdominal aortic aneurysm. Additional factors that place women at risk include smoking, advancing age, hypertension, obesity, physical inactivity, poor nutrition, family history of early heart disease (generally agreed upon as occurring before age 55 in first-degree relative males and before age 65 in first-degree relative women), collagen vascular disease, polycystic ovarian syndrome [women with polycystic ovarian syndrome (PCOS) have insulin resistance, impaired glucose tolerance, higher incidence of diabetes, and metabolic syndrome] and a history of gestational diabetes, preeclampsia, or pregnancy-induced hypertension.[9] All of these conditions increase CV risk and contribute to the development of CVD.[10]

Preeclampsia is historically characterized by new-onset hypertension (greater than or equal to 140/90) accompanied by proteinuria of greater than 300 mg per 24 hours after 20 weeks gestation.[11] New criteria by the American College of Obstetricians and Gynecologists (ACOG) remove the proteinuria requirement in order to identify the disease process earlier. Instead new-onset hypertension and end-organ dysfunction characterized by any one of the following

Office Care of Women, ed. Martin E. Olsen and Botros Rizk. Published by Cambridge University Press.

meets the criteria for preeclampsia: thrombocytopenia, renal insufficiency, impaired liver function, pulmonary edema, or cerebral or visual symptoms.[12] The disease is associated with endothelial dysfunction, atherogenesis, and elevated levels of TC, LDL-C, and triglycerides during the first, second, and third trimesters in women who develop preeclampsia compared to women who remain normotensive during pregnancy. Additi-$onally, maternal high-density lipoprotein cholesterol (HDL-C) levels are lower during the third trimester than found in normotensive parturients. Preeclampsia also promotes a maternal inflammatory response that could be reflected in an elevated high-sensitivity c-reactive protein (hsCRP), which augments the endothelial dysfunction and atherogenesis. Early screening of lipid levels may identify those at risk for development of preeclampsia.[11] Development of preeclampsia doubles the risk for ischemic heart disease, stroke, or thromboembolic events approximately 5–15 years after pregnancy; women with this history, therefore, should have further assessment for CV risk and risk amelioration with periodic monitoring.[12]

Women with systemic lupus erythematosus and rheumatoid arthritis have an increased relative risk for CVD; women with these autoimmune disorders should be screened for additional CV risk factors with appropriate preventive strategies implemented if indicated by the presence of prior CV events.[12]

Although screening recommendations are generalized to all women, certain ethnic groups have higher prevalence of certain CV risks such as hypertension in African-American women and diabetes in Hispanic women. In fact, mortality from coronary artery disease is similar in African-American women to that of Caucasian men. Gender and ethnic disparities highlight the need for greater preventive measures, CV risk assessment, and management of identified CV risk that are amenable to intervention and treatment.[12]

Many professional organizations have generated or adopted lipid screening strategies in order to identify those who could benefit from targeted lipid therapy as a means of primary prevention of coronary heart disease or secondary prevention of future CV events. Table 43-1 lists screening recommendations by major organizations.[14–20] Research has determined that atherogenesis occurs early in childhood and is progressive throughout life; therefore, two of the organizations have developed screening guidelines for children, adolescents, and young adults. Concentrations of lipids reach levels seen in young adults by age 2, so screening is not recommended before that age.[17]

The evaluation of women for CV risk assessment should include a medical history to identify symptoms of CVD. Family history assessment for evidence of premature CVD is indicated. Social history should identify tobacco use, alcohol consumption, nutrition, and physical activity. The obstetrical history should identify pregnancy complications. Physical examination includes blood pressure and body mass index (BMI) assessment at a minimum. Laboratory tests to be performed as part of the risk assessment in addition to lipids include blood glucose levels, renal function tests, and possibly hsCRP to evaluate for inflammation.[8, 9] Women at intermediate risk for CVD who have an elevated hsCRP might benefit from targeted therapy through discussion and shared decision making between patient and physician.[18, 20] Screening is recommended for first-degree relatives of persons who have been diagnosed with familial hypercholesterolemia.[8]

Hormonal contraceptives and hormone therapy

Although the consensus is strong that oral contraceptive (OC) agents are associated with adverse vascular events, it is not unanimous; the use of oral contraceptives and injectable progestogens were found to have no significant increases in overall risk estimates for stroke, venous thromboembolism, or acute myocardial infarction in the general population of women in a World Health Organization study.[21] One study did show that the presence of obesity or hypercholesterolemia increased the risk of stroke, but the contraceptive-associated odds ratio (OR) was based on small numbers.[22] Another study showed increased incidence of myocardial infarction in women on OCs who also had hyperlipidemia.[23]

Third-generation OCs (desogestrol, gestodene, and norgestimate) are commonly believed to have less effect on lipid profiles than second-generation OCs, but these medications can elevate lipid levels;[24] no consensus exists that these medications have a lower risk of myocardial infarction than second-generation agents.[23] Steady increases in triglycerides, VDL, and HDL were noted over a three-year period of third-generation OC use with the greatest increase occurring after the first six months of use. These medications are protective against abnormally low HDL levels.[24] A literature review indicates that lipid changes are *not* progressive and lipids revert to their pretreatment levels after patients have stopped taking the OCs.[25]

Table 43-1 Lipid screening recommendations for women and girls

Organization	Recommendation
USPSTF [14]	Women ≥45 yo and at increased risk for CHD Women 20–45 yo at increased risk of CHD Women ≥20 yo with no increased risk of CHD
AAFP [15]	Women ≥45 yo and at increased risk for CHD Women 20–45 yo at increased risk of CHD Insufficient evidence for or against screening women 20 or older not at increased risk for CHD Insufficient evidence for or against routine screening of children or young adults to age 20
ACOG [16]	Ages ≥13 at high risk for CHD (FH hyperlipidemia, early CHD <50 men and <60 women, personal history of ASCVD, obesity, diabetes, hypertension, tobacco use); routine at age 45 and every 5 years
AAP [17]	Children age 2 with FH hyperlipidemia or early CHD (≤55 yo male, ≤65 yo women); unknown FH; or with CHD risk factors, such as obesity, hypertension, cigarette smoking, or diabetes; retesting in 3–5 years if lipids within reference ranges initially
ACC/AHA [20]	Assess 10-year risk of ASCVD by calculating risk via Pooled Cohort Equations between ages 40–79 with no CHD and then every 4–6 years by assessing risk factors; 30-year risk assessment in ages 20–59 with 10-year risk of ASCVD <7.5%
NICE [18]	Assess 10-year risk of ASCVD by calculating risk via QRISK2 ages 25–84 every 5 years, excluding type 1 diabetes, CKD (GFR <60 mL/min/1.73 m^2), and familial hypercholesterolemia
AACE [19]	Assess 10-year risk of ASCVD by calculating risk via Reynolds risk score at ages 20–55 years, every 1–2 years ages 55–65, and annually >65 years; screen annually in patients with diabetes and FH of early CHD (myocardial infarction or sudden death before age 55 male or before age 65 female) Children older than 2 years every 3–5 years FH early CHD or hyperlipidemia, obesity, insulin resistance syndrome, or when no FH available Adolescents older than 16 years every 5 years or more often if have FH early CHD, obesity, or components of metabolic syndrome

USPSTF – United States Preventive Services Task Force, AAFP –American Academy of Family Physicians, ACOG – American College of Obstetrics and Gynecology, ACC – American College of Cardiology, AHA – American Heart Association, NICE – National Institute for Health and Care Excellence, AACE – American Association of Clinical Endocrinologists
CHD – coronary heart disease, FH – family history, ASCVD – atherosclerotic cardiovascular disease (abdominal aortic aneurysm, carotid stenosis, peripheral artery disease, stroke), CKD – chronic kidney disease, GFR – glomerular filtration rate

Depo-medroxyprogesterone acetate (DMPA) has been shown to have small, temporary, and reversible effects on the lipid profile. One small study postulates that long-term DMPA use could impair arterial endothelial function and thereby increase coronary vascular disease risk.[26]

Although it may be prudent to encourage patients with hyperlipidemia to avoid hormonal contraception, there is a lack of evidence to show that this intervention has an evidence-based positive effect for patients.

See Chapter 31 for a full discussion of hormone therapy (HT). Consensus exists that HT does not lower overall risk of coronary vascular disease (CVD). But in one review of combined data from the Women's Health Initiative (WHI) and the Heart and Estrogen/progestin Replacement Study (HERS), women who initiated HT within 10 years of menopause had a nonsignificantly lower risk of coronary heart disease while those who initiated HT more than 10 years after menopause had an increased risk.[27] It was thus suggested that optimal candidates for HT include age less than 60, recent onset of menopause, absence of metabolic syndrome, absence of factor V Leiden genotype, and favorable lipid panel.[27] There is no recommendation that lipid screening be performed before initiating HT, but it would be reasonable for the practitioner to ensure that a patient's lipid screening is up to date prior to initiation of therapy. This may be especially true in patients with vasomotor symptoms at older ages.[28] Statins may attenuate any risk of increased CVD associated with HT.[27]

Familial hypercholesterolemia

Familial hypercholesterolemia (FHC) is one of the most common metabolic genetic disorders. It is an autosomal dominant condition that is characterized by elevated levels of LDL-C. There are two forms of FHC, a heterozygous (heFHC) or homozygous (hoFHC) form. The heFHC form is more common, with an estimated prevalence of 1:200–500; the hoFHC is extremely rare, with a prevalence of 1:1,000,000.[29] FHC is more common in specific ethnic groups. In descending order of prevalence, the populations are French Canadian, Tunisian, Christian Lebanese, South African Afrikaners, and South African Ashkenazi Jews.[30] The most common mutation is at the low-density lipoprotein receptor (LDLR) gene on the short arm of chromosome 19. This results in elevated levels of LDLC due to impaired or absent binding of the apolipoprotein (APO-B-100) protein of the LDL particle, thereby causing failure of the LDL particle to be internalized into the hepatocyte. Not all persons with FHC carry the LDLR mutation, but they may have other mutations that affect the uptake of the LDL particle (see Table 43-2).[31]

Familial hypercholesterolemia is a major determinant of premature CVD and accounts for approximately 5% of myocardial infarctions under the age of 60 and about 20% of those that occur in individuals under the age of 45.[31] There are an estimated 620,000 individuals with FHC in the United States; many families, however, are undiagnosed and remain at risk for early coronary artery disease.[33, 34] It is estimated that only 20% of patients with FHC have been identified.[31] Unfortunately, many are diagnosed after the occurrence of a CV event.

Total cholesterol and LDL-C levels are higher and the disease more severe in the homozygous form of the congenital disorder than in the heterozygous form (see Table 43-3).[31] Those with the hoFHC will experience clinical CHD in adolescence and young adulthood, including severe aortic stenosis, coronary artery disease, and coronary bypass surgery or even death. The elevated cholesterol levels lead to atherogenesis, especially in coronary arteries, but cholesterol is also deposited in other tissues.[30]

During general lipid screening, markedly elevated levels of LDL-C should prompt further evaluation to determine the possibility of FHC (see Table 43-4). Family history should identify premature coronary heart disease and hypercholesterolemia in first-degree relatives. Cholesterol screening should begin at age 2 for children with a positive family history of early CHD or hypercholesterolemia.[32]

FHC is characterized by three major features: (1) elevated LDL-C, (2) xanthomas of tendon and skin, and (3) premature CAD.[35] Xanthomas are depositions of cholesterol in tendons or skin; they are cues to the clinical diagnosis of FHC. Xanthomas of the skin frequently occur on extensor surfaces exposed to mechanical stimuli such as the knees, elbows, wrist, or gluteus. Tendon xanthomas are often at the Achilles tendon; these may require palpation to detect. Tuberous xanthomas or xanthelasma under the age of 20–25 are highly suspicious for FHC. The absence of xanthomas does not exclude the diagnosis of FHC as xanthomas become more evident with aging. Corneal arcus is a white, gray, or blue opaque ring in the corneal margin that is particularly suspicious for FHC in patients less than age 45; it becomes more common in the general population

Table 43-2 Common FHC genetic mutations [29]

Genetic mutation	Inheritance	FHC cases
LDL receptor defect	Autosomal dominant	>95%
Familial defective APO-B	Autosomal dominant	2%–5%
Proprotein convertase subtilisin/kexin type 9 (PCSK9)	Autosomal dominant	<1%

Table 43-3 Lipid levels in FHC [31]

FHC form	Total cholesterol (mg/dL)	LDL levels (mg/dL)
Heterozygous	350–600	200–400
Homozygous	650–1,000	>600

Table 43-4 At-risk baseline lipid levels for FHC [32]

Age	LDL cholesterol (mg/dL)	Non-HDL cholesterol * (mg/dL)
Adults (≥20 years)	≥190	≥220
Children (<20 years)	≥160	≥190

* Non-HDL cholesterol = TC – HD

with aging.[29, 30, 35] These physical findings should prompt the clinician to assess lipid levels. The probability of FHC is approximately 80% in the general population with certain age-specific LDL-C concentrations necessitating a thorough family history and thorough evaluation (see Table 43-5).[32]

Increased CHD is inherent with the diagnosis of FHC; patients should undergo an assessment for additional cardiac risk factors that are amenable to modification and treated aggressively when present, such as smoking, hypertension, and diabetes.[31] Women have a 30% increased risk of CHD by age 60, as compared to male development of CHD earlier with an approximately 50% increased risk of CHD by age 50.[34]

It is important that physicians providing primary care to women identify hypercholesterolemia and FHC, assess cardiac risk factors, and be able to provide lipid management along with primary and secondary prevention of cardiac events through risk assessment and modification. They must be aware of physical signs of FHC and diagnostic criteria.[33] Secondary causes of hyperlipidemia should be explored during the evaluation of elevated LDL-C. Hypothyroidism, diabetes, and hepatic and renal disease should be excluded before making the diagnosis of FHC.[35]

The identification of clinical signs is the first step in diagnosis; these include a positive family history, tendon/skin xanthomas, corneal arcus, and elevated lipid concentrations; the absence of any of these findings, however, does not eliminate FHC.[31] A clinical diagnosis may be made when at least two first-degree relatives have the marked age-specific LDL-C elevations; a child in the family carries the diagnosis of FHC; or when a patient or close relative has tendon xanthomas. A formal diagnosis may be made by using a validated set of criteria. The most commonly accepted are the US Make Early Diagnosis Prevent Early Death (MEDPED), Dutch Lipid Clinic Network, and the UK Simon-Broome Registry. The MEDPED criteria for diagnosing heFHC use age and consanguinity along with TC and LDL-C levels (see Table 43-6).[31, 34]

Once an individual has been identified as having FHC, cascade screening is recommended. Cascade screening is the screening of close family members in an attempt to detect the genetic disease. There is an approximately 50% chance of finding the disease in first-degree relatives, 25% in second-degree relatives, and 12.5% in third-degree relatives. The screening involves obtaining lipid levels.[32] Genetic testing may be a part of cascade screening when the diagnosis is indeterminate. The gold standard for diagnosis of FHC is DNA results confirming evidence of an LDLR, APO-B, or PCSK9 gene; as many as 20% of individuals with a clinical diagnosis of FHC will not, however, have a mutation found on DNA testing. A negative genetic test does not fully eliminate the diagnosis of FHC; with the elevated LDL-C levels and high CV risk, treatment should be instituted regardless of the results.[32] Some have advocated limiting cascade screening to those individuals who have been found to have a mutation defect identified on genetic testing in order to be cost-effective.[36] Some suggest prenatal counseling and genetic testing for those

Table 43-5 High-probability FHC age-specific lipid levels (32)

Age	LDL cholesterol (mg/dL)
≥30 years	≥250
20–29 years	≥220
<20 years	≥190

Table 43-6 MEDPED criteria* for FHC [31, 34]

Age (years)	Total cholesterol (and LDL-C) levels in mg/dL			
	First-degree relative	Second-degree relative	Third-degree relative	General population
<18	220 (155)	230 (165)	240 (170)	270 (200)
20	240 (170)	250 (180)	260 (185)	290 (220)
30	270 (190)	280 (200)	290 (210)	340 (240)
≥40	290 (205)	300 (225)	310 (225)	360 (260)

* Criteria points set for 80% probability of individual having FHC.

affected by or at risk for the congenital disease. This could offer the opportunity to discuss potential risks to future offspring as well as provide an opportunity for preconceptual and contraceptive counseling. Prenatal testing is controversial, however, since the disease does not affect cognitive ability and a treatment is available, particularly if the testing is requested for pregnancy termination rather than for early diagnosis.[30] Prenatal testing would necessitate a thorough conversation between clinician and patient to explore the implications of the decision to undergo prenatal testing.

Lifestyle management

Regardless of the reason for hyperlipidemia, lifestyle management serves as the foundation for primary and secondary prevention of CVD. Unfortunately many clinicians do not adequately perceive the CV risk of women and therefore do not recommend appropriate interventions to improve CHD care.[2] Women also lack awareness of their own CVD risk.[1] Education is needed to reduce gender disparity to improve CHD preventive care. One of the most inclusive guidelines addressing lifestyle interventions for preventive care was recently published by the American Heart Association (AHA) and the American College of Cardiology (ACC); this targets reductions in LDL-C and non-HDL and blood pressure. The guideline emphasizes a diet containing vegetables; fruit; whole grains; low-fat dairy products; protein from fish, poultry, and legumes; and limited intake of sweets and red meat. Sodium restriction to about 2 g per day is recommended in most cases, although further reductions in sodium could reduce blood pressure further. Physical activity recommendations are for at least 150 minutes per week of moderate aerobic activity in a minimum of 10-minute increments spread throughout the week. Finally, a healthy weight is recommended (see Table 43-7).[37] Similar recommendations have been made by the National Institute for Health and Care Excellence and the American Association of Clinical Endocrinologists (see Table 43-8).[18, 19] Behavioral counseling is recommended for those individuals with at least one risk factor for CHD and those who are overweight or obese in order to promote a healthy diet and physical activity.[38] Cardiovascular risk reduction also should include smoking cessation and tobacco avoidance education along with education and encouragement of moderate alcohol consumption.[18, 19, 37, 39]

The greatest diet evidence exists for the Dietary Approaches to Stop Hypertension (DASH), which has

Table 43-7 Lifestyle recommendations – ACC/AHA [37]

Recommendations	Level of evidence
Lipids (lowering of LDL-C)	A
1. Diet of vegetables, fruits, and whole grains; low-fat dairy; poultry, fish, legumes; nontropical vegetable oils and nuts; limit sweets, sugar-containing beverages, and red meat	A
2. Adapt calories to healthy weight, personal and cultural preferences	A
3. 5%–6% calories from saturated fat	A
4. Reduce calories from trans fat	A
5. Physical activity of 3–4 aerobic sessions/wk lasting an average of 40 minutes per session of moderate to vigorous activity	
Blood pressure (lowering of BP)	A
1. Diet of vegetables, fruits and whole grains; low-fat dairy, poultry, fish, legumes, nontropical vegetable oils and nuts; limit sweets, sugar-containing beverages, and red meat	A
2. Adapt calories to healthy weight, personal and cultural preferences	A
3. Follow food plans such as AHA Diet, DASH Diet, or USDA Food Pattern	B
4. Consume ≤2400 mg/d sodium; further reductions to 1,500 mg/d lowers BP further; lowering sodium by 1,000 mg/d still lowers BP	A
5. Combine DASH diet with lower sodium intake	A
6. Physical activity of 3–4 aerobic sessions/wk lasting an average of 40 minutes per session of moderate to vigorous activity	

AHA – American Heart Association, DASH – Dietary Approaches to Stop Hypertension, USDA – United States Department of Agriculture

Table 43-8 Lifestyle recommendations – NICE and AACE [18, 19]

NICE	AACE
Diet	
1. Reduce total fat to <30% of total calories; saturated fats <10% and dietary cholesterol to <300 mg/day a. replace saturated fats with monounsaturated or polyunsaturated fats b. replace with olive oil or grapeseed oil or spreads 2. Reduce intake of sugar and products containing refined sugars 3. Eat 5 servings of fruit and vegetables daily 4. Eat 2 servings of fish weekly (at least one an oily fish such has salmon, trout, mackerel, sardines, or herring) 5. Eat 4–5 servings of unsalted nuts, seeds, or legumes weekly 6. Choose whole grains when eating starches 7. No plant sterols or sterol esters for primary prevention	1. Reduce total fat to 25%–35% of total calories; saturated fats to <7% and trans fats to <1% of total calories and cholesterol to <200 mg/day 2. Reduce caloric intake for healthy weight 3. At least 5–6 servings of fruits and vegetables daily 4. At least 6 servings of grains daily a. 1/3 of those as whole grains 5. Eat legumes, high-fiber cereals, low-fat dairy products 6. Eat fish, lean meats, and skinless poultry 7. Include 10 g–25 g of soluble fiber daily 8. Include about 2 g of plant stanol esters daily
Physical activity	
1. 150 minutes of moderate intensity aerobic sessions/wk lasting an average of 30 minutes per session or 75 minutes of vigorous intensity aerobic sessions or use a mixture of both 2. Muscle-strengthening exercises that involves legs, hips, arms, shoulders, chest, back and abdomen 2 or more days per week 3. Exercise at maximum safety range when unable to attain moderate intensity due to chronic medical conditions	1. 30 minutes of moderate intensity aerobic activity 3–6 times per week, expending at least 200 kcal/day 2. Goals can be met in single sessions or in multiple 10-minute sessions 3. Muscle-strengthening activity at least 2 days a week
Weight management	
1. Maintain a healthy weight 2. Offer weight reduction if overweight or obese	1. Offer weight loss education if obese
Alcohol	
1. No more than 2–3 units a day of alcohol (1 unit equals 1.5 oz of liquor, 5 oz of wine or 12 oz of beer) 2. No binge drinking	No distinct recommendation made
Smoking	
1. Avoid tobacco products 2. Offer tobacco cessation advice and intensive support	1. Support smoking cessation efforts through education, behavioral therapy, and/or pharmacotherapy

NICE – National Institute for Health and Care Excellence, AACE – American Association of Clinical Endocrinologists

been shown to reduce LDL-C in adult men and women including African Americans and non–African Americans. Additionally, with replacement of 10% of the calories from carbohydrates with proteins or unsaturated fats, BP is lowered by an additional 1 mmHg–3 mmHg and the LDL-C by 3 mg/dL, HDL-C by 1 mg/dL, and triglycerides by 16 mg/dL relative to the DASH diet alone. Saturated fats should preferentially be substituted for polyunsaturated fats, followed by monounsaturated fats and then whole grains or carbohydrates. Reduction of saturated fats lowers LDL-C and HDL-C. Reduction of LDL-C occurs consistently with reduction in trans fat, which usually comes from the intake of meat and dairy products. Reducing red meat and using low-fat dairy products therefore will add to fat reduction. Reduction of sodium lowers blood pressure in all stages of hypertension in adults older than 25 years of age. Evidence exists for a reduction in CV events by 30% with a reduction in sodium by 1,000 mg/day.[37] Smart, subtle dietary changes can lead to significant reduction in CV risk by reducing LDL-C and blood pressure. Behavioral counseling has been shown to be an effective means to effect these changes. A meta-analysis found that intensive behavioral counseling in those identified with CHD risk factors had favorable effects on dietary and physical activity behaviors, reduced cholesterol levels, lowered blood pressure, weight reduction, and lowered glucose levels, thus enhancing CHD risk reduction.[38]

Several diet variations have been studied to determine their effect on the lipid profile and blood pressure. Substitution of low-glycemic foods for high-glycemic foods in one five week trial in the context of the DASH diet had no effect on LDL-C or systolic blood pressure; therefore, using glycemic index for carbohydrate selection may not improve CV risk.[40] A pilot randomized controlled trial (RCT) by Foraker et al. in premenopausal women, the Lifestyle Eating and Fitness (LEAF) study, investigated the effect of a low-fat versus low-carbohydrate diet on body weight as well as changes in blood pressure and lipids. The low-fat diet had 20% total calories from fat, 20% from protein, and 60% from carbohydrates. Alternatively, the low-carbohydrate diet recommended 40% total calories from carbohydrates, 30% from fats, and 30% from protein. All women in the RCT received physical activity prescriptions to promote weight loss. This study included primarily Caucasian women (75%) with an average age of 41 years. Only about 10% of the women were hypertensive or had high total cholesterol levels. Despite initial reductions in blood pressure and TC and LDL-C, at study end there was no difference between the two dietary groups in sustained lipid reductions; however, there was a sustained reduction of 11 mmHg in hypertensive patients and 6 mmHg in normotensive patients. A low adherence to both the diets and physical activity may have affected the outcome.[41] Another study explored the effect of low-carbohydrate and low-fat diets in men and women on weight and CV risk factors with about 50% African-American participants. Those following the low-carbohydrate diet were instructed to maintain total carbohydrates minus total fiber of less than 40 g/day. Those in the low-fat diet arm were instructed to maintain less than 30% daily total fat intake and 55% total intake from carbohydrates. In this study those in the low-carbohydrate diet arm had significant weight loss, increased levels of HDL, reductions in non-HDL cholesterol, and reductions in serum triglycerides. Additionally, there were significant reductions in hsCRP and the 10-year CV risk via the Framingham risk score in the low-carbohydrate group; a low-carbohydrate diet may therefore be an option to reduce CHD with further study.[42]

Lifestyle management is recommended for CV risk reduction in persons with familial hypercholesterolemia. Behavioral counseling for dietary and lifestyle modification for adults is required to assist in management of the disease. Attention is paid to reduction of fats and cholesterol with increased fiber in the diet, avoidance of tobacco and alcohol products, and the incorporation of regular physical activity (see Table 43-9).[30, 43] Management of weight is very important. Dietary cholesterol should be limited to 100 mg per 1,000 kcal per day, not to exceed 300 mg. Additional health professionals such as registered dieticians may be necessary to assist with monitoring and counseling. Lifestyle management is useful in reducing CV risk, but it is ineffective as monotherapy in reducing LDL-C to target levels.[35, 44]

Medical management

Current guidelines incorporate treatment of hyperlipidemia within an overall program to reduce CV risk. Statins, which inhibit 3-hydroxy-3-methylglutaryl coenzyme A (HMG-CoA) reductase, are the drugs of choice for the management of hyperlipidemia and CV risk. They also improve endothelial function and reduce inflammation. The guidelines recommend calculating the 10-year CV risk to determine if the risk suggests primary prevention would be beneficial. In general, each of the CV risk algorithms incorporates age and gender along with components of the lipid profile, blood pressure, tobacco use, and weight. Examples include the

Framingham Risk Assessment Tool developed from the historic Framingham Heart Study used in the National Cholesterol Education Program (NCEP); Adult Treatment III (ATP3) guideline;[45] the QRISK2 algorithm developed in the United Kingdom and used by the National Institute for Health and Care Excellence (NICE);[18] the Reynolds Risk Score recommended for women used in the guideline by the American Association of Clinical Endocrinologists (AACE) based on the Framingham Risk Assessment Tool adding two additional components, the hsCRP and a family history of early CV disease, to identify more at-risk women;[19] and the Pooled Cohort Equation used in the guideline recently released by American College of Cardiology (ACC) and American Heart Association (AHA).[20] Notably the ACC/AHA guideline represents a clinical practice update of the NCEP ATP3 guideline, using a strict evidence-based approach and basing recommendations on high-quality RCTs and systematic reviews. It also expanded the definition of CHD to include stroke, peripheral arterial disease, stable and unstable angina, abdominal aortic aneurysm, and transient ischemic attack in addition to acute coronary syndrome and myocardial infarction. Pretreatment cholesterol values should preferentially be used in these tools to obtain a more accurate risk score. Some of the tools are not validated with treatment levels of cholesterol, for example the Pooled Cohort Equation.[20]

Table 43-9 Lifestyle modifications in familial hypercholesterolemia [29, 30, 43]

1. Reduce intake of daily saturated fats and cholesterol
    a. 25%–35% total fat
    b. <7% saturated fats
    c. cholesterol <200 mg
2. Consume 2 grams of plant sterols and sterol esters per day*
3. Consume soluble fiber of 10 g–20 g per day
4. Practice weight control through physical activity and appropriate caloric intake
5. Limit alcohol consumption
6. Avoid tobacco products

* Plant sterols and esters are found in some nuts, corn, soy, whole grains, fortified foods and oils, spreads, and dressings.

Statin medications are classified based on the ability of the drug to lower cholesterol. The dosages, classifications, and intensity level are based on systematic reviews showing the percentage reduction of LDL-C that resulted in an improved CV risk. Table 43-10 details statin intensity and the dosages at those levels.[20]

Cardiovascular risk is usually classified as high, moderate, or low risk. Recommendations for statin selection incorporate determined CV risk. In the NICE guideline, it is recommended those 40–84 years old have a QRISK2 score calculated and if it reveals a 10-year CHD risk of ≥10%, then a full CHD is warranted as well as initiation of a statin for primary prevention. This includes individuals with type 2 diabetes; however, for those aged 85 and older or with type 1 diabetes or chronic kidney disease (CKD), QRISK2 score is necessary and therapy should be offered. High intensity statin therapy is recommended for all those with CVD for secondary prevention. The NICE guidelines do not specify a LDL-C target, but rather target a 40% reduction of the non-HDL cholesterol. In general, combination therapy with other lipid-lowering agents is not recommended.[18]

Table 43-10 Statin characteristics [20]

Low intensity LDL ↓ 30%	Moderate intensity LDL ↓ 30%–50%	High intensity LDL ↓ ≥50%
Simvastatin 10 mg Pravastatin 10–20 mg Lovastatin 20 mg Fluvastatin 20–40 mg Pitavastatin 1 mg	Rosuvastatin 5–10 mg Atorvastatin 10–20 mg Simvastatin 20–40 mg Lovastatin 40 mg Pravastatin 40–80 mg Fluvastatin 40 mg BID Fluvastatin XL 80 mg Pitavastatin 2–4 mg	Rosuvastatin 20–40 mg Atorvastatin 40–80 mg

BID = twice daily

In the AACE guideline, CV risk should be calculated in women using the Reynolds Risk Tool and if the ASCVD risk is >10%, then statin therapy is recommended along with a full CV risk assessment. Goals of therapy are based on CV risk. The LDL-C goal in women with high CV risk, with diabetes, and at least one additional CV risk factor, and those with CVD A LDL-C is less than 70 mg/dL. AACE guideline also details goals for other components of the lipid profile but particularly HDL to >40 mg/dL and triglycerides to <150 mg/dL in men and women. Statins remain the initial drugs of choice for reducing LDL-C because of its beneficial effect on reducing CV morbidity and mortality. The AACE alternatively recommend fibrates for primary prevention of CHD in those with both hypertriglyceridemia (>200 mg/dL) and for primary and secondary prevention in those with low HDL-C (<40 mg/dL) concentrations. Niacin is recommended for reducing LDL-C and triglycerides and increasing HDL-C. Bile acid sequestrants are recommended for reducing LDL-C and APO-B and mildly increasing HDL-C as well as potentially increasing triglycerides. Cholesterol absorption inhibitors are recommended as combination therapy with a statin for reduction of LDL-C and APO-B although there is no evidence that ezetimibe, the only drug in this class of medications, has beneficial effects on reducing CV risk. Combination therapy with statins is recommended in certain clinical situations. Examples are as follows: therapeutic targets are not achieved with statin monotherapy, mixed dyslipidemias, and patients with hypertriglyceridemia and low HDL-C.[19]

The ACC/AHA guideline recommends calculation of ASCVD risk using the Pooled Cohort Equation and identifies four groups in which the potential to benefit from CV risk reduction exceeds the potential for adverse effects. These are (1) those with ASCVD, (2) those ≥21 years old with primary elevations of LDL-C ≥190 mg/dL, (3) individuals 40–75 years old with diabetes and an LDL-C of 70 mg/dL–189 mg/dL, and (4) those aged 40–75 without ASCVD or diabetes with a LDL-C 70 mg/dL–189 mg/dL. No targets for LDL-C or non-HDL are recommended for primary or secondary prevention of CHD but rather the use of either a high or moderate intensity statin based on CVD risk. Statin therapy is indicated for primary prevention in diabetics aged 40–75 with and without a ≥7.5% 10-year ASCVD risk using the Pooled Cohort Equation. Women with LDL-C levels between 89 mg/dL and 189 mg/dL without clinical ASCVD or diabetes should have their ASCVD risk calculated to determine if statin therapy is a consideration. This guideline recognizes the use of additional factors to consider statin therapy if there is clinical suspicion that the patient may benefit from it and the individual does not fit into any one of the four categories. Examples are an LDL-C of 160 mg/dL or greater or other evidence of hyperlipidemia; family history of premature heart disease; hsCRP ≥2 mg/dL; arterial-brachial index <0.9; a coronary calcium score of 300 Å or higher or at the seventy-fifth percentile for age, gender, and ethnicity; and patient preference. These additional parameters could be considered along with clinical judgment to discuss the potential benefits of statin therapy with women. No other recommendations are made for use of other lipid-lowering mediations except the use of fibrates for triglyceride levels >500 mg/dL to address the risk of pancreatitis before instituting statin therapy.[20] Table 43-11 summarizes key points of the ATP 3, ACC/AHA, NICE, and AACE guidelines.

Statin use and selection should take into consideration not only CV risk, but also clinical judgment for CV risk, patient preference, and statin properties along with the ability of the statin to lower LDL-C and total cholesterol.

Statins are classified based on their hydrophilic or lipophilic properties. Examples of lipophilic statins are atorvastatin, lovastatin, and simvastatin. Lipophilic statins penetrate muscle cells to a higher degree and place patients at a greater risk for rhabdomyolysis. They also cross the blood-brain barrier more easily which can lead to insomnia and adversely affect cognition. Hydrophilic statins, pravastatin, rosuvastatin, and fluvastatin, have greater hepatic selectivity creating the potential for hepatic toxicity and have less effects on muscle. Additionally, lovastatin absorption is increased with food while atorvastatin, fluvastatin, and pravastatin are decreased when taken with food. Simvastatin and rosuvastatin are not affected by food. Pravastatin and rosuvastatin have less drug interactions due to less interaction with metabolic degradation pathways. Rosuvastatin and atorvastatin have the longest half-life.[46]

A notable adverse effect of statins is the potential for increasing fasting blood glucose. In the Justification for the Use of Statins in Prevention: An Intervention Trial Evaluating Rousavastatin (JUPITER) trial, men

Table 43-11 Summaries of key elements of treatment guidelines

	ATP3 (2002) [45]	ACC/AHA (2013) [20]
Risk assessment	Based on counting of risk factors and estimating 10-year CHD risk (Framingham)	Pooled Cohort Equation (http://clincalc.com/Cardiology/ASCVD/PooledCohort.aspx?example)
Pharmacotherapy	Recommends statins, BASs, nicotinic acid, fibric acids depending on extent of lipid lowering needed	Focuses on statins. Other cholesterol lowering therapy does not provide acceptable CVD risk reduction for their potential adverse effects
Goals	LDL-C: <160, <130, <100 (maybe <70) depending on risk	No LDL-C goals
Terms	CVD and CHD	ASCVD
Nonstatins	It is reasonable to add nonstatin cholesterol-lowering drugs to statins if necessary	Only consider nonstatin cholesterol-lowering drugs if patients cannot tolerate statins
Monitoring: lipids **Monitoring: ALT**	Monitor for 6–8 weeks after statin initiation or dose change, then every 4–6 months Baseline, 12 weeks after statin initiation and then annually or as indicated	Monitor 4–12 weeks after statin initiation, then every 3–12 months Baseline and if normal, repeat with signs of hepatotoxicity
	NICE (2014) [18]	**AACE (2012) [19]**
Risk assessment	Based on counting of risk factors and estimating 10-year CHD risk (QRISK2): exclude T1DM, FHC, and GFR <60 mL/min/1.73 m^2 Age 85	Based on counting of risk factors and estimating 10-year CHD risk (Framingham, men; Reynolds, women)
Pharmacotherapy	Recommends statin (atorvastatin 20 mg or 80 mg)	Focuses on statins; other cholesterol-lowering therapy does not provide acceptable CVD risk reduction for their potential adverse effects
Goals	No LDL goals	LDL-C: <160, <130, <100 (maybe <70) depending on risk; APO-B <90 mg/dL primary, <80 mg/dL secondary. TG <150; HDL >40
Terms	CVD	CHD (Male); CHD, Stroke, ASCVD (Female)
Nonstatins	No nonstatins for prevention of CVD; ezetimibe considered for Familial Hypercholesterolemia	Recommends statins as drug of choice for LDL lowering, BAS, nicotinic acid, fibric acids dependent on other lipid modifications needed
Monitoring: lipids **Monitoring: ALT**	Nonfasting lipids at baseline and then at 3 months (40% reduction non-HDL goal) Baseline, 12 weeks after statin initiation then at 12 months; not again unless indicated	Baseline fasting lipids and every 6 weeks to target, then at 6–12 month intervals; more often if DM worsens, weight gain, new CAD risk factor, adverse lipid change Baseline and 3 months after initiation, repeat "periodically e.g. semiannually"

and women at low to moderate risk of CVD, normal LDL-C levels, but an elevated hsCRP, given rousavastatin had marked reductions of LDL-C and lowered hsCRP but more importantly had fewer major CV events compared to placebo. During the trial, however, those on rosuvastatin had a greater chance of developing diabetes.[47] This adverse effect was duplicated in women with PCOS given atorvastatin in a RCT. Lipid levels and hsCRP were reduced compared to placebo but those on atorvastatin developed impaired glucose tolerance and insulin sensitivity thereby increasing the potential for the development of diabetes.[10] For most, the benefits of CV reduction will outweigh the risk of elevated fasting blood glucose; however, statin labeling carries the risk for an increase in fasting blood glucose and the hemoglobin A1c. This effect should be a part of the shared decision making when discussing statin therapy. Aggressive lifestyle changes must be a part of CV risk reduction as a means to offset this effect.

Other populations of women deserve special consideration. Women of childbearing age require extensive preconceptual counseling to decide the timing and management of hyperlipidemia if pregnancy is desired. Most lipid-lowering medications are contraindicated in pregnancy due to the risk of fetal anomalies. Discontinuation of lipid-lowering medications such as statins, ezetimibe, and niacin ideally should be discontinued 4–12 weeks prior to discontinuation of contraception. If unintended pregnancy occurs, lipid-lowering medications should be discontinued immediately with immediate physician consultation. Statins, ezetimibe, and niacin are contraindicated during lactation as well. Bile acid sequestrants (BAS) that bind intestinal bile acids, particularly colesevelam which is pregnancy class B, can be used in pregnancy with physician guidance but many women discontinue the medication due to gastrointestinal side effects, namely dyspepsia and constipation. Caution should be exercised when using BAS with elevated triglyceride levels ≥300 mg/dL; they are contraindicated with levels ≥400 mg/dL. BASs increase the synthesis of triglycerides and at these levels the risk of developing pancreatitis increases.[35, 43, 48]

Management of hyperlipidemia in premenopausal and pregnant women is extremely important especially in those diagnosed with familial hypercholesterolemia. LDL-C and total cholesterol are normally increased in pregnancy; however, in those with FHC those levels can be much greater. There is a potential for fetal compromise due to atherosclerosis of utero-placental arteries as well as maternal preeclampsia and hypertension. Management includes BAS, cholesterol-restricted diets, and close physician monitoring; however, LDL apheresis may be considered during pregnancy when there is already significant maternal ASCVD or with homozygous FHC. LDL apheresis is the process of selectively removing LDL particles from the circulation through extracorporeal binding to dextran sulfate or heparin. The procedure must be repeated every one to two weeks but removes 50%–70% of LDL-C that can last for two weeks. Adverse events are uncommon with LDL apheresis but can include hypotension, nausea, headache, anemia, and arrhythmias.[29, 31, 48]

Pharmacotherapy for adults with FHC begins with aggressive high-intensity statin therapy with a target of >50% reduction in LDL-C from baseline. Those with clinical CHD or multiple cardiac risk factors should have a more aggressive target for LDL-C reduction. Combination therapy with ezetimibe is recommended as the next medication to be added followed by bile acid sequestrants and possibly niacin. Exetimibe inhibits cholesterol absorption in the small intestine and niacin decreases LDL production, decreases hepatic triglyceride production, and increases lipoprotein lipase activity. Some sources recommend LDL apheresis instead of adding niacin if the LDL-C target level has not been reached after the addition of BASs.[39, 43] Statins are preferred when pharmacotherapy is indicated in girls experiencing menarche. Strong indications include LDL-C >190 mg/dL or >160 mg/dL with a family history of early cardiac disease or those with two or more cardiac risk factors. Ezetimibe and BASs may be added but LDL-C reductions are much lower and compliance with BASs is low.[29, 35]

LDL apheresis is an approved therapy for adults and children who have not achieved adequate LDL-C reduction with maximal medical therapy after six months of treatment or intolerance of the therapy, not on any medical therapy, or have continued symptomatic disease. Referral is indicated in patients with hoFHC and LDL ≥300 mg/dL, heFHC and LDL ≥300 mg/dL, or LDL ≥200 mg/dL and more than two additional cardiac risk factors, or ≥160 mg/dL and clinical cardiac disease or a cardiac equivalent such as diabetes. It is estimated that more than 2% of those with FHC in the United States are eligible for LDL apheresis.[43, 49]

Severe cases require more drastic measures. Surgical procedures may be necessary in an effort to affect the lipid profile and the development of atherosclerosis. Liver transplantation is an alternative in severe cases as well as portacaval shunt surgery to limit cholesterol absorption and promote bile acid loss.[31] More novel therapies are currently in development to reduce the cumulative lifetime risk of CHD to attain target LDL-C levels as monotherapy or in addition to traditional statin therapy. New medications in development target PCSKP, APO-B, microsomal triglyceride transfer protein inhibitors, and cholesteryl ester transfer protein inhibitors.[50] The effectiveness, tolerability, and safety of these new therapies are currently uncertain.

Despite the recommendations, there will be women that will be intolerant to statins or other therapies, do not desire pharmacotherapy, or do not fully understand their risk associated with hyperlipidemia. It is imperative in the context of the doctor-patient relationship to provide proper education and tailor hyperlipidemia therapy to patient preferences through informed consent and shared decision making.

Concluding remarks

Office health-care providers who are responsible for preventative treatment of female patients should be familiar with the assessment and management of hyperlipidemia. In the developed world, CVD is the most frequent cause of death for women. Appropriate screening of women is essential because adequate management can decrease CV risk and diminish the morbidity and mortality of women patients.

References

1. Mosca L, Ferris A, Fabunmi R, Robertson RM. Tracking women's awareness of heart disease: An American Heart Association National Study. *Circulation.* Available at: www.circulationha.org. DOI: 10.1161/01.CIR.0000115222.69428.C9 2004; Feb 4; 573–579. (Accessed Nov. 17, 2014.)
2. Mosca L, Linfante AH, Benjamin EJ, et al. National study of physician awareness and adherence to cardiovascular disease prevention guidelines. *Circulation.* Available at: www.circulationha.org. DOI: 10.1161/01.CIR0000154568.43333.82 2005; **111**: 499–510. (Accessed Nov. 17, 2014.)
3. Abuful A, Gidron Y, Henkin Y. Physicians' attitudes toward preventive therapy for coronary artery disease: Is there a gender bias? *Clin Cardiol* 2005 Aug;**28**: 389–393.
4. Rosamond W, Flegal K, Furie K, et al. (Writing group). Heart disease and stroke statistics – 2008 update: a report from the American Heart Association Statistics Committee and Stroke Statistics Subcommittee. *Circulation.* Available at: http://circ.ahajournals.org. DOI: 10.1161/CIRCULATIONAHA.107.187998. 2008; **117**: e25–e146. (Accessed Nov. 17, 2014.)
5. Kim AM, Tingen CM, Woodruff TK. Sex bias in trials and treatment must end. *Nature* 2010 June 10; **465**: 688–689.
6. Mosca L, Benjamin EJ, Berra K, et al. Effectiveness-based guidelines for the prevention of cardiovascular disease in women—2011 Update: A guideline from the American Heart Association. *J Am Coll Cardiol* 2011 Mar 22; **57**(12): 1404–1423. DOI:10.1016/j.jacc.2011.02.005.
7. WomenHeart: The National Coalition for Women with Heart Disease. Women & Heart Disease Fact Sheet. Available at: www.womenheart.org/resources.cvdfactsheet.cfm. (Accessed Nov. 20, 2014.)
8. Gotto AM, Moon JE. Management of cardiovascular risk: the importance of meeting lipid targets. *Am J Cardiol* 2012; **110**(suppl): 3A–14A.
9. Wenger NK. Prevention of cardiovascular disease in women: highlights for the clinician of the 2011 American Heart Association guidelines. *Adv Chronic Kidney Dis* 2013 Sep; **20**(5): 419–422.
10. Puurunen J, Piltonen T, Puukka K, et al. Statin therapy worsens insulin sensitivity in women with polycystic ovary syndrome (PCOS): a prospective, randomized, double-blind, placebo-controlled study. *J Clin Endocrinol Metab* 2013 Dec; **98**(12): 4798–4807.
11. Spracklen CN, Smith CJ, Saftlas AF, et al. Maternal hyperlipidemia and the risk of preeclampsia: a meta-analysis. *Am J Epidemiol* 2014 Aug; **180**(4): 346–358.
12. Mosca L, Benjamin EJ, Berra K, et al. Effectiveness-based guidelines for the prevention of cardiovascular disease in women-2011update: a guideline from the American Heart Association. *Circulation* 2011; **123** (11): 1243–1262.
13. Roberts JM, August PA, Bakris G, et al. Hypertension in pregnancy: report of the American College of Obstetricians and Gynecologists' task force in hypertension in pregnancy. *Obstet Gynecol* 2013 Nov; **122**(5): 1122–1131.
14. US Preventive Services Task Force. Lipid disorders in adults (cholesterol, dyslipidemia): screening. Recommendation Summary. September 2014. Available at: www.uspreventiveservicestaskforce/Page/Topic/recommendation-summary/lipid-disorders-in-adults-cholesterol-dyslipidemia-screening. (Accessed Dec. 30, 2014).

15. American Academy of Family Physicians. Summary of recommendations for clinical preventive services. November 2014. Available at: www.aafp.org/dam/AAFP/documents/patient_care/clinical_recommendations/cps-recommendations.pdf. (Accessed Dec. 30, 2014).
16. The American College of Obstetricians and Gynecologists. Well-woman care: assessments & recommendations. July 2013. Available at: www.acog.org/-/media/Departments/Annual-Womens-Health-Care/PrimaryAndPreventiveCare.pdf. (Accessed Dec. 30, 2014).
17. Daniels SR, Greer FR, Committee on Nutrition. Lipid screening and cardiovascular health in childhood. *Pediatrics* 2008; **122**: 198–208.
18. National Institute for Health and Care Excellence. Lipid modification: cardiovascular risk assessment and the modification of blood lipids for the primary and secondary prevention of cardiovascular disease. *NICE Clinical Guideline 181* 2014 July; 1–50.
19. Jellinger PS, Smith DA, Mehta AE, et al. American Association of Clinical Endocrinologists' guidelines for management of dyslipidemia and prevention of atherosclerosis. *Endocr Pract* 2012; **18**(suppl 1): 1–77.
20. Stone NJ, Robinson J, Lichtenstein AH, et al. 2013 ACC/AHA guideline on the treatment of blood cholesterol to reduce atherosclerotic cardiovascular risk in adults: a report of the American College of Cardiology/American Heart Association task force on practice guidelines. *Circulation* 2013 Nov. Available at: http://circ.ahajournals.org/content/early2013/11/11/11/01.cir.0000437738.63852.7a. citation. (Accessed May 15, 2015.)
21. World Health Organization Collaborative Study of Cardiovascular Disease and Steroid Hormone Contraception. Cardiovascular disease and use of oral and injectable progestogen-only contraceptives and combined injectable contraceptives. *Contraception* 1998; **57**: 315–324.
22. Kemmeren JM, Tanis BC, van den Bosch MAAJ, et al. Risk of arterial thrombosis in relation to oral contraceptives (RATIO) study: oral contraceptives and the risk of ischemic stroke. *Stroke* 2002; **33**: 1202–1208.
23. Tanis BC, van den Bosch MAAJ, Kemmeren JM, et al. Oral Contraceptives and the risk of myocardial infarction. *N Engl J Med* 2001 Dec; **345**(25): 1787–1793.
24. Berenson AB, Rahman M, Wilkinson G. Effect of injectable and oral contraceptives on serum lipids. *Obstet Gynecol* 2009 Oct; **114**(4): 786–94.
25. Fotherby K. Oral contraceptives and lipids. *BMJ*. 1989; **298**(6680): 1049–1050.
26. Sorensen MB, Collins P, Ong PJL, et al. Long-term use of contraceptive depot medroxyprogesterone acetate in young women impairs arterial endothelial function assessed by cardiovascular magnetic resonance. *Circulation* 2002; **106**: 1646–1651.
27. Bassuk SS, Manson JE. Menopausal hormone therapy and cardiovascular disease risk: utility of biomarkers and clinical factors for risk stratification. *Clin Chem*. 2014; **60**(1): 68–77.
28. Rossouw JE, Prentice RL, Manson JE, et al. Postmenopausal hormone therapy and risk of cardiovascular disease by age and years since menopause. *JAMA* 2007; **297**: 1465–1477.
29. Goldberg AC, Hopkins PN, Toth PP, et al. Familial hypercholesterolemia: screening, diagnosis and management of pediatric and adult patients: clinical guidance from the National Lipid Association expert panel on familial hypercholesterolemia. *J Clin Lipidol* 2011; **5**: S1–S8.
30. Youngblom E, Knowles JW. Familial hypercholesterolemia. 2014 Jan 2. In: Pagon RA, Adam MP, Ardinger HH, et al., editors. *GeneReviews©* [Internet]. Seattle, WA: University of Washington, Seattle; 1993–2014. Available from: www.ncbi.nlm.nih.gov/books/NBK174884. (Accessed Dec. 29, 2014.)
31. Hovingh GK, Davidson MH, Kastelein JJP, O'Connor AM. Diagnosis and treatment of familial hypercholesterolaemia. *Eu Heart J* 2013; **34**: 962–971.
32. Hopkins PN, Toth PP, Ballantyne CM, Rader DJ. Familial hypercholesterolemia: prevalence, genetics, diagnosis and screening recommendations from the National Lipid Association expert panel on familial hypercholesterolemia. *J Clin Lipidol* 2011; **5**: S9–S17.
33. Goldberg AC, Robinson JG, Cromwell WC, et al. Future issues, public policy, and public awareness of familial hypercholesterolemias: recommendations from the National Lipid Association Expert panel on familial hypercholesterolemia. *J Clin Lipidol* 2011; **5**: S46–S51.
34. Yudi M, Omera L, McCubbery N, et al. Suboptimal consideration and management of potential familial hypercholesterolaemia in patients with suspected premature coronary artery disease. *Singapore Med J* 2012; **53**(3): 174–178.
35. Harada-Shiba M, Arai H, Oikawa S, et al. Guidelines for the management of famiulial hypercholesterolemia. *J Atheroscler Thromb* 2012; **19**: 1043–1060.
36. Talmud P, Shah S, Whittall R, Futema M, Howard P, Cooper JA et al. Use of low density lipoprotein cholesterol gene score to distinguish patients with polygenic and monogenic familial hypercholesterolaemia: a case-control study. *Lancet* 2013; **381**: 1293–1301.
37. Eckel RH, Jakicic JM, Ard JD, et al. 2013 AHA/ACC guideline on lifestyle management to reduce cardiovascular risk: a report of the American College of Cardiology/American Heart Association task force on

practice guidelines. *Circulation* 2014; **129**(suppl 2): S76–S99.

38. Lin JS, O'Connor E, Evans CV, et al. Behavioral counseling to promote a healthy lifestyle in persons with cardiovascular Risk factors: a systematic review for the US Preventive Services Task Force. *Ann Intern Med* 2014; **161**: 568–578.
39. Robinson JG, Goldberg AC. Treatment of adults with familial hypercholesterolemia and evidence for treatment: recommendations from the National Lipid Association expert panel on familial hypercholesterolemia. *J Clin Lipidol* 2011; **5**: S18–S29.
40. Sacks FM, Carey VJ, Anderson CAM, et al. Effects of high vs low glycemic index of dietary carbohydrate on cardiovascular disease risk factors and insulin sensitivity. *JAMA* 2014; **312**(23): 2531–2541.
41. Foraker RE, Pennell M, Sprangers P, et al. Effect of a low-fat or low-carbohydrate weight-loss diet on markers of cardiovascular risk among premenopausal women: a randomized trial. *J Womens Health (Larchmt)* 2014 Aug; **23**(8): 675–680.
42. Bazzano LA, Hu T, Reynolds K, et al. Effects of low-carbohydrate and low-fat diets. *Ann Intern Med* 2014; **161**: 309–331.
43. Ito MK, McGowan MP, Moriarty PM. Management of familial hypercholesterolemias in adult patients: recommendations from the National Lipid Association expert panel on familial hypercholesterolemia. *J Clin Lipidol* 2011; **5**: S38–S45.
44. Broekhuizen K, van Poppel MNM, Koppes LL, et al. No significant improvement of cardiovascular disease risk indicators by a lifestyle intervention in people with familial hypercholesterolemia compared to usual care: result of a randomised controlled trial. *BMC Research Notes* 2012; **5**: 181. DOI: 10.1186/1756-0050-5-181.
45. National Cholesterol Education Program. *Third report of the expert panel on detection, evaluation, and treatment of high blood cholesterol in adults (adult treatment panel III). NIH Pub. No. 02-5215.* Bethesda, MD: National Heart, Lung, and Blood Institute, 2002; 284 pages.
46. McKenney JM. Pharmacologic characteristics of statins. *Clin Cardiol* 2003 Apr; **26**(4 suppl 3): III 32–38.
47. Ridker PM. The JUPITER trial: results, controversies, and implications for prevention. *Circ Cardiovasc Qual Outcomes* 2009; **2**: 279–285.
48. Eapen DJ, Valiani K, Reddy S, Sperling L. Management of familial hypercholesterolemia during pregnancy: case series and discussion. *J Clin Lipidol* 2012; **6**: 88–91.
49. Vishwanath R, Hemphill LC. Familial hypercholesterolemia and estimation of US patients eligible for low-density lipoprotein apheresis after maximally tolerated lipid-lowering therapy. *J Clin Lipidol* 2012; **8**: 18–28.
50. Nordestgaard BG, Chapman MJ, Humphries SE, et al. Familial hypercholesterolaemia is underdiagnosed and undertreated in the general population: guidance for clinicians to prevent coronary heart disease. *Eu Heart J* 2013; **34**: 3478–3490.

Chapter 44

Osteoporosis and osteopenia

Ronald C. Hamdy

Introduction

Osteoporosis is a disease characterized by reduced bone strength leading to an increased fracture risk. It is not part of the normal aging process and affects both genders and all ethnic groups. About 50% of Caucasian women aged 50 years and older are expected to sustain an osteoporotic fracture.[1] It is silent; patients have no warning symptoms and are not aware of having osteoporosis until a fracture occurs.

Impact of osteoporosis

Fracture is the main complication of osteoporosis; any bone may fracture and the impact of fractures depends on the fractured bone. Hip fractures are associated with the worst prognosis whereas vertebral fractures are often silent. All osteoporotic fractures, however, even silent vertebral fractures, are associated with increased mortality and morbidity.[2] They also increase the risk of subsequent fractures, thus triggering a vicious cycle as more fractures are sustained.[3]

Hip fractures

Osteoporotic hip fractures are catastrophic life-changing events: about 20% of women who sustain an osteoporotic hip fracture are expected to die within a year of the fracture, 20% become so disabled as to need long-term institutional care, 20% are not able to resume their daily activities, and only 40% are able to resume their prefracture daily activities.[4–6]

Vertebral fractures

Vertebral fractures are the most common type of osteoporotic fractures. Most occur while the patient is carrying on her daily activities and are not due to trauma.[7] The typical manifestations include sudden onset of severe, incapacitating, localized back pain often occurring spontaneously with no precipitating trauma.[8] These are referred to as clinical vertebral compression fractures to differentiate them from the morphometric vertebral compression fractures which do not have acute pain.

Morphometric vertebral fractures are diagnosed when the patient is having imaging studies for a condition not related to osteoporosis (opportunistic diagnosis). Unfortunately, in many instances, these fractures are not reported in the x-ray summary and as a result may go unnoticed.[9] About two-thirds of vertebral compression fractures are morphometric (i.e., silent) fractures.

Both clinical and morphometric vertebral compression fractures lead to height loss, kyphosis, protuberant abdomen, deformed body image, decreased lung capacity, sleep disorders, loss of self-esteem, depression, and increased mortality.[9]

Fractures of the proximal humerus

Fractures of the proximal humerus are usually the result of a fall.[10] Management is difficult and many patients are unable to resume their prefracture level of functioning because of pain and limitation in the range of motion. Many require prolonged hospitalization.[11] Mortality is increased.[12]

Fractures of the distal radius

Fractures of the distal radius are the earliest osteoporotic fractures to occur; most are the result of a fall on the outstretched forearm. Six months after sustaining the fracture, more than half the patients report difficulties performing their daily activities. Persistent pain, degenerative arthritis, and reflex sympathetic dystrophy are complications.[4]

Overall economic burden

It is estimated that in the United States, every year there are about 2 million osteoporotic fractures

Office Care of Women, ed. Martin E. Olsen and Botros Rizk. Published by Cambridge University Press.

leading to about 432,000 hospitalizations, 2.5 million office visits, and 180,000 admissions to nursing homes. Every year, in the United States, among Caucasian women there are more cases of osteoporotic fractures than cases of breast cancer, heart attacks, and strokes. The cost of managing osteoporotic fractures is increasing and estimated to exceed $25 billion by 2025. Hip fractures account for about 80% of this cost.[13]

Some interesting trends

Encouraging trends exist in the United States: the number of hip fractures has decreased from about 600 per 100,000 in 1997 to 400 per 100,000 in 2007.[14] Similar findings have been reported in other countries.[15–20] This coincides with the introduction of bisphosphonates: alendronate became commercially available in 1995.

Many patients who have sustained osteoporotic fractures are neither diagnosed nor treated for osteoporosis. This is unfortunate given the availability of medications that can reduce the risk of hip fractures by about 50% and the risk of multiple vertebral fractures by about 90%.[21] Treatment cost is low; a three-month supply of alendronate cost less than $10.00 in 2014.

A general apathy about osteoporosis exists. The American Orthopedic Association launched the "Own the Bone Program" to encourage orthopedic surgeons to assume responsibility for patients with osteoporotic fractures. Unfortunately the program received a lukewarm reception. A 2012 initiative involves hiring "fracture liaison officers" to ensure patients with osteoporotic fractures are diagnosed and treated.[22] It is too early to evaluate this program.

Diagnosis

Fragility fractures

Fragility fractures are diagnostic of osteoporosis regardless of densitometric findings.[1] They are defined as fractures occurring after a fall from a standing position or precipitated by trauma that ordinarily would not be expected to lead to a fracture. When they occur spontaneously they are referred to as atraumatic fractures.

Fragility vertebral compression fractures are sometimes silent and accidentally discovered during an imaging study done for an unrelated condition. This gives patients an opportunity for treatment of silent osteoporosis to prevent further fractures.

Densitometric diagnosis

In the absence of fragility fractures, osteoporosis can be diagnosed by bone densitometry.[1, 23] During this procedure the patient's bone is exposed to two waves of x-rays, hence the name dual energy x-ray absorptiometry: DXA or DEXA. As the two waves are absorbed to different extents by bone and soft tissue, it is possible to calculate the bone mineral content and bone surface area. The former is divided by the latter to calculate the bone mineral density (BMD). The patient's BMD is compared to that of a normal young healthy adult reference population and the number of standard deviations the patient's BMD is versus that of the reference population is designated as the T-score.

T-scores are used to establish the diagnosis based on the World Health Organization guidelines: patients with a T-score of −2.5 or lower are classified as having "osteoporosis"; those with a T-score of −1.0 or higher are classified as "normal" and patients with a T-score higher than −2.5, but lower than −1.0 are classified as "osteopenia."[24] It must be emphasized that this classification only applies to postmenopausal women and is restricted to the T-scores of the femoral neck, total hip, and lumbar vertebrae. Sometimes it is not possible to scan any of these sites as may occur in patients with bilateral hip replacements, gross osteophytes, multiple vertebral compression fractures, extra-vertebral calcifications, deformities or grossly overweight patients. In these instances the distal one-third of 33% radius can be used. Also a minimum of two lumbar vertebrae should be included in the calculation of the T-score for diagnostic purposes.[24–26] Although the T-scores of other bone sites are routinely derived, they cannot be used for diagnostic purposes. T-scores can also be used to estimate the fracture risk.

The patient's BMD can be compared to that of an age-matched reference population and the number of standard deviations between patient's and reference population is designated as the Z-score. Z-scores are useful in premenopausal women, children, and adolescents. In these populations the term "osteoporosis" is not recommended unless the patient has sustained a fragility fracture. Those with a Z-score −2.0 or lower are referred to as having a "low bone mineral density for given age."[25, 27–29]

Laboratory tests – identifying secondary causes of osteoporosis

Laboratory tests are useful to identify secondary causes of osteoporosis. An assay of the serum 25-hydroxy-vitamin level is usually done to identify vitamin D deficiency.

A comprehensive metabolic profile is usually routinely done: an elevated serum calcium level may indicate hyperparathyroidism, a moderately elevated serum alkaline phosphatase level may suggest vitamin D deficiency, fracture repair or neoplasia; a grossly elevated alkaline phosphatase suggests Paget's disease of bone; low albumin may be due to malnutrition or malabsorption, elevated protein may be due to multiple myeloma. Evidence of impaired renal and hepatic functions may trigger further investigations. Caution should be exercised when prescribing bisphosphonates to patients with renal dysfunction or low serum calcium levels. Similarly denosumab and parenteral bisphosphonates should not be administered to patients with hypocalcemia. A complete blood count may identify anemia or malnutrition.

Other potential tests include tissue transglutaminase if celiac disease is suspected, ionized serum calcium and parathyroid hormone (intact molecule) if hyperparathyroidism is suspected, 24-hours urinary calcium and sodium excretion if hypercalciuria is suspected, serum and urine protein electrophoresis if multiple myeloma is suspected and serum magnesium, pre-albumin and phosphate levels if malnutrition is suspected.

Assay of bone markers is not usually indicated in the initial workup; it is used as a parameter to determine whether the patient is adhering to the prescribed antiresorptive medication.

Assessing fracture risk

Although BMD/T-scores are important factors affecting fracture risk, many other factors modulate this risk. A number of assessment scales are available to estimate the patient's fracture risk. At present the most widely used one is the FRAX algorithm.[30–32] It has been validated in a number of countries and is available free of charge on the web.

FRAX takes into consideration the patient's ethnic group, age, gender, weight, height, and seven risk factors: history of parental hip fracture, personal history of fracture, glucocorticoid therapy, cigarette smoking, alcohol abuse, rheumatoid arthritis, and secondary osteoporosis. It can be calculated with or without the BMD/T-score of the femoral neck. Once the information is uploaded, the patient's 10-year probability of sustaining a hip or major fracture is calculated and expressed as a percentage.

FRAX is particularly useful in patients with osteopenia. One of the main uses of the FRAX algorithm is to help clinicians decide which patient with osteopenia should be offered treatment. The National Osteoporosis Foundation recommends that pharmacological treatment be considered in patients with osteopenia whose FRAX score reaches/exceeds 3% and 20% for the risk of a hip or major fracture, respectively.[1]

FRAX has a number of limitations. It does not take into account the risk of falling. The answer to the seven risk factors included in the permutation can only be either yes or no; the answer will be the same if the patient smokes one or twenty cigarettes a day, is on a very small or very large dose of corticosteroids and has sustained one fracture or multiple fractures. Another major drawback is that it cannot be used to monitor the patient's response to therapy.

Assessing fall risk

Most osteoporotic fractures are preceded by a fall; most patients fall a few times before sustaining a fracture. It is important to assess the patient's fall risk because increased fall risk is an independent risk factor. Causes of falls can be grouped into four main groups.[23] First are intrinsic pathologies such as arrhythmias, orthostatic hypotension, vertebro-basilar insufficiency, sensitive carotid sinus, Parkinson's disease, peripheral neuropathies, strokes, cerebellar insufficiency, arthropathies, and myopathies. Second are medications (either prescribed or over the counter), especially hypnotics, sedatives, hypotensives, diuretics, and psychotropic medications. Alcohol may increase medication risk.

Third, environmental hazards may increase fall risk such as trailing wires; loose worn-out, ill-fitting carpets; small rugs; obstacles and poorly visualized decorative furniture. Fourth, the patient may have difficulty perceiving the environment as in cases of excessive glare, poor lighting or excessive lighting. Bifocal glasses are a major cause of falls. Patients with mental impairment may take increased risks and hence sustain a fall. Finally abuse by omission or commission should be considered in some instances.

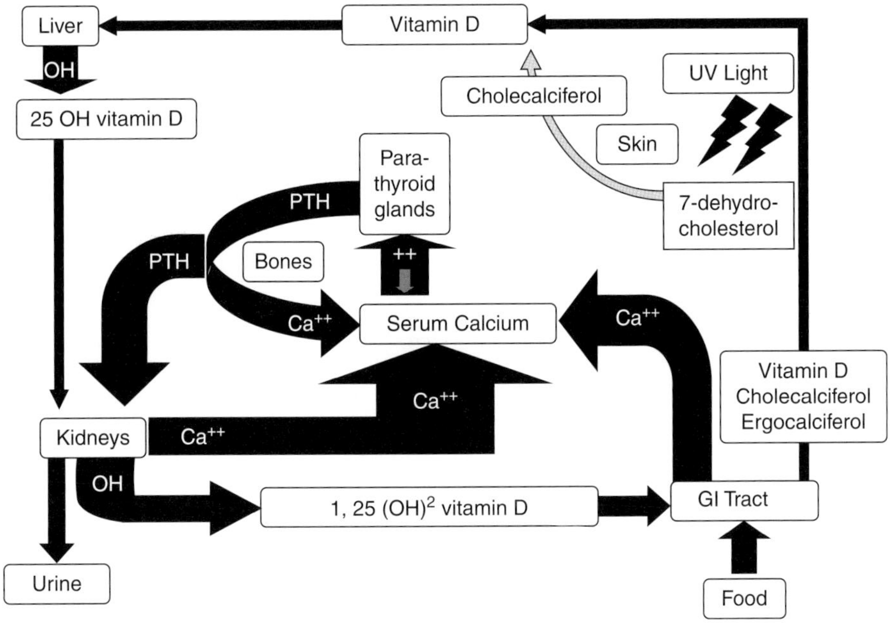

Figure 44-1 Hypocalcemia triggered homeostatic mechanisms.

A number of functional tests are available to evaluate the patient's risk of falling. Although the get-up-and-go test has some limitations, it is a convenient, quick test with excellent reproducibility.[33] It is the time the patient takes to get up from a chair without using the arm rests, walk 10 feet, and return to the chair. The patient may use a cane or walking frame. Most "healthy" people should be able to complete the task in less than 12 seconds. Patients who take more than 14 seconds to complete the task are at increased risk of falling.

Initiating pharmacologic treatment for osteoporosis

Background – bone turnover

Bone is a dynamic tissue: osteoclasts resorb "old bone" and osteoblasts deposit new bone which then becomes mineralized. Two main stimuli increase bone resorption: a decreasing serum calcium level and an increased mechanical stress.

Decreasing serum calcium level is a potent stimulus to increased bone resorption mediated through calcium sensing cells in the parathyroid glands, which when stimulated by the decreasing ionized serum calcium level trigger the release of parathyroid hormone (PTH) from vesicles containing PTH (see Figure 44-1). Within seconds of release, PTH reaches bones and kidneys. In the bones PTH stimulates the osteoclasts to increase bone resorption. In the kidneys PTH increases renal tubular calcium resorption thus preserving calcium serum levels. PTH also stimulates the 1-alpha-hydroxylase enzyme in the kidneys to hydroxylate 25-hydroxy-vitamin D to 1,25-di-hydroxy-vitamin D, the most active vitamin D metabolite which increases calcium absorption through the intestines.

Estrogen, by reducing the activation of osteoclasts, plays a major role in maintaining a healthy skeletal mass. At menopause, more osteoclasts are activated, bone resorption is increased, and the bone mass decreases. In the early postmenopausal period the rate of bone loss may reach 3%–5% of the skeletal mass annually for three to five years and then stabilizes at an annual rate of 0.5%–1.0%.

Available medications

There are essentially two groups of medications available for the treatment of osteoporosis: antiresorptives and osteoanabolics. Antiresorptives inhibit osteoclastic activity and bone resorption. As they have no direct effect on osteoblasts, the rate of bone formation continues unaffected, and the net result of the bone resorption/bone formation equation is an increase in bone formation. Antiresorptives include

Table 44-1 Major studies with various medications for osteoporosis

Medications	Study acronym	Fracture risk reduction		Postmenopausal osteoporosis		Reference numbers
		Hip	Verte-bral	Treat-ment	Prevention	
Alendronate	FIT-CFA; FIT-VIA; 10 SIT	Yes	Yes	Yes	Yes	36– 8
Ibandronate	BONE	No*	Yes	Yes	Yes	42
Risedronate	HIP: VERT (NA) VERT (MN)	Yes	Yes	Yes	Yes	39–41, 48
Zoledronic acid	Horizon-PIT Horizon-RhT	Yes	Yes	Yes	Yes	43–47
Calcitonin	PROOF	No*	Yes	Yes	No	60, 61
Denosumab	FREEDOM	Yes	Yes	Yes	No	54–57
Raloxifene.,	MORE	No*	Yes	Yes	Yes	58
Teriparatide	PT; EFOS	**	Yes	Yes	No	62–64

* The lack of demonstrable effect may be due to studies not being powered to this end point.
** The pivotal study had to be prematurely terminated to evaluate the osteosarcoma risk.

bisphosphonates, denosumab, raloxifene, and calcitonin. Osteoanabolics directly stimulate osteoblasts and increase the rate of bone formation and hence bone mass. They include teriparatide.

Antiresorptive medications

Bisphosphonates

Bisphosphonates increase bone mass and reduce the risk of hip, vertebral, and other bone fractures to different degrees (Table 44-1).[23, 34–48] All bisphosphonates share the same basic chemical structure: two phosphonic acid molecules joined by a carbon atom and two side chains. The side chains determine the pharmacokinetic and pharmacodynamic profile of the various bisphosphonates.[34, 35]

Bisphosphonates can be administered orally or intravenously. The main advantage of intravenously administered bisphosphonates is that there are no adverse GI effects. The main adverse effect of intravenously administered bisphosphonate is the acute phase reaction which affects about 18% of bisphosphonate naïve patients, but only 9% of patients receiving their second annual infusion. The acute phase reaction is less commonly seen in patients receiving the monthly or weekly oral dose. The acute phase reaction manifests itself as fatigue, lethargy, generalized aches and pains and at times a low-grade temperature that may last a few days. It is not an allergic reaction. Severity can be reduced by acetaminophen or nonsteroidal anti-inflammatory compounds. Before the infusion patients should be encouraged to increase fluid intake. It might be prudent to avoid taking diuretics, especially loop diuretics, before and for a couple of hours after the infusion if feasible.

The absorption of oral bisphosphonates is very low: only 0.6%–3% of the orally administered dose is absorbed.[49] In order to maximize absorption the bisphosphonate has to be administered in the fasting state. It should not be taken with any fluid except with water. Some clinicians recommend it be taken with distilled water, which is free of additives that may interfere with the bioavailability of the orally administered bisphosphonates.

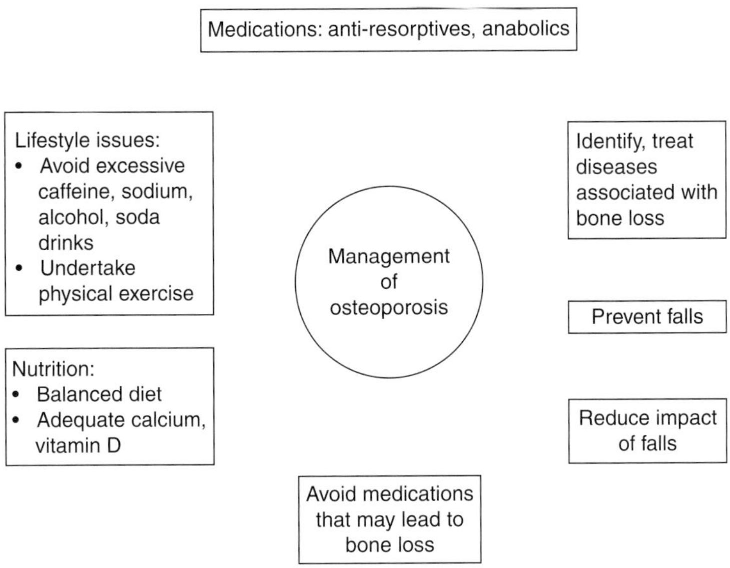

Figure 44-2 Management of osteoporosis.

Side effects include heartburn, low abdominal pain, cramps, and sometimes diarrhea. The medication may irritate the small intestinal mucosa and induce peristaltic contractions, which can result in abdominal pain, cramps and/or diarrhea one to two hours after taking the medication. Symptomatic patients should eat a high-fiber food 30 minutes after taking the medication so that the food coats the unabsorbed bisphosphonate particles in the stomach.

Bisphosphonates are excreted unchanged by the kidneys. Intravenously administered ones should not be administered if the creatinine clearance is lower than 35 mL/min and the dose of orally administered ones should be adjusted when prescribed to patients with impaired renal functions.

A formulation of risedronate (delayed release risedronate) can be administered non-fasting after breakfast. The active ingredient (risedronate) is surrounded by a chelating agent and the tablet is coated by a pH-sensitive layer unaffected by gastric acidity. Studies have documented comparable effects of this preparation to conventional risedronate.[48]

Arrhythmias, especially atrial fibrillation, have been associated with bisphosphonate therapy, particularly intravenously administered bisphosphonates. In most instances the onset of the arrhythmia is about a month after the IV administration making a cause and effect relationship unlikely.[50]

Rarely patients may develop ocular complications including scleritis and uveitis. These potentially serious conditions may occur weeks, months, or even years after initiating bisphosphonate therapy and should be treated as emergencies.[51] Nonspecific conjunctivitis and photophobia also have been reported. They are usually benign, self-limiting conditions, but need to be addressed as they may herald more serious complications.[52]

Skin reactions have rarely been reported with bisphosphonates including rash, pruritus, toxic epidermal necrolysis, and Stevens-Johnson syndrome.[53] Rare possible adverse events of bisphosphonates are discussed later, including atypical femoral shaft fractures and osteonecrosis of the jaw.

Denosumab

Denosumab reduces the risk of hip, vertebral, and nonhip fractures.[54–56] It is a monoclonal immunoglobulin antibody with high affinity and specificity to the receptor activator of nuclear factor kappa-B ligand (RANK-L) thus reducing the formation, activation, maturation and activity of osteoclasts. The effect on RANK-L is reversible. Furthermore, its potential for eliciting an antibody response is very low.[57] As it is not excreted by the kidneys, it can be safely administered to patients with impaired renal function.

Denosumab is administered by subcutaneous injections at 6-monthly intervals and is well tolerated.

An increased risk of infections seen in initial studies was not seen subsequently casting doubt on a causal relationship.[56, 57] The main adverse effect is flatulence lasting up to a few weeks after the injection affecting about 2% of patients.

Estrogen

Estrogen replacement therapy prevents and reverses the menopause-associated loss of bone mass and reduces fracture risk, including the risk of hip fractures. In the United States estrogen is no longer approved for the management of osteoporosis because when administered de novo to women 60 years of age or older, it is associated with a number of adverse events. However, estrogen is still approved for the prevention of osteoporosis, provided it is given in the smallest possible dose for the shortest period of time.

Selective estrogen receptor modulators

Raloxifene is a selective estrogen receptor modulator. It reduces the risk of vertebral fractures and in the United States is approved for the management of osteoporosis.[58] It has not been shown to reduce the risk of hip fractures. Its main adverse effects include hot flashes (especially if started within the first five years after menopause) and deep venous thrombosis, which are increased to about the same level induced by estrogen. Patients on raloxifene should refrain from taking the medication for about two weeks prior to an anticipated period of immobilization such as a long trip or elective surgery.

Calcitonin

Calcitonin is a hormone secreted by the C-cells of the thyroid gland. The main stimulus for its secretion is an increase in the serum calcium level. It directly inhibits the osteoclasts by binding to surface calcitonin receptors, thus interfering with their activity and therefore bone resorption. As a result, the balance between bone resorption and bone formation is improved. Calcitonin also increases the renal calcium excretion.

Calcitonin can be administered by intranasal insufflation or subcutaneously. Attempts to market an oral formulation have been abandoned.[59] Calcitonin reduces the risk of vertebral, but neither hip nor other nonhip fractures.[60] The main adverse effect is nasal irritation when administered intranasally. Although antibodies to calcitonin develop, they seldom interfere with its activity. Calcitonin has an analgesic effect, possibly associated with beta-endorphins.[61] It is sometimes used after an acute vertebral compression fracture to control pain.

Osteo-anabolic medication

Teriparatide (recombinant human parathyroid hormone 1–34) is the only osteo-anabolic medication commercially available in the United States. Another compound, the entire PTH 1–84, also has been studied, but at the time of this book's publication is not commercially available in the United States. Teriparatide stimulates bone formation and bone turnover, increases bone mineral density and reduces the risk of fractures.[62] It is administered for a maximum of two years. At the end of this course an antiresorptive agent should be administered to maintain the increases in BMD; if teriparatide is discontinued and no antiresorptives medication prescribed, the gains in BMD gradually fade away.[63] It is administered by daily subcutaneous injections. It is associated with relatively few adverse effects. An increased risk of osteosarcoma was noted in rats; this finding was not replicated in other experimental animals. Osteosarcoma rates in patients on teriparatide do not exceed the general population.[64] Contraindications to teriparatide therapy include hyperparathyroidism and radiation exposure.

Nonpharmacologic management of osteoporosis – lifestyle changes

Nonpharmacologic management of osteoporosis should be an essential and integral part of the management strategy. It consists mostly of lifestyle changes.

Daily calcium intake

The recommended daily calcium intakes,[23] as well as the upper limit of intake as per the Institute of Medicine (IOM) are shown in Table 44-2.[65] It is preferable to get the recommended calcium intake from food as opposed to tablets. If calcium supplements and antacids must be taken, calcium citrate is preferred to calcium carbonate as the citrate compound does not need gastric acidity to be dissolved.

Many foods either contain calcium or are fortified with calcium. Calcium fortified orange juice for instance has the same content of calcium as milk

Table 44-2 Recommended calcium and vitamin D daily intake and upper limit intake for various age groups

Age group (years)	Calcium RDA mg/day	ULI mg/day	Vitamin D RDA IU/day	ULT IU/day
1–3	700	2,500	600	2,500
4–8	1,000	2,500	600	3,000
9–18	1,300	3,000	600	4,000
19–50	1,000	2,500	600	4,000
51–70	1,200	2,000	600	4,000
>70 years	1,200	2,000	800	4,000

RDA – recommended dietary allowance, ULI – upper level intake
Source: Adapted from Institute of Medicine (US) Committee to Review Dietary References Intake for Vitamin D and Calcium. Ross AC, Taylor CL, Yagjm. AL, et al. *Dietary Reference Intakes for Calcium and Vitamin D*. Washington, DC: National Academies Press (US); 2011.

(300 mg per 8 ounces). The food content of some select food is shown in Table 44-3. Drinking chocolate in particular could be rich in calcium. Readers are advised to check the food labels as different brands of the same product may contain different amounts of calcium.

Food labels often do not indicate the mg amount of calcium available in that particular food, but instead indicate the percentage of calcium. This percentage is based on the recommended daily intake of women between the ages of 19 and 50 years: 1,000 mg. For example, a label showing a serving contains 20% of the recommended daily calcium intake, means it contains 200 mg of calcium.

Vitamin D

Vitamin D is essential for the absorption of calcium through the intestinal mucosa. When there is adequate exposure to sunlight, it is formed in the skin: ultraviolet light converts 7-dehydro-cholesterol to cholecalciferol. Vitamin D can also be obtained from food: ergocalciferol from plant products and cholecalciferol from animal products. Vitamin D deficiency results in a negative calcium balance because of the decreased calcium absorption through the intestinal tract.

Vitamin D deficiency is common. As the skin ages it is less efficient at producing vitamin D, and dietary vitamin D intake is often low.

The diagnosis of hypovitaminosis D is established by assaying the serum 25-hydroxy-vitamin D level. There is no consensus on the optimum management of vitamin D deficiency. Common regimens include: cholecalciferol 4,000 units daily or ergocalciferol 50,000 units once a week for 12 weeks. Assaying the serum 25-hydroxy-vitamin D is recommended at the end of the 12-week course to determine whether the patient needs another course of vitamin D. Most patients respond to a 12-week course of vitamin D supplementation, but some need several courses to correct vitamin D deficiency.

A well-balanced nutritious diet

A well-balanced nutritious diet is important for a healthy skeleton.[66–68] Cognitively intact, physically independent older women living on their own are least likely to develop malnutrition: men living on their own are the most vulnerable population. However, women with cognitive dysfunction are susceptible to the development of malnutrition. Older people with dental problems often avoid difficult to chew protein-rich food. Poor dental health is a major cause of malnutrition in developed countries.

Sodium and caffeine intake

Excessive sodium and caffeine intake may lead to a negative calcium balance by increasing renal

Table 44-3 Calcium content (mg) per portion size of selected foods

	Serving size	Calcium (mg)
Milk		
Whole, skim, 2%, 1%	8 oz	300
Calcium fortified	8 oz	500
Almond milk	8 oz	450
Chocolate drink with:		
Water	8 oz	300
Milk	8 oz	600
Calcium fortified milk	8 oz	800
Yogurt	6 oz	300
Orange juice:		
Regular	8 oz	0
Calcium fortified	8 oz	300
Vegetables:		
Broccoli	8 oz	100
Collard greens	8 oz	200
Tip C-ze-ms	8 oz	200
Spinach	8 oz	120
Bread fortified with calcium	1 slice	100
CI & EYE		
Ice cream	6 oz	120

* Readers should check the food label as calcium contents often vary according to brand.

calcium excretion.[69] Sodium is ubiquitous in our diet; preserved and canned foods tend to be rich in sodium. Soda drinks contain sodium and may contain phosphoric acid which binds to calcium and interferes with its absorption.[70] But as long as the individual consumes the recommended calcium intake, she may safely consume three soda drinks or cups of coffee daily without jeopardizing her calcium homeostasis.

Cigarette smoking

Cigarette smoking increases the risk of osteoporosis and fractures.[71] A number of mechanisms are responsible including stimulation of osteoclastic activity and the lifestyle many smokers adopt including leading sedentary lifestyles and consuming a diet that is not well balanced and often deficient in protein, calcium, and vitamin D.

Alcohol abuse

Although alcohol intake in moderation tends to be associated with positive effects on skeletal health, regular consumption of two or more drinks a day has deleterious effects on the bone health through its effects on osteoblasts, osteoclasts, and osteocytes.[72–74] Regular excessive alcohol intake is also often associated with nutritional deficiencies, body composition changes, and a number of pathologies that increase the risk of falls and hence fractures.[72–74]

Physical exercise

There is ample evidence to show that a physically active lifestyle is associated with a healthier skeleton and that physical exercise at any age is associated with an increased bone mass and reduced risk of falls and possibly fractures.[75–77] Unfortunately most studies on exercise do not include fractures as end points. Bones respond best to a combination of endurance or aerobic exercises and resistive exercises.

Walking with light weights attached to each wrist and ankle is a useful physical exercise combining endurance and resistive exercises. In order to decrease the risk of injuring adjacent joints and fatigue, heavy weights should be avoided. Unfortunately the positive effects of exercise on bone mass last only as long as the individual exercises.

Monitoring patients on treatment

Given that osteoporosis is an asymptomatic silent disease until a fracture occurs, adherence with medication regimens is problematic, a patient must be motivated to maintain adherence. She must understand the nature of the disease, its potential complications, and its pharmacologic and nonpharmacologic management. She also must be fully aware of potential complications, and should understand the risk-benefit ratio of the medication. She must be convinced that it is in her best interest to take a medication and change her lifestyle.

Supporting the patient is important to ensure adherence. Support staff may play a crucial role in contacting the patient at regular intervals. Patients benefit from feedback, but the patient and treating clinician may have to wait two years for the next DXA scan before knowing whether the medication is effective.

For patients on oral medications, assay for markers of bone resorption such as urine or serum N-telopeptide (NTX) or C-telopeptide (CTX) before initiating treatment and about three months later may provide some feedback and reassurance that the medication is effective. A change of at least 40% needs to be observed to determine that the rate of bone resorption has decreased. Many insurers do not reimburse the cost of assaying these markers twice.

When the medication is administered parenterally, the patient can be reassured that it is effective at altering the bone turnover rate as its bioavailability is assured.

Possible rare complications of treatment

Atypical femoral shaft fractures

Concerns have been raised about a few patients on long-term antiresorptive therapy (bisphosphonate and denosumab) sustaining fragility fractures of the femoral shaft. The present evidence suggests these fractures are insufficiency fractures that have progressed and involve the entire cortex.[78] Although these fractures share many common features with osteoporotic fragility fractures, there are some basic differences between them. They are referred to as atypical femoral shaft fractures (AFSF) to differentiate them from the "typical" osteoporotic femoral shaft fractures.

Whereas typical osteoporotic fractures are usually comminuted, atypical fractures are noncomminuted and tend to be transverse or have a short oblique configuration. Atypical femoral shaft fractures are often preceded for several weeks by prodromal symptoms such as pain and tenderness along the femoral shaft.

It may be argued that by inhibiting bone turnover, antiresorptives may interfere with the healing of insufficiency fractures and therefore lead to a complete "atypical" fracture. A causal relationship between atypical fractures and antiresorptive therapy, however, could not be established especially given the large disproportion between the number of patients on antiresorptive therapy and the number of patients sustaining these fractures. Besides, some patients who sustained atypical fractures have not been on any antiresorptive medication. A review of pivotal studies could not document an increased incidence of these fractures in patients treated with antiresorptive medication.[79]

The risk of patients on bisphosphonates sustaining atypical femoral shaft fractures is low: 3–50 cases per 100,000 person-years.[78] Given the potential beneficial effects of antiresorptive medication, the rarity of atypical femoral shaft fractures, especially during the first three to five years of initiating treatment and given the frequent presence of prodromal symptoms that should alert patient and treating clinician of an impending fracture, health-care providers should not deny antiresorptive therapy to patients with osteoporosis. Patients and health-care providers, however, need to be vigilant.

Osteonecrosis of the jaw

There have been several reports of patients on antiresorptive therapy developing osteonecrosis of the jaw (ONJ).[80] Most of these instances developed in patients who underwent tooth extraction or invasive dental work. The majority of these patients were on bisphosphonates administered in large doses for malignant conditions, and many patients were simultaneously on other medications that may interfere with the healing process. Also, many patients had poor dental hygiene and were cigarette smokers.

A plausible link exists between antiresorptives and osteonecrosis of the jaw: antiresorptives decrease bone turnover to such an extent that injured or necrotic bone is not removed. But the sheer number of patients who have received antiresorptives medications and those who develop osteonecrosis of the jaw are such that it is not possible to establish a direct cause-and-effect relationship. At most antiresorptive therapy may contribute to the development or worsening of the condition.

Four different stages of ONJ have been described: in stage I a cavity with bone tissue at its base is visible, but it is largely asymptomatic. In stage II the lesion is painful and there are signs of inflammation. In stage III fistulae and purulent discharges are seen. A stage 0 has been added to describe patients who experience jaw pain, have some of radiological features of ONJ, and have been on antiresorptive medication.[81]

The essence of management is scrupulous oral hygiene and frequent use of oral antiseptics. Eventually most stage I cases of ONJ heal spontaneously. Rarely surgical intervention by a specialist with experience managing ONJ is needed. The fear of ONJ should not deter clinicians from prescribing antiresorptives. The risk-benefit ratio is very much in favor of taking the antiresorptives medication.

Screening for osteoporosis

Given the prevalence of osteoporosis, its silent nature until a fracture occurs, the ease of diagnosing it, and the availability of effective, relatively cheap medication that can significantly reduce the risk of fractures, it behooves clinicians to screen patients for osteoporosis. Osteoporotic fractures are life-changing events. Screening of the following is recommended: [1, 82–84]

1. Women aged 65 and older regardless of the presence of risk factors.
2. Women between the ages of 50 and 65 years if they have risk factors. There is no consensus on which risk factors should be taken into consideration. The US Preventive Services Task Force recommends screening women if their risk of sustaining a fracture exceeds that of a hypothetical woman 65 years of age with no risk factors as determined by the FRAX algorithm.
3. Adults who have sustained fractures.
4. Adults diagnosed with diseases that may lead to bone demineralization.
5. Adults on long-term medication likely to induce bone demineralization.

Prevention

The balance between bone formation and bone resorption goes through three phases. First is a phase of bone accretion in children and adolescents. During this period bone formation exceeds bone resorption and the skeleton grows bigger. The second phase is that of bone consolidation: the skeleton does not grow bigger, but the bones become stronger and denser. This phase culminates into the peak bone mass, reached by different bones at different ages. About 80% of the peak bone mass is genetically determined and 20% determined by the individual's lifestyle. The third phase is bone loss, which starts around the age of 35 when bone resorption exceeds bone formation. Initially the loss is 0.5%–1% annually. In some women it is accelerated after menopause, reaching 3%–5% annually during the first five years post menopause. It then slows down to 0.5%–1% annually.

Prevention is two-pronged: maximizing peak bone mass and minimizing bone loss. The former can be achieved in childhood, adolescence, and early adulthood. The latter is addressed after the age of 35 years and especially after menopause.

Maximizing peak bone mass and minimizing bone loss can be done by ensuring a well-balanced nutritious diet and a good daily calcium and vitamin D intake; by avoiding excessive sodium, caffeine, and carbonated drinks intake; and by avoiding cigarette smoking and alcohol abuse. Regular physical exercise enhances skeletal growth and slows bone loss.

Estrogen replacement therapy reduces bone loss in postmenopausal women and reduces fracture risk. Although approved by the FDA in the United States for the prevention of osteoporosis, it is with the proviso that it be given in the smallest possible dose and for the shortest period of time. It is important to have a clear strategy when initiating hormone replacement therapy in postmenopausal women because whenever it is stopped it may induce a phase of excessive bone resorption.

Concluding remarks

Osteoporosis is a very common condition. It is silent until a fracture occurs. Osteoporotic fractures are life-changing events associated with a poor prognosis and increased morbidity and mortality. About half the female Caucasian population aged 50 years and older is expected to sustain an osteoporotic fracture. The availability of effective and relatively cheap and safe medication that can significantly reduce the risk of fractures mandates that health-care professionals identify and treat patients with osteoporosis as soon as possible before a fracture occurs.

References

1. National Osteoporosis Foundation. *Clinician's Guide to Prevention and Treatment of Osteoporosis.* Washington, DC: National Osteoporosis Foundation (www.nof.org); 2014.

2. NIH Consensus Development Panel on Osteoporosis Prevention, Diagnosis, and Therapy. Osteoporosis prevention, diagnosis, and therapy. *JAMA.* 2001 Feb 14;**285**(6):785–95.
3. Klotzbuecher CM, Ross PD, Landsman PB, et al. Patients with prior fractures have an increased risk of future fractures: a summary of the literature and statistical synthesis. *J Bone Miner Res.* 2000;**15**(4): 721–39.
4. Harvey N, Dennison E, Cooper C. Epidemiology of osteoporotic fractures. In: Rosen CJ ed. *Primer on the Metabolic Bone Diseases and Disorders of Mineral Metabolism.* 7th edition. Hoboken, NJ: John Wiley & Sons, Inc.; 2008:198–203.
5. Chrischilles EA, Butler CD, Davis CS, et al. A model of lifetime osteoporosis impact. *Arch Intern Med.* 1991;**151**(10):2026–32.
6. Office of the Surgeon General (US). *Bone Health and Osteoporosis: A Report of the Surgeon General.* Rockville, MD: Office of the Surgeon General (US); 2004.
7. Lauritzen JB. Osteoporotic fractures. In: An YH ed. *Orthopaedic Issues in Osteoporosis.* Boca Raton: CRC Press LLC; 2003:171–3.
8. Cooper C, Atkinson EJ, O'Fallon WM, et al. Incidence of clinically diagnosed vertebral fractures: a population-based study in Rochester, Minnesota, 1985–1989. *J Bone Miner Res.* 1992;**7**(2): 221–7.
9. Gehlbach SH, Bigelow C, Heimisdottir M, et al. Recognition of vertebral fracture in a clinical setting. *Osteoporos Int.* 2000;**11**(7):577–82.
10. Palvanen M, Kannus P, Parkkari J, et al. The injury mechanisms of osteoporotic upper extremity fractures among older adults: a controlled study of 287 consecutive patients and their 108 controls. *Osteoporos Int.* 2000;**11**(10):822–31.
11. Lübbeke A, Stern R, Grab B, et al. Upper extremity fractures in the elderly: consequences on utilization of rehabilitation care. *Aging Clin Exp Res.* 2005;**17**(4): 276–80.
12. Shortt NL, Robinson CM. Mortality after low-energy fractures in patients aged at least 45 years old. *J Orthop Trauma.* 2005;**19**(6):396–400.
13. Burge R, Dawson-Hughes B, Solomon DH, et al. Incidence and economic burden of osteoporosis-related fractures in the United States, 2005–2025. *J Bone Miner Res.* 2007 Mar;**22**(3):465–75.
14. Nieves JW, Bilezikian JP, Lane JM, et al. Fragility fractures of the hip and femur: incidence and patient characteristics. *Osteoporos Int.* 2010;**21**(3):399–408.
15. Leslie WD, Sadatsafavi M, Lix LM, et al. Secular decreases in fracture rates 1986–2006 for Manitoba, Canada: a population-based analysis. *Osteoporos Int.* 2011;**22**(7):2137–43.
16. Lippuner K, Popp AW, Schwab P, et al. Fracture hospitalizations between years 2000 and 2007 in Switzerland: a trend analysis. *Osteoporos Int.* 2011;**22** (9):2487–97.
17. Chevalley T, Guilley E, Herrmann FR, et al. Incidence of hip fracture over a 10-year period (1991–2000): reversal of a secular trend. *Bone.* 2007;**40**(5):1284–9.
18. Kannus P, Niemi S, Parkkari J, et al. Nationwide decline in incidence of hip fracture. *J Bone Miner Res.* 2006;**21**(12):1836–8.
19. Fisher A, Martin J, Srikusalanukul W, et al. Bisphosphonate use and hip fracture epidemiology: ecologic proof from the contrary. *Clin Interv Aging.* 2010;**5**:355–62.
20. Pasco JA, Brennan SL, Henry MJ, et al. Changes in hip fracture rates in southeastern Australia spanning the period 1994–2007. *J Bone Miner Res.* 2011;**26**(7): 1648–54.
21. Black DM, Cummings SR, Karpf DB, et al. Randomised trial of effect of alendronate on risk of fracture in women with existing vertebral fractures. Fracture Intervention Trial Research Group. *Lancet.* 1996;**348**(9041):1535–41.
22. Eisman JA, Bogoch ER, Dell R, et al. Making the first fracture the last fracture: ASBMR task force report on secondary fracture prevention. *J Bone Miner Res.* 2012 Oct;**27**(10):2039–46.
23. Hamdy RC, Lewiecki EM. Diagnosis In: *Osteoporosis.* New York: Oxford University Press; 2013: chapter 4.
24. Kanis JA, Melton LJ 3rd, Christiansen C, et al. The diagnosis of osteoporosis. *J Bone Miner Res.* 1994;**9** (8):1137–41.
25. Hans D, Downs RW Jr, Duboeuf F, et al. Skeletal sites for osteoporosis diagnosis: the 2005 ISCD Official Positions. *J Clin Densitom.* 2006;**9**(1):15–21.
26. Hamdy RC, Petak SM, Lenchick L, International Society for Clinical densitometry Position Development Panel and Scientific Advisory Committee. Which central dual x-ray absorptiometry skeletal sites and regions of interest should be used to determine the diagnosis of osteoporosis? *J Clin Densitom.* 2002;**5**(Suppl):S11–S18.
27. Lewiecki EM. Premenopausal bone health assessment. *Curr Rheumatol Rep.* 2005;**7**(1):46–52.
28. Heaney RP, Abrams S, Dawson-Hughes B, et al. Peak bone mass. *Osteoporos Int.* 2000;**11** (12):985–1009.
29. Katzman DK, Bachrach LK, Carter DR, et al. Clinical and anthropometric correlates of bone mineral acquisition in healthy adolescent girls. *J Clin Endocrinol Metab.* 1991;**73**(6):1332–9.

30. Kanis JA, Hans D, Cooper C, et al. Interpretation and use of FRAX in clinical practice. *Osteoporos Int.* 2011 Sep;**22**(9):2395–411.

31. Lewiecki EM, Compston JE, Miller PD, et al. Official Positions for FRAX® Bone Mineral Density and FRAX® simplification from Joint Official Positions Development Conference of the International Society for Clinical Densitometry and International Osteoporosis Foundation on FRAX®. *J Clin Densitom.* 2011;**14**(3):226–36.

32. Hans DB, Kanis JA, Baim S, et al. Joint official positions of the International Society for Clinical Densitometry and International Osteoporosis Foundation on FRAX®. Executive summary of the 2010 Position Development Conference on Interpretation and use of FRAX® in clinical practice. *J Clin Densitom.* 2011;**14**(3):171–80.

33. Schoene D, Wu SM, Mikolaizak AS, et al. Discriminative ability and predictive validity of the timed up and go test in identifying older people who fall: systematic review and meta-analysis. *J Am Geriatr Soc.* 2013 Feb;**61**(2):202–8.

34. Rizzoli R. Bisphosphonates for post-menopausal osteoporosis: are they all the same? *QJM.* 2011;**104** (4):281–300.

35. Nancollas GH, Tang R, Phipps RJ, et al. Novel insights into actions of bisphosphonates on bone: differences in interactions with hydroxyapatite. *Bone.* 2006;**38**(5): 617–27.

36. Cummings SR, Black DM, Thompson DE, et al. Effect of alendronate on risk of fracture in women with low bone density but without vertebral fractures: results from the Fracture Intervention Trial. *JAMA.* 1998;**280** (24):2077–82.

37. Black DM, Thompson DE, Bauer DC, et al. Fracture risk reduction with alendronate in women with osteoporosis: the Fracture Intervention Trial. FIT Research Group. *J Clin Endocrinol Metab.* 2000;**85**(11): 4118–24.

38. Pols HA, Felsenberg D, Hanley DA, et al. Multinational, placebo-controlled, randomized trial of the effects of alendronate on bone density and fracture risk in postmenopausal women with low bone mass: results of the FOSIT study. Fosamax International Trial Study Group. *Osteoporosis Int.* 1999;**9**(5):461–8.

39. McClung MR, Geusens P, Miller PD, et al. Effect of risedronate on the risk of hip fracture in elderly women. Hip Intervention Program Study Group. *N Engl J Med.* 2001;**344**(5):333–40.

40. Watts NB, Josse RG, Hamdy RC, et al. Risedronate prevents new vertebral fractures in postmenopausal women at high risk. *J Clin Endocrinol Metab.* 2003;**88** (2):542–9.

41. Harris ST, Watts NB, Genant HK, et al. Effects of risedronate treatment on vertebral and nonvertebral fractures in women with postmenopausal osteoporosis: a randomized controlled trial. Vertebral Efficacy with Risedronate Therapy (VERT) Study Group. *JAMA.* 1999;**282**(14):1344–52.

42. Chesnut III CH, Skag A, Christiansen C, et al. Effects of oral ibandronate administered daily or intermittently on fracture risk in postmenopausal osteoporosis. *J Bone Miner Res.* 2004;**19**(8):1241–49.

43. Black DM, Delmas PD, Eastell R, et al. Once-yearly zoledronic acid for treatment of postmenopausal osteoporosis. *N Engl J Med.* 2007;**356**(18):1809–22.

44. Black DM, Reid IR, Boonen S, et al. The effect of 3 versus 6 years of zoledronic acid treatment of osteoporosis: a randomized extension to the HORIZON-Pivotal Fracture Trial (PFT). *J Bone Miner Res.* 2012;**27**:243–54.

45. Boonen S, Black DM, Colón-Emeric CS, et al. Efficacy and safety of a once-yearly intravenous zoledronic acid 5 mg for fracture prevention in elderly postmenopausal women with osteoporosis aged 75 and older. *J Am Geriatr Soc.* 2010;**58**(2):292–9.

46. Lyles KW, Colón-Emeric CS, Magaziner JS, et al. Zoledronic acid and clinical fractures and mortality after hip fracture. *N Engl J Med.* 2007;**357**:1799–1809.

47. Eriksen EF, Lyles KW, Colón-Emeric CS, et al. Antifracture efficacy and reduction of mortality in relation to timing of the first dose of zoledronic acid after hip fracture. *J Bone Miner Res.* 2009;**24**(7): 1308–13.

48. McClung MR, Miller PD, Brown JP, et al. Efficacy and safety of a novel delayed-release risedronate 35 mg once-a-week tablet. *Osteoporos Int.* 2012;**23**(1):267–76.

49. Chapurlat RD, Delmas PD. Drug insight: bisphosphonates for postmenopausal osteoporosis. *Nat Clin Pract Endocrinol Metab.* 2006;**2**(4):211–19.

50. Barrett-Connor E, Swern AS, Hustad CM, et al. Alendronate and atrial fibrillation: a meta-analysis of randomized placebo-controlled clinical trials. *Osteoporos Int.* 2012;**23**(1):233–45.

51. Papapetrou PD. Bisphosphonate-associated adverse events. *Hormones (Athens).* 2009;**8**(2):96–110.

52. Procianoy F, Procianoy E. Orbital inflammatory disease secondary to a single-dose administration of zoledronic acid for treatment of postmenopausal osteoporosis. *Osteoporos Int.* 2010;**21**(6):1057–8.

53. Abrahamsen B. Adverse effects of bisphosphonates. *Calcif Tissue Int.* 2010;**86**(6):421–35.

54. Cummings SR, San Martin J, McClung MR, et al. Denosumab for prevention of fractures in postmenopausal women with osteoporosis. *N Engl J Med.* 2009;**361**(8):756–65.

55. Boonen S, Adachi JD, Man Z, et al. Treatment with denosumab reduces the incidence of new vertebral and

hip fractures in postmenopausal women at high risk. *J Clin Endocrinol Metab.* 2011;**96**(6):1727–36.

56. Brown JP, Bone HG, Chapurlat R, et al. *Six years of denosumab treatment in postmenopausal women with osteoporosis: results from the first three years of the FREEDOM extension.* Presented at ACR; Chicago; November 2011.

57. Singer A, Gruaer A. Denosumab for the management of postmenopausal osteoporosis. *Postgrad Med.* 2010;**122**:176–87.

58. Ettinger B, Black DM, Mitlak BH, et al. Reduction of vertebral fracture risk in postmenopausal women with osteoporosis treated with raloxifene: results from a 3-year randomized clinical trial. Multiple Outcomes of Raloxifene Evaluation (MORE) Investigators. *JAMA.* 1999;**282**(7):637–45.

59. Hamdy RC, Daley DN. Oral calcitonin. *Int J Women's Health.* 2012:**4**;471–9.

60. Chesnut CH 3rd, Silverman S, Andriano K, et al. A randomized trial of nasal spray salmon calcitonin in postmenopausal women with established osteoporosis: the prevent recurrence of osteoporotic fractures study. PROOF Study Group. *Am J Med.* 2000;**109**(4):267–76.

61. Ofluoglu D, Akyuz G, Unay O, et al. The effect of calcitonin on beta-endorphin levels in postmenopausal osteoporotic patients with back pain. *Clin Rheumatol.* 2007;**26**(1):44–9.

62. Neer RM, Arnaud CD, Zanchetta JR, et al. Effect of parathyroid hormone (1–34) on fractures and bone mineral density in postmenopausal women with osteoporosis. *N Engl J Med.* 2001;**344**(19):1434–41.

63. Leder BZ, Neer RM, Wyland JJ, et al. Effects of teriparatide treatment and discontinuation in postmenopausal women and eugonadal men with osteoporosis. *J Clin Endocrinol Metab.* 2009;**94**(8): 2915–21.

64. Andrews EB, Gilsenan AW, Midkiff K, et al. The US postmarketing surveillance study of adult osteosarcoma and teriparatide: study design and findings from the first 7 years. *J Bone Miner Res.* 2012 Dec;**27**(12):2429–37.

65. Ross AC, Taylor CL, Yaktine AL, Del Valle HB, editors. *Dietary Reference Intakes for Calcium and Vitamin D. Institute of Medicine (US) Committee to Review Dietary Reference Intakes for Vitamin D and Calcium.* Washington, DC: National Academies Press (US); 2011.

66. Rivlin RS. Keeping the young-elderly healthy: is it too late to improve our health through nutrition? *Am J Clin Nutr.* 2007;**86**(5):1572S–6S.

67. Munger RG, Cerhan JR, Chiu BC. Prospective study of dietary protein intake and risk of hip fracture in postmenopausal women. *Am J Clin Nutr.* 1999;**69**(1): 147–52.

68. Body JJ, Bergmann P, Boonen S, et al. Non-pharmacological management of osteoporosis: a consensus of the Belgian Bone Club. *Osteoporos Int.* 2011;**22**(11):2769–88.

69. Kiel DP, Felson DT, Hannan MT, et al. Caffeine and the risk of hip fracture: the Framingham Study. *Am J Epidemiol.* 1990;**132**(4):675–84.

70. Tucker KL, Morita K, Qiao N, et al. Colas, but not other carbonated beverages, are associated with low bone mineral density in older women: The Framingham Osteoporosis Study. *Am J Clin Nutr.* 2006;**84**(4):936–42.

71. Yan C, Avadhani NG, Iqbal J. The effects of smoke carcinogens on bone. *Curr Osteoporos Rep.* 2011;**9**(4): 202–9.

72. Maurel DB, Boisseau N, Benhamou CL, Jaffre C. Alcohol and bone: review of dose effects and mechanisms. *Osteoporos Int.* 2012 Jan;**23**(1):1–16.

73. Maurel DB, Boisseau N, Benhamou CL, et al. Alcohol and bone: review of dose effects and mechanisms. *Osteoporos Int.* 2012;**23**(1):1–16.

74. Abukhadir SS, Mohamed N, Mohamed N. Pathogenesis of alcohol-induced osteoporosis and its treatment: a review. *Curr Drug Targets.* 2013 Dec;**14** (13):1601–10.

75. Nikander R, Sievänen H, Heinonen A, et al. Targeted exercise against osteoporosis: A systematic review and meta-analysis for optimising bone strength throughout life. *BMC Med.* 2010;**8**:47–63.

76. Howe TE, Shea B, Dawson LJ, et al. Exercise for preventing and treating osteoporosis in postmenopausal women. *Cochrane Database Syst Rev.* 2011 Jul;**6**(7):CD000333.

77. Langsetmo L, Hitchcock CL, Kingwell EJ, et al. Physical activity, body mass index and bone mineral density-associations in a prospective population-based cohort of women and men: the Canadian Multicentre Osteoporosis Study (CaMos). *Bone.* 2012;**50**(1): 401–8.

78. Shane E, Burr D, Abrahamsen B, et al. Atypical subtrochanteric and diaphyseal femoral fractures: second report of a task force of the American Society for Bone and Mineral Research. *J Bone Miner Res.* 2014;**29**(1):1–23.

79. Black DM, Kelly MP, Genant HK, et al. Bisphosphonates and fractures of the subtrochanteric or diaphyseal femur. *N Engl J Med.* 2010;**362**(19): 1761–71.

80. Khosla S, Burr D, Cauley J, et al. Bisphosphonate-associated osteonecrosis of the jaw: report of a task force of the American Society for Bone and Mineral Research. *J Bone Miner Res.* 2007;**22**(10):1479–91.

81. Advisory Task Force on Bisphosphonate-Related Osteonecrosis of the Jaws. American Association of

Oral and Maxillofacial Surgeons. American Association of Oral and Maxillofacial Surgeons position paper on bisphosphonate-related osteonecrosis of the jaws. *J Oral Maxillofac Surg.* 2007;**65**(3):369–76.

82. US Preventive Services Task Force. Screening for Osteoporosis: US Preventive Services Task Force Recommendation Statement. *Ann Intern Med.* 2011;**154**:356–64.

83. Lim LS, Hoeksema LJ, Sherin K, et al. Screening for osteoporosis in the adult US population: ACPM position statement on preventive practice. *Am J Prev Med.* 2009;**36**(4):366–75.

84. Watts NB, Bilezikian JP, Camacho PM, et al. American Association of Clinical Endocrinologists medical guidelines for clinical practice for the diagnosis and treatment of postmenopausal osteoporosis. *Endocr Pract.* 2010 Nov–Dec;**16**(Suppl 3):1–37.

Chapter

45 Office care of substance abuse patients

Lee Dresang, Randall Brown, and Elizabeth J. Kvach

Introduction

Epidemiology, diagnosis, and treatment of alcohol and other substance abuse disorders differ for women and men. Hazardous drinking can lead to accelerated morbidity in women compared to men, and women are screened for alcohol use disorder less frequently than men. Ten percent of nonpregnant women and 4% of pregnant women report illicit drug use. The costs to health care of substance abuse disorders in women go beyond the care of individual patients since drug-exposed newborns also require treatment.

This chapter will review (1) comorbid mental illness in women with substance abuse disorders, (2) alcohol use disorder in nonpregnant women, (3) illicit substance use disorders in nonpregnant women, (4) preconception care for both, and (5) legal and ethical issues. For alcohol and other drug disorders, evidence-based recommendations will be made for office screening and treatment.

Comorbid mental illness in women with substance use disorders

Women with mental health disorders are at risk for substance use disorders (SUD) and vice versa. Comorbid mental illness has strong association with alcohol use disorder (AUD). In addition, SUDs are strongly correlated to incidence of gender-based violence (GBV). To be successful, treatment for SUDs needs to comprehensively incorporate care of comorbid mental illness and response to GBV. Additionally, women with AUD have a higher prevalence of somatization disorder than men, and women with polysubstance use have a higher prevalence of major depression, anxiety, PTSD, eating disorders, and personality disorders.[1]

Intimate partner violence (IPV) is strongly associated with AUD.[2] Two-thirds of women entering drug treatment programs report having experienced sexual or physical abuse, including life-threatening IPV.[3]

Female adolescents with drug use problems are more likely to suffer from disruptive behavior disorders, major depression, and anxiety disorders.[4]

AUD in nonpregnant women

Approximately 30% of people in the United States use alcohol excessively, leading to more than 85,000 deaths per year.[5] Excessive alcohol use includes binge drinking, heavy drinking, and any drinking by pregnant women and persons under the age of 21. *Binge drinking* is defined for women as ≥4 drinks on a single occasion (≥5 drinks for men), and *heavy drinking* is defined as ≥8 drinks/week for women (≥15 drinks for men).[6]

A study of 345,076 US women aged 18–44 from 2006 to 2010 found that 51.5% of nonpregnant women and 7.6% of pregnant women reported drinking alcohol and 15.0% of nonpregnant women and 1.4% of pregnant women reported binge drinking.[7] Binge drinking was reported twice as often among nonpregnant women aged 18–24 years (20.5%) as those aged 35–44 years (11.8%).[7]

The *American Psychiatric Association's Diagnostic and Statistical Manual*, Fifth Edition (DSM-5), published in May 2013, combined the 1994 DSM-IV criteria for the diagnoses of alcohol abuse and alcohol dependence with the term AUD. With the DSM-5 definition, legal criteria were removed and craving was added (see Table 45-1). AUD is categorized as mild if patients meet two or three criteria, moderate if there are four or five, and severe if there are six or more. DSM-5 terminology will be used throughout this chapter.[8]

Although AUDs are more common in men than women, there is evidence that hazardous drinking can lead to accelerated morbidity in women due to physiologic differences in alcohol absorption and metabolism.

Office Care of Women, ed. Martin E. Olsen and Botros Rizk. Published by Cambridge University Press.

Table 45-1 DSM-5 criteria for alcohol use disorder [9]

1. Alcohol is often taken in larger amounts or over a longer period than was intended
2. There is a persistent desire or unsuccessful efforts to cut down or control alcohol use
3. A great deal of time is spent in activities necessary to obtain alcohol, use alcohol, or recover from its effects
4. Craving, or a strong desire or urge to use alcohol
5. Recurrent alcohol use resulting in a failure to fulfill major role/obligations at work, school, or home
6. Continued alcohol use despite having persistent or recurrent social or interpersonal problems caused or exacerbated by the effects of alcohol
7. Important social, occupational, or recreational activities are given up or reduced because of alcohol use
8. Recurrent alcohol use in situations in which it is physically hazardous
9. Alcohol use is continued despite knowledge of having a persistent or recurrent physical or psychological problem that is likely to have been caused or exacerbated by alcohol
10. Tolerance, as defined by either of the following:
    a. A need for markedly increased amounts of alcohol to achieve intoxication or desired effect
    b. A markedly diminished effect with continued use of the same amount of alcohol
11. Withdrawal, as manifested by either of the following:
    a. The characteristic withdrawal syndrome for alcohol (refer to criteria A and B of the criteria set for alcohol withdrawal)
    b. Alcohol (or a closely related substance, such as a benzodiazepine) is taken to relieve or avoid withdrawal symptoms

This includes accelerated and increased risk of heart disease, liver disease, hypertension, obesity, anemia, malnutrition, gastrointestinal (GI) hemorrhage, GI ulcers, cancer (mouth, throat, esophagus, liver, colon, and breast), and loss of brain volume.[10–12]

Although the risk of heart disease is higher with heavy drinkers, it appears to be lower with light to moderate drinkers compared with both those who abstain and heavy drinkers. Light to moderate drinking has not only been associated with decreased risk of coronary artery disease, but also with decreased risk of total mortality, diabetes mellitus, congestive heart failure, and stroke.[13]

Table 45-2 Screening tools for AUD

AUDIT

1. How often do you have a drink containing alcohol?
2. How many standard drinks containing alcohol do you have on a typical day when drinking?
3. How often do you have six or more drinks on one occasion?
4. During the past year, how often have you found that you were not able to stop drinking once you had started?
5. During the past year, how often have you failed to do what was normally expected of you because of drinking?
6. During the past year, how often have you needed a drink in the morning to get yourself going after a heavy drinking session?
7. During the past year, how often have you had a feeling of guilt or remorse after drinking?
8. During the past year, have you been unable to remember what happened the night before because you had been drinking?
9. Have you or someone else been injured as a result of your drinking?
10. Has a relative or friend, doctor, or other health worker been concerned about your drinking or suggested you cut down?

AUDIT-C

1. How often do you have a drink containing alcohol?
2. How many units of alcohol do you drink on a typical day when you are drinking?
3. How often have you had six or more units if female, or eight or more if male, on a single occasion in the last year?

Screening for AUD

Studies using simulated patients show that women are screened and referred less often than men.[14] The US Preventive Services Task Force (USPSTF) recommends "that clinicians screen adults aged 18 years or older for alcohol misuse and provide persons engaged in risky or hazardous drinking with brief behavioral counseling interventions to reduce alcohol misuse. (Grade B recommendation)."[5] Evidence is insufficient to recommend for or against screening those less than 18 years old.[5]

Tools recommended for screening by USPSTF include the Alcohol Use Disorders Identification Test (AUDIT), AUDIT-Consumption (AUDIT-C), or single-question screening tools (see Table 45-2).[1]

Table 45-3 Recommended FDA-approved pharmacotherapies for alcohol use disorder

	Naltrexone (oral)	Naltrexone (injectable)	Acamprosate
Dosage	50 mg daily	380 mg monthly	333 mg TID for 5 days, then 666 mg TID
Contraindications	Opioid physical dependence	Opioid physical dependence	Severe renal dysfunction (CrCl <30)
	Cirrhosis	Cirrhosis	
	Transaminase elevation >3 times upper limit of normal	Transaminase elevation >3 times	
Monitoring	Liver function at baseline, month 1, month 3, month 6, and annually thereafter	Liver function at baseline, month 1, month 3, month 6, and annually thereafter	Renal function as clinically indicated
Pregnancy category	C	C	C

AUDIT is the most widely studied and has good sensitivity and specificity for detecting alcohol use among multiple populations. It contains 10 questions and takes two to five minutes to administer. The abbreviated AUDIT-C involves three questions and takes one to two minutes to administer. The single-question screening asks: "How many times in the past year have you had five [for men] or four [for women and all adults older than 65] or more drinks in a day?" The AUDIT and AUDIT-C tools with scoring and interpretation can be accessed for free at www.integration.samhsa.gov/clinical-practice/screening-tools.

Although many providers may be familiar with the "CAGE" questions for alcohol misuse screening (**c**ut down desire/attempts, **a**nnoyance when confronted about use, **g**uilt about use, and **e**ye-opener or morning use to calm nerves or withdrawal symptoms), this tool is not time sensitive; it does not assess current use or consequences, but, rather, the use/consequences over the patient's lifetime. Hence, tools such as the AUDIT and AUDIT-C are preferable.

Pharmacotherapy

The following FDA-approved pharmacotherapies can help prevent relapse in early recovery when used as adjuncts to behavioral treatment: oral naltrexone (Revia), long-acting injectable naltrexone (Vivitrol), and acamprosate (Campral) (see Table 45-3). Topiramate (Topamax), though not specifically FDA-approved for this indication, has also reduced heavy drinking (target daily dose 200 mg–300 mg).[15] Gabapentin early in treatment (target dose 1,600 mg–2,400 mg total dose daily, divided three times daily) has also been found to be helpful in reducing withdrawal/abstinence symptoms.[16]

There is no evidence-based order in which drugs should be tried. Combination therapy has not been superior to monotherapy.[15] Similar to depression and other mental illnesses, counseling should take place in conjunction with medication.

Although disulfiram (Antabuse) is also FDA-approved for adjunctive treatment of AUDs (dosing 250 mg–500 mg daily), its lack of relative effectiveness under typical prescribing conditions, potentially serious toxicities, several contraindications, and common interaction with other prescribed medications and over-the-counter products makes it less preferred to other approved therapies and a more challenging regimen to manage. When used, it is generally preferable for dosing to be witnessed.[17]

Duration of pharmacotherapy should be individually tailored. Longer retention in treatment is associated with improved outcomes.[18] If pharmacotherapy continues to facilitate retention in care (or if a trial of medication discontinuation is followed by relapse), continued pharmacotherapy and monitoring is likely indicated.

Brief intervention

The USPSTF found that "brief multi-contact behavioral counseling seems to have the best evidence of effectiveness; very brief behavioral counseling has limited effect."[5] Brief multicontact behavioral counseling is 6–15 minutes each; very brief behavioral counseling is less than five minutes.[5]

A meta-analysis of 19 RCTs including 5,639 women found that primary care brief interventions resulted in a decrease in weekly alcohol consumption [−38 g/wk (approximately 4 drinks); 95% CI −51 to −24 g/wk]. The decrease was sustained at 6 and 12 months.[19]

Components of brief interventions which have been found to be effective include giving feedback on drinking behavior, advising change, setting goals, multiple visits, patient follow-up, provider training, and the use of additional staff or system supports for screening or assessment. Shame and criticism are ineffective for self-evident reasons. Instead, counseling should respect autonomy, support self-efficacy, and offer hope and resources.

The National Institute on Alcohol Abuse and Alcoholism (NIAAA) published an evidence-based guide, *Helping Patients Who Drink Too Much*. Drinking behaviors are divided into five categories, and an appropriate intervention is recommended for each.[15]

Referral for treatment

When a woman's needs are greater than what a clinic can offer, referral is indicated. Unfortunately, referral options are scarce in many settings. Even when referral to a treatment program is not indicated or not an option, a team approach can be helpful. The broader care team can include social workers, nurses, peer educators, community organizations, clergy, family members, and friends. Women with AUD often struggle with comorbid mental illness; it can make sense to combine alcohol treatment with other mental health services.

Financial stress and unemployment can be a factor in alcohol and other substance use. Employment can help with maintenance of drug or alcohol abstinence.[20] Inclusion of job and housing assistance in alcohol-treatment plans increases the chance of long-term success.

Adolescents

The approach to screening and treatment of AUD in adolescents deserves special attention. At preventive health visits, providers should speak with adolescents alone in addition to with their parents/guardians. Confidentiality should be respected unless there is a perceived threat to themselves or others.

Although adolescent alcohol use rates have been declining since the 1970s, use is still high: in 2011, about one in four eighth-graders, one in two tenth-graders, and almost two of three twelfth-graders reported drinking alcohol in the preceding month.[21] Binge drinking was reported by 6.4%–21.6% of this age group.[21]

In a study of 533 adolescents aged 14–18, providers' clinical impression underestimated substance abuse problems. None of the 36 with alcohol or drug dependence were identified.[22] Of 86 adolescents diagnosed with SUDs, providers identified 75% as using, but for 50% they estimated use as "minimal."[22] A recommendation was made to use structured screening tools.

The screening tools AUDIT, POSIT, CAGE, and CRAFFT all have useful sensitivity and specificity in screening for AUDs in adolescents. Sensitivities were as follows: AUDIT 0.88 (95%CI 0.83–0.93), POSIT 0.84 (95%CI 0.79–0.90), CAGE 0.37 (95%CI 0.29–0.44), and CRAFFT 0.92 (95%CI 0.88–0.96). Specificities were: AUDIT 0.81 (95%CI 0.77–0.85), POSIT 0.89 (95%CI 0.86–0.92), CAGE 0.96 (95%CI 0.94–0.98), and CRAFFT 0.64 (95%CI 0.59–0.69).[23] Many prefer the CRAFFT tool with adolescents (see Table 45-4). The commonly used CAGE tool has a low sensitivity with adolescents.

Prevention

Universal prevention through public awareness campaigns, billboards, and mandatory warning labels on alcoholic beverages are all effective strategies for

Table 45-4 CRAFFT screening for illicit drug use in adolescents

C – Have you ever ridden in a Car driven by someone [including yourself] who was high or had been using alcohol or drugs?
R – Have you ever used alcohol or drugs to Relax, feel better about yourself, or fit in?
A – Have you ever used alcohol or drugs while you are by yourself, Alone?
F – Do you ever Forget things you did while using alcohol or drugs?
F – Does your Family or do your Friends ever tell you that you should cut down on your drinking or drug use?
T – Have you ever gotten in Trouble while you were using alcohol or drugs?

increasing awareness of alcohol issues and changing social and cultural norms.[24]

The World Health Organization suggests best practices for limiting alcohol problems including minimum legal age purchase regulations, restricted hours or days of sales, outlet density restrictions, increase in alcohol taxes, sobriety check points, lowered blood alcohol content limits, driver's license suspension, graduated licensing for novice drinkers, and brief interventions for hazardous drinkers.[24]

Other substance use, nonpregnant women

Among women of childbearing age (15–44), 10% of nonpregnant women and 4% of pregnant women report illicit drug use.[25] Drug use disorders cost more than $180 billion annually, including $605 million in health costs for drug-exposed newborns.[14]

In a study of more than 336,000 files from the National Survey on Drug Use and Health 2005–2010, men and women with substance use with or without comorbid depression described similar barriers to care with attitudinal factors being the greatest; 42%–55% did not feel that treatment would help.[26]

A meta-analysis of 35 trials showed that psychosocial interventions have a moderate effect in the treatment of SUDs.[27] Factors that have been identified as important in substance abuse programs for women include "diminishing client ambivalence, instilling hope, establishing trust-based provider-client relationships, individualizing treatment, and establishing and maintaining personal dignity and respect."[28]

USPSTF does not recommend for or against screening for illicit drug use due to lack of evidence regarding benefits and risks.[25] However, given the significant morbidity and mortality associated with SUDs, it is good practice for clinicians to screen patients and offer treatment.

Opiates

Epidemiology

Opiates may be swallowed, injected, sniffed, and smoked. They include heroin, methadone, OxyContin®, Vicodin®, codeine, morphine, and fentanyl. Street names include big H, black tar, brown sugar, Dover's powder, hillbilly heroin, horse, junk, lean or purple drank, MPTP (new heroin), mud, OC, ox, oxy, oxycotton, paregoric, sippin syrup, and smack looks.[29]

The societal cost of opiate use disorder is great, and is associated with rising morbidity and mortality related to drug overdose. In 2010, more than 15,000 deaths were attributable to drug overdose in women, of which 60% were related to prescription opioids. From 1999 to 2010, rates of death from opioid pain relievers in women have increased fivefold. In fact, since 2007, more women have died from opioid overdose than from motor vehicle accidents.[30]

Symptoms of intoxication/withdrawal

Signs and symptoms of narcotic use include drowsiness, lethargy, slurred speech, incoordination, pupil constriction, constipation, nausea, and decreased respiration. Withdrawal symptoms include irritability, anxiety, yawning, watery eyes, pupil dilation, diarrhea, sweating, nausea, vomiting, tremors, hypertension, and tachycardia.[29]

Pharmacotherapy

Women tend to start treatment earlier in their opiate addiction than men and therefore have fewer years of opiate use.[31] The most successful outpatient treatment approaches for opiate use disorders are opiate replacement therapy, of which only methadone and buprenorphine/naloxone (Suboxone), and buprenorphine (Subutex) have been approved by the FDA.

Methadone is a long-acting opiate utilized as opioid agonist therapy (OAT) which allows patients to stop using heroin, avoid legal issues related to illicit narcotic use, and maintain a job and family. It is an agonist that blocks the mu receptor and decreases heroin use by cross-tolerance. Women are less likely to use heroin with methadone doses of 80 mg per day or higher.[20] Methadone can only be prescribed for opiate replacement in a certified methadone clinic, which can be an advantage to patients who need a more structured recovery program, but it can be a disadvantage to those who have restrictive work schedules, limited transportation, or difficulty with child care.

Buprenorphine is a partial mu opioid receptor agonist, making it less likely to produce a euphoric effect and lead to life-threatening overdose. In the United States, it comes in two forms: buprenorphine alone (Subutex) and in combination with naltrexone (Suboxone). Buprenorphine can be administered in the office setting as long as the prescribing provider is certified with an eight-hour online training course (www.buppractice.com). Suboxone is considered a safer formulation because the naltrexone is inactive in the sublingual/oral administration route, but it is active if injected intravenously, so it will counter the effects of the IV opiate. Both formulations have advantages over methadone in that they can be administered in the office-based settings, are safer, and will lead to less neonatal abstinence syndrome if taken in pregnancy.[32] However, only Subutex is FDA-approved for use with pregnant women.

Clonidine helps with some of the autonomic signs/symptoms of opiate withdrawal, such as anxiety, hot/cold flushes, and hypertension.[20] It should, however, be monitored closely because it can cause oversedation and hypotension. It may be used in combination with other medicines such as benzodiazepines and in detoxification regimens.

Other medications including nonsteroidal anti-inflammatory drugs (NSAIDs), anti-emetics, anti-diarrheals, and sleep aids may be helpful in treating withdrawal symptoms.

Behavioral therapy

In general, OAT alone is effective treatment for opiate use disorders. A 2011 meta-analysis showed no comparative advantage in retention in treatment or abstinence rates for patients randomized to OAT alone versus OAT with psychosocial interventions.[33] Options for psychosocial interventions include individual or group addiction counseling; peer-support groups (i.e., Narcotics Anonymous); abstinence-based therapy; and structured, standardized approaches such as contingency management, relapse prevention, and cognitive behavioral therapy (CBT). A 2008 meta-analysis found that combined contingency management and CBT, and contingency management alone had better outcomes than other interventions.[27]

Cocaine

Epidemiology

Cocaine can be absorbed through any mucous membrane. Most commonly, it is injected intravenously or intramuscularly, snorted, or smoked (crack). It may be taken with tobacco, THC, or opiates (referred to as speed-balling). Street names include coca, coke, crack, flake, snow, and soda cot.[29]

Crack has been popular since mid-1980s because it is cheaper than powder cocaine and comes in a usable unit. A study of 312 men and 312 women found that although women utilize health-care services more than men, this is less true for women who use crack.[34]

Symptoms of intoxication/withdrawal

Signs and symptoms of cocaine intoxication include increased alertness, irritability, anxiety, hypertension, tachycardia, palpitations, chest pain, seizures, unilateral weakness, dilated pupils, erosion of the nasal cavity, insomnia, and decreased appetite.[29]

Cocaine withdrawal involves more psychological than physical symptoms. Women withdrawing from cocaine may experience depression and fatigue. Craving can last for weeks.[20]

Pharmacotherapy

There are no FDA-approved pharmacotherapies currently for cocaine use disorders. Pharmacotherapy, therefore, is commonly guided by treatment of psychiatric comorbidity. Medications that may help include benzodiazepines, dopamine agonists, antidepressants, and anticonvulsants.[20]

Behavioral therapy

An RCT of 145 cocaine-dependent women compared three approaches to cocaine addiction: contingency management (CM) (e.g., money if negative drug screens), CBT, and community reinforcement approach (CRA). CM led to longer proportion of cocaine-free days, fewer positive drug tests, and higher rates of abstinence through 12 months than other approaches.[35]

Cannabis

Epidemiology

Marijuana from the *Cannabis sativa* plant is smoked, eaten, and brewed in tea. Marijuana contains more than 400 chemicals; delta-9-tetrahydrocannabinol (THC) is thought to be the main psychoactive ingredient. Street names include aunt mary, BC bud, blunts, boom, chronic, dope, gangster, ganja, grass, hash, herb, hydro, indo, joint, kif, mary jane, mota, pot, reefer, sinsemilla, skunk, smoke, weed, and yerbalooks. Blunts are cigars that are emptied of tobacco and filled with marijuana. Hashish and hashish oil, also from the cannabis plant, have effects similar to but stronger than marijuana.[36]

Marijuana has been legalized in some states. The implications for women need further research.

Symptoms of intoxication/withdrawal

Signs and symptoms of marijuana intoxication include problems with perception, memory, motivation, and coordination; increased appetite; bloodshot eyes; tachycardia; hypotension; and cough. Risk of various cancers is increased. Withdrawal can cause irritability, insomnia, decreased appetite, headache, shakiness, sweating, stomach pain, and nausea.[36]

Pharmacotherapy

No medicine has been approved specifically for treatment of marijuana intoxication. Behavioral therapy is the mainstay of treatment. Benzodiazepines and atypical antipsychotics may be used if a woman is having extreme agitation or psychosis due to marijuana.[37] N-acetylcysteine has provided some relief from withdrawal symptoms in subjects motivated to abstain.[38]

Behavioral therapy

Psychosocial interventions were more effective in decreasing THC usage than opiate usage.[27]

Other drugs

There are many substances of abuse. A detailed discussion of each is beyond the scope of this chapter. For more information, please access www.justice.gov/dea/druginfo/factsheets.shtml for other stimulants (including amphetamines, methamphetamines, and methylphenidate), hallucinogens (including Ecstasy/MDMA, K2/Spice, Ketamine, LSD, Peyote & Mescaline, and Psilocybin), benzodiazepines, and bath salts/synthetic stimulants/designer cathinones.[29]

Adolescents

A study of 538 adolescents aged 14–18 found that a CRAFFT score of 2 or higher was a good screening test for identifying any substance use problem [sensitivity, 0.76; specificity, 0.94; positive predictive value (PPV), 0.83; and negative predictive value (NPV), 0.91], any substance abuse disorder (sensitivity, 0.80; specificity, 0.86; PPV, 0.53; and NPV, 0.96), and dependence (sensitivity, 0.92; specificity, 0.80; PPV, 0.25; and NPV 0.99).[39] The CRAFFT screening was equally valid for males and females.[39] A study of 525 primary care patients aged 12–17 found that CRAFFT with a cutoff of two positive responses has excellent sensitivity and specificity for SUDs using DSM-5 criteria.[40]

Preconception/interconception care

Birth control

In the United States, 40%–50% of pregnancies are unintended; in some low-income communities, 80% of pregnancies are unplanned.[41]

An intervention for women with alcohol and drug use disorders in Seattle resulted in an increase in regular use of birth control from 5% to 61% over a 12-month period.[42]

Providing access to contraception is important for all women, particularly those with substance abuse disorders. Long-acting reversible contraception (LARCs), including Nexplanon and IUDs, may be an attractive option because they are effective, do not require daily action, and may be discontinued.[43] Because women with SUDs are less likely to use contraception and are more likely to experience abuse, emergency contraception should be made available along with education about when and how to use it.[44]

Hormonal methods that are metabolized by the liver may be contraindicated for women with cirrhosis due to AUD. Nonhormonal methods – including IUDs, condoms, tubal ligation, or occlusion – and vasectomy may be the best options for women with cirrhosis.

Sexually transmitted infection screening

Women with SUDs are at increased risk for sexually transmitted infections (STIs). Interconception visits should include appropriate screening. The USPSTF recommends screening for chlamydia, gonorrhea, syphilis, and HIV. For women engaged in high-risk behaviors, additional screening for hepatitis B and C should be considered.[45] The American Congress of Obstetricians and Gynecologists (ACOG) and Centers for Disease Control and Prevention (CDC) recommend HIV testing for all women aged 13–63 once in their lifetime and annually for high-risk women, assessing risk factors annually and making annual HIV testing available to all women regardless of risk factors.[46]

Cervical cancer screening

As women with substance abuse disorders are at increased risk for STIs, they are at risk for human papillomavirus (HPV) and cervical dysplasia. American

Society of Colposcopy and Cervical Pathology and ACOG guidelines can direct cervical cancer screening and management of cervical dysplasia.[47]

Vaccinations

Interconception care is an opportunity to make sure women with SUDs are up to date on their immunizations. The HPV vaccine is recommended for women aged 11–26; cervical screening guidelines are not different for women who have been vaccinated. Care between pregnancies allows vaccination with live vaccines including MMR and varicella, which are contraindicated in pregnancy. National vaccine recommendations are made by the Advisory Committee on Immunization Practices (www.cdc.gov/vaccines/acip).

Other high-risk behaviors

Women with SUDs often are not up to date on routine health maintenance issues and commonly engage in other high-risk behaviors such as high-risk sexual partners or exchanging sex for drugs/money. Office visits provide an opportunity to detect and address these issues.

Tobacco abuse is common among women with substance abuse. Options for cessation aids are greater when addressed before pregnancy. Many women quit smoking during pregnancy, and postpartum/interconception care provides an opportunity to promote maintenance of cessation.

Fetal alcohol spectrum disorder prevention

Alcohol is used more commonly than tobacco in women of childbearing age.[25] Fetal alcohol spectrum disorder (FASD) is estimated to affect more than 1% of infants born in the United States.[7] FASD is defined as "the range of effects that can occur in a person whose mother drank alcohol during pregnancy, including physical, mental, behavior, and learning disabilities, with possible lifelong implications."[48] FASD is the leading cause of preventable developmental delay in the United States.[41]

A 2005 recommendation from the surgeon general, the American Academy of Pediatrics (AAP), and ACOG recommended alcohol abstinence for all women of childbearing age who are not using reliable birth control.[7] According to one study, 7.6% of women of childbearing age are sexually active without birth control.[25] Many women cut down or quit drinking alcohol when they know they are pregnant but drink through the first weeks of pregnancy. Women of childbearing age see a physician on average three times per year, allowing ample opportunity for preconception alcohol counseling.[41]

The CDC currently funds regional training centers to help health-care providers identify, manage, and prevent FASD.[7] Screening and brief interventions are recommended. These were discussed in earlier in the chapter. The USPSTF recommends screening and treatment in the primary care setting to prevent alcohol use in pregnancy.

Risk assessment may be a way to focus FASD prevention efforts on the highest risk patients. Risk factors include smoking and illicit drug use, partner with a pattern of heavy drinking, mental health problems, history of sexual or physical abuse, and loss of custody of other children.[41] Questionnaires to assess alcohol and other drug use can save time and improve documentation.

Opiates

There are no differences in maternal outcomes between methadone and buprenorphine in pregnancy, but the incidence of neonatal absence syndrome is lower with use of buprenorphine.[32]

Preconception care allows a safer transition from methadone to buprenorphine. It is preferable to be on buprenorphine rather than methadone during pregnancy, in part, because the incidence of neonatal withdrawal syndrome is less.[31] It is not recommended to transition from methadone to buprenorphine *during* pregnancy because a woman would need to go through methadone withdrawal in the process.

Women who have a history of opiate use disorder and are planning pregnancy should be given as much psychosocial support as possible in addition to biomedical care.

Cocaine

Cocaine has been linked to low-birth weight, prematurity, stillbirth, placental abruption.[25] Developmental issues in children exposed to cocaine in utero are hard to separate from those exposed to alcohol, tobacco, and other drugs.[49]

Other drugs

It is recommended to stop all drug use prior to becoming pregnant, so efforts should be made to support women in treatment programs and offer free or low-cost contraception to prevent unintended pregnancy while in recovery.

Adolescents

Teenagers have the highest rates of unintended pregnancies.[41] Preventive care visits always need to include discussion of sexual activity, contraception, STI prevention and screening, but particularly if patients screen positive for drug use.

Legal and ethical issues

Legal issues

In 2005, more than 1 million women in the United States were incarcerated, twice as many as in 1990.[28] Approximately 60% of these women have alcohol or other drug use issues.[28] Alcohol and other drug treatment is often court mandated. Incarceration alone is ineffective and often more expensive than treatment. In fact, jail often allows ongoing access to drugs but not treatment. It may be more effective to sentence someone to choose drug treatment versus incarceration than to mandate drug treatment.[20]

Because of socioeconomic factors, crack is used more commonly by African Americans and powder cocaine by whites. Mandatory sentencing for crack cocaine has led to a disproportionate incarceration of African Americans, which affects African-American women in many negative ways. Positive drug screens for methamphetamines and opiates, principally used by Caucasians, are more often referred to social services than the courts.[14]

Women who have children may be affected not only by substance use but also by associated legal issues. They may delay or avoid treatment because they fear they may lose custody of their children. Mandatory reporting laws often require that child protective services be notified when a parent is struggling with alcohol or other substance use issues; however, substance use does not prove inadequate parenting or neglect.

To influence legal issues that affect women on a broader scale, motivated providers may desire involvement at a legislative level locally, statewide, and/or nationally. Laws regarding substance abuse are often not applied equally across racial and economic lines.

Ethical issues

Complex ethical issues may arise in addressing AUD in women. Children and mental health issues are two factors that result in difficult decision making. Ethics committees are sometimes available to help.

Lack of insurance may limit treatment options. Drug abuse has a similar heritability, course, and response to treatment as other chronic medical illnesses including diabetes, hypertension, and asthma.[50] This fact can be used to argue that insurance should cover costs of ongoing monitoring and treatment as with other chronic diseases.[50]

Concluding remarks

Alcohol and substance use disorders may present differently and require different approaches in women and men. The quantity of alcohol that can be safely consumed is lower for women than men. AUDIT and AUDIT-C are effective tools for detecting AUD in adults. CRAFFT is particularly useful with adolescents. Comorbid mental health issues, gender-based violence, contraception, and STI issues play an important role in treating women with AUD and SUD. Addressing AUD and SUD before and between pregnancies can improve outcomes not only for women but also their children.

References

1. Landheim A, Bakken K, Vaglum P. Gender differences in the prevalence of symptom disorders and personality disorders among poly-substance abusers and pure alcoholics. Substance abusers treated in two counties in Norway. *Eur Addict Res.* 2003;**9**:8–17.
2. Devries K, Child J, Bacchus L, et al. Intimate partner violence victimization and alcohol consumption in women: a systematic review and meta-analysis. *Addiction.* 2014;**109**:379–91.
3. Gil-Rivas V, Fiorentine R, Anglin M. Sexual abuse, physical abuse, and posttraumatic stress disorder among women participating in outpatient drug abuse treatment. *J Psychoactive Drugs.* 1996;**28**:95–102.
4. Latimer W, Stone A, Voight A, Winters K, August G. Gender differences in psychiatric comorbidity among adolescents with substance use disorders. *Exp Clin Psychopharmacol.* 2002;**10**:310–15.
5. Moyer V, Preventive Services Task Force. Screening and behavioral counseling interventions in primary care to reduce alcohol misuse: US Preventive Services Task Force recommendation statement. *Ann Intern Med.* 2013 Aug 6;**159**(3):210–18.
6. Centers for Disease Control and Prevention. Alcohol and Public Health. Last updated February 4, 2016.

Available at: www.cdc.gov/alcohol/fact-sheets/alcohol-use.htm. Accessed on February 19, 2016.

7. Centers for Disease Control and Prevention (CDC). Alcohol use and binge drinking among women of childbearing age–United States, 2006–2010. *MMWR Morb Mortal Wkly Rep.* 2012;**61**:534–8.
8. American Psychiatric Association. Diagnostic and Statistical Manual of Mental Disorders. 5th edition. Washington, DC: American Psychiatric Association; 2013.
9. National Institute on Alcohol Abuse and Alcoholism. Alcohol Use Disorder: A Comparison between DSM–IV and DSM–5. Available at: http://pubs.niaaa.nih.gov/publications/dsmfactsheet/dsmfact.pdf. Accessed on February 19, 2016.
10. Ashley M, Olin J, le Riche W, et al. Morbidity in alcoholics: evidence for accelerated development of physical disease in women. *Arch Intern Med.* 1977;**137**: 883–7.
11. Hommer D, Momenan R, Kaiser E, Rawlings R. Evidence for a gender-related effect of alcoholism on brain volumes. *Am J Psychiatry.* 2001;**158**:198–204.
12. Loft S, Olesen K, Døssing M. Increased susceptibility to liver disease in relation to alcohol consumption in women. *Scand J Gastroenterol.* 1987;**22**:1251–6.
13. O'Keefe J, Bhatti S, Bajwa A, et al. Alcohol and cardiovascular health: the dose makes the poison . . . or the remedy. *Mayo Clin Proc.* 2014;**89**:382–93.
14. American College of Obstetricians and Gynecologists. ACOG Committee Opinion No. 422: at-risk drinking and illicit drug use: ethical issues in obstetric and gynecologic practice. *Obstet Gynecol.* 2008;**112**: 1449–60.
15. Willenbring M, Massey S, Gardner M. Helping patients who drink too much: an evidence-based guide for primary care clinicians. *Am Fam Physician.* 2009;**80**:44–50.
16. Anton R, Myrick H, Wright T, et al. Gabapentin combined with naltrexone for the treatment of alcohol dependence. *Am J Psychiatry.* 2011;**168**:709–17.
17. Jonas D, Amick H, Feltner C, et al. Pharmacotherapy for adults with alcohol use disorders in outpatient settings: a systematic review and meta-analysis. *JAMA.* 2014;**311**:1889–90.
18. Moos R, Moos B. Long-term influence of duration and intensity of treatment on previously untreated individuals with alcohol use disorders. *Addiction.* 2003;**98**:325–37.
19. Bertholet N, Daeppen J, Wietlisbach V, et al. Reduction of alcohol consumption by brief alcohol intervention in primary care: systematic review and meta-analysis. *Arch Intern Med.* 2005;**165**:986–95.
20. Kleber H. Pharmacologic treatments for heroin and cocaine dependence. *Am J Addict.* 2003;**12**(Suppl 2): S5–S18.
21. Patrick M, Schulenberg J. Prevalence and predictors of adolescent alcohol use and binge drinking in the United States. *Alcohol Res.* 2013;**35**:193–200.
22. Wilson C, Sherritt L, Gates E, Knight J. Are clinical impressions of adolescent substance use accurate? *Pediatrics.* 2004;**114**:e536–40.
23. Knight J, Sherritt L, Harris S, et al. Validity of brief alcohol screening tests among adolescents: a comparison of the AUDIT, POSIT, CAGE, and CRAFFT. *Alcohol Clin Exp Res.* 2003;**27**:67–73.
24. Barry K, Caetano R, Cheng G, et al. Reducing Alcohol-Exposed Pregnancies. A Report of the National Task Force on Fetal Alcohol Syndrome and Fetal Alcohol Effect. Available at: www.cdc.gov/ncbddd/fasd/documents/redalcohpreg.pdf. Accessed on February 19, 2016.
25. Floyd R, Jack B, Cefalo R, et al. The clinical content of preconception care: alcohol, tobacco, and illicit drug exposures. *Am J Obstet Gynecol.* 2008;**199**: S333–9.
26. Chen L, Strain E, Crum R, Mojtabai R. Gender differences in substance abuse treatment and barriers to care among persons with substance use disorders with and without comorbid major depression. *J Addict Med.* 2013;7:325–34.
27. Dutra L, Stathopoulou G, Basden S, et al. A meta-analytic review of psychosocial interventions for substance use disorders. *Am J Psychiatry.* 2008;**165**: 179–87.
28. Finfgeld-Connett D, Johnson E. Substance abuse treatment for women who are under correctional supervision in the community: a systematic review of qualitative findings. *Issues Ment Health Nurs.* 2011;**32**: 640–8.
29. Drug Enforcement Agency. Drug fact sheets. Available at: www.justice.gov/dea/druginfo/factsheets.shtml. Accessed on February 19, 2016.
30. Centers for Disease Control and Prevention. Vital signs: overdoses of prescription opioid pain relievers and other drugs among women – United States, 1999–2010. *MMWR (Morb Mortal Wkly Rep).* 2013;**62**: 537–42.
31. Unger A, Jung E, Winklbaur B, Fischer G. Gender issues in the pharmacotherapy of opioid-addicted women: buprenorphine. *J Addict Dis.* 2010;**29**: 217–30.
32. Jones H, Kaltenbach K, Heil S, et al. Neonatal abstinence syndrome after methadone or buprenorphine exposure. *N Engl J Med.* 2010;**363**: 2320–31.

33. Amato L, Minozzi S, Davoli M, Vecchi S. Psychosocial combined with agonist maintenance treatments versus agonist maintenance treatments alone for treatment of opioid dependence. *Cochrane Database Syst Rev.* 2011 Oct 5;**10**:CD004147.
34. Metsch L, McCoy H, McCoy C, et al. Use of health care services by women who use crack cocaine. *Women & Health.* 1999;**30**:35–51.
35. Schottenfeld R, Moore B, Pantalon M. Contingency management with community reinforcement approach or twelve-step facilitation drug counseling for cocaine dependent pregnant women or women with young children. *Drug Alcohol Depend.* 2011;**118**:48–55.
36. Drug Enforcement Agency. Drug fact sheet: marijuana. Available at: http://www.dea.gov/druginfo/drug_data_sheets/Marijuana.pdf. Accessed on February 19, 2016.
37. Danovitch I, Gorelick D. State of the art treatments for cannabis dependence. *Psychiatr Clin North Am.* 2012;**35**:309–26.
38. Gray K, Carpenter M, Baker N, et al. A double-blind randomized controlled trial of N-acetylcysteine in cannabis-dependent adolescents. *Am J Psychiatry.* 2012;**169**:805–12.
39. Knight J, Sherritt L, Shrier L, et al. Validity of the CRAFFT substance abuse screening test among adolescent clinic patients. *Arch Pediatr Adolesc Med.* 2002;**156**:607–14.
40. Mitchell S, Kelly S, Gryczynski J, et al. The CRAFFT cut-points and DSM-5 criteria for alcohol and other drugs: a reevaluation and reexamination. *Subst Abus.* 2014;**35**(4):376–80.
41. Das S, Rao V, Chaudhuri J. Preconception counseling in the prevention of fetal alcohol syndrome: a unique window of opportunity. *Clin Ter.* 2009;**160**:315–22.
42. Grant T, Ernst C, Streissguth A. An intervention with high-risk mothers who abuse alcohol and drugs: the Seattle Advocacy Model. *Am J Public Health.* 1996;**86**: 1816–17.
43. American College of Obstetricians and Gynecologists. ACOG Practice Bulletin No. 121: long-acting reversible contraception: Implants and intrauterine devices. *Obstet Gynecol.* 2011;**118**:184–96.
44. American College of Obstetricians and Gynecologists. ACOG Practice Bulletin No. 112: emergency contraception. *Obstet Gynecol.* 2010;**115**:1100–9.
45. Meyers D, Wolff T, Gregory K, Marion L, Moyer V, Nelson H, et al. USPSTF recommendations for STI screening. *Am Fam Physician.* 2008;**77**:819–924.
46. American college of Obstetricians and Gynecologists: ACOG Committee Opinion no 596: Committee on Gynecologic Practice: Routine human immunodeficiency virus screening. *Obstet Gynecol.* 2014;**123**(5): 137–139.
47. Massad L, Einstein M, Huh W, et al. 2012 updated consensus guidelines for the management of abnormal cervical cancer screening tests and cancer precursors. *Obstet Gynecol.* 2013 Apr;**121**(4):829–46.
48. Calhoun F, Attilia M, Spagnolo P, et al. National Institute on Alcohol Abuse and Alcoholism and the study of fetal alcohol spectrum disorders. The International Consortium. *Ann Ist Super Sanita.* 2006;**42**:4–7.
49. Frank D, Augustyn M, Knight W, et al. Growth, development, and behavior in early childhood following prenatal cocaine exposure: a systematic review. *JAMA.* 2001;**285**:1613–25.
50. McLellan A, Lewis D, O'Brien C, Kleber H. Drug dependence, a chronic medical illness: implications for treatment, insurance, and outcomes evaluation. *JAMA.* 2000;**284**:1689–95.

Chapter 46

Office care of geriatric patients

Anita Blanchard and Adrianne Dade

Introduction

We are an aging nation. According to the US census data, it is estimated that the number of Americans over the age of 65 will almost double from 43.1 million in 2012 to 83.7 million by 2050. The proportion of this age group to the general population is also estimated to grow from 13.7 percent to 20.9 percent.[1] Similar trends in life expectancy are predicted in other countries (see Figure 46-1). Female life expectancy exceeds male life expectancy.[1] Women now live one-third of their lives after menopause. Health care strategies that specifically focus on the needs of older women are essential.

Addressing the problems of an aging population has become a central part of health care. More than 75 million people cope with two or more chronic medical conditions in the United States.[2] Geriatric patients compose the highest proportion with multiple medical comorbidities. Although functional decline related to chronic disease is characteristic of the aging process, new innovations in preventive care have led to longer healthier lives.

This chapter will focus on current guidelines and considerations in this population including screening and prevention practices, special gynecologic considerations in geriatric patients, frailty, and end-of-life decision making.

Screening and prevention strategies in the geriatric population

Preventive care and good lifestyle practices have significant impact on longevity. Box 46-1 identifies some of the parameters considered in preventive care.

Nutrition

Optimal nutrition in the elderly has important relevance to stabilize the added demands of comorbid diseases and functional impairment. Research indicates

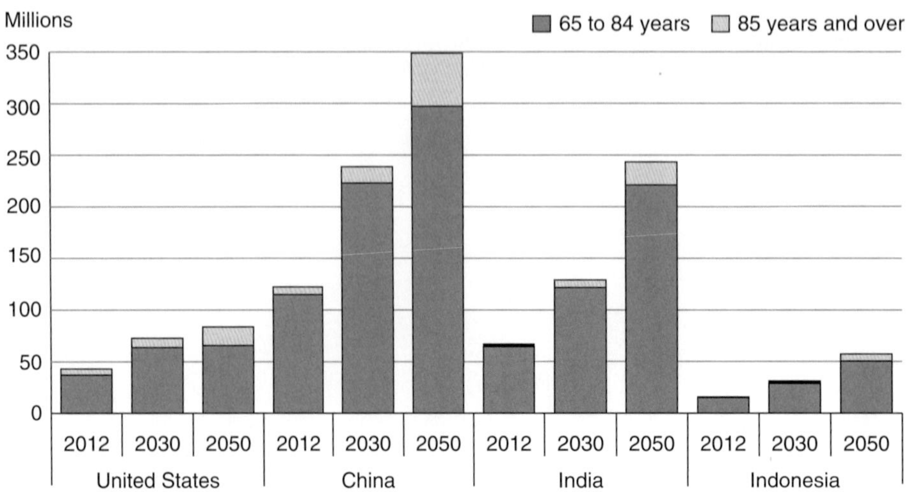

Figure 46-1 Life expectancy trends (from US Census Bureau [1]).

Office Care of Women, ed. Martin E. Olsen and Botros Rizk. Published by Cambridge University Press.

BOX 46-1 Preventive care strategies

Nutrition
Exercise
Immunizations
Visual acuity
Hearing acuity
Dental health
Cardiovascular health
Mental health/cognitive assessment
Bone health
Fall prevention
Risk reduction in smoking, alcohol, and habit habit-forming substances
Cancer screening:
- Skin
- Breast
- Gynecological
- Colon
- Lung

that the traditional Mediterranean diet that is high in vegetables, fruits, fish, whole grains, and monounsaturated oil can be protective against cognitive decline and dementia.[3] Diet also influences development of cardiovascular disorders, endocrine diseases including type 2 diabetes and some types of cancer. Health-care teams must recognize factors influencing nutrition, review dietary intake, identify dietary deficiencies and establish nutritional balance (Figure 46-2).[4] Determinants of nutrition are multifactorial including food access, physical and mental health status, habits affecting nutrition, and socioeconomic status.[4] Physical limits may include gastrointestinal disorders affecting swallowing and absorption. Poor dentition also contributes to the ability of chew food. Osteoarthritis can impact the ability to prepare food. Depressed mood and cognitive function may affect appetite and routine patterns of meals. Older patients who are not able to adequately care for themselves and who live in isolated housing are particularly at risk of poor nutrition. Smoking, alcohol, and illicit drug use also affect nutrition. Nutritional deficiencies can be both the cause and result in the cycle of elder care

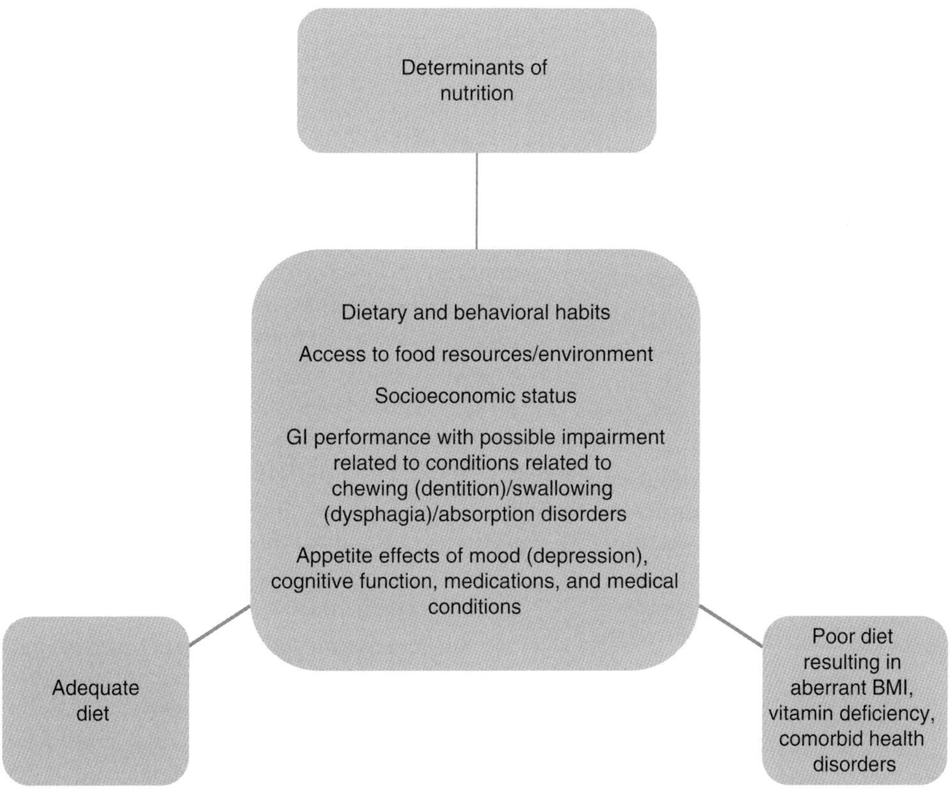

Figure 46-2 Nutritional balance.

challenges. Poor nutrition can result in opposite extremes of malnutrition or obesity.

Cachexia is a metabolic disorder associated with underlying chronic medical conditions such as cancer and HIV/AIDS; it is characterized by loss of muscle and fat mass.[5] Malnourishment can be unrecognized by health-care practitioners. One method of evaluation is the mini nutrition assessment tool; its short form can be easily used as an initial screen for malnutrition.[6] Malnutrition has many consequences including longer hospitalization, increased fall risk, decreased physical function, poor quality of life, and increased morbidity and mortality.[5] Interventions to correct undernourishment include multidisciplinary support, nutritional education, counseling with individualized diet plans prepared by registered dieticians, and follow-up home visits.[5]

Obesity is associated with a number of medical disorders including hypertension, diabetes, and hyperlipidemia. From 1980 to 2008, obesity has doubled in adults.[7] In patients over 60, 31% are obese.[8] (See Chapter 39 for additional discussion on obesity.) Older patients who are obese are also more likely to report chronic joint pain, back pain, indigestion, depressed mood, anxiety, fatigue, and insomnia.[9] Weight loss strategies in older adults should be implemented gradually with a combination of calorie restriction and individualized resistance exercise regimen. It is important to maintain adequate protein and vitamin requirements including calcium, vitamin D, and B12 throughout the weight loss process.[10] The role of bariatric surgery in severe or morbidly obese patients over 65 is unclear. In general, lifestyle modifications that can be maintained are the best initial strategies for weight control.

Exercise

Physiologic changes related to exercise can counter morbidity related to health disorders. These overall effects may be found in many organ systems seen in Table 46-1.[11] The Centers for Disease Control and Prevention (CDC) offers guidelines for older adults who are generally fit with no limiting health conditions (see Figure 46-3).[12] Exercise regimens must be adapted and closely supervised for individuals with health disorders.

Table 46-1 Overall effects of exercise in the elderly organ systems

Cardiovascular system	Decreased arterial stiffness Increased arterial compliance Improved blood pressure in hypertensive patients Reduction in hemoglobin AIC in diabetic patients Reduction in obesity related complications Decreased risk of developing coronary heart disease
Respiratory system	Improved pulmonary function including increased FEV 1 and FVC Improved quality of life
Cerebrovascular system	Improved cognitive function Decreased depressive symptoms Improved mood Enhanced neurogenesis Enhanced brain volume
Skeletal system	Improved balance Improved gait Improved muscle strength Improved functional independence Reduced risk of falls

Source: Adapted from reference 11.

Immunizations

All health-care providers should review immunization history and establish recommendations for vaccines based on the patient's need. The following list is a summary of the CDC-recommended vaccines that should be considered for geriatric office patients:[13]

- influenza inactivated vaccine (IIV, includes recombinant influenza vaccine), given intramuscularly or intradermally
- influenza, live attenuated influenza vaccine (LAIV), given intranasally

Adults aged 65 and older can be given the standard-dose IIV or, alternatively, high-dose IIV. Patients who are severely immunocompromised should receive the IIV rather than the LAIV. The dosage should be given every year in the fall or winter as soon as the vaccine is available.

- pneumococcal polysaccharide, given intramuscularly or subcutaneously
- pneumococcal conjugate, given intramuscularly

This vaccine is recommended for people aged 65 and older. Patient should receive one dose if unvaccinated or if the vaccination history is unknown. If the first dose was given before age 65 and five years have elapsed, a second dose should be administered.

- measles, mumps, rubella, given subcutaneously

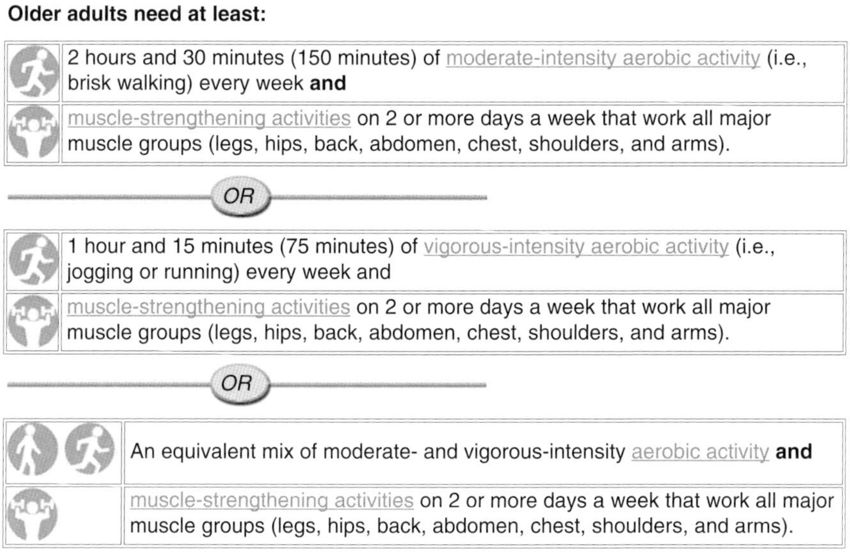

Figure 46-3 CDC guidelines on exercise: If you're 65 years of age or older, are generally fit, and have no limiting health conditions, you can follow the guidelines listed.

Patients who are born before 1957 are considered to be immune, but assessment of immunity through serology or documentation should be obtained by health-care professionals.

- varicella, given subcutaneously

All patients without evidence of immunity should be vaccinated. The vaccine should be given in two doses, four to eight weeks apart.

- hepatitis A, given intramuscularly

This is recommended for all adults who desire protection even without risk factors. For those patients older than 40 and within a two-week exposure to the virus, immune globulin is preferred over the vaccine. Other work, travel, and medical criteria may be considered for vaccine administration. The vaccine is given in two does, 6–18 month apart.

- hepatitis B, given intramuscularly

This is recommended for all adults who desire protection even without risk factors. Geriatric patients with HBs-Ag positive household contacts and sexual partners, other high-risk sexual behavior, health-care professionals, and people with chronic liver disease should receive the vaccine. The vaccine is given in three doses at zero, one, and six months.

- haemophilus influenza type b, given intramuscularly or subcutaneously

The vaccine is recommended only in those geriatric patients with a high risk for haemophilus infection such as asplenic patients and recipients of hematopoietic stem cell transplant (HSCT).

- meningococcal conjugate vaccine, given intramuscularly
- meningococcal polysaccharide vaccine, given subcutaneously

This vaccine should be given to geriatric patients with anatomic or functional asplenia or persistent complement component deficiency. Booster doses are given to these patients every five years.

- tetanus, diphtheria, pertussis, given intramuscularly (tetanus toxoid cannot be used in place of Tdap or Td)

This vaccine is recommended for patients who lack documentation of previous immunization. A Td booster is repeated every 10 years.

- zoster, given subcutaneously

This vaccine is recommended in patients 60 years and older. Patients are given a one-time dose if unvaccinated or even if they had a previous history of herpes zoster or chickenpox.

Visual acuity

The prevalence of visual acuity impairment is approximately 9% among older adults and can lead to significant risk for falls and a reduction in life quality. The most common reasons for visual impairment are refractive error, cataracts, and age-related macular degeneration. Risk factors for most forms of visual impairment are age. Other risk factors for cataracts include smoking, corticosteroid use, alcohol use, diabetes, exposure to ultraviolet light, and

African-American race. Smoking, family history, and Caucasian race are associated risk factors for age-related macular degeneration.

Screening for visual acuity impairment with a validated visual test is a method that can be performed in the primary care office. The American Congress of Obstetrics and Gynecology (ACOG) recommends evaluation and counseling about visual acuity screening for all women aged 65 and older.[14]

Hearing acuity

The most common cause of hearing loss is aging. Prevalence rates of up to 30% are found in the age group 65–74, and up to 45% in adults 75 years and older.[15, 16] Hearing loss can be due to a variety of reasons including congenital and various acquired reasons such as infection, loud noise, ototoxic medications, and head injury. Tinnitus or problems understanding speech are early signs. In the geriatric patient, presbycusis usually happens slowly over time and in both ears.

Screening tests can be utilized in the office. Visual inspection looking for anatomical abnormalities and signs of infection should be the first step. Additional assessment of the patient's hearing can be accomplished with physical diagnostic tests such as the whispered voice and finger rub near the ears. Screening questionnaires such as the Self-assessment of Communication (SAC) or the Hearing Handicap Inventory for the Elderly Screening Version (HHIE-S) may be used.[17] Screening should occur every three years.

Dental health

Geriatric patients are at risk for chronic oral conditions such as dental caries, periodontitis, benign mucosal lesions, and oral cancer. Increasing evidence exists that poor oral health can be associated with diabetes, cardiovascular disease, pneumonia, rheumatologic diseases, and wound healing.[18] Dental visits should be encouraged during gynecologic office visits.

Preventative screening for early detection of oral cancer may identify individuals with pre-cancerous lesions such as leukoplakia. Screening can be targeted to high-risk populations including individuals with a history of tobacco and alcohol usage. The most common screening method is visual inspection. There is no evidence that the use of adjunctive technologies such as toluidine blue, brush biopsy, or fluorescence imaging are useful to reduce oral cancer mortality.[19] The Cochrane review concluded some evidence exists that visual inspection might reduce the death rate in this high-risk population.[20]

Cardiovascular health

Cardiovascular disease is the leading cause of mortality and accounts for 42% of all deaths in people over 65. Preventive strategies to avoid development and complications of cardiovascular disease, including management of hypertension and lipid disorders, are most effective in prolonging the lifespan of the elderly.

Hypertension

High blood pressure is defined as systolic blood pressure of 140 mmHg or higher, or a diastolic pressure of 90 mmHg or higher. The diagnosis of hypertension is made when the elevated blood pressure measurements are taken at least during two visits over a period of one to several weeks.

Patients with a blood pressure less than 120/80 should be screened every two years; patients with a systolic blood pressure of 120 mmHg–139 mmHg or a diastolic blood pressure of 80 mmHg–90 mmHg should be screened every year.[21] See Chapter 42.

Dyslipidemia

Increased total cholesterol, increased low-density lipoprotein-cholesterol, and decreased high-density lipoprotein-cholesterol are significant risk factors for coronary heart disease. These changes in lipid profile can be genetic or acquired. Screening in asymptomatic women aged 45 years and older is recommended. The optimal screening interval is unknown, but it is reasonable to provide testing every five years or sooner if prior test results are close critical values requiring treatment.[22] See Chapter 43.

Coronary heart disease

Coronary heart disease is the leading cause of death in the United States in both men and women, accounting for nearly 16% of all deaths each year. The US Preventive Services Task Force (USPSTF) recommends against routine screening for coronary heart disease with an electrocardiography in patients who are asymptomatic.[23] However, the American College of Cardiology Foundation and the American Heart Association agree that the resting ECG evaluation is a reasonable tool for cardiovascular risk assessment in asymptomatic adults with hypertension or diabetes.

Asymptomatic carotid artery stenosis

Although asymptomatic carotid artery stenosis is a risk factor for stroke, it causes a relatively small proportion of strokes. There are no validated and reliable methods to determine risk for carotid artery stenosis. The USPSTF recommends against screening the general adult population.[24]

Abdominal aortic aneurysm

Abdominal aortic aneurysms affect about 1.0%–1.3% of women aged 50 years or older. The USPSTF recommends against routine screening for abdominal aortic aneurysm in asymptomatic women who never smoked. There is insufficient evidence to assess value of screening in women aged 65–75 years old who ever smoked.[25]

Mental health and cognition

After age 75 formal functional and cognitive status screening should be assessed, and a team approach should be utilized to make age appropriate decisions regarding care.[26] There is some cognitive decline in all patients as they age. Memory changes are the most commonly reported cognitive complaint in elderly patients; however, remote memory is relatively preserved. Older patients report less ability to learn or retain new information compared to younger individuals. History taking should be slow paced and follow-up instructions should be written for geriatric patients.

Many forms of dementia exist. Alzheimer's disease is the most prevalent of the primary neurodegenerative disorders. It is characterized by progressive memory decline in the absence of other medical or psychiatric causes. Confirmation of Alzheimer's disease is proven by neuropsychological testing with significant deficiency in two or more areas of cognition.[27] In addition to Alzheimer's disease, other medical conditions may impact cognitive function, including hypertension, diabetes, nutritional deficiencies, delirium, and medical problems resulting in oxygen deprivation including chronic obstructive pulmonary disease and obstructive sleep apnea. Depression is common in the elderly and can affect mental function. Medications including opiates, benzodiazepines, anticonvulsants, and antidepressants may also affect cognitive status. Mini cognition tests, six item screener test, and naming test have all been proposed as initial assessment tools in geriatric gynecology.[28] Reversible causes should be identified and treated, and medical conditions should be optimized.

Bone health

Osteoporosis

Bones are living dynamic structures with continued building, breakdown, and reformation. With osteoporosis, the balance of breakdown is greater than replacement. Health-care costs related to fragility fractures are reported in the billions of dollars and is a leading contributor to medical expense. Impact on quality of life is substantial. The relative risk of death following osteoporotic fractures of the hip and vertebrae are six- to ninefold greater in women aged 55–81. Half of patients who suffer hip fractures never regain full functional recovery, and 33% require long-term care.[29] Chapter 44 provides details on osteoporosis.

An essential component of bone health is fall prevention. Prior history of falling, gait and balance disturbances, and medications contribute to fall risk. Psychotropic, anticonvulsant, and antihypertensive drugs can also contribute to fall risk.[30] When an at-risk patient has been identified, referral for physical therapy assessment, home health consultation, and long-term geriatric specialist follow-up are recommended.

Avoiding bad habits, risk reduction strategies

Avoiding behavior with adverse health consequences is also important during the aging process. In the Nurses Health Study, middle-aged women who were normal weight, with a healthy diet and exercise routine, who did not smoke and consumed only moderate amounts of alcohol, had a significant reduction in their risk of coronary events compared to their counterparts.[31, 32]

Smoking cessation is discussed in Chapter 40. Moderate alcohol consumption, not exceeding two 8-ounce drinks per day, may have some survival benefit in relation to cardiovascular disorder. Excessive consumption can be associated with organ system dysfunction, including gastrointestinal effects (GI bleeding, esophageal and liver disorders), cardiovascular compromise (cardiomyopathy), and neurologic impairment (seizures, cerebellar degeneration, peripheral neuropathy, and cognitive disorders).[32]

Polypharmacy or the use of multiple medications in which some are redundant or not clinically indicated is a common problem in elderly populations.

Table 46-2 Skin disorders in the elderly

Common neoplasm	Appearance
Seborrheic keratosis (benign)	"Stuck-on appearance" brown/black papules or plaques, multiple, commonly found on face, trunk, and back
Skin tags (benign)	Flesh colored, multiple, usually 1-4 mm in size
Cherry angiomas (benign)	Small 1–4 mm in size, bright red or purple rounded lesions mostly found on upper extremities or trunk
Leukoplakia (premalignant)	White patches on mucosal surface, associated with alcohol/ tobacco
Malignant melanoma	Brown/black plaques with asymmetry, irregular borders, variegated color,
Basal cell carcinoma	Pearly papules, rolled edges, telangiectasia
Squamous cell carcinoma	Irregular growths with an indurated base
Keratoacanthoma (subtype of squamous cell carcinoma)	Erythematous dome-shaped,1–10 cm nodule with a keratin plug center

Source: Adapted from reference 34.

Recognition of this problem and coordinated care across medical disciplines can help avoid harmful drug interaction or overtreatment of medical conditions.

Avoidance of other risky behaviors should also be advised. Exposure to ultraviolet light may increase risk of cataracts and skin cancer. Sleep deprivation, cell phone use while driving, impaired reaction time, and lack of seat belt use may contribute to injury in motor vehicle accidents.

Cancer screening

Care regarding cancer detection is on a continuum with prevention, risk assessment, screening, diagnosis, intervention, recurrence surveillance, survivorship, and end-of-life decision making. The usefulness of cancer screening must be weighed against the ability to intervene and the relevance of other competing medical disorders that may also impact morbidity and mortality related to treatment. Upper age limits for screening vary by organizational guidelines. Life expectancy of less than five years may also dictate the relevance of screening for malignancy.

Skin cancer screening

Natural skin changes occur with the aging process such as loss of elasticity, dryness, fragility, and increased vascularity. Other skin changes such as wrinkling in areas other than smile lines, discoloration of skin, and rough textural changes can be due to environmental factors such as smoking, sun exposure, and excessive substance abuse.[33] It is important for clinicians to help educate patients about normal and abnormal skin changes. Assessing risk factors and screening for premalignant and malignant skin neoplasms is essential. There are many benign and malignant neoplasms that can afflict the geriatric population.[34] See Table 46-2.

Skin cancer is the most commonly diagnosed cancer. Melanoma accounts for only 5%–6% of skin cancer, but approximately 75% mortality from skin cancer.[33] Screening should begin with a history and discussion of risk factors. Specific risk factors for melanoma include family history, significant sun exposure, sunburns, fair-skinned patients over the age of 65, patients with atypical moles, and patients with 50 or more moles. According to the USPSTF, the evidence is insufficient to make a recommendation for screening; many advocate whole body examination as the best modality for screening.[35] The American Cancer Society recommends a monthly self-examination and a skin examination by a physician for people over 20 years at the periodic health encounter.

Cervical cancer screening

Cervical cancer is the third most common gynecologic cancer in the United States. In 2010, 11,818 women in the United Stated were diagnosed with cervical cancer.[36] Symptoms can include irregular vaginal bleeding or spotting, postcoital bleeding, and vaginal discharge.[37] Screening in the elderly varies according to medical organization, but in the general healthy screening population, pap testing can be discontinued at age 65.[38]

ACOG recommends in low-risk patients that screening be discontinued at age 65–70 if the patients have had three or more consecutive negative Pap smears and no abnormal results in 10 years; if the patient has risk factors such as immunosuppression, HIV, multiple sexual partners, DES in utero, continue screening at least 20 years after CIN 2–3 results. See Chapter 8 for cervical cancer screening.

Breast cancer screening

Breast cancer is the second most common malignancy in women. It is estimated that American women have a one in seven lifetime risk of breast cancer with a life expectancy of 85 years. In 2010, 206,966 women in the United States were diagnosed with breast cancer; 40,996 women in the United States died from breast cancer in 2010.[36] Breast cancer screening regimens vary among different organizations. USPTF recommendations indicate that biennial screening mammography in women aged 50–74 years has moderate certainty that the net benefit exists. For screening mammography in women 75 years or older, evidence is lacking and the balance of benefits and harms cannot be determined.[39]

Colon cancer screening

Colon cancer is the third most common cancer in women. In early disease patients may be asymptomatic. Weight loss, occult blood loss, and abdominal pain are all possible symptoms. In a postmenopausal woman with anemia, colon cancer must be considered highly in the differential.

The USPSTF recommends screening for colorectal cancer using fecal occult blood testing, sigmoidoscopy, or colonoscopy in adults beginning at age 50 years and continuing until age 75 years. The risks and benefits of these screening methods vary.[40]

The USPSTF recommends against routine screening for colorectal cancer in adults aged 76–85 years or older. There may be considerations that support colorectal cancer screening in an individual patient. The USPSTF concludes that the evidence is insufficient to assess the benefits and harms of computed tomographic colonography and fecal DNA testing as screening modalities for colorectal cancer.

ACOG recommends colonoscopy as the preferred method of colon cancer screening.

Lung cancer screening

The USPSTF recommends annual screening for lung cancer with low-dose computed tomography (LDCT) in adults aged 55–80 years who have a 30 pack-year smoking history and currently smoke or have quit within the past 15 years. Screening should be discontinued once a person has not smoked for 15 years or develops a health problem that substantially limits life expectancy or the ability or willingness to have curative lung surgery.[41]

Geriatric gynecology

Menopause

Most definitions of geriatric patients use 60–65 years as the age marker. The average age of menopause is 51 years, so menopause transition is typically complete in the geriatric population.

One study, however, noted that 7.8% of women continued to experience hot flushes, 20 years or more since menopause.[42] It is important to rule out other etiologies in the elderly including panic attack, hyperthyroidism, and drug-induced symptoms associated with selective estrogen receptor modulators.

Cochrane review of randomized trials suggests that antidepressants, gabapentin, and clonidine are nonhormonal pharmacologic interventions that may reduce hot flushes.[43] Limited prospective trials are available about the use of nonpharmacologic interventions to relieve these symptoms. Treatment of vasomotor symptoms is discussed in Chapter 31.

Vulvitis

Vulvar symptoms including pruritis, burning, and pain may be categories into infection (including candida), dermatoses (including contact dermatitis and lichen sclerosus), neurologic origin, or manifestations of systemic disorders. Vulvovaginal atrophy is a very common but treatable cause of vulvitis. Lesions of the vulva should be biopsied to rule out malignancy; pruritic lesions should engender concern about potential vulvar dysplasia. Vulvar swelling that is global may be associated with herpes simplex virus (HSV). Bartholin gland abscesses in the elderly should be investigated with a higher incidence of adenocarcinoma of the Bartholin gland occurring more commonly after menopause.

Vaginal bleeding

Benign causes of vaginal bleeding include vaginal atrophy, cervicitis, cervical polyps, endometrial polyps, and other endometrial pathology including endometrial hyperplasia. Precursors to cancer and frank malignancies including vulvar, vaginal, endometrial and cervical cancers are more prominently considered in elderly patients and should be adequately assessed. Ninety percent of cases of endometrial cancer are diagnosed after menopause. Assessment of the endometrium with either ultrasound solely or in combination with endometrial biopsy is warranted when unexplained bleeding occurs. (For more information about abnormal uterine bleeding, refer to Chapter 16.)

Abdominal pain

Assessment of abdominal pain in the elderly can be challenging. Presentations may be atypical and history taking may be challenged due to cognitive impairment. Elderly patients may have a blunted response reflected in vital signs. They can present late in the disease process.

Chronicity, location, and characteristics of the pain including alleviating and aggravating factors should be elicited to aid in the diagnosis. Physical exam including vital signs, abdominal exam, and rectovaginal exam support the narrowed differential. In the elderly population, leiomyomata cease increasing in size, adenomyosis and endometriosis are also quiescent. Pelvic masses of uterine or adnexal origin should be investigated. Gastrointestinal disorders including gastroenteritis, gastric/peptic ulcer, esophagitis diverticular disorders, appendicitis, biliary disorders, liver masses, irritable bowel syndrome (IBS), irritable bowel disease (IBD), pancreatitis, incarcerated hernia, bowel obstruction, and malignancy should also be considered. Colon cancer is the third most common cancer in women. Urinary etiologies including cystitis, pyelonephritis, and renal stones should also be considered. Dermatome-related pain may be associated with herpes zoster. Atypical causes of abdominal pain should be investigated, including aortic dissection, mesenteric ischemia, pericarditis, myocardial infarction, and lower lobe pneumonia and diabetic ketoacidosis.

Laboratory testing and imaging should be geared to assess broad scope of intraabdominal processes. If the patient is in acute distress regardless of age, hospitalization and acute surveillance is needed. A final diagnosis sometimes takes multiple office visits, so it is important to construct an ordered differential diagnosis with special attention to rule out life-threatening disorders such as vascular disorders and surgical emergencies.

Incontinence and pelvic organ prolapse

The causes and risk factors of urinary incontinence can include reversible conditions such as urinary tract infection (UTI), atrophic vaginitis, stool impaction, medication effect, caffeine, and alcohol. One of the main risk factors is older age that is associated with a hypoestrogenic state. There is a weakening of the levator ani and coccygeus muscles of the pelvic floor. Bladder capacity can also be decreased, which favors urge incontinence. Other associated factors that have been linked to incontinence include childbirth, obesity, smoking, diabetes, chronic cough, and cognitive impairment. Chapters 20 and 21 discuss incontinence and pelvic prolapse thoroughly.

Urinary incontinence can have a profound effect on a patient's quality of life. The prevalence increases with age. The general prevalence in elderly women is 30%–50%. Mixed and urge incontinence are more common in older women, whereas middle-aged women more frequently report stress incontinence. In the United States, the prevalence is higher among white women when compared to African-American, Hispanic, or Asian women.

Often patients are not forthcoming regarding urinary incontinence as many believe it is a "normal" aspect of aging with limited options for management. The first step in screening is to ask a direct question about urinary incontinence. An exploration of the patient's medical history and medication usage should be conducted to determine if these contribute to the incontinence.

There are no evidence-based screening guidelines for screening. However, there are several questionnaires that can be used for screening patients for urinary incontinence. For example, the Questionnaire for Urinary Incontinence Diagnosis (QUID) is a validated screening questionnaire used to diagnose stress or urge incontinence in women. A shorter questionnaire that can be used if time is a factor is the Bladder Control Self-Assessment Questionnaire (B-SAQ), which was designed as a screening tool for the presence of bothersome lower urinary tract symptoms in women.[44, 45]

Sexual health

Postmenopausal patients may report decreased libido or dyspareunia. It is important to take a careful history including assessment for depressed mood or marital discord. It is also essential to rule out sexual assault and elder abuse.

Dyspareunia may often be associated with vaginal atrophy. Nonhormonal lubricants are a first line of therapy. Often a maturation index is not indicated, and physical appearance alone may confirm the diagnosis. Testing to rule out fungal or bacterial infection should also be considered. In addition careful inspection of the vulva and vagina should be performed to rule out fissures from friction trauma and to assess for vulvar dermatoses including lichen sclerosus and lichen planus which can cause vulvar architectural changes including introital narrowing and scarring of the clitoral hood. If no physical changes beyond atrophy are noted and with no contraindications, a vaginal estrogen preparation can be used in the form of cream, pill, or ring. Patients must be counseled that the therapy takes time to have results. If the caliber of the vaginal introitus is small or vaginismus is noted, vaginal dilators can be prescribed.

Frailty

Frailty is defined as an age-associated progressive decline in physiologic systems resulting in low functional reserve with decreased ability to cope with chronic and acute health stressors.[46] The risk of frailty increases with age and can be found in up to 25% of patients over 85 years old.[47] It is twice as common in African-American than in Caucasian or Hispanic patients. Women are more predisposed than men.[45] Common manifestations of frailty include deterioration of function, mobility, cognition, nutrition, and endurance. Outcomes may include increased risk of falling, injury, hospitalization, disability, dependence, and overall mortality. The Fried criteria for recognizing frailty can be assessed in the office, including weight loss, muscle weakness, low physical activity, slow gait, and poor endurance (see Table 46-3). Other medical conditions are associated with the presence and rate of progression of frailty. Prevention, early intervention, and recognition of frailty should be a part of the gynecologic care plan for the elderly. Observation of the patient and her function over time can also provide useful clues. If frailty is suspected, the patient should be referred to a geriatrician for comprehensive investigation.

End-of-life decision making

The end-of-life decision discussion with patients can be daunting and time-consuming for physicians and patients. At first glance, it is masked in the overall theme of death, which makes this a difficult conversation. However, the end-of-life decision making is not just about terminal illness. It is more about the last phase of the human life cycle.[40]

The discussion should include making the patient aware that she has a right to decide about the amount of future medical treatment. It should be stressed that putting medical decisions in place early avoids conflicts and can decrease the burden of decision making for family members. Patients may want to choose a proxy in case there is a development of patient incompetence in the future. Physicians should clarify that their job in the discussion revolves around education and facilitation of medical care, and a physician cannot make decisions on a patient's behalf.

In a busy practice, the discussion of end-of-life decision making can be done over a few visits. The conversation may begin as a part of the intake form. The form can ask direct questions about the patient's desire to have the discussion; it could ask direct questions about current illnesses and the extension of care she wants provided. The form can also address questions of proxy. Assuming competence,

Table 46-3 Frailty defined as three or more of the listed criteria

Determinant	Description	
Weight loss	Unintentional weight loss of 10 or more pounds in one year	
Exhaustion/poor endurance	Exhaustion defined by self-report Everything I did was an effort last week I could not get going in the last week	
Low physical activity	Less than 270 kcals expenditure per week on the activity scale based on the short form of the Minnesota leisure time activity questionnaire	
Muscle weakness	Body mass index (BMI) to grip strength comparison	
	BMI	Grip strength (kg)
	≤23	≤17
	23.1 to 26	≤17.3
	26.1 to 29	≤18
	>29	≤21
Slow gait (female criteria)	Walk time for 15 feet:	
	Height ≤159 cm	≥7 seconds
	Height >159 cm	≥6 seconds

direct questioning of patients can be utilized at the routine visit. Patient reflection can be initiated with such question as "This is a minor problem, but if you become seriously ill one day, would you hope that I tell you directly or that I tell your spouse?" or "How do you fell about what I have just said about problem X or Y? Does it make you think of the future and how you would like physicians to treat you?"[48]

Although the end-of-life decision making discussion should ideally be made prior to the onset of a significant illness, it is often not until patients are faced with decisions about management of these medical conditions that the conversation occurs with the physician and family members. Findings suggest that advance directives and physician-patient discussions that focus on acceptable health states and valued life activities may be better suited to patients' end-of-life care goals than those that focus on specific medical interventions, such as cardiopulmonary resuscitation.[49] Overall, older patients and their families may benefit the most from a conversation regarding end-of-life decisions prior to illness.

References

1. Ortman JM, Velkoff VA, Hogan H. *An Aging Nation: The Older Population in the United States*, Current Population Reports. Washington, DC: US Census Bureau. 2014, P25-1140.
2. Parekh AK, Burton MB. The challenge of multiple comorbidity for the US health care system. *JAMA.* 2010;**303**:1303–1304.
3. Morris M. Nutritional determinants of cognitive aging and dementia. *Proceedings of the Nutrition Society.* 2012 Feb;**71**(1):1–13.
4. Bermudez O, Dwyer J. Identifying Elders at Risk of Malnutrition: A universal challenge. United Nations Standing Committee on Nutrition. SCN News, Number 19 Nutrition and Healthy Agents 1999.
5. Agarwal E., Miller M, Yaxley A, Isenring E. Malnutrition in the elderly: A narrative review. *Maturitas* 2013;**76**:296–302.
6. Rubenstein L, Harker J, Salva A, et al. Screening for undernutrition in geriatric practice: developing the short form mininutritional assessment (MNA-SF). *J Gerontol A Biol Sci Med Sci.* 2001 Jun;**56**(6):M366–72.
7. National Center for Chronic Disease Prevention and Health Promotion. *Obesity: Halting the Epidemic by Making Health Easier.* Atlanta, GA: Centers for Disease Control and Prevention; 2011. Available at: www.cdc.gov/chronicdisease/resources/publications/aag/pdf/2011/Obesity_AAG_WEB_508.pdf. Accessed September 25, 2013.
8. Hedley AA, Ogden CL, Johnson CL, et al. Prevalence of overweight and obesity among US children, adolescents and adults, 1999–2002. *JAMA.* 2004;**291**(23):2847–2850.
9. Patterson RE, Frank LL, Kristal AR, et al. A comprehensive examination of health conditions associated with obesity in older adults. *Am J Prev Med.* 2004;**27**(5):385–390.
10. Jarosz PA, Bellar A. Age-appropriate obesity treatment. *Nurse Practitioner.* 2008:**33**(5):24–31.
11. Ackerman JP, Heckman GA, McKelvie RS. Exercise capacity and aging. *American Journal of Lifestyle Medicine.* 2014 July. Available at: http://ajl.sagepub.com/content/9/4/252.abstract?rss=1. Accessed December 23, 2015.
12. CDC physical activity basics. Available at: www.cdc.gov/physicalactivity/basics/older_adults. Accessed December 23, 2015.
13. CDC guidelines on immunization. Available at: www.cdc.gov/vaccines/schedules/hcp/adult.html#recs. Accessed December 23, 2015.
14. US Preventive Services Task Force. Screening for impaired visual acuity in older adults: recommendation letter. *Ann Intern Med.* 2009;**151**:37–43.
15. Lin F. One in five Americans has a hearing loss. [Press release]. (November 2011). Available at: www.hopkinsmedicine.org/news/media/releases/one_in_five_americans_has_hearing_loss. Accessed December 23, 2015.
16. National Institute on Deafness and Other Communication Disorders. National Institutes of Health. Quick statistics. Available at: www.nidcd.nih.gov/health/statistics/Pages/quick.aspx. Accessed December 23, 2015.
17. US Preventive Services Task Force. Screening for hearing loss in older adults: recommendation letter. *Am Fam Physician.* 2013 Jan 15;**87**(2). Available at http://www.aafp.org/afp/2013/0115/od1.html. Accessed December 23, 2015.
18. Gonsalves W, Wrightson A, Henry R. Common oral conditions in older persons. *Am Fam Physician.* 2008 Oct 1; **78**(7):845–852.
19. US Preventive Services Task Force. Screening for oral cancer: final recommendation statement. 2013. Available at: www.uspreventiveservicestaskforce.org/uspstf13/oralcan/oralcanfinalrec.htm. Accessed December 23, 2015.
20. Brocklehurst P, Kujan O, O'Malley LA, et al. Screening programmes for the early detection and prevention of oral cancer. The Cochrane Library. Available at: http://onlinelibrary.wiley.com/doi/10.1002/14651858.CD004150.pub4/abstract. Accessed December 23, 2015.

21. US Preventive Services Task Force. Screening for high blood pressure: US Preventive Services Task Force reaffirmation recommendation statement. AHRQ Publication No. 08-05105-EF-2, December 2007. *Ann Intern Med.* 2007 Dec 4;**147**(11):783–786.
22. US Preventive Services Task Force. Screening for lipid disorders in adults: US Preventive Services Task Force Recommendation Statement. June 2008. Available at: www.uspreventiveservicestaskforce.org/uspstf08/lipid/lipidrs.htm. Accessed December 23, 2015.
23. US Preventive Services Task Force. Screening for coronary heart disease with electrocardiography: recommendation statement. AHRQ Publication No. 11-05158-EF-2. July 2012. Available at: www.uspreventiveservicestaskforce.org/uspstf11/coronarydis/chdfinalrs.htm. Accessed December 23, 2015.
24. US Preventive Services Task Force. Screening for asymptomatic carotid artery stenosis: recommendation statement. AHRQ Publication No. 13-05178-EF-2. Available at: www.uspreventiveservicestaskforce.org/uspstf13/cas/casfinalrs.htm. Accessed December 23, 2015.
25. US Preventive Services Task Force. Screening for abdominal aortic aneurysm: final recommendation statement. AHRQ Publication No. 14-05202-EF-2. Available at: www.uspreventiveservicestaskforce.org/uspstf14/abdoman/abdomanfinalrs.htm. Accessed December 23, 2015.
26. Reuben DB. Medical care for the final years of life: "when you're 83, it's not going to be 20 years." *JAMA.* 2009;**302**(24):2686–2694.
27. Craft S, Cholerton B, Reger M. Cognitive changes associated with normal and pathological aging. In: *Hazzard's Geriatric Medicine and Gerontology*, sixth edition. New York: McGraw-Hill, 2009; chapter 62. Available at: http://accessmedicine.mhmedical.com/content.aspx?bookid=371&sectionid=41587676. Accessed December 23, 2015.
28. Miller KL, Baraldi CA. Geriatric gynecology: promoting health and avoiding harm. *Am J Obstet Gynecol.* 2012 Nov;**207**(5):355–367.
29. Wells GA et al. Alendronate for the primary and secondary prevention of osteoporotic fractures in postmenopausal women. *Cochrane Reviews.* 2008 Jan 23;**1**:CD001155. DOI: 10.1002/14651858. 30. CD001155.pub2.
30. Tinetti ME, Kumar C. The patient who falls: "it's always a trade off." *JAMA.* 2010;**303**(3):258–266.
31. Colditz GA, Manson JE, Hankinson SE. The Nurses' Health Study 20-year contribution to the understanding of health among women. *Journal of Women's Health.* 1997 Feb;**6**(1):49–62.
32. Phelan EA, Paniagua MA, Hazzard WR. Preventive gerontology: strategies for optimizing health across the lifespan. In: *Hazzard's Geriatric Medicine and Gerontology*, sixth edition. New York: McGraw-Hill, 2009: chapter 9. Available at: http://accessmedicine.mhmedical.com/content.aspx?sectionid=41587612&bookid=371&Resultclick=2&q=chapter%209. Accessed December 23, 2015.
33. Gordon ML, Hecker MS. Care of the skin at midlife: diagnosis of pigmented lesions. *Geriatrics* 1997;**52**(8):67–69.
34. Jafferany M, Huynh TV, Silverman MA, Zaidi Z. Geriatic dermatoses: a clinical review of skin diseases in an aging population. *Int J Dermatol.* 2012 May;**51**(5):509–522.
35. US Preventive Services Task Force. Screening for skin cancer: recommendation letter. *Ann Intern Med.* 2009;**150**:188–193.
36. US Cancer Statistics Working Group. *United States Cancer Statistics: 1999–2010 Incidence and Mortality Web-based Report.* Atlanta, GA: Department of Health and Human Services, Centers for Disease Control and Prevention, and National Cancer Institute; 2013.
37. Miller KL, Baraldi CA. Geriatric gynecology: promoting health and avoiding harm. *Am J Obstet Gynecol* 2012;**207**(5):355–367.
38. US Preventive Services Task Force. Screening for *cervical cancer*, topic page. April 2012. Available at: www.uspreventiveservicestaskforce.org/uspstf/uspscerv.htm. Accessed December 23, 2015.
39. US Preventive Services Task Force. Screening for breast cancer, topic page. July 2010. Available at: www.uspreventiveservicestaskforce.org/uspstf/uspsbrca.htm. Accessed December 23, 2015.
40. US Preventive Services Task Force. Screening for colorectal cancer, topic page. Available at: www.uspreventiveservicestaskforce.org/uspstf/uspscolo.htm. Accessed December 23, 2015.
41. US Preventive Services Task Force. Screening for lung cancer, topic page. Available at: www.uspreventiveservicestaskforce.org/uspstf/uspslung.htm. Accessed December 23, 2015.
42. Huang AJ, Grady D, Jacoby VL, et al. Persistent hot flushes in older postmenopausal women. *Arch Intern Med.* 2008;**168**(8):840–846.
43. Rada G, Capurro D, Pantoja T, et al. Non-hormonal interventions for hot flushes in women with a history of breast cancer. *Cochrane Database Syst Rev.* 2010 Sep 8;**9**:CD004923. DOI: 10.1002/14651858.CD004923.pub2.
44. Deng DY. Urinary incontinence in women. *Med Clin North Am.* 2011;**95**(1):101–109.
45. Rakel R. *Textbook of Family Medicine: Presentation of Urinary Incontinence.* Philadelphia: Elsevier, 2014.

46. Xue QL. The frailty syndrome: definition and natural history. *Clin Geriatr Med.* Feb 2011;**27**(1):1–15.
47. Fried LP, Tangen CM, Walston J, et al. Frailty in older adults: evidence for a phenotype. *J Gerontol A Biol Sci Med Sci.* 2001;**56**(3):M146–M157.
48. Nazerali N. Counseling the elderly on decision making for the end of life: practical issues for physicians. *Can Fam Physician.* 1995;**41**:829–833.
49. Rosenfeld KE. End-of-life decision making: a qualitative study of elderly individuals. *J Gen Intern Med.* 2000;**15**(9):620–625.

Chapter 47

Office care of disabled patients

Natalie E. Roche, Lena Nguyen, and Ondrea McKay

Introduction

The definition of "disability" varies, but a common meaning as reported by the US Department of Health and Human Services in 2010 is the inability to perform activities of daily living. Activities of daily living include walking, standing, sitting, climbing steps, carrying items without assistance. The limitations in activities can be caused by physical and or by mental diseases. The most common cause of disability in women is arthritis or rheumatism.[1]

The World Health Organization (WHO) published the International Classification of Functioning, Disability, and Health (ICF) in 2001. The ICF defines disability as an umbrella term for impairments, activity limitations, and restrictions. ICF describes disability as the interaction between a person's health condition, personal status, and their environment.[2]

The total percentage of people in the United States with some disability is 20%. According to the US Census, the number of disabled females reported in 2005–2010 census data is 28.6 million, representing 18.3% of the total population of Americans.[3, 4] The number of disabled females is rising as the survival rates improve for many illnesses. Additionally, the population of elderly women is increasing; at 65 years or greater more than 50% of women have some disability.[5]

Women with disabilities need the same general health care as women without disabilities with the addition of care to address their specific needs. Women with disabilities may not receive regular health screening within the recommended guidelines.

Scope of the problem

The presence of a disability does not exclude the possibility of good health for a patient. Disabled persons should have an expectation of good health and should be encouraged to achieve the most optimal health status possible.

The prevention of disease and promotion of good health should be a basic goal in our health-care system for all women. The access to preventive and treatment services should be available to all women regardless of their status as able or disabled. Preventive services should include counseling, patient education, and screening for diseases. The goal is to prevent disease or to diagnose and treat disease in the early stages to minimize health consequences.

Disabled females can find it difficult to complete prevention milestones and to achieve maximum health promotion when compared to their able counterparts.

In the years 2008 to 2009, the Centers for Disease Control and Prevention (CDC) reported a higher inactivity rate for adults with disabilities of 22% compared to 10% in the able population. There were higher percentages of obesity in the disabled population at 37.6% versus 23.8% for the able population.

Women with disabilities may be more vulnerable to secondary conditions (urinary tract infection, pressure ulcers); comorbid conditions (increased diabetes in schizophrenic patients), increased health risk behaviors (sedentary lifestyle, obesity) and lower life expectancy from certain diseases. The need for adequate screening and early diagnosis in this population is without question however the patients may experience a range of barriers to health care.[6, 7]

Physical accessibility to care is the most obvious barrier to disabled women with physical limitations. [6] Physical barriers include stairs, inaccessible parking areas and doorways, poor signage, inadequate toilet facilities and public phones.

Patients may also encounter health-care providers with inadequate skills to meet their needs and are four times more likely to report bad treatment and three

Office Care of Women, ed. Martin E. Olsen and Botros Rizk. Published by Cambridge University Press.

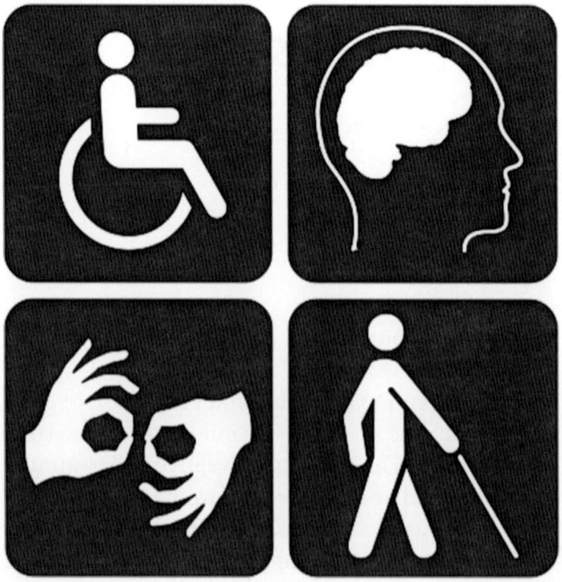

Figure 47-1 Handicapped signs.

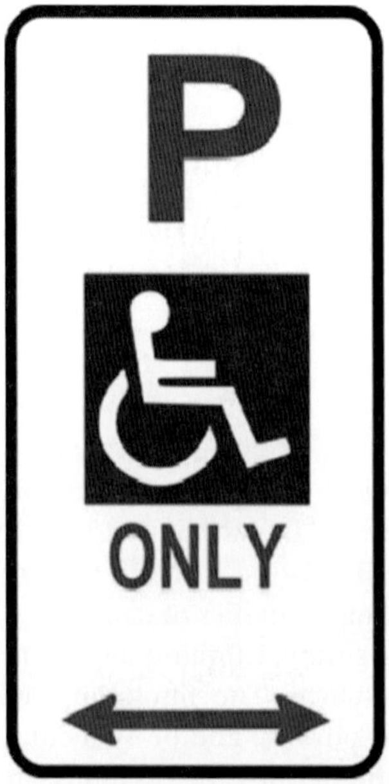

Figure 47-2 Handicapped parking signs.

times more likely to be denied care according to the WHO.[6]

Requirements of the American Disabilities Act of 1990

The US federal government requires through the America Disabilities Act (ADA) of 1990 that barriers to access be removed. Such barriers might prevent a patient with a disability from obtaining services that are available to individuals in the absence of a disability. The law states:

> A public accommodation shall take those steps that may be necessary to ensure that no individual with a disability is excluded, denied services, segregated or otherwise treated differently than other individuals because of the absence of auxiliary aids and services, unless public accommodation can demonstrate that taking those steps would fundamentally alter the nature of goods, services, facilities, privileges, advantages or accommodation being offered or would result in undue burden (i.e. significant difficulty or expense).[8]

Private hospitals and medical offices are covered by Title III of the ADA as places of public accommodation. Public hospitals, clinics, and medical offices operated by state and local governments are covered by Title II of the ADA as programs of the public entities.

Both Title II and Title III of the ADA require that health-care providers give individuals with disabilities:

> Full and equal access to their health care services and facilities; and Reasonable modifications to policies, practices, and procedures when necessary to make health care services fully available to individuals with disabilities, unless modifications would fundamentally alter the nature of the services.

(See Figures 47-1, 47-2, 47-3, and 47-4.)

All buildings are subject to accessibility requirements. Under Title III facilities are required to remove architectural barriers where achievable. If barrier removal is not readily achievable the entity must make service available through alternative methods if those methods are achievable.

Doctors' offices are required to have:

- accessible exam rooms including doorways with a width of at least 32 inches when the door is open 90 degrees and clear floor and turning space
- accessible medical equipment including adjustable height exam tables and chairs
- elements to stabilize and support patients for transfer to the exam table
- safety and comfort measures on the exam table such as rails, strops, stabilization cushions, wedges or rolled towels
- adequate staff training to aid patient in transfer to and from exam tables [9]

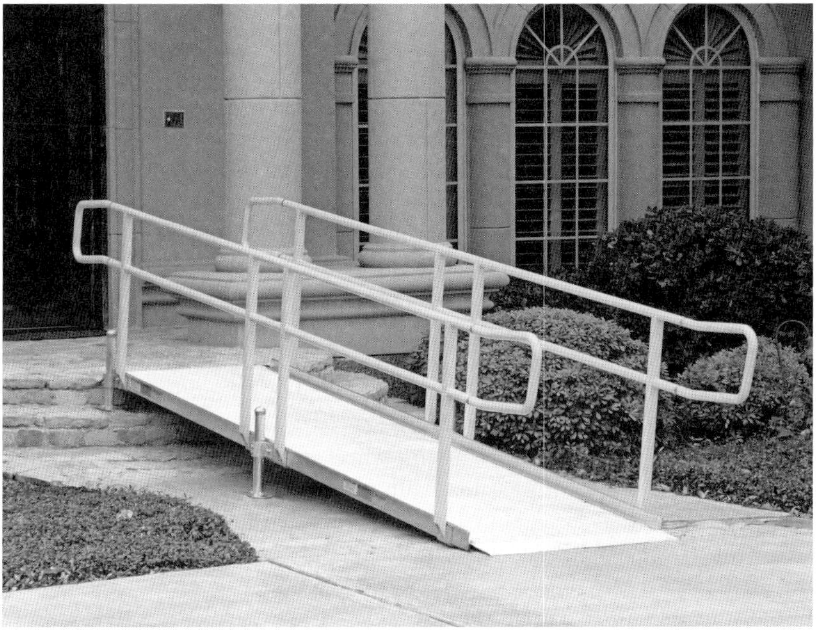

Figure 47-3 Handicapped access ramp.

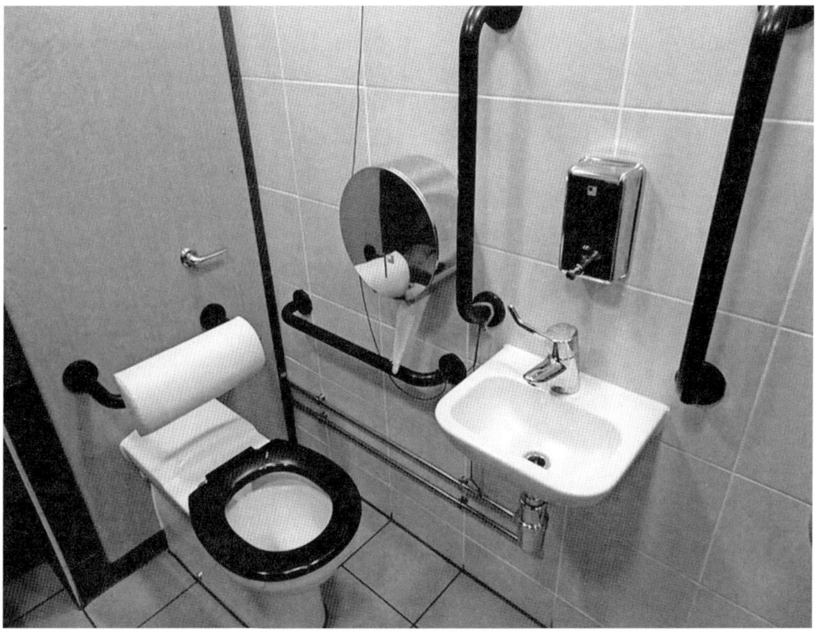

Figure 47-4 Handicapped toilet.

Failure to comply with ADA requirements can lead to stiff penalties. The Department of Justice can file lawsuits in federal court to enforce the ADA law. Under Title III of the ADA civil penalties of up to \$55,000 for the first violation and \$110,000 for subsequent violations can be levied.

Primary and preventive gynecologic care for the disabled women

The care of all women has to be tailored to the needs of the individual patient. The care of the disabled women is more challenging because of the additional areas that need to be addressed for a successful patient visit.

The care is also more challenging because 27.4% of disabled patients reported financial barriers to obtaining health care. This patient population has lower employment and wages; this is associated with greater reliance on public health insurance (Medicaid and Medicare in the United States) and has a higher number of uninsured patients.[7]

The care of the disabled patient begins prior to the actual patient visit. The office must have scheduling capability that will allow the hearing impaired patients to make appointments using a telecommunication device for the deaf (TDD) or teletypewriter (TYY) or telephone relay service (TTY). (See Box 47-1.)

The staff should inquire about special needs at the time an appointment is scheduled so that arrangements can be made to assist the patient with deaf interpreters, transportation, directions for use of handicapped accessible entrances, elevators to accommodate stretchers, and recommendation to empty the bladder, rectum, and ostomy bags before the visit in patients with neurogenic dysfunction/stomas, etc. (See Figures 47-2, 47-3, and 47-4.) The staff should determine if the disabled patient gives consent for exam and treatment. If the patient does not give consent the guardian or authorized caregiver should be instructed to accompany the patient. The guardian will be required to give written consent for the care provided to the patient.[10, 22]

BOX 47-1 Auxiliary aids and services

Qualified interpreters on-site or through video remote interpreting (VRI) services; note takers; real-time computer-aided transcription services; written materials; exchange of written notes; telephone handset amplifiers; assistive listening devices; assistive listening systems; telephones compatible with hearing aids; closed caption decoders; open and closed captioning, including real-time captioning; voice, text, and video-based telecommunications products and systems, including text telephones (TTYs), videophones, and captioned telephones, or equally effective telecommunications devices; videotext displays; accessible electronic and information technology; or other effective methods of making aurally delivered information available to individuals who are deaf or hard of hearing.

American with Disabilities Act of 1990 (ADA) 42 USC §§ 36.303 (2000).

Upon arrival, the staff should make inquiries regarding the level of assistance required by the patient. Transportation difficulties are common for patients with disabilities and flexibility regarding appointment time should be considered at the time the appointment is made. Some patient's will need assistance completing registration and history forms and this should be done in a way that is private for each patient. The reception desk should have a location with wheel chair height to facilitate communication with wheel chair bound patients.

Some patients will need help when called to the consultation or examination room in the office. The staff should ask for guidance from the patient regarding the type of assistance she would like to receive. (See Table 47-1.)

The history for a new patient should be comprehensive with special attention to a complete medication history. A dialogue should occur between the patient and provider regarding chronic medical problems and the type and severity of the disability, past gynecologic exams and the patient's concerns about the current visit. The health-care providers may need to familiarize themselves with the patient's disability prior to the visit to allow for maximum efficiency on the day of the visit. Patients who require an interpreter or the help of an assistant for the history should be addressed by the provider and care should be taken to avoid focus on the interpreter/assistant.

Visually impaired patients should be asked for guidance regarding their method of orientation to a new environment. They will need help to find the exam room and the exam gown.

The staff should be trained in safe methods for transfer from wheelchair or stretcher to the examination table. Positioning of patients for the pelvic exam will be a challenge for patients with joint restrictions, contractures, and spasticity. The use of water resistant pads, draw sheets, padded stirrups, bootleg stirrups, rolled pillows/towels, and wedge may be helpful. Positioning other than the standard lithotomy position may be needed to comfortably position some patients. Use of diamond, knee chest, M-shape, V-shape, lateral, elevation of hips on a roll, and McRoberts positioning may be helpful in facilitating

Table 47-1 Gyn visit flowsheet for examination of the disabled woman

1. Schedule visit
   a) Schedule appointment using TDD, TY, TTY for hearing impaired
   b) Interpreter, transportation
   c) Give instructions for accessible parking and entrance ramps
   d) Schedule additional time and book at low volume session
   e) Determine if patient signs consents if not advise of need for guardian written consent
   f) Advise medical staff of impending visit so patient contact can be initiated for special instructions to empty stomas, bladder, rectum if indicated
2. Visit intake
   a) Inquire about type of assistance needed, provide help with registration forms if needed
   b) Accompany patient to consult or exam room if requested
   c) Give assistance with patient history forms if requested
   d) Accompany patient to exam room if requested and give assistance with gowning, transfer to exam table
   e) Provide help with positioning on exam table as directed by patient
   f) Assist with dressing and transfer off exam table as directed by patient
3. End visit
   a) Get feedback from patient about visit experience
   b) Schedule follow-up
   c) Give patient appropriate educational materials (e.g., large print, braille)

the pelvic exam. (See Figure 47-5.) Some patients with negative previous experiences or spasticity may benefit from a small dose of an anxiolytic or analgesic before the pelvic examination. Pap smear and genital polymerase chain reaction (GC Chlamydia PCR) can be obtained without a speculum. Some patients have to be examined on a stretcher or bed and the pelvic exam can be performed with the hips elevated on a roll or bedpan with the speculum inverted to facilitate visualization of the cervix. A subset of patients may require pelvic examination under sedation or general anesthesia.

BOX 47-2 Assistive listening devices and alerting systems

There are many assistive listening devices and alerting systems available for those in need. These systems often work by amplifying an existing tone, using flashing lights or vibrations to alert people with hearing loss to environmental sounds. Examples of some of these devices include:

- *Baby cry signaler:* It has an adjustable sensitivity dial to pick up the softest sound and send a signal.
- *Doorbell signaler*
- *Smoke alarm signaler:* Some alarms have built in strobe lights.
- *Telephone signaler:* One type of signaler plugs directly into the telephone line and electrical outlet. Another type can be attached to the side of the telephone to pick up the sound of the bell.
- *Wake-up alarm signaler:* Signalers vary from portable alarm clocks with built-in strobe lights to alarm clocks with a build-in outlet where a lamp or vibrating alert can be plugged in.

Care is indicated to choose the appropriate-sized warm speculum and the selective use of lidocaine gel will facilitate the pelvic examination.

Patients with cognitive impairment, past sexual abuse, or previous painful pelvic examinations may need the annual gynecologic visit separated into two or three visits. The history followed by a general physical examination can be done as a single visit, leaving the pelvic exam for a separate visit. Multiple visits may allow the patient to develop familiarity and comfort with the office environment and staff.[22]

Examination of the perineum for signs of poor hygiene, vulvovaginitis, and signs of sexually transmitted diseases (STD) and for cuts, burns, and bruises is indicated; these may be suggestive of sexual abuse.[11] Sexually transmitted disease (STD) screening should be done in the same frequency as for able females. Women who are disabled may have limitations in barrier method use and may be therefore be at increased risk for STD acquisition. Urine STD screens are helpful in women for whom speculum exam are difficult or impossible in the office setting. Education about STD prevention should be a priority. Prior education may be suboptimal due to false assumptions about the sexual behavior of disabled women.

BOX 47-3 Telecommunications devices

There are a number of telecommunications devices that are available for use, including:

- *Amplified ringers:* Various types of ringers can be attached to a telephone line to inform a person who is hard of hearing that the telephone is ringing.
- *Amplified telephone:* Numerous telephones have built-in amplifiers that vary in range from 25 to 55 decibels. Many of these telephones have variable tone selectors and loud ringers.
- *Portable phone amplifier:* A lightweight battery operated device with an adjustable volume control that fits over the listening end of the handset.
- *TTY (sometimes referred to as TDD):* Has keyboard with a visual display screen that allows people to communicate with each other over the telephone lines by typing and reading their conversations. With appropriate software and equipment, computers can function as TTYs. Portable and wireless TTYs are also available.
- *Voice carry over (VCO) telephone:* For people who are unable to hear over the telephone but prefer to use their voice to communicate VCO telephone calls must be made through a relay service.
- *Braille embossers:* These transfer computer-generated text into embossed Braille output.

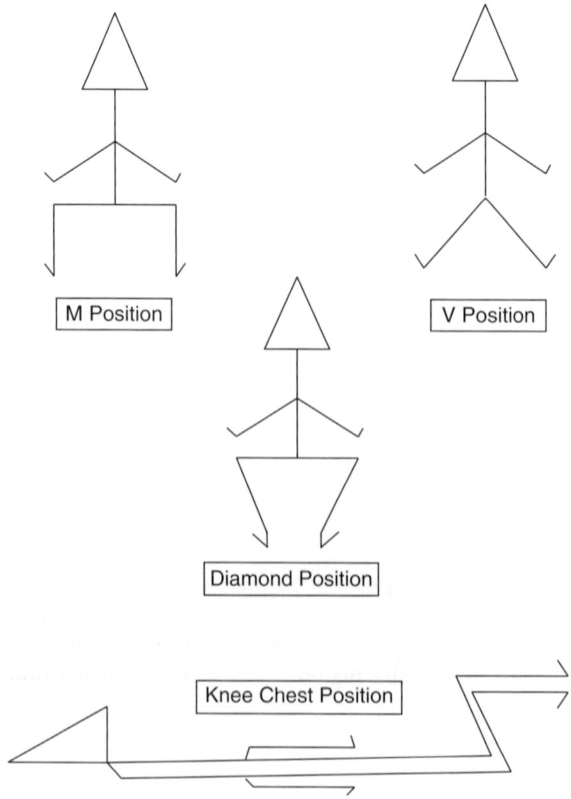

Figure 47-5 Positions for gynecological exam of the disabled woman.

Cancer screening is performed less often in women with disabilities. Fewer Pap smears and slightly fewer mammograms are performed (a 72.3% prevalence of mammography screening has been reported) in this patient population. Changes in Pap smear screening recommendations decrease the number of pap smears required for most women. The schedule of the three-to-five-year cervical cancer screening falls in line with the recommendation of ACOG's Special Issues in Womens' Health which suggests a pelvic exam every three years for patients with disabilities that require general anesthesia for the pelvic examination.[12, 13]

Breast cancers are the leading cause of cancer-related deaths among all women in the United States. Many women with disability face substantial barriers in obtaining mammograms. According to the CDC, women 50–74 years of age with a disability were less likely to obtain breast cancer screening due to limited health literacy, less self-efficacy, lack of provider recommendation, lack of access to the service, and communication barriers. The primary reasons for failure to receive a mammogram were physical limitations, lack of referral, and patient underestimation of risk. Mammography equipment is now available that can facilitate mammogram examination in women with mobility issues. The equipment is not available in all locations, but resources can be identified at www.bhawd.org. Patients with mobility issues that prevent breast self-exam have the option of having a partner or caregiver trained to perform the examination.

Autonomic stress syndrome/ autonomic dysreflexia

Patients with high spinal cord injuries present a special challenge for health-care providers because of the risk of autonomic dysreflexia.[9]

Autonomic dysreflexia (AD) is a syndrome where afferent impulses triggered by painful stimuli enter the spinal cord and start reflex arcs that are not modulated by higher centers. The syndrome occurs in patients with spinal cord lesions at or above T10 particularly those above T6. Lesions at these levels prevent the normal hypothalamic control over sympathetic spinal reflexes.[14]

Symptoms include severe hypertension with headache, respiratory distress, bradycardia, arrhythmia, diaphoresis, tingling, flushing, piloerection in dermatomes above the spinal cord lesions and nasal stuffiness.

Blood pressure can be affected by AD. The severity of the hypertension can be extreme with blood pressure elevations in excess of 300/150. Untreated AD can lead to intracranial hemorrhage, coma, and death.

Multiple stimuli can trigger AD including any manipulation of the cervix, bladder or rectum, as well as strong suprapubic pressure, bladder distention, disimpaction of the rectum, excessive deep breathing, and immersion of the feet in cold water.

The best management of this syndrome is avoidance. The best ways to prevent AD is to have the patient empty the bladder to avoid over distention and to empty the rectum to avoid fecal impaction.

The pelvic examination can be performed using a speculum coated with anesthetic jelly and the use of nifedipine 30 mg sublingual before office procedures that can elicit AD.

Treatment of AD involves the use of rapid acting antihypertensive, cardiac and blood pressure monitoring and transfers from the ambulatory facility to the hospital setting.

Violence and abuse

Patients with disabilities have higher rates of abuse by partners than their able counterparts and have a risk of abuse by caregivers. Women with disabilities who are abused experience longer durations of abuse. Patients may experience fear of loss of assistance if they report abuse by caregivers. The standard screening used for detection of abuse of women in the office setting does not address withholding assistance or assistive devices such as canes, wheel chairs, and teletypewriters. The patients may also experience neglect, inadequate provision of care, withholding of medications in addition to physical, emotional and sexual abuse. The American College of Obstetrics and Gynecology (ACOG) has an abuse assessment screen that addresses the issues specific to disabled women. Patients who want to leave abusive relationships may have difficulty finding accessible shelters to accommodate their disabilities. The use of state resources to find shelter placement may be needed. State reporting requirements for abuse of disabled persons vary from state to state and health-care providers will need to familiarize themselves with state law.[11, 15]

Sexuality

Health-care providers often views disabled women as asexual; this is a common misconception. Sexual desire is similar to able women. Rates of sexual activity in disabled women vary with age of onset of the disability, degree of social isolation, and the amount of social support available.

The gynecologic visit is an opportunity to identify issues related to sexual function, contraception, STD diagnosis and treatment, and fertility issues.[14, 30]

Sexual dysfunction

Women with disabilities can experience the same range of sexual dysfunction as the able population. There are special concerns about the effect of medications for chronic illness and physical limitations on sexuality in this population. Medications such as tranquilizers, antidepressants, antispasmodics, and antihypertensive may negatively affect sexual satisfaction and performance.

Sexual adaptations and adjustments may be needed for patients with physical disabilities that limit mobility. The health-care providers can be instrumental in giving guidance that will promote communication between sexual partners and encourage the creativity and experimentation that will be needed to develop a satisfactory sexual experience.

Contraception

Sexually active disabled women who are at risk for pregnancy will need contraceptive counseling and management. The special considerations in this population include the difficulty with barrier contraception for developmentally delayed women and women with mobility issues. The recommendation that all women have their male partners use condoms to prevent STD if not in a monogamous relationship is standard. In the absence of condom use, education about risk reduction and a schedule for STD testing should be established. Long-acting reversible contraception (LARC), including intrauterine device (IUD) and contraceptive implants, offers the highest effectiveness and lowest failure rates. The ease of placement will vary depending on the disability of the individual woman. If sedation or general anesthesia is needed for the placement, the risk versus benefit of LARC must be weighed against alternative contraceptive. Oral contraceptives are safe and effective and have the added benefit of decreasing menstrual flow and the number of bleeding episodes per year. The pills should be used with caution in wheelchair bound patients if there is a higher risk of DVT. Patients on anticonvulsant therapy will need a dose adjustment of their anticonvulsant medication; consultation with the physician managing that aspect of the patient's care may be required. The use of Nuvaring® will be limited in patients with mobility issues that inhibit or prevent placement. The use of the contraceptive patch is safe and effective form of contraception but the patch may be removed by developmentally delayed patients. Progestin only contraception in the form of depo provera injection and progestin only pills can be used by all women. The side effects of irregular bleeding, mood changes, and weight gain should be considered. All patients and caregivers should be made aware of post-coital contraception.[20, 22, 28, 30]

Sterilization

A request for sterilization may be initiated by a disabled woman or by her care guardian. The ACOG Committee Opinion No. 371 recommends that the presence of a mental disability justifies neither acceptance nor rejection of sterilization.[19] The autonomy of the patient, patient participation in counseling and consent by the patient is required. If the patient cannot participate in the counseling and consent process an attempt should be made to restore or improve the patient's ability to participate. This can be achieved by medication adjustment, education at a level appropriate to the patient's ability and the use of a stress-free environment. If all efforts to improve the patient's ability to participate in the consent process fail then it is important to determine if the failure is temporary or permanent. The patient's guardian, family, and caregivers should be consulted about the request for sterilization. The origin of the request and reason for the request should be determined. Consideration of alternative methods of fertility control should be undertaken, and there should be a discussion of parenting. The risk of child abuse and neglect should be considered given the possibility that the patient becomes pregnant and delivers a child. The final decision regarding plans for sterilization must consider the patient's needs and desires first and foremost. The use of consultation with an ethics committee may be very helpful to safeguard the patient's interests in cases where there is a disagreement among the participants in the decision making process. State laws vary regarding the involvement of the court system in the approval of sterilization of patients who cannot give consent. State laws vary in the process and procedure for making a determination of patient competence. Health-care providers must familiarize themselves with the laws of their jurisdiction.[24]

Infertility

There is no good estimate of the number of reproductive-aged women with disabilities who are infertile. The percentage of infertile women who are disabled is unlikely to differ from the general population where 10.9% of women aged 15–44 were infertile as reported by the CDC for 2006–2010.[16] The common causes of female infertility are anatomic and hormonal. Tubal occlusion is usually a late complication of pelvic infection. Some disabled women with limited pelvic sensation, or visual impairments may have a delay in diagnosis and treatment. The delays can be exacerbated by low index of suspicion for the diagnosis of pelvic infection on the part of health-care providers. Some disabled women have a higher rate of hormonal derangement because of brain injury, autoimmune disease, and exposure to medications that can interfere with ovulation. Disorders of sexual function place some disabled women at risk for infertility secondary to inadequate frequency of coitus and the use of lubricants that can impair sperm motility. As with all patients, the infertility evaluation should be conducted in an organized and cost effective manner. A detailed preconception evaluation should precede any infertility evaluation and treatment. Some components of the infertility evaluation may be difficult for some disabled women. Determination of tubal patency by hysterosalpingogram or sonohysteroscopy may be difficult or impossible for patients with physical limitations that inhibit the pelvic examination. There is also risk of autonomic dysreflexia in patients with high spinal cord injuries. An alternative approach is more invasive testing using hysteroscopy or laparoscopy under anesthesia. Ovulation kits can be difficult to use in patients with irregular cycles and in patients with visual impairment. For patients with severe physical limitations where the adequacy of intercourse is unknown, post coital testing can be used to document intravaginal intromission. Patients who require the use of lubricants should use products that do not inhibit sperm motility such as egg white, vegetable oil, and Replens®. Disabled women with sedentary lifestyles may become obese; this can impair ovulation and the responsiveness to ovulation induction agents. Weight loss is a difficult problem for most adults but can be severe for the disabled patient. Multiple gestations can increase pregnancy risk for disabled women with severe musculoskeletal disorders and chronic illnesses that affect vital organs, so a discussion of selective reduction should be undertaken before infertility treatment begins in high-risk patients.[23]

Gynecologic care of the disabled adolescent

The management of adolescents requires patience, sensitivity, and knowledge of developmental milestones.

The health-care provider may be called upon to provide gynecologic care to adolescents with physical and/or mental disabilities. Adolescents with complex medical problems and severe disabilities are generally best managed using a team approach. Inclusion of the pediatrician or adolescent medicine specialist in team care of complicated adolescents will usually give the best clinical outcome. General preventive care milestones such as vaccination are generally managed by the pediatrician. Specific issues related to sexuality may be referred for management to the gynecology health-care provider. The gynecology visit may be initiated by the patient, her caregiver or by the pediatrician. Basic components of care addressed during a gynecology visit include abuse prevention, contraception, and STD prevention and screening. Abuse is common in the disabled population, and education for prevention should be given at a level appropriate to the individual patient. The No Go Tell model is simple and easily explained, but adjustments have to be made for adolescents with mobility impairments who have a difficult time removing themselves from dangerous situations. The provider must have a high index of suspicion for abuse and assess physical and behavioral signs. It is mandatory to report all suspected abuse.

Menstruation can present a hygiene problem for patients who cannot manage personal hygiene because of limited mobility, cognitive impairment, communication problems, or extreme obesity. Adolescents that can toilet themselves can usually be taught to manage menstrual hygiene.[21] Menstrual disorders in adolescents with disabilities should follow the same guideline for evaluation and management as their able counterparts. Treatment must be tailored to the diagnosis and the desires of the patient. If she is incapable of communication her guardian's input is even more critical. The contraceptive needs of the patient should be addressed with as much privacy and patient autonomy as possible. The full range of contraceptive options can be used by most patients with limitations on barrier methods and Nuvaring® if there are severe physical limitations. Some adolescents with cognitive impairments will remove patches and alternative methods of contraception may be appropriate. The need for sedation or general anesthesia to place contraceptive implants and IUD has to be balanced against the contraceptive benefits and the availability of alternative forms of contraception. Adolescent patients with behavioral problems, especially mood disturbances, may have better outcomes if progestin only pills are used for one month prior to administration of depo provera, which has mood disturbance as a side effect.[10, 20, 28]

Concluding remarks

Gynecologic care of the disabled women must provide the patient with the same high quality preventive care and gynecologic treatment as all women. The disabled patient may need additional time and thought to achieve a successful outcome. The health-care provider who takes the time and the interest to gain education can provide excellent care to this patient population and correct a vitally important deficiency in care for women.

References

1. US Department of Health and Human Services HRaSA. Women's Health USA 2010, Preventive Care [April 6, 2016]. Available from: http://mchb.hrsa.gov/whusa10/pdfs/w08.pdf. Accessed 5 Dec 2015.
2. World Health Organization. *Towards a Common Language for Functioning, Disability and Health*, Geneva: ICF; 2002. Available from: http://WHO.
3. Centers for Disease Control and Prevention. Differences in Health Status among People with Disabilities Compared to People without Disabilities. Available from: www.cdc.gov/ncbddd/disabilityandhealdh/health status.html.

4. US Department of Health and Human Services HRaSA. Women's Health USA 2010, Self-Reported Health Status [April 2, 2014]. Available from: http://mchb.hrsa.gov/whusa10/hstater/hi/pages/206srhs.html.
5. US Department of Health and Human Services HRaSA. Women's Health USA 2010, Activity Limitations. Available from: http://mchb.hrsa.gov/whusa10/hstat/hi/pages206srhs.html.
6. WHO Disability and Health. Fact Sheet No. 352, Reviewed Sept. 2013 [May 1, 2014]. Available from: www.who.int/mediacentre/factsheets/fs352/en.
7. Reichard A, FMH. Using population-based data to examine preventive services by disability type among dually eligible (Medicare/Medicaid) adults. *Disability and Health Journal*. 2013(**6**):5–86.
8. American Disabilities Act 1990. [April 2, 2014]. Available from: www.ada.gov/ada.htm.
9. Welner SL, Foley CC, Nosek MA, Holes A. Practical considerations in the performance of physical examinations on women with disabilities. *Obstet Gynecol Surv*. 1999; **54**(7):457–62.
10. Owens K, Honebrink A. Gynecologic care of medically complicated adolescents. *Pediatr Clin North Am*. 1999; **46**(3):631–42.
11. Plummer SB, FPA. Women with disabilities' experience with physical and sexual abuse: review of the literature and implications for the field. *Trauma Violence & Abuse*. 2012; **13**(1):15–19.
12. Welner SL, Simon JA, Welner B. Maximizing health in menopausal women with disabilities. *Menopause* 2002 May;**9**(3):208–19.
13. Welner SL. Screening issues in gynecologic malignancies for women with disabilities: critical considerations. *Journal for Women's Health*. 1998; **7**(3): 281–5.
14. ACOG. Obstetrics & Gynecology, Women with Disabilities 2014 [April 2, 2014]. Available from: www.acog.org.
15. Rosen DB. Violence and exploitation against women and girls with disability. *Annals of the New York Academy of Sciences*. 2006; **1087**(1):170–7.
16. US Census Bureau CD. Age-Adjusted and Unadjusted Disability Rates by Gender, Race, Hispanic Origin, 2005 and 2010. Available from: www.census.gov/people/disability/publications/disab10.
17. ACOG. Benefits to women of Medicaid expansion through the Affordable Care Act. *ACOG Committee Opinion*. 2013; **552**:1–3.
18. Chescheir NC. Global obesity and the effect on women's health. *Obstetrics & Gynecol*. 2011; **117**(5):1213–22.
19. ACOG. Sterilization of Women, Including Those with Mental Disabilities. Update of "Sterilization of Women, Including Those with Mental Disabilities" in Ethics in Obstetrics and Gynecology. *ACOG Committee Opinion, Committee on Ethics*. 2007; **371**:1–4.
20. ACOG. Adolescents and Long-Acting Reversible Contraception: Implants and Intrauterine Devices. *ACOG Committee Opinion*. 2012; **539**:1–7.
21. ACOG. Menstrual Manipulation for Adolescents with Disabilities. *ACOG Committee Opinion, Committee on Adolescent Health Care*. 2009; **448**:1–4.
22. Wilkinson JE, Cerreto MC. Primary care for women with intellectual disabilities. *J Am Board Fam Med*. 2008; **21**(3):215–22.
23. Welner S, Haseltine F (eds.). *Welner's Guide to the Care of Women with Disabilities*. Philadelphia: Lippincott Williams & Wilkins. 2004.
24. ACOG. Special Ethical Considerations Inherent with Sterilization Procedures. ACOG News Release. 2007.
25. Erekson EA, Ratner ES, Walke LM, Fried TR, Gynecologic surgery in the geriatric patient. *Obstetrics & Gynecol*. 2012; **119**(6).
26. Kovesdy CP, Molnar MZ. Restricting kidney transplant wait-listing for obese patients: let's stop defending the indefensible. *Seminars in Dialysis*. 2014; **27**(1):1–3.
27. ACOG Department of Government Affairs. Health Care for Women, Health Care for All, A Reform Agenda. 2008 Feb. Available from: www.acog.org/-/media/Departments/Resource-Center/HCFWHCFA.
28. ACOG. CDC Report: We Needs Better Efforts to Prevent Teen Pregnancy, ACOG Announcements, [cited 2014]. Available from: www.acog.org.
29. ACOG. Annual Women's Health Care. Tests and Immunication for High-Risk Women 2012. Available from: www.acog.org.
30. McCarthy M. Prescribing contraception to women with intellectual disabilities: general practitioners' attitudes and practices. *Sex Disabil*. 2011; **29**:339–49.
31. Kaplan C. Special issues in contraception: caring for women with disabilities. *J Midwifery Womens Health*. 2006; **51**(6):450–6.
32. ACOG. Merck Research Fellowship in Reproductive Healthcare Needs within a Disabled Population. ACOG Research Fellowships and Awards. 2014.
33. ACOG. Health Care for Homeless Women. *ACOG Committee Opinion, Committee on Health Care for Underserved Women*. 2013; **576**:1–5.
34. ACOG. Reproductive Health Care for Adolescents with Disabilities, Supplement to Guidelines for Adolescent Health Care, 2nd Edition [cited 2014]. Available from: www.acog.org.
35. ACOG. Special Issues in Women's Health, ACOG Resources and Publications, [January 27, 2014]. Available from: www.acog.org.

36. Centers for Disease Control. Racial/Ethnic Disparities in Self-Rated Health Status among Adults with and without Disabilities – United States, 2004–2006. Available from: www.cdc.gov/mmwr/preview/mmwrhtml/mm5739a1.htm

37. Schopp LH KH, Sanford TC, Hagglund KJ, Wongvatunyu S. Impact of Comprehensive Gynecologic Services on Health Maintenance Behaviours among Women with Spinal Cord Injury 2002. Available from: www.ncbi.nlm.nih.gov/pubmed/12519485.

38. Sterilization of Women and Girls with Disabilities. Available from: www.stoptortureinhealthcare.org

39. ACOG. Access to Reproductive Health Care for Women with Disabilities, Special Populations, Special Issues in Women's Health [April 6, 2014]. Available from: www.acog.org/Resources_And_Publications

40. Lagu T HN, Rotherberg MB, Green KL, et al. Access to Subspecialty Care for Patients with Mobility Impairment: Survey 2013. Available from: http://annals.org/article.aspx?articleid=1667265.

41. Schopp L ST, Hagglund K, Gay J, Coatney M. Removing service barriers for women with physical disabilities: promoting accessibility in the gynecologic care setting. *J Midwifery Womens Health* 2002 Mar–Apr; **47**(2):74–9.

Chapter 48

Domestic violence

Martin E. Olsen

Introduction

Violence against women has significant adverse effects against the health and well-being of women and their children. Intimate partner violence (IPV) is a form of abuse perpetrated by a person who was, is, or wishes to be in an intimate relationship with the target of the abuse. Elements of intimate partner violence include injury, psychological abuse, forced social isolation, stalking, deprivation, intimidation, threats, aggression, and reproductive coercion.[1, 2] Intimate partner violence can occur among heterosexual or same sex couples and can be found in all communities regardless of age, race, religion, ethnicity, educational background, or economic status.[3]

Scope of the problem

Health-care providers frequently encounter women who are targets of intimate partner violence. More than one in three US women have experienced rape, physical violence, or stalking by an intimate partner.[4] The lifetime prevalence of rape by intimate partners of US women is 8.8%. Nearly 16% of women have experienced other forms of sexual violence; severe physical violence has been experienced by 22.3% and stalking by 9.2% of female US citizens.[5] Women with a history of IPV are more likely to seek health care than patients without such a history.[6] Providers express uncertainty in their abilities to screen and counsel patients who suffer from domestic violence.[7]

Intimate partner violence can include many violent and controlling behaviors.[8] See Table 48-1 for descriptions of the types of abuse associated with intimate partner violence.

Effects of IPV on pregnancy include poor weight gain, late entry into prenatal care, infection, anemia, alcohol use, tobacco use, and low birth weight.[9] Acute consequences of assault for the pregnant patient may include stillbirth, pelvic fracture, placental abruption, fetal injury, and preterm delivery.[10]

Approximately 240,000 emergency room visits occur annually in United States as a result of IPV.[11] Intangible costs of IPV include decreased quality of life, undiagnosed depression, and lowered self-esteem.[3] Intimate partner violence can undermine the family unit with subsequent diminished economic resources; domestic and sexual violence is the leading cause of homelessness for women and families.[12] Abused women are higher users of mental health services even after the abuse ends.[6]

Characteristics of intimate partner violence

No particular psychological or cultural profile defines the targets of IPV. Increased risk of IPV is found in single, separated, or divorced women, women between the ages of 17 and 24, women who abuse alcohol or drugs, and women who are pregnant.

Intimate partner violence frequently involves a cycle. An episode of abuse is followed by a honeymoon phase. In this phase, the perpetrator will frequently demonstrate a very caring attitude. The next phase is the escalating tensions phase, which can be a very stressful interval for the target of IPV. The escalating tensions phase is followed by the next episode of abuse. Over time, the honeymoon phase shortens and the level of violence becomes more severe. The clinician must remember that the patient who suffers from IPV is at risk for homicide. Women are nine times as likely to be killed by an intimate partner than by a stranger. Research shows the risk is increased if the following characteristics are present: partner has access to a gun, estrangement, threats to kill, threats with a weapon, nonfatal strangulation, and stepchild in the home.[13] Other health consequences of IPV are seen in Table 48-2.[3]

Office Care of Women, ed. Martin E. Olsen and Botros Rizk. Published by Cambridge University Press.

Table 48-1 Types of intimate partner violence

Physical violence	Slapping Pushing Shaking Biting Scratching Choking Burning Hitting Use of a knife Use of a gun Use of another weapon
Sexual violence	Any nonconsensual or unwanted sexual contact Attempted or completed penetration of vagina Attempted or completed penetration of oral cavity Attempted or completed penetration of anus Unwanted touching Unwanted fondling
Psychological or emotional violence	Humiliation Name-calling Profanity Deliberate embarrassment Financial manipulation and control Isolation from friends and family Withholding information and resources Controlling movement and activities Threats
Reproductive coercion	Sabotaging birth control pills Poking holes in condoms Destroying contraceptives Intentionally exposing the patient to STI Removal vaginal rings Removal contraceptive patch Removal IUD Failure to engage in withdrawal as previously agreed

Table 48-2 Health consequences of intimate partner violence

Acute injuries	Head Face Breast Abdomen Genitalia and reproductive system
Nonacute presentations	Chronic headaches Sleep disturbance Appetite disturbances Palpations Chronic pelvic pain Urinary frequency or urgency Irritable bowel syndrome Sexual dysfunction Abdominal symptoms Recurrent vaginal infections

Reproductive coercion

Reproductive coercion is a form of power maintenance. The experience of violence increases a woman's risk of unintended pregnancy.[14] Reproductive coercion occurs when a partner sabotages efforts at contraception, reuses to practice safe sex, intentionally exposes the patient to sexually transmitted infection, controls the outcome of a pregnancy, forbids sterilization, or controls access to reproductive health services.[3]

Intimate partner violence has been shown to reduce the rates of both condom use and oral contraceptive use.[15] Birth control sabotage is a planned interference with the woman's contraceptive efforts in an attempt to promote pregnancy in the female partner. Examples include hiding, withholding, or destroying a partners oral contraceptives; breaking or poking holes in a condom or removing a condom during sexual activities; failure to withdraw the penis when that was the agreed-upon method of contraception, and removing vaginal rings, contraceptive patches, or intrauterine devices.[14]

Pregnancy coercion involves behavior such as threats or violence if the woman does not comply with the male partner's wishes regarding the decision to terminate or continue a pregnancy.[16]

One study reported that 15% of patients with a history of abuse who were seeking care in family planning clinics reported birth control sabotage.[17] A different study showed one-third of patients who experienced IPV also reported reproductive control by their partners.[17] Intimate partner violence is three times more likely in patients seeking elective abortion than in patients who continue a pregnancy;[18] routine screening for IPV in patients seeking abortion is justified.[19] One-fourth of adolescent females reported that their male partners were trying to get them pregnant through interference with planned contraception.[19]

Health-care providers can provide interventions which address reproductive coercion. Discrete methods of contraception such as IUDs, emergency contraception, and depo-medroxyprogesterone acetate injections can be offered to these patients.[3] Etonogestrel implants have also been mentioned as possible long-acting options for patients undergoing reproductive coercion, but it should be remembered that a large bruise may occur after implant insertion and that the implants are frequently palpable.

Other practical considerations for the provider dealing with patients who are experiencing reproductive coercion include (1) giving the patient a plain envelope for emergency contraceptive pills since emergency oral contraception is often packaged in a box with bold labeling, (2) offering a copper IUD instead of oral agents for emergency contraception to provide long-term protection, (3) realizing that some partners who perpetrate IPV may monitor the woman's menstrual cycle, so a copper IUD may be a better choice than a hormone containing IUD that could cause amenorrhea, (4) possibly cutting IUD strings inside the cervical loss to ensure the strings are undetectable and to prevent removal by a partner.[14]

Information cards about reproductive coercion can be discreetly made available for patients, but providers must realize it may not be safe for some patients to take these information cards home. The display of educational posters that address IPV and reproductive coercion may be helpful. The posters should be multicultural, multilingual, and can be placed in restrooms, reception areas, examination rooms, hallways, and other highly visible areas.[16]

Vulnerable populations

Adolescents

Younger women experience a substantial proportion of IPV.[5] Ten percent of female high school students have reported physical violence from dating partners in the previous year.[20, 21] Adolescents who experience dating violence are less likely to use condoms. [21] It is hypothesized that fear impacts the condom negotiation process; the risks of sexually transmitted infections including human immunodeficiency virus (HIV) are thus increased. The incidence of multiple sexual partners over the last three months was also increased in adolescents who experienced dating violence. Pregnancy is about twice as high in dating violence targets as in the general adolescent female population.[21] Substance abuse before the last episode of intercourse is also increased in those who experienced dating violence.[21] School based dating violence interventions have show success in high-income countries. Long-term programs have higher success than single awareness-raising or discussion sessions.[22]

Immigrant women

Immigration is associated with stresses and challenges that may increase the risk of IPV.[23] Recent immigrant women may have a lower rate of IPV than non-recent immigrant women.[24] Immigrant women may fear deportation and can be hesitant to report IPV. These women may be unaware that, in many jurisdictions, regulations may allow immigrants who have been subjected to physical or mental abuse caused by IPV to legally remain in the country of immigration if it is justified on humanitarian grounds.

Disabled women

Women with disabilities are more likely to be abused than women without disabilities or men with disabilities.[25] The most common perpetrators are former or current intimate partners, but family members, caregivers, and strangers may also be perpetrators.[25, 26] Unfortunately, disabled women are sometimes seen by health-care providers as asexual or undesirable as intimate partners; this belief may result in a failure to identify IPV in these individuals. Ballan et al. found that half of the disabled patients who were experiencing intimate partner violence were married and two-thirds had children.[25]

Disabled women who are targets of domestic violence may be even less likely to report the abuse due to fears of subsequent isolation. Although the fear of losing custody of children is a deterrent to the reporting of abuse, disabled women with children were found to be significantly more likely to obtain an order of protection.[25] Disabled women frequently rely very significantly upon their partners or other caregivers for help; abusers may therefore be in a position to deny needed support, withhold medication, prevent the use of medical equipment such as wheelchairs, or sabotage other personal needs such as help with bathing, toileting, or eating. Unfortunately, many domestic violence shelters are unable to accept women with disabilities,[3] and those that do offer shelter may not be equipped to provide adequate transportation to those disabled individuals who need this assistance.[27] The majority of disabled women exposed to IPV may also have a psychiatric disability of some type;[25] only about half of shelters are able to provide mental health assistance.[27]

Elder abuse

Elder abuse occurs in all social, racial, educational, economic, and cultural settings. Patients who suffer elder abuse know their perpetrators 90% of the time. Abuse may be physical, sexual, or psychological. Psychological abuse includes neglect, abandonment, and financial exploitation. For all types of abuse combined, two-thirds of the abusers are partners or adult children; also 53% are male and 47% are female.[28] Nonphysical abuse tends to escalate or intensify later in life, whereas physical and sexual violence decline; elderly women in abusive relationships consider the nonphysical abuse to be more damaging than the physical abuse over time.[29] The financial and emotional risks of leaving relationships late in life are amplified by increased financial dependence, deep social ties to neighborhoods, and strong sentimental attachments to home and community.[30] In the United States, all jurisdictions have laws authorizing the provision of human protective services in cases of child abuse, elder abuse, or the abuse of individuals with disabilities.

Screening and diagnosis

The American Congress of Obstetrics and Gynecology (ACOG) advocates for universal screening of female patients for IPV. Such screening could occur during annual examinations, family-planning visits, prenatal care, and other follow-up visits for ongoing care.[3]

The World Health Organization (WHO) does not recommend universal screening but instead recommends targeted screening. The WHO recommendation is that health-care providers be aware of the mental and physical health indicators associated with violence and ask about violence when these indicators are present.[31] It should be noted that in settings or countries where rates of violence are high and referral options are scarce, universal inquiry might bring little benefit to women. Unfortunately, screening for intimate partner violence does pose a risk to the target of IPV. For those regions that have few resources to assist patients exposed to intimate partner violence, the risk of discussion may very well outweigh any potential benefit. At the minimum, therefore, a provider who screens patients for IPV should have an action plan for those patients who are found to be targets of intimate partner violence.

Screening for IPV in pregnant women should occur at the first panel visit, at least once per trimester, and at the postpartum check-up.[3] Most patients are comfortable with domestic violence screening and patient self-administered screenings are as effective as clinician interviewing in the areas of disclosure, patient comfort, and time.[32, 33] For screening to occur, confidentiality must be assured, a protocol for dealing with the issues must be present, the provider should be trained in methods to ask and respond to concerns about intimate partner violence, and a referral system must be in place.[31]

History must be obtained in a sensitive and nonjudgmental fashion. The partner must not be present. An opening statement such as, "Because abuse and violence are so common I ask about this routinely," is appropriate.[34] The provider's concern may make a positive impression on the patient even if she is not yet ready to discuss the violence in her life. When asking about specific details, it may be helpful to remember that the term "rape" may not be a word that will resonate with the patient because the events are occurring with her partner. The woman may see a more general term such as "forced sex" as a better description. The approach to the patient must be supportive and nonjudgmental. If the patient has injuries that are inconsistent with the history provided, the provider should strongly suspect IPV and initiate patient education on the topic if it is safe for the patient to have this conversation.

Management

Women generally want their health-care providers to provide first-line support for IPV. Such support includes attentive listening, sensitive nonjudgmental inquiry about needs, validation of the disclosure without pressure, provision for safety of the woman and her children, and identification of and help with access to resources.[35]

A critically important initial step is to assess the immediate safety concerns of the patient for herself and for any children who may rely upon her for their care. Clinicians must remember that an IPV patient may be at risk for homicide;[36] if it is not safe for the patient return home, she will need to be placed in contact with an alternative option such as a domestic violence shelter. Some legal jurisdictions do not mandate reporting of domestic violence to law-enforcement officials but the vast majority of jurisdictions do mandate reporting of child abuse; providers must be aware of the risk that violence may be directed toward both the female patient and her children. The violence is also likely reportable if the target of the intimate partner is an adolescent. The controversies involved in mandatory reporting are discussed later in the chapter.

Patients experiencing abuse should be given the opportunity to receive assistance in contacting in law enforcement agencies as well as assistance in obtaining restraining orders if indicated.[37] If a patient is not ready to leave the abusive environment, a discussion of a safety plan should be considered. The safety plan includes elements such as securing and hiding money, obtaining an extra house or car key, collecting important documents such as birth certificates, social security numbers, and marriage licenses. It may be appropriate to develop a code to use with family and friends to signal the need for assistance.

Certain elements or objects such as keys, money and documents, may be hidden in an empty tampon container along with other sanitary products or with a trusted friend, neighbor, or relative. A safety plan may also include procedures to remove weapons from the house. The patient can be encouraged to mentally plan her escape, for example, using a window if the door is blocked and avoiding areas such as the kitchen where objects that can be used as weapons may be present.[38] Potential supportive actions by clinicians are listed in Table 48-3.

Table 48-3 Potential actions by health-care providers to support the patient experiencing intimate partner violence

- Identify intimate partner violence
- Provide supportive response to patient disclosure
- Provide indicated clinical care including post-sexual assault care or injury treatment when needed
- Educate patient about elements of an exit plan
- Educate patient about shelter options
- Initiate referral to support groups or mental health providers if appropriate
- Ensure patient is aware of legal options and contact law enforcement if patient desires this protection
- Assess for reproductive coercion
- Discuss contraceptive needs

The vast majority of patients with IPV will end up returning home after their contact with the health-care system. This fact can be very frustrating to physicians. A woman will not accept help until she is aware that what she is experiencing is abuse. This change in perception may take months to years and is characterized by a series of incidents, factors, or circumstances that significantly change how a woman views the violence; these events are characterized as turning points.[39] Physicians should remember that their continuing support is very important in allowing the patient to experience such a turning point which may then help her to eventually take the step of leaving an abusive relationship permanently. Intimate partner violence is a long-standing problem and it is therefore unlikely that any single intervention will result in a permanent change, but over time the care and support of multiple health-care providers may allow and encourage a patient to improve her life by gaining safety and healing. The discussion of IPV in a caring manner may be improved by the provision of educational materials.[3]

Clinicians should not make any effort to force patients to accept assistance; it must be remembered that the patient is facing a very real potential for violence and remembrance of the caveat "first do no harm" is essential. Providers should not place information into a patient's purse or bag as the perpetrator may find that material and increase aggression. Perpetrators may monitor the patient's cell phone usage; therefore, it may be appropriate to offer the patient access to a private phone. If the practice's discharge routine includes a paper summary with a list of diagnoses, it must be remembered that the perpetrator may see this documentation.

Interventions to increase safety behaviors of abused women are effective if the intervention occurs within a close time interval after the event. The increase in safety behaviors remains large at three months and continues to be substantial at six months; repeat interventions may therefore have benefit.[40] Intervention by health-care providers may increase patients' abilities to exit abusive situations.[41]

Cognitive behavioral therapy has been recommended for women with post-traumatic stress disorder who are no longer experiencing violence.[31]

Intimate partner violence and the health-care system

Many national health-care policies and budgets fail to provide any attention to the topic of violence against women. In some countries, no data exists, although in others the issue is not a priority. Recognition of IPV is an important first step to improve the lives of women facing intimate partner violence.[42]

Patients who experience intimate partner violence may be afraid to notify their partners of a sexually transmitted infection (STI). A diagnosis of an STI may initiate violence toward the woman. Women who are targets of IPV are significantly more likely to know or be suspicious of nonmonogamous partner sexual activity with another person.[43] This situation may cause the reporting of STIs to health departments to become a risk to IPV targets.

Many jurisdictions have mandatory reporting laws that must be followed by health-care providers. These laws do not necessarily protect the survivors of intimate partner violence and they create ethical dilemmas for clinicians when patients do not want their cases reported.[44] Advantages of mandatory reporting include enabling women to get help without being responsible for the report, making the targets feel less alone and less to blame, and teaching perpetrators the seriousness of the situation. Disadvantages include concerns about retaliation, fear that children will be taken away, anxiety about interactions with authority figures, and concerns over autonomy and confidentiality. The WHO has concluded that the evidence does not support mandatory reporting of intimate partner violence to law-enforcement agencies.[31]

Health-care systems have a role in the primary prevention of IPV through the documentation of violence against women. An emphasis can be placed on understanding the health burden and also coordinating action with other sectors.[42] Patients may benefit from contact with resources including legal services, law enforcement protection, housing assistance, financial services, psychological care, and educational components.[42] Since much of IPV is experienced at an early age, prevention efforts must begin when patients are young.[5]

Women-centered interventions use a combination of factors including psychosocial support, advocacy, counseling, and home visitation to improve the physical and psychological health and well-being of those who have experienced IPV. Literature review shows that some interventions have positive outcomes such as reductions in depression. A minority of studies shows significant decreases in violence.[41, 42, 45] Most studies on programs designed to reduce recidivism in male perpetrators have been unable to demonstrate effectiveness.[45]

Concluding remarks

Intimate partner violence is unfortunately a common problem faced by patients who access the health-care system. When this diagnosis is made, the most important action is to address the safety of the patient. Health-care providers should subsequently educate the patients about the dangers of their environments and the steps that patients can take to maintain their personal safety and that of any children who might be involved. Although most patients will elect to return to the environment in which they are experiencing IPV, the clinicians' efforts may bear fruit in the future as the patients, over time, come to realize that positive options exist for them to constructively change their lives.

References

1. Black MC, Basile KC, Breiding MJ, et al. *The National Intimate Partner and Sexual Violence Survey (NISVS): 2010 Summary Report.* Atlanta, GA: National Center for Injury Prevention and Control, Centers for Disease Control & Prevention; 2011. Available at: www.cdc.gov/violenceprevention/nisvs. Accessed Dec 5, 2015.
2. Family Violence Prevention Fund. *Reproductive health and partner violence guidelines: an integrated response to intimate partner violence and reproductive coercion.* San Francisco: FVPF; 2010. Available at: www.futureswithoutviolence.org/userfiles/file/HealthCare/Repro_Guide.pdf. Accessed Dec 5, 2015.
3. Intimate Partner Violence: Committee on Health Care for Underserved Women. Committee Opinion Number 518. *Obstet Gynecol* Feb. 2012.

4. Black MC, Basile KC, Breiding MJ, et al. *The National Intimate Partner and Sexual Violence Survey (NISVS): 2010 Summary Report.* Atlanta (GA): National Center for Injury Prevention and Control, Centers for Disease Control and Prevention; 2011. Available at: www.cdc.gov/ViolencePrevention/pdf/NISVS_Report2010-a.pdf. Accessed Dec 5, 2015.

5. Breiding MJ, Smith SG, Basile KC, et al. Prevalence and characteristics of sexual violence, stalking, and intimate partner violence victimization – national intimate partner and sexual violence survey, United States, 2011. *MMWR Surveill Summ* 2014 Sep 5; **63**(8):1–18.

6. Bonomi AE, Anderson ML, Rivara FP, Thompson RS. Health care utilization and costs associate with physical and nonphysical-only intimate partner violence. *Heal Serv Resear (HSR)* 2009 June **44**;(3):1052–67.

7. Rhodes KV, Frankel RM, Levinthal N, et al. "You're not a victim of domestic violence, are you?" Provider-patient communication about domestic violence. *Ann Intern Med* 2007 Nov 6;**147**(9):620–7.

8. Deshpande NA, Lewis-O'Connor, A. Screening for intimate partner violence during pregnancy. *Rev Obstet Gynecol* 2013;**6**(3–4):141–8.

9. Parker B, McFarlane J, Soeken K. Abuse during pregnancy: effects on maternal complications and birth weight in adult and teenage women. *Obstet Gynecol* 1994;**84**:323–8.

10. El Kady De, Gilbert WM, Xing G, Smith LH. Maternal and neonatal outcomes of assaults during pregnancy. *Obstet Gynecol* 2005;**105**:357–63.

11. National Center for Injury Prevention and Control. *Costs of intimate partner violence against women in the United States.* Atlanta, GA: Centers for Disease Control and Prevention; 2003. Available at: www.cdc.gov/violence prevention/pdf/IPVBook-a.pdf. Accessed Dec 5, 2015.

12. Health care for homeless women. Committee Opinion No. 454. American College of Obstetricians and Gynecologists. *Obstet Gynecol* 2010;**115**:396–9.

13. Campbell JC, Class N, Sharps P, et al. Intimate partner homicide: review and implications of research and policy. *Trauma Violence Abuse* 2007;**8**:246–69.

14. Reproductive and sexual coercion. Committee Opinion No. 554. American College of Obstetricians and Gynecologists. *Obstet Gynecol* 2013 Feb;**121**:411–5.

15. Bergmann JN, Stockman JK. How does intimate partner violence affect condom and oral contraceptive use in the United States? A systematic review of the literature. *Contraception* 2015 Feb 21. doi:10.10161 j. contraception.2015.02.009.

16. Chamberlain L, Levenson R. *Addressing intimate partner violence, reproductive and sexual coercion: a guide for obstetric, gynecologic and reproductive health care settings.* 2nd ed. Washington, DC: American College of Obstetricians and Gynecologists; San Francisco: Futures Without Violence; 2012.

17. Miller E, Decker MR, McCauley HL, et al. Pregnancy coercion, intimate partner violence and unintended pregnancy. *Contraception* 2010;**81**:316–22.

18. Bourassa D, Berube J. The prevalence of intimate partner violence among women and teenagers seeking abortion compared with those continuing pregnancy. *J Obstet Gynaecol Can* 2007;**29**:415–23.

19. Miller E, Decker MR, Reed E, et al. Male partner pregnancy-promoting behaviors and adolescent partner violence: findings from a qualitative study with adolescent females. *Ambul Pediatr* 2007;**7**:360–6.

20. Grunbaum JA, Kann L, Kinchen SA, et al. Youth risk behavior surveillance: United States, 2001. *MMWR Surveill Summ* 2002;**51**(4):1–62.

21. Silverman JG, Raj A, Clements K. Dating violence and associated sexual risk and pregnancy among adolescent girls in the United States. *Pediatrics* 2004;**114**:e220–5.

22. Lundgren R, Amin A. Addressing intimate partner violence and sexual violence among adolescents: emerging evidence of effectiveness. *J Adolesc Health* 2015;**56**:S42–50.

23. Hazen AL, Soriano FI. Experiences with intimate partner violence among Latina women. *Violence Against Women* 2007 Jun;**13**(6):562–82.

24. Hyman I, Forte T, Du Mont J, et al. The association between length of stay in Canada and intimate partner violence among immigrant women. *Am J Pub Health April* 2006;**96**(4):654–9.

25. Ballan MS, Freyer MB, Marti CN, et al. Looking beyond prevalence: a demographic profile of survivors of intimate partner violence with disabilities. *J Interpersonal Viol* 2014;**29**(17):3167–79.

26. Young ME, Nosek MA, Howland C, et al. Prevalence of abuse of women with physical disabilities. *Arch Phys Med Rehabil* 1997 Dec;**78**(12 Suppl 5):S34–8.

27. Douglas EM, Hines DA. The reported availability of US domestic violence services to victims who vary by immigration status, primary language, and disability. *Partner Abuse* 2011 Nov 4;**2**:427–51.

28. National Center for Elder Abuse. *The national elder abuse incidence study: final report.* Washington, DC: NCEA; 1998. Available at: http://aoa.gov/AoA_Programs/Elder_Rights/Elder_Abuse/docs/ABuseReport_Full.pdf. Accessed Dec 5, 2015.

29. Seff LR, Beaulaurier RL, Newman FL. Nonphysical abuse: findings in domestic violence against older women study. *J Emotional Abuse* 2008;**8**: 355–74.

30. Hightower J, Smith MJ, Hightower HC. Hearing the voices of abused older women. *J of Gerontological Soc Work* 2006;**46**:20527.

31. World Health Organization. Responding to intimate partner violence and sexual violence against women: WHO clinical and policy guidelines. 2013.

32. Chen PH, Rovi S, Washington J, et al. Randomized comparison of 3 methods to screen for domestic violence in family practice. *Ann Fam Med* 2007;**5**:430–5.

33. Ahmad F, Hogg-Johnson S, Stewart DE, et al. Computer-assisted screening for intimate partner violence and control: a randomized trial. *Ann Intern Med* 2009;**151**:93–102.

34. American Medical Association. *Diagnostic and treatment guidelines on domestic violence*. Chicago: AMA; 1992.

35. Feder GS, Hutson M, Ramsay J, Taket AR. Women exposed to intimate partner violence: expectations and experiences when they encounter health care professionals: a meta-analysis of qualitative studies. *Arch Intern Med* 2006;**166**:22–37.

36. Campbell JC, Webster D, Glass N. The danger assessment: validation of a lethality risk assessment instrument for intimate partner femicide. *J Interpers Violence* 2009;**24**:653–74.

37. Choo EK, Houry DE. Managing intimate partner violence in the emergency department. *Ann Emerg Med* 2015 Apr;**65**(4):447–51. Epub 2014 Dec 20.

38. McFarlane J, Parker B, Soeken K, et al. Safety behaviors of abused women after an intervention during pregnancy. *J Obstet Gynecol Neonatal Nurs* 1998;**27**:64–9.

39. Chang JC, Dado D, Hawker L, et al. Understanding turning points in intimate partner violence: factors and circumstances leading women victims toward change. *J of Women's Health* 2010;**19**(2):251–9.

40. McFarlane J, Malecha A, Gist J, et al. An intervention to increase safety behaviors of abused women: results of a randomized clinical trial. *Nurs Res* 2002;**51**:347–54.

41. Assessing intimate partner violence in health care settings leads to women's receipt of interventions and improved health. *Public Health Reports July–Aug.* 2006;**121**:435–44.

42. Garcia-Moreno C, Hegarty K, d'Oliveria AF, et al. The health-systems response to violence against women. *Lancet* 2015 Apr;**385**(9977):1567–79. Epub 2014 Nov 21.

43. Bauer HM, Gibson P, Hernandez M, et al. Intimate partner violence and high-risk sexual behaviors among female patients with sexually transmitted diseases. *Sex Transm Dis* 2002;**29**:411–16.

44. Hyman A, Schillinger D, Lo B. Laws mandating reporting of domestic violence. Do they promote patient well-being? *JAMA* 1995;**273**:1781–7.

45. Ellsberg M, Arango DJ, Morton M, et al. Prevention of violence against women and girls: what does the evidence say? *Lancet* 2015 Apr;**385**(9977):1555–66. Epub 2014 Nov 21.

Chapter 49

Sexual assault

Martin E. Olsen

Introduction

Sexual assault is a common issue faced by female patients. Unfortunately, a majority of sexual assault survivors do not seek acute medical care.[1] Those who do seek acute care most often present to emergency facilities for evaluation, but they may present to their primary care providers or gynecologists. Follow-up care after initial evaluation and treatment, or in the absence of acute treatment, is important. It is therefore necessary that providers of health care to women be familiar with the evaluation and management of sexual assault survivors.

Sexual assault is a fast-growing, frequently committed, and under-reported crime. It is a crime of violence and aggression that encompasses a range of activity from sexual coercion to unwanted sexual contact to forcible rape.[2]

Sexual assault subsets include acquaintance rape, date rape, statutory rape, child sexual abuse, and incest. Acquaintance and date rape refer to sexual assaults committed by someone known to the victim. Incest refers to a close familial relationship between the victim and the perpetrator. Statutory rape refers to consensual sexual intercourse with an individual older than a specified age.[3] The age at which an adolescent may consent to sexual intercourse varies by legal jurisdiction and, in the United States, ranges from 14 years to 18 years.[3] This chapter will confine itself to adult female patients assaulted by male perpetrators.

Scope of the problem

In the United States, approximately 190,000 sexual assaults occur every year.[4] More than 90% of survivors are female.[5] Eighteen percent of women in a large US study reported victimization via a complete or attempted rape in their lifetime.[6] The assaults are under-reported; less than 20% may be reported to law enforcement agencies.[1]

Sexual assault survivors may experience life-threatening injuries as a component of the attack. The risk of injury increases if the perpetrator is a current or former intimate partner; if the rape occurs in the survivor's or perpetrator's home; if the rape is completed; if harm to the survivor or another is threatened by the perpetrator; if a gun, knife, or other weapon is used during the assault; or if the perpetrator is using drugs or alcohol at the time of the assault.[6]

Long-term health effects associated with female sexual assault include diminished levels of functional capacity, alterations in health perception, and decreased quality of life.[7] Many women will not be forthright with their health-care providers about a history of either adult sexual assault or childhood sexual abuse. Sexual assault survivors are more likely to present to their health-care providers with chronic pelvic pain, dysfunctional uterine bleeding, dysmenorrhea, and sexual dysfunction than patients without a history of adult sexual assault; the presence of more than one of these diagnoses further increases the odds that the patient is a sexual assault survivor.[8]

The presence of alcohol abuse in a patient has a long-term association with sexual assault. More than half of women seeking abuse treatment were found to have a history of completed rape.[9]

Approach to the recently assaulted patient

The patient's recovery from a sexual assault can begin during the evaluation if the medical experience is sensitive and caring. When evaluating a sexual assault survivor, the provider is both a health-care provider with an injured patient as well as a forensic evaluator with

Office Care of Women, ed. Martin E. Olsen and Botros Rizk. Published by Cambridge University Press.

significant legal responsibilities. Empathy, sensitivity, a nonpatronizing attitude, and listening skills are paramount in dealing with people who have been sexually assaulted. Most patients seen after sexual assault will demonstrate no genital injuries, but a majority experience extra-genital injuries.[1, 10] Head injuries are the most dangerous extra-genital injury.[10]

Hospital-based programs to provide an acute medical and forensic examination are present in a large number of locations. In some US cities, trained sexual assault nurse examiners (SANE) can fulfill this role. In many regions, however, gynecologists or primary health providers will be the first point of contact for patients after sexual assault. Gynecologists will therefore need to be familiar with the forensic examination procedure.[3]

If the patient communicates with the health-care provider prior to the evaluation, she should be educated on efforts to preserve forensic evidence. This includes avoidance of eating, drinking, smoking, chewing gum, oral hygiene, defecation, urination, and showering.[11] She should not bathe, change her clothes, or clean her fingernails prior to the evaluation.

Before initiating a sexual assault forensic evaluation, the health-care provider must first confirm the absence of any life-threatening injuries. Physical injuries must be dealt with as a priority, and the forensic medical examination should be carried out only after the patient has been stabilized. If the patient has altered intellectual capacity due to intoxication from alcohol or drugs the examination should be deferred until the capacity to consent has returned.[11]

Emergencies that may occur after sexual assaults include anxiety, panic attacks, asthma attacks, seizures, hyperglycemia or hypoglycemia in diabetics, alcohol or drug intoxication, withdrawal, and head injury. The use of foreign objects in a sexual assault attack may cause lacerations to the vaginal or anal canals with resulting rectal or vaginal lacerations or intraperitoneal injury.

History

The provider must ask sensitive questions in a respectful and professional manner. If the provider appears uncomfortable, the patient may sense the discomfort and experience diminished confidence in her care. An explanation of the medical and forensic evaluation should occur prior to initiation of history taking with an opportunity for the patient to ask questions about the process. Assessment for risk of self-harm should be undertaken as the assault may trigger self-harming behavior.[12]

Table 49-1 Important historical items in the assessment of sexual assault patients

- Are any severe bodily injuries present?
- When did the event occur?
- Where did the event occur?
- Who was the perpetrator(s)?
- Were weapons, restraints, or other types of force used?
- Were drugs or alcohol involved?
- Contraceptive method?
- Was there oral, anal, or vaginal violation?
- What nongenital acts (such as licking or spitting) occurred?
- Did the rapist use a condom?
- Did the victim shower, change clothes, or otherwise cleanse herself?
- When was the last tetanus shot?
- Did activities after the assault include eating, vomiting, urination, douching, defecation, showering, bathing, or changing clothes?
- When was the last consensual intercourse?
- Will the patient be safe upon discharge?

Comprehensive history taking is similar to that for patients with other disease processes. Some of the questions specific to this condition are listed in Table 49-1.

Physical exam of the sexual assault survivor

The medical portion of the exam includes a detailed examination of the entire body in order to assess all potential areas of trauma and rule out life-threatening injuries. In addition to genitalia, the breast is a common target of assault; facial injuries or head trauma may also occur. The forensic evaluation may include photographs or drawings of the injuries.

If the patient consents to contact with a law enforcement organization, evidence will be placed in the sexual assault evidence collection kit per the protocol of the legal jurisdiction. A representative sexual assault evidence collection kit is pictured in Figures 49-1 and 49-2. These kits contain instructions and envelopes for specific evidence components.

The health-care provider should document the emotional condition of the patient. Specific components of the physical examination are listed in Table 49-2.

Table 49-2 Physical exam of sexual assault survivors

- Full body survey for injuries. Face and breasts are frequent targets of extra-genital attack. If oral violation, inspect mouth for injuries. Confirm the patient is medically stable.
- Obtain an informed consent for any forensic exam.
- Document all injuries; consider drawings or photographs.
- Assess patient for alcohol or drug intoxication.
- Obtain specimens for forensic evaluation if patient permission has been obtained for legal involvement and fulfill requirements of sexual assault evidence collection kit.
- Inspect vulva for injuries. Excellent light is essential and magnification may be considered.
- In case of foreign object assault, be aware and inspect for potential vaginal laceration and subsequent intraperitoneal injury.
- Obtain vaginal secretions and perform microscopic evaluation for motile sperm and trichomonas.
- Obtain specimens for gonorrhea and chlamydia.
- Inspect anus for injury.

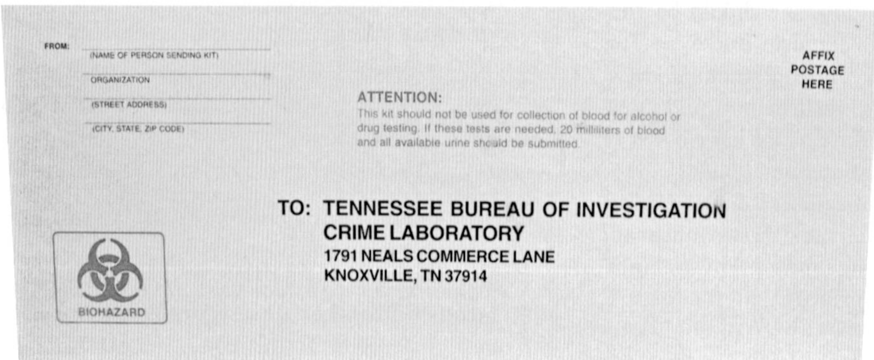

Figure 49-1 Sexual assault evidence collection kit unopened.

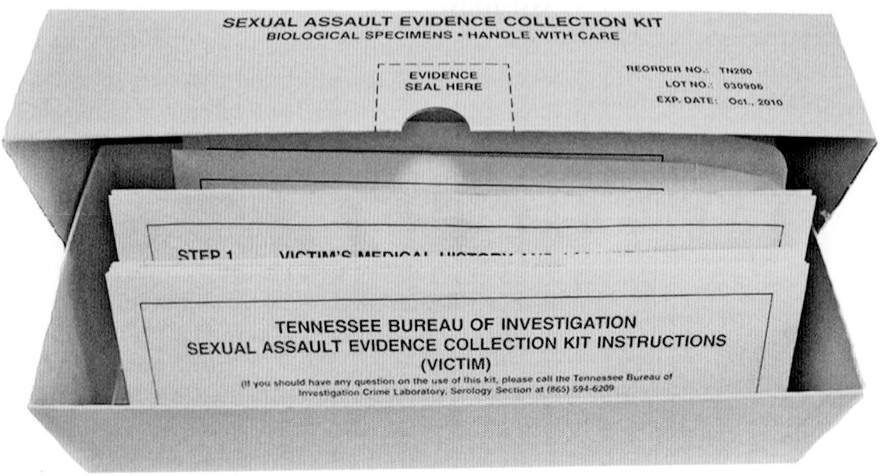

Figure 49-2 Sexual assault evidence collection kit opened.

Laboratory analysis

Acute laboratory assessment includes a pregnancy test. If the test is positive, the victim will know that the father of the fetus is *not* the recent rapist.

Testing for *N. Gonorrhea* and *C. Trachomatis* should be considered. A wet mount should be analyzed for *T. vaginalis*. The Centers for Disease Control and Prevention (CDC) recommends a serum specimen for evaluation of human immunodeficiency virus (HIV), hepatitis B, and syphilis, but some authors disagree with this recommendation.[13, 14] The evaluator should keep in mind the possibility that a future defense attorney may use any positive result from these tests as a mechanism to promote a concept that the assault was consensual.

Drug-facilitated sexual assault is felt to be increasing.[15] In drug-facilitated rapes, the victims are incapacitated and unable to resist sexual contact. Memory may be impaired. Date rape drugs are often consumed with alcohol and their effects may be erroneously identified as alcohol intoxication. Rapid toxicological analysis is indicated; over fifty drugs have been known or suspected of involvement in drug-facilitated sexual assault.[16] If the provider is concerned about date rape drugs, a separate drug screen for such substances may be required. Traditional drug panels test for drugs of abuse; date rape drugs do not fit into this category.

Treatment

Components of treatment include post-coital contraception, sexually transmitted disease prevention and psychologic follow-up. The evaluator must confirm that the patient has a safe place to go upon discharge.

The national rape-related pregnancy rate is believed to be approximately 5% per rape among females aged 12–45 years.[17] Emergency contraception is available in multiple forms:

- hormonal methods include high dose levonorgestrel (Plan B®) or ulipristal acetate (Ella®) or high doses of standard birth control pills (Yuzpe method)
- intrauterine device (IUD)
- mifepristone is available as a post-coital contraceptive in some regions, although in the United States it is only available as an abortifacient.

The levonorgestrel oral emergency contraceptive reduces a woman's chances of pregnancy to 2.6% when used within 72 hours compared to the ulipristal acetate medication, which reduces a woman's chances of pregnancy to 1.8% if used within 120 hours.[18]

Although it is difficult to quantify the risk of acquiring a new sexually transmitted infection after sexual assault, a literature review showed the risk of acquiring Neisseria gonorrhea infection after sexual assault is 0%–26%, while the rate of acquiring *Chlamydia trachomatis* infection is 4%–17%. Acquisition of *Trichomonas vaginalis* infection is 0%–19%.[19] Prophylaxis for *Chlamydia trachomatis, Neisseria gonorrhea,* and *trichomonas vaginalis* is recommended; three medications will be required. For *Neisseria gonorrhea*, the recommended treatment regimen is a single dose of ceftriaxone 250 mg IM *or* a single dose of cefixime 400 mg orally. For *trichomonas vaginalis*, a single dose of metronidazole 2 g orally should be given. For *Chlamydia trachomatis*, a single dose of azithromycin 1 g orally or doxycycline 100 mg orally twice a day for seven days is prescribed.[20]

Appropriate antibiotic prophylaxis is often omitted for sexual assault survivors; approximate treatment rates as low as 6.7% have been recorded.[21] Implementation of a standardized electronic order entry system for sexual assault victims in the emergency room has been show to improve adherence to CDC sexually transmitted disease prophylaxis guidelines.[11]

HIV seroconversion secondary to sexual assault has occurred but the frequency seems to be low for vaginal assault and slightly higher for rectal assault.[13] The risk of HIV transmission is estimated to be 1 or 2 cases per 100,000 for vaginal assault and 2 or 3 cases per 10,00 for anal assault.[14] If the perpetrator's HIV status is known to be positive, the victim should be offered HIV prophylaxis. If the HIV status is unknown, the risks and benefits of nonoccupational post-exposure prophylaxis must be considered on a case-by-case basis.

Although a definitive statement of benefit cannot be made regarding post-exposure prophylaxis against HIV, post-exposure prophylaxis should be offered, in the author's opinion, to those patients who request it. Additional risk factors that may encourage the use of HIV post-exposure prophylaxis include known high-risk behaviors by the assailant, multiple assailants, presence of mucosal lesions in the survivor or assailant, or the presence of lacerations or abrasions. If the survivor has been violated via receptive anal sex, HIV prophylaxis has been recommended.[22]

Post-exposure prophylaxis to HIV within 72 hours of the assault is likely to be effective.[23]

Options for HIV prophylaxis after sexual exposure include:

- Kaletra one tablet per day and tenofovir two tablets twice per day for 28 days. This regimen may require symptomatic treatment with loperamide for the diarrhea associated with the prophylaxis. Nausea and vomiting may also be side effects that require additional medication.[12]
- Tenofovir plus emtricitabine (Truvada) once a day for 28 days.[14]
- Lamivudine plus zidovudine (Combivir) one tablet twice a day for 28 days.

HIV prophylactic medications can have varying and significant side effects including gastrointestinal upset, liver enzyme elevations, neutropenia, anemia, and renal toxicity.[14] These side effects may have a deleterious effect on patient completion of the prescribed regimen.

Acquisition of hepatitis after sexual assault has been reported.[24] Hepatitis B vaccination has been recommended and at minimum should be considered in areas where a high prevalence of this infection exists.[22, 25] A rapid course of vaccination may prevent acute hepatitis B infection if given for up to six weeks after exposure.[26] If the assailant is known to be at risk for hepatitis B, prophylaxis with immunoglobulin and subsequent rapid immunization may be considered.[12]

It seems reasonable to consider tetanus prophylaxis or a booster of tetanus toxoid if bodily abrasions or other wounds are present and the patient's prior tetanus administration date is remote. The offering of a shower and provision of fresh clothes would be appropriate.

Due to the high emotional intensity of a sexual assault experience, patients may have difficulty remembering information provided by health-care providers. Instructions and plans should therefore be provided in writing and a visit for clinical and psychological follow-up should be scheduled in one to two weeks. Sexual assault treatment goals are summarized in Table 49-3.

Table 49-3 Medical management of the sexual assault patient

- Assure patient safety and privacy
- Treat physical injuries
- Discuss results of evaluation with patient
- Discuss results pregnancy test
- STD testing is recommended by the CDC but not by all experts
- Emergency contraception if patient is at risk of pregnancy from the assault and pregnancy test is negative
- Tetanus booster if indicated
- Prophylaxis against chlamydia with azithromycin or doxycycline
- Prophylaxis against gonorrhea with ceftriaxone
- HIV prophylaxis if anal assault or high -risk assailant
- Hepatitis B prophylaxis could be considered in areas at high risk for transmission
- Confirm patient has a safe home environment prior to discharge
- Provide initial counseling and arrange for follow-up counseling and assess for risk of self-harm
- Arrange for follow-up medical care
- Arrange for follow-up psychologic care and/or refer to local victim advocacy group
- Provide prevention of self-harm and suicide
- Confirm safeguards are in place for vulnerable patients

Short-term medical follow-up

The patient must receive follow-up counseling. Follow-up medical evaluations provide opportunities to detect post-assault infections, complete hepatitis B immunization if indicated, confirm ongoing counseling, and monitor post-exposure prophylactic medication.

A follow-up pregnancy test three weeks after emergency contraception should be considered. If emergency contraception did not prevent the pregnancy, the patient should be offered the option of termination of pregnancy. Products of conception may have forensic significance.

Repeat examination for sexually transmitted diseases (*C. trachomatis*, *N. gonorrhea*, and *T. vaginalis*) is recommended in one to two weeks. Serologic testing for syphilis and HIV are recommended at six weeks, three months, and six months after the assault.[13]

The physician and legal responsibility

The health-care provider's initial legal responsibilities are summarized in Table 49-4.

Less than 20% of rape victims report the assault to law enforcement, and less than half of these cases are successfully prosecuted.[1, 27, 28] On those occasions that a case goes to court, the examining health-care

Table 49-4 Sexual assault – brief summary of legal responsibilities

- Provide accurate medical record of events.
- Document injuries.
- Collect samples as indicated by local or state regulations using the evidence collection kit.
- Microscopically analyze vaginal fluids and identify the presence or absence of sperm.
- Complete law enforcement reports as required.
- Ensure chain of evidence.
- Be prepared to offer testimony if subpoenaed.

provider may be subpoenaed to testify about the evaluation. The health-care provider is usually a witness for the prosecution but on occasion may be subpoenaed as a witness for the defense.

In medico-legal cases such as prosecutions for sexual assault, the physician or other health-care provider's responsibility is to the truth. In the author's experience, defense attorneys have attempted to demonstrate a lack of competence on the part of the physician. It is the physician's responsibility to do his or her part to ensure that the judge and/or jury receive complete and unprejudiced information. It is not the medical expert's job to convict anyone.

It is reasonable for the physician to decline an invitation to meet with the defense attorney prior to the trial or deposition unless a representative from the prosecutor's office is also present. If the physician is unfamiliar with the trial process, it is reasonable to request a meeting with the agency (usually the prosecutor's office) that issued the subpoena prior to the court appearance in order to plan ahead for his/her responsibility.

In a survey of Sexual Assault Nurse Examiners (SANE), more than half of these knowledgeable professionals indicated that their most recent trial experience had been challenging. The challenges included (a) providing testimony was emotionally unnerving, (b) difficulties were present with the defense attorney regarding the victim, (c) difficulties with the defense attorney were present regarding the exam and/or evidence, (d) difficulty with the defense attorney were present regarding qualifications of the SANE examiner, and (e) the prosecutor was poorly prepared.[29]

Long-term consequences of sexual assault

Post-traumatic stress disorder may be a long-term consequence of sexual assault. The symptoms of this disorder include reexperiencing the trauma, avoidance, and a state of hyper arousal.[30] One-third of sexual assault survivors develop post-traumatic stress disorders; assault survivors are three times more likely than the general population of women to be currently experiencing a major depressive disorder.[27] Individuals who have been a target of sexual assault have an increased chance of attempted suicide compared to individuals who have not been sexually assaulted.[31] Not all unwanted sexual experiences are labeled as assaults by patients; labeling should not be considered as a criterion for determining who has experienced sexual victimization.[32]

After sexual assault, rape trauma syndrome is common. Rape trauma syndrome consists of an acute phase and long-term reorganization process that is seen after forcible rape or attempted forcible rape. The syndrome includes behavioral, somatic, and psychologic reactions to the life-threatening situation experienced by the survivor. The acute phase of the syndrome shows a disorganization of the patient's lifestyle with a predominant feeling of fear. Self-blame may be a component. The second, or reorganization, phase is a longer-term process that can include phobic reactions, nightmares, and sexual dysfunction.[33]

Screening

Health-care providers should routinely screen all patients for a history of sexual assault, paying particular attention to those who report sexual dysfunction, pelvic pain, and dysmenorrhea.[34] Although sexual assault screening appears to be more common than in the past, less than half of patients recalled ever being screened for sexual assault in one study.[35] Women felt comfortable being screened and felt that information about sexual victimization was helpful.

Clinicians should screen for substance abuse when evaluating patients with a history of sexual assault. Conversely, clinicians should screen for a history of sexual assault in patients with a history of substance abuse.[3]

Prevention

Several patient categories include women who are at increased risk of sexual assault. Women with disabilities that severely limit activities of daily living are at increased risk of sexual assault. Women with cognitive defects may also be at increased risk but abuse in this population is difficult to assess.[36] Lesbian and bisexual or transgendered patients and alcohol/ drug abusers are also at increased risk.[37, 38] Younger women report sexual assault more than do older women.[39] Individuals who have never been married or are separated or divorced are more likely to experience unwanted sexual activity.[39] Alcohol use increases the victim's vulnerability to sexual assault; alcohol and drugs have long been recognized as important risk factors for sexual assault.[39–40] As many as 20%–25% of college women may be sexually assaulted during their college years, making individuals in this demographic group potential beneficiaries of prevention programs.[42]

Only a few studies on sexual assault prevention exist. Success was described in two of five publications on college sexual assault prevention programs.[43] The author was unable to identify any studies on the efficacy for any medical office sexual assault prevention program. It seems reasonable to suggest, however, that health-care providers for women, and especially those who care for women in vulnerable categories, should educate patients about the high incidence of sexual assault, the linking of sexual assault with drug and alcohol abuse, the existence of "date rape" drugs which can be placed into beverages, and the need to be aware of personal safety at all times.

Sexual assault and society

An in-depth study of sexual assault survivors' contact with the health-care system concluded that health-care providers who provide suboptimal care to sexual assault survivors can impede the recovery of these patients.[44] Factors associated with impediments to the recovery process include health-care provider inexperience, adherence to rape myths, acceptance of stereotypes, and disrespectful or inconsiderate treatment of survivors. Survivor participants' accounts conveyed a wish for health professionals to receive more training in dealing with women who have experienced sexual assault. Participants generally wanted to disclose the assault and be encouraged to do so, but instead their experience showed that health professionals failed to inquire about sexual assault. Study subjects reported concerns of not being believed or even blamed by health-care professionals. Participants desired respectful treatment; they wanted to be offered medical services and treatment but did not want to be forced into accepting these services or treatments. Subjects reported the failure of health professionals to attend to or believe disclosures of their sexual assault prevented them from receiving necessary medical care and trivialized the survivor's experiences.[44]

Clinicians often need training in the provision of sexual assault care.[45] Additionally, health-care providers have been exposed to the same rape myths as the general population and their acceptance of such myths may negatively impact patient care. Such myths include that rape is provoked by the victim, that promiscuous women are raped, that rape can be avoided by resistance, that women respect men for overpowering them, and that rapists are not responsible for their acts.[46]

Many communities have developed programs to support sexual assault victims. Studies suggest that sexual assault treatment-based settings attract more sexual assault survivors than forensic-based settings. The involvement of all relevant stakeholders including the voluntary and community sectors is felt to be important to ensure appropriate referral and follow-up mechanisms. It is felt imperative that this care be available free of charge to anyone who wishes it.[11]

Sexual assault nurse examiners (SANE) are specially trained medical professionals who provide care documentation and collect evidence from sexual assault victims. Research has shown that SANE-trained providers collect more effective biological evidence than non-SANE providers.[47]

For many survivors, the emergency department is the first and only opportunity to receive both immediate therapeutic care and care for emotional trauma. Since many components of complete post assault care can be missed, it is important that health-care providers ensure that those patients seen in follow-up have received the appropriate initial care. Health-care providers should be aware of many deficiencies frequently observed in the management of sexual assault victims. Less than one-fifth of hospitals provide complete comprehensive medical care management services.[48] Only 50% of hospitals provide onsite emergency contraception, and only 40% of hospitals provide both acute rape crisis counseling and referrals for longer-term care.[48] Eighteen percent of hospitals fail to always provide prophylaxis for some sexually transmitted infections.[48]

Those who wish to improve the provision of services to sexual assault victims in their own communities may wish to initiate training programs; simulation training has been shown to enhance the education of sexual assault forensic examiners.[5]

Concluding remarks

Sexual assault is a prevalent issue that is managed as a medical condition using the principles mentioned above. Effects of sexual assault on the patient are both acute and chronic. Resources external to the practitioner's office are important in successful management. Many sexual assault victims report suboptimal experiences with the health-care system. It is appropriate for health-care providers to work with their communities to improve the care of these patients.

References

1. Tjaden PG, Thoennes N. *Extent, nature, and consequences of rape victimization: findings from the National Violence against Women Survey.* Washington, DC: National Institute of Justice, 2006. (NCJ 210346.)
2. Dunn SFM, Gilchrist VJ. Sexual assault. *Prim Care* 1993; **20**:359–73. Bibliographic Links [Context Link].
3. ACOG Committee Opinion No. 499. Sexual Assault. American College of Obstetricians and Gynecologists. Committee on Health Care for Underserved Women. *Obstet Gynecol* 2011 Aug;**118**(2 Pt 1):396–9.
4. US Department of Justice, Office of Justice Programs, Bureau of Justice Statistics. Criminal victimization in the United States – statistical tables, 2005. Available at: http://bjs.ojp.usdoj.gov/index.cfm?ty=pbdetai l&iid=1095. Accessed November 20, 2009.
5. Fitzpatrick M, Ta A, Lenchus J, Arheart KL, Rosen LF, Birnbach DJ. Sexual assault forensic examiners' training and assessment using simulation technology. *J Emerg Nurs* 2012 Jan;**38**(1):85–90.
6. Tjaden P, Thoennes N. *Full report of the prevalence, incidence, and consequences of violence against women: findings from the National Violence against Women Survey.* NCJ 183781. Washington, DC: US Department of Justice, Office of Justice Programs; 2000. Available at: http://www.ncjrs.gov/pdffiles1/nij/183781.pdf. Retrieved May 5, 2010.
7. Dickinson LM, de Gruy FV 3rd, Dickinson WP, Candib LM. Health-related quality of life and symptom profiles of female survivors of sexual abuse. *Arch Fam Med* 1999 Jan–Feb;**8**(1):35–43.
8. Golding JM, Wilsnack SC, Learman LA. Prevalence of sexual assault history among women with common gynecologic symptoms. *Am J Obstet Gynecol* Oct; **179**(4):1013–19.
9. Dansky BS, Saladin ME, Coffey SF, Brady KT. Use of self-report measures of crime-related posttraumatic stress disorder with substance use disordered patients. *J Subst Abuse Treat* 1997 March;**14**(5):431–7.
10. Bowyer L, Dalton ME. Female victims of rape and their genital injuries. *Br J Obstet Gynaecol* 1997 May;**104**(5):617–20.
11. Eogan M, McHugh A, Holohan M. The role of the sexual assault centre. *Best Pract Res Clin Obstet Gynaecol* 2013 Feb;**27**(1):47–58.
12. Cybulska B. Immediate medical care after sexual assault. *Best Pract Res Clin Obstet Gynaecol* 2013 Feb;**27**(1):141–9.
13. Centers for Disease Control. Sexually Transmitted Diseases Treatment Guidelines, 2006. Sexual Assault and STDS. Available at: www.cdc.gov/mmwr/preview/mmwrhtml/rr5511a1.htm. Accessed Dec 5, 2015.
14. Linden JA. Care of the adult patient after sexual assault. *N Engl J Med* 2011;**369**(9):834–41.
15. Beynon CM, McVeigh C, McVeigh J, et al. The involvement of drugs and alcohol in drug-facilitated sexual assault: a systematic review of the evidence. *Trauma Violence & Abuse* 2008;**9**:178–88. Available at: http://tva.sagepub.com/content/9/3/178. Accessed Dec 5, 2015.
16. Dinis-Oliveira RJ, Magalhães T. Forensic toxicology in drug-facilitated sexual assault. *Toxicol Mech Methods* 2013 Sep;**23**(7):471–8.
17. Holmes MM, Resnick HS, Kilpatrick DG, Best CL. Rape-related pregnancy: estimates and descriptive characteristics from a national sample of women. *Am J Obstet Gynecol* 1996 Aug;**175**(2):320–5.
18. Glasier AF, Cameron ST, Fine PM, et al. Ulipristal acetate versus levonorgestrel for emergency contraception: a randomized non-inferiority trial and meta-analysis. *Lancet* 2010 Feb;**375**:555–62.
19. Reynolds MW, Peipert JF, Collins B. Epidemiologic issues of sexually transmitted diseases in sexual assault victims. *Obstet Gynecol Surv* 2000 Jan;**55**(1):51–7.
20. Workowski KA, Berman S, Centers for Disease Control and Prevention (CDC). Sexually Transmitted Diseases Treatment Guidelines 2010. *MMWR Recomm Rep* 2010 Dec 17;**59**(RR-12):1–110.
21. Straight JD, Heaton PC. Emergency department care for victims of sexual offense. *Am J Health-Syst Pharm* 2007 Sep 1;**64**:1845–50.
22. Cybulska B. Immediate medical care after sexual assault. *Best Pract Clin Obstet Gynaecol* 2013 Feb; **27**(1):141–9.
23. McCarty EJ, Quah S, Maw R, et al. Post-exposure prophylaxis following sexual exposure to HIV: a seven-year retrospective analysis in a regional centre. *Int J STD AIDS* 2011 Jul;**22**(7):407–8.
24. Crowe C, Forster GE, Dinsmore WW, Maw RD. A case of acute hepatitis B occurring four months after multiple rape. *Int J STD AIDS* 1996 Mar–Apr; 7(2):133–4.

25. Association for Genitourinary Medicine, Medical Society for the Study of Venereal Disease. 2001 National Guidelines on the Management of Adult Victims of Sexual Assault. Available at: http://www.bashh.org/documents/54/54.pdf. Accessed Dec 5, 2015.
26. Ahmed SM, Volpellier M, Forster G. The use of the super accelerated hepatitis B vaccination regimen in a north London sexual assault referral centre (SARC). *Jour For Legal Med 14* 2007;72–74.
27. National Victim Center. Crime Victims Research and Treatment Center. Rape in America: A report to the nation. 1992 April 23;1–16. Available at: www.victimsofcrime.org/docs/Reports%20and%20Studies/rape-in-america.pdf?sfvrsn=0. Accessed Dec 5, 2015.
28. Campbell R, Patterson D, Bybee D, Dworkin ER. Predicting sexual assault prosecution outcomes: The role of medical forensic evidence collected by sexual assault nurse examiners. *Criminal Justice and Behavior* 2009 July;**36**(7):712–27. Available at: http://cjb.sagepub.com/content/36/7/712. Accessed Dec 5, 2015.
29. Campbell R, Long SM, Townsend SM, et al. Sexual assault nurse examiners' experiences providing expert witness court testimony. *J Forsensic Nurs* 2007 Spring;**3**(1):7–14.
30. Nakell L. Adult post-traumatic stress disorder: screening and treating in primary care. *Prim Care Clin Office Pract* 2007;**34**:593–610.
31. Ullman SE, Najdowski CJ. Correlates of serious suicidal ideation and attempts in female adult sexual assault survivors. *Suicide Life-Threat Behav* 2009 Feb;**39**(1):47–57.
32. Harned MD. Does it matter what you call it? The relationship between labeling unwanted sexual experiences and distress. *J Consult Clin Psychol* 2004 Dec;**72**(6):1090–9.
33. Burgess AW, Holmstrom LL. Rape trauma syndrome. *Am J Psychiatry* 1974 Sep;**131**(9):981–6.
34. Council on Scientific Affairs, AMA (1992) Violence against women: relevance for medical practitioners. *JAMA* 1992 June;**267**(23): 3184–9.
35. Littleton HL, Bereenson AB, Breitkopf CR. An evaluation of health care providers' sexual violence screening practices. *Am J Obstet Gynecol* 2007;**196**:564. el–e7.
36. Castell C, Martin SL, Smith JB, et al. National study of physical and sexual assault among women with disabilities. *Inj Prev* 2008 Apr;**14**(2):87–90.
37. Balsam KF, Rothblum ED, Beauchaine TP. Victimization over the life span: a comparison of lesbian, gay, bisexual, and heterosexual siblings. *Jour Consult Clin Psych* 2005;**73**(3):477–87.
38. Horvath M, Brown J. The role of drugs and alcohol in rape. *Med Sci Law* 2006 Jul;**46**(3):219–28.
39. Basile KC, Chen J, Black MC, Saltzman LE. Prevalence and characteristics of sexual violence victimization among US adults, 2001–2003. *Viol & Vict* 2007;**22**(4):437–48.
40. Golan A, Dishi-Galitzk M, Barda J, Lurie S. The care of sexual assault victims: the first regional center in Israel –10 years experience. *Isr Med Assoc J* 2012 Nov; **14**(11):658–61.
41. Beynon CM, McVeigh C, McVeigh J, et al. The involvement of drugs and alcohol in drug-facilitated sexual assault: a systematic review of the evidence. *Trauma, Violence, & Abuse* 2008 July;**9**(3):178–88.
42. Fisher BS, Cullen FT, Turner MG. *The sexual victimization of college women*. Washington, DC: US Dept of Justice. National Institute of Justice; 2000. Publication NCJ 182369.
43. Rothman E, Silverman J. The effect of a college sexual assault prevention program on first-year students' victimization rates. *J Am Coll Health* 2007 Mar–Apr; **55**(5):283–90.
44. Ranjbar V, Speer SA. Revictimization and recovery from sexual assault: implications for health professionals. *Violence Vict* 2013;**28**(2):274–87.
45. Martin SL, Young SK, Billings DL, Bross CC. Health care-based interventions for women who have experienced sexual violence: a review of the literature. *Trauma, Violence, & Abuse* 2007;**8**:3–18.
46. Heinrich LB. Care of the female rape victim. *Nurse Pract* 1987 Nov;**12**(11):9–12, 16–18, 23–7.
47. Sievers V, Murphy S, Miller JJ. Sexual assault evidence collection more accurate when completed by sexual assault nurse examiners: Colorado's experience. *J Emer Nurs* 2003 Dec;**29**:511–14.
48. Patel A, Roston A, Tilmon S, et al. Assessing the extent of provision of comprehensive medical care management for female sexual assault patients in US hospital emergency departments. *Int J Gynaecol Obstet* 2013 Jul;**10**:1–5.

Chapter 50

Ethics in office practice

Elizabeth A. Ferries-Rowe

Introduction

Health-care providers recognize the necessity of practicing ethical care and generally believe they provide it. As such, devoting a chapter of an office practice textbook to bioethics may seem superfluous. Certainly, some of the more egregious errors in medical ethics are now a thing of the past. The infamous Tuskegee syphilis experiment of 1932–1972 has become a cautionary tale about informed consent and justice in medical care,[1] and many states now have laws to protect patients from compulsory sterilization as a direct response to the eugenics movement of the early twentieth century.[2] Without belittling these efforts to advance respectful patient care, it is important to recognize the many ethical challenges that still present during the care of obstetric and gynecologic patients in the office setting. High-stakes issues including domestic violence, respect for privacy, abortion care, and informed consent are likely to initiate consideration of ethical concerns by their very nature, but less contentious decisions also require a facility with basic medical ethics as a platform on which to construct a range of appropriate treatment options and to communicate those options effectively to patients.

This chapter will first review the four traditional pillars of bioethics and discuss the application of those concepts to common obstetric and gynecologic clinical situations. The evolution of patient-provider communication styles as it applies to these tenets of medical ethics will then be discussed. The chapter will conclude with case scenarios to illustrate the type of ethically fraught decisions obstetricians and gynecologists may regularly encounter during office care. The process of intentionally considering ethical concerns as part of routine patient care will be described. Just as in the operating room, where repetition of operative technique develops "muscle memory" that allows good practice to become routine, conscious consideration of medical ethics in standard practice will allows providers to become comfortable with these issues and capable of regularly providing the type of patient-centered care required for patients.

The four pillars of bioethics

Tom Beauchamp and James Childress introduced the four traditional pillars of bioethics in their textbook *Principles of Biomedical Ethics* in 1977.[3] Prior to the publication of this text, bioethics had been described as "a mixture of religion, whimsy, exhortation, legal precedents, various traditions, philosophies of life, miscellaneous moral rules and epithets."[4] Beauchamp and Childress recognized the shortcomings of this ad hoc approach and developed a more systematic framework to standardize the discussion of bioethics and to allow for a common starting point for conversation and decision making in the provision of medical care. The four concepts introduced were *beneficence*, *non-maleficence*, *autonomy*, and *justice*. After discussing each of these concepts separately, the interaction of these pillars will be considered along with conflict resolution when conflicts arise.

Beneficence

The first principle of bioethics to consider is beneficence, which refers to the obligation to actively pursue the well-being of others.[5] Efforts to promote health, whether through preventative care (e.g., cervical and breast cancer screening) or active treatment of illness (e.g., medical management or surgical care), are grounded in the principle of beneficence. Treatment choices are made with the goal of meeting obligations to advance the well-being of patients.

Office Care of Women, ed. Martin E. Olsen and Botros Rizk. Published by Cambridge University Press.

Of course, all potentially beneficial options come with associated risks. The obligation to beneficence is counterbalanced by next tenet of bioethics – non-maleficence.

Non-maleficence

Contrary to the active pursuit of the good that defines beneficence, non-maleficence restrains action in order to avoid doing harm. The medical concept of "First, do no harm" is built on the concept of non-maleficence.[5] Providers have the responsibility to avoid acting in ways that would place patients in positions of lesser health than if no intervention had occurred. It is easy to see how beneficence and non-maleficence may conflict. Consider the common situation in which a provider discusses treatment options for menorrhagia related to fibroids. Hysterectomy offers the benefit of definitive resolution of bleeding, which seems most consistent with the duty to beneficence. On the other hand, it also carries the greatest risk of potential morbidity and mortality. As such, hysterectomy may run afoul of the duty to non-maleficence. The provider must consider whether the potential risk for harm and opportunity for benefit of a particular therapy are such that he or she better promotes the well-being of the patient by expectant management, medical therapy, or surgical treatment.

Each clinical scenario is different, of course, and the unique opportunity for understanding that exists within the clinical encounter both allows and obligates providers to consider those unique details in order to help patients make medical decisions that best meet their needs.

Autonomy

The third pillar, autonomy, refers to the principle that a competent patient has the right to determine what happens to her during the course of medical therapy. As Beauchamp and Childress define it, autonomy requires two conditions: "1) *liberty* (independence from controlling influences) and 2) *agency* (capacity for intentional action)."[5] At first, this tenet seems pretty straightforward and the obligation to it relatively easy to meet. So long as a patient is deemed competent (i.e., possessing agency), providers are generally comfortable not treating patients in ways that they have expressly refused. However, it is important to consider what is meant by liberty. Do providers risk inappropriately controlling patients by selectively including or excluding data from counseling? Are appeals to authority or emotion used in ways that limit patients' abilities to exercise autonomy?

It seems important to include objective, relevant information in a nondirective way in order to promote autonomous decision making, but the realities of a busy office practice can make this a daunting – if not impossible – task. Interest in providing ethical care requires development of ways to support patient autonomy within the confines of short visit times and highly varied levels of both patient education and desire for information. Later the various approaches to patient-provider communication will be assessed in order to optimize autonomy in a practicable way.

Justice

Distribution of limited resources in health care necessitates a discussion of justice. This final principle in this construct of bioethics can be defined as "fair, equitable, and appropriate treatment in light of what is due or owed to persons."[5] By its very nature, justice is more abstractly relevant to the individual than are the other three pillars of bioethics are, and it falls upon providers to consider the manner in which health-care decisions impact the distribution of and access to health care at the community level. Although there are many different philosophical theories of justice, the relevant constant thread that runs through them is recognition of the necessary tradeoffs that are made in circumstances of limited resources. Whereas for some, considerations of justice may lead to political participation or work with underserved populations, it remains relevant in even the most basic clinical encounter. Judicious use of imaging and expensive medications, participation in insurance plans of varying reimbursement levels, and division of clinical work between various venues and populations are part and parcel of the obligation to justice.

Competing obligations

If these four pillars can all be satisfied at once, then there is not much ethical angst to resolve. Of course, medical decisions are rarely so straightforward. As the aforementioned hysterectomy scenario illustrates, competing obligations often must be weighed against each other to determine the right course of action. This illustrates the prima facie nature of these four ethical obligations. Prima facie obligations are those that are owed when all other things are equal, but *actual* duties are those that we are obligated to perform in a particular situation.[5] That is, actual duty

Table 50-1 Theoretical application of prima facie obligations to hysterectomy in a relatively healthy patient

Beneficence	Non-maleficence
Supports hysterectomy	Weakly opposes hysterectomy
Autonomy	**Justice**
Supports hysterectomy	Weakly supports hysterectomy

Table 50-2 Theoretical application of prima facie obligations to hysterectomy in a patient with multiple comorbidities

Beneficence	Non-maleficence
Weakly supports hysterectomy	Strongly opposes hysterectomy
Autonomy	**Justice**
Supports hysterectomy	Weakly opposes hysterectomy (increased burden to the health-care system given risk of complications)

to the patient is the decision made after weighing prima facie obligations and resolving conflicts between them with the patient's well-being and expressed desires at the heart of decision making.

The value of this framework for medically ethical decision making is its universal applicability. Developing a comfort with these tenets and with the resolution of conflicts between them is the foundation for ethics in the clinical setting. For example, consider the choice to perform a hysterectomy for fibroids on an otherwise healthy patient with a good understanding of the risks and benefits of her options. The matrix in Table 50-1 provides a visual structure within which to consider treatment options.

Using this framework, it seems easy to conclude that hysterectomy is an ethical choice for this patient. Consider, though, what the framework might look like for a patient with small, subserosal fibroids who is requesting a hysterectomy for heavy periods. If this patient has a history of prior bowel injury due to adhesive disease, a hemoglobin of 14 g/dL, and a recent hemoglobin A1c of 12%, the algorithm may look more like Table 50-2. In this case, it would seem that declining to perform a hysterectomy for this patient is the more ethical decision.

Autonomy has played the dominant role in recent years – largely in response to the egregious assaults on autonomy in the first part of the century. As such, it can be challenging for a provider to refuse to perform a procedure that a patient requests. It is a mistake, though, to conclude that autonomy trumps the other three pillars of medical ethics.[5] There is a sound foundation for the ethical avoidance of certain treatments, even though the patient has expressed a desire for a particular therapy. Providers are not obligated to act simply because a competent patient expresses a desire that such be done. Further, providers are not required to provide care that is found to be futile, harmful, or morally objectionable.[5–7] Respect for autonomy does dictate that a patient's competent, voluntary decision making is recognized and that providers be forthright with reasons for refusing to provide the requested therapy. In some circumstances, it may also be appropriate to refer the patient to another provider.

Competing obligations in obstetric care

Obstetric care provides a unique challenge to medical ethics. Not only must obligations to the mother as the patient be considered, but prenatal care presumes the fetus is considered a separate patient to which an obligation is also owed. The notion of fetal personhood is ambiguous and politically fraught,[8] but in practice many recommendations and treatments offered to pregnant women are designed to promote the health of the fetus. Further, the avoidance of some therapies in pregnancy that may otherwise benefit the mother is a reflection of the obligation to non-maleficence to the fetus. Obligations to both parties get muddy when the obligation to one is in conflict with the obligation to the other. From abortion to substance abuse by pregnant women to medically indicated preterm delivery, conflicts between obligations to the mother and to the fetus are pervasive. It can be overwhelming, if not impossible, to try to resolve these conflicts without some method of systematically considering and weighing prima facie obligations to each. The preceding matrix of the four tenets of bioethics can be modified to include both maternal and fetal obligations for each, which provides a logical framework for determining actual obligations and determining right action. See Table 50-3. This is not a perfect model, since autonomy is not a concept that can be usefully applied to a fetus. The basic process of weighing various prima facie obligations is comparable to the earlier hysterectomy example, though, and can be used to help guide decision making in the care of pregnant patients.

Patient–physician communication

The provision of medical care is not a one-sided academic exercise. Effective patient-provider communication is both a means to the end of ethical decision making and an end in itself that creates an environment of patient-centered care.[9, 10] Ezekiel and Linda Emanuel characterized four different models of physician-patient communication in the *Journal of the American Medical Association* in 1992: (1) *the paternalistic model*, (2) *the informative model*, (3) *the interpretive model*, and (4) *the deliberative model*.[11] This construct is a useful way to describe the range of approaches to medical decision making in the clinical context, and it also illustrates the evolution of decision making from paternalism to consumerism to, hopefully, the optimal balance of expertise brought to the table by both the provider and the patient. (See Table 50-4 for a summary of these models.)

Table 50-3 Theoretical application of prima facie obligations to obstetric care

Beneficence		**Non-maleficence**	
Woman	Fetus	Woman	Fetus
Autonomy		**Justice**	
Woman	Fetus	Woman	Fetus

The paternalistic model

The paternalistic model includes communication patterns in which the provider uses his or her medical skills to identify the patient's condition, determines the treatment most likely to relieve that condition, and presents selected information to encourage the patient to choose the treatment the he or she has deemed best for the patient. In the extreme, paternalism involves the provider enacting a course of treatment without attending to the patient's understanding of the diagnosis or options and without eliciting the patient's desires. In this model, the provider acts as the patient's guardian with an emphasis on identifying the patient's best interests and making decisions to promote those interests. Beneficence and, to a lesser degree non-maleficence, are prioritized in this model.

Because providers have completed medical training and patients generally have not, it can be easy to fall into paternalistic patterns that rely on appeal to authority to determine treatments. The difficulty with this model, of course, is that "best treatment" often cannot be objectively identified. Consider the menorrhagia scenario presented earlier. The physician may believe that hysterectomy is the superior course of action because it conclusively addresses the medical condition, but the patient may prioritize future fertility or desire for uninterrupted employment. The paternalistic decision to perform surgery would not meet the patient's criteria for what is best.

Although the paternalistic model was once the most common approach to patient-provider

Table 50-4 Summary of patient-provider communication styles

	Provider obligation	Provider role	Conception of autonomy
Paternalism	Promoting patient well-being independent of patient preferences	Guardian	Assenting to objective values
Informative	Proving information and implementing patient plan	Technical expert	Control over medical care
Interpretive	Elucidating and interpreting patient values and implementing patient plan	Counselor	Self-understanding relevant to medical care
Deliberative	Articulating patient values, persuading patient to choose admirable values, and implementing patient plan	Teacher/friend	Moral self-development relevant to medical care

Source: Adapted from Emanuel and Emanuel (1992, p. 2222).[11]

communication, the example above illustrates its major weakness and prompts a look for alternative communication styles.

The informative model

Unlike the paternalistic model, the informative model emphasizes patient authority. The role of the provider is to supply all relevant information, and the patient then chooses from all options for diagnosis and treatment. The provider is then obligated to carry out the patient's expressed preferences. In a sense, the provider acts as technical advisor, providing medical expertise that the patient lacks to allow the patient to make decisions consistent with her values. This consumer model of health care places greater emphasis on patient autonomy than on the other three pillars of medical ethics.

At first glance, this model seems appealing and consistent with current norms for informed consent. Closer inspection demonstrates important weaknesses. It is not possible for a health-care provider to relay all relevant information to a patient because the entirety of medical training combines to produce the medical expertise that the provider brings to the table. Even if it were possible to truly relay all necessary facts to a patient, her role as patient can make it impossible for her to be entirely objective regarding her medical care. After all, if it is considered a conflict of interest to care for family members because of lack of separation necessary for objectivity, surely it is even more so for a patient acting as her own health-care provider.

The informative model clearly serves as a reaction to the paternalistic model, but it swings so far to the other side of the balance of power and responsibility that it is equally imperfect. In a sense, the informative model invites provider abdication of his or her responsibility to the patient – "because the patient wants it" becomes the trump card for medically inadvisable therapy, and this model has no counterbalance for that risk. Emanuel and Emanuel offer two additional models designed to address the weaknesses of both the paternalistic and informative models.

The interpretive model

As described by the authors, the goal of the interpretive model is "to elucidate the patient's values and what he or she actually wants, and to help the patient select the available medical interventions that realize these values."[11] The provider is again expected to offer information on possible diagnoses, available testing, and risks and benefits of various treatment options. Initially, this seems very similar to the informative model. The interpretive model, however, assigns an additional responsibility to the provider. It asks the provider to assist his or her patient to understand her own goals for her health care and to help the patient identify the options most consistent with those stated goals. The provider serves not only as provider of health care, but also as counselor to assist the patient in values clarification. The provider's full medical expertise can then come to bear in determining which course of action best serves those values.

Clearly, this model of communication seeks to address the subjectivity inherent in determining "best treatment" that plagues the paternalistic model. Like the informative model, it maintains the patient as the central figure in determining her own health care. It offers more than the informative model does because it does not place unreasonable expectations on the patient to make decisions without the benefit of provider judgment and expertise.

The deliberative model

Given the apparent advantages of the interpretive model, one may wonder why further work should be done to advance patient-provider communication. There is a weakness in the interpretive model, though, that should be addressed. Although the interpretive model allows for the elucidation of patient values, it does not leave room for the provider to discuss the quality and worth of those values or to introduce new values. Allowing the provider to weigh in on the worth of the patient's values sounds dangerously close to paternalism, but the meaningful difference is that the provider seeks to persuade, not to induce the patient to any particular action. In fact, a meaningful part of providing medical care is working to convince patients of the superiority of some values over others. Efforts to encourage smoking cessation, increased physical activity, or condom use all hinge on the notion that health-care providers should rightly attempt to convince patients about the relative value of respiratory health, cardiovascular health, and sexual health.

The deliberative model attempts to address this provider responsibility omitted in the interpretive model by providing a mechanism for the provider to attempt to persuade the patient that some values are superior to others. Unlike paternalism, which uses selective information and appeals to authority to impose the provider's will on the patient, the deliberative model uses full disclosure and values clarification through peer to peer discussion to advocate for optimal health care that meets patient needs and is consistent with best medical practices.

Choice of communication model

Each model has its advantages and disadvantages, and in practice each model has its place. A patient with a urinary tract infection, for example, may be well satisfied with a relatively paternalistic approach that quickly and efficiently addresses her concerns. Contraceptive counseling is something for which we often employ the informative approach. A patient facing a new cancer diagnosis will need significantly more assistance with values clarification, information provision, and weighing the risks and benefits of alternative therapies that would be better suited to the deliberative model. Patient preference also plays into the choice of style.

Both the interpretive and deliberative models require a significant amount of time to develop the type of relationship that allows for the discussion needed to achieve clarity of values. The continuity of care inherent in the practice of obstetrics and gynecology serves us well in these types of value-rich discussions because the natural development of the patient-provider relationship provides background that saves time when difficult decisions must be made. The biggest challenge that providers face with the interpretive and deliberative models is rapidly developing this type of relationship when a new patient presents with a complicated condition in need of care. The solution is twofold: (1) as providers become more facile with these styles through repeated use, they are used more efficiently, and (2) communication styles must be varied throughout the clinic day in order to efficiently care for patients with less complicated issues on any given day, so that the time necessary for more complicated patients can be devoted when they present.

At present, the informative model is the dominant model, and many providers are unprepared to participate in the discussion of values necessary to utilize the interpretive or deliberative models.[11] Given the advantages of these models, it will be important for medical training in the future to include more structured instruction on patient-provider communication approaches.

Case studies

In order to better illustrate the interplay of traditional bioethics, communication, and informed consent, consider the following case studies.

Case 1

> You are seeing a 31-year-old G1P0 at 12 weeks of pregnancy for routine new obstetric exam. She has no personal or family history of heritable medical conditions, but reports that her online mom-to-be group has been discussing prenatal testing and asks you if she should have testing in this pregnancy. What would you recommend?

Discussion

With the advent of noninvasive testing for fetal anomalies, patients are now faced with the decision about when and what sort of testing they would like to pursue in an effort to identify fetal anomalies. Early testing poses little risk to the mother, and it can be performed as part of routine blood testing with little additional effort. The ease of testing, though, is deceptive. It is easy for patients to undergo screening tests with little or no discussion of the implications of those tests.[12, 13] In 1997, Press and Browner reported the findings of a survey that investigated parents' reasons for choosing prenatal testing.[14] The following responses illustrate the potential for misunderstanding and confusion that can serve as pitfalls for patients and providers:

"... the more information I have about my baby the better."[14]
"How can it hurt to know?"[14]
"I think you should do whatever you can to help the baby."[14]

The first two responses suggest that there is value to more knowledge, but the value is general and nonspecific. Further, there is no apparent consideration of the choices that may present themselves based on that knowledge. The last statement demonstrates a belief that testing will somehow benefit the baby. Generally speaking, testing has the capacity to identify abnormalities, but very few of those abnormalities are amenable to intrauterine therapy. The preceding statements suggest that the patients may not fully understand the potential risks and benefits of testing, and may be unprepared to handle abnormal results based on insufficient preparatory counseling.

The case for prenatal testing also irrevocably involves a consideration of the question of abortion.[15] For some patients, a diagnosis of a serious anomaly may lead them to choose elective termination of their pregnancies, and for these women the relevance of prenatal testing is clear. For women who express an unwillingness to terminate a pregnancy, regardless of any identified abnormalities, the role of testing is more controversial. Some women may choose to undergo testing anyway, based on the belief that the ability to prepare for a sick child will be of benefit. Other women, though, may decline testing based on a belief that abnormal findings will not change the management of the pregnancy and will only cause anxiety. Without appropriate counseling before testing, though, many patients may opt for a simple blood test without considering the implications of that test.

Consider the provider's obligation to the four pillars of bioethics in the context of prenatal testing. In what situations is beneficence to the mother met by testing? When might it be met by not testing? Might the possibility of abortion be considered to pit beneficence for the mother against non-maleficence for the fetus? What does the obligation to justice require of providers, in light of variable access to either high-risk prenatal care or elective pregnancy termination based on socioeconomic status? These questions do not have straightforward answers, and the answers will vary by patient, provider, and circumstance. They demonstrate, though, the role of bioethics in even seemingly routine outpatient obstetric and gynecologic care. The challenge for providers is to develop a way to address these complicated questions that is efficient and effective and that assists patients in actively participating in their care.

The way that providers communicate with patients and the way that they assess and support patient autonomy are the tools with which providers tackle these difficult questions. The paternalistic model is not a helpful model in this circumstance, because it substitutes provider values for patient values and does not consider how the patient may choose to use the results of testing. The informative model may be better suited, but it seems unrealistic to expect a patient to fully understand the implications of uncertain testing or the expected lifetime outcome for children with identified medical conditions. The interpretive model allows the provider to explore patient values and help the patient to identify whether testing or declining testing is more consistent with those values. As such, it is better suited to counseling about prenatal testing than either the paternalistic or informative models. It does not, however, allow for the provider to introduce new values or encourage the weighing of new values against identified values.

Imagine that the patient in this case has expressed that the most important thing for her is that her child be mentally "normal," and that she would terminate her pregnancy if there were an increased risk for Down syndrome. Although it is not the provider's role to criticize the patient's values, it is incumbent upon the provider to ensure that the patient has considered alternate values – including the value of health and happiness for any offspring and the possibility of relatively happy, healthy lives for children with Down syndrome – so that she can make an autonomous, well-informed decision. By the same token, a provider is obligated to discuss realistic expectations for duration and quality of life with a woman carrying a fetus diagnosed with a significant fetal anomaly, particularly when a patient states that she wants "everything done for the baby." These theoretical patients may make different decisions about testing based on this counseling or they may not, but the provider's responsibility to his or her patients is best met by helping them to consider various aspects of these important decisions so that they are able to make them based on full disclosure. This example demonstrates the value of the deliberative model in assisting patients to consider the various bioethical components of routine medical care. Further, it illustrates how medical ethics and communication models are intimately related, with ideal communication supporting and promoting patient-centered care.

Case 2

You are seeing a 23-year-old G0 for routine annual exam when she asks you about having her "tubes tied." She tells you that she has never found any birth control she likes, and she does not want children. She does not have a partner at this time, but her sisters have many children and she does not believe children would ever fit into her plans. How do you counsel her? Would you perform a sterilization procedure?

Discussion

This seemingly straightforward patient request highlights a number of issues, both ethical and communication related. There are, of course, some providers who do not offer sterilization under any circumstances for personal and religious reasons, but studies suggest that many providers would be hesitant to offer this patient elective sterilization. Harrison and Cooke (1988) conducted a survey of physicians assessing willingness to perform sterilization in a number of clinical scenarios.[16] They identified of number of factors that contributed to willingness, with the following factors identified as highly significant ($P < 0.0005$): age, parity/timing, and race. Additional significant factors were marital status, income, education, and medical comorbidities. Providers were less likely to offer sterilization to women who were young, nulliparous, and single, largely due to concerns for later regret of the procedure.[17, 18] Given this individual's risk for regret based on her demographics, data would suggest many gynecologists may not initially be comfortable offering this elective procedure.

Consider the ethical issues systematically, though. First consider how Beauchamp and Childress's tenets of bioethics may apply. From a technical standpoint, tubal ligation is a relatively low-risk procedure, so the prima facie obligation to non-maleficence does not strongly discourage the procedure. The potential for regret, though, does indicate that sterilization may pose a risk for future harm to the patient, suggesting that the obligation to non-maleficence may support a refusal to perform the procedure. The obligation to beneficence suggests that those providers who are not opposed to sterilization in general are right to offer a procedure to prevent pregnancy in a relatively safe way for a woman who desires to avoid pregnancy. Assuming that the patient is competent to make her own medical decisions, the obligation to autonomy would also support performing the procedure. Issues of race and socioeconomic status play into the obligation to justice, and providers should examine themselves to determine whether or not their own judgments about a particular patient's ability to parent impact their willingness to perform the procedure. Apparently, beneficence and autonomy are supported by offering the procedure, while non-maleficence is supported by not offering it. Assuming the provider is able to refrain from making value judgments about the worth of this patient as a parent, how does her or she resolve this conflict and identify his or her actual obligation to the patient?

Again, the provider relies on his or her communication with the patient in the context of the clinical encounter. Although once the norm, paternalism is no longer recognized as appropriate medical care in this circumstance, and outright refusal to perform the procedure may not be appropriate. The informative model would allow the provider to present data regarding concern for regret, as well as to discuss alternative long-acting reversible contraception, and may lead the patient to choose another route of care. Exploring the patient's priorities, though, would allow both the patient and provider to better understand her reasoning and to discuss treatment options in keeping with those priorities. The interpretive model and deliberative model both encourage this sort of values clarification, and both would be better suited to this scenario. As the provider explores possible futures with the patient, including the possibility of future improved financial circumstances, relationships, and health status, the deliberative model would allow for a more robust discussion of previously unconsidered values, ideally leading to shared decision making that meets the needs of the patient and is consistent with the provider's understanding of appropriate care for this particular patient. The patient may be persuaded to use alternative contraception, or the provider may be persuaded that the patient is an appropriate candidate for sterilization, but it is only through this type of communication that those decisions can be made in a mutually satisfying way.

Concluding remarks

The two case studies in this chapter, although varied in their specifics, both demonstrate the method in which an organized approach to considering the ethics of office practice can help providers to better care for patients. The studies further emphasize the importance of effective communication to not only to relay facts, but also to explore values and create a care plan that is consistent with patient values without sacrificing the expertise that the provider offers. Sometimes these conversations are time-consuming, and the temptation to take shortcuts is real as providers face busy office schedules. There are relatively few clinical situations, though, for which the rapid decision making made possible by the paternalistic model is appropriate. Both the informative and interpretive models are potentially useful in some situations, but the deliberative model is best suited to true shared decision making. In the interest of meeting obligations to the basic tenets of bioethics, providers are responsible for becoming comfortable with communication styles that effectively maximize the contributions of both providers and patients. As with any skill, more proficiency occurs with practice. The reader may consider employing values clarification into a simple office encounter to begin to develop the skills necessary to effectively use the deliberative model when more difficult shared decision making becomes necessary. Given the opportunity to improve not only the care offered, but also the relationship with patients and the confidence they have in health care, it behooves health-care providers to make an effort to incorporate intentional consideration of medical ethics into routine office practice.

References

1. US Public Health Service Syphilis Study at Tuskegee 2013 [updated September 24, 2013]. Available from: www.cdc.gov/tuskegee/timeline.htm.
2. Reilly PR. Involuntary sterilization in the United States: a surgical solution. *Quarterly Review of Biology* 1987;**62** (2):153–70.
3. Beauchamp T, Childress J. *Principles of Biomedical Ethics*. New York: Oxford University Press; 1977.
4. Clouser K. Bioethics and philosophy. *Hastings Center Report* 1993;**23**(6):S10e1.
5. Beauchamp T, Childress J. *Principles of Biomedical Ethics*. New York: Oxford University Press; 2009: 417 p.
6. Emanuel E, Pearson S. Physician autonomy and health care reform. *JAMA* 2012;**307**(4):367–8.
7. Pope T. Legal briefing: conscience clauses and conscientious refusal. *Journal of Clinical Ethics* 2010;**21** (2):163–80.
8. Johnson D. The creation of fetal rights: conflicts with women's constitutional rights to liberty, privacy, and equal protection. *Yale Law Journal* 1986;**95**:599–625.
9. Street R, Makoul G, Arora N, Epstein R. How does communication heal? Pathways linking clinician-patient communication to health outcomes. *Patient Education and Counseling* 2008;**74**:295–301.
10. Duggan A, Thompson T. Provider-Patient Interactions and Related Outcomes. In: Thompson T, Parrott R, Nussbaum J (eds.). *Routledge Handbook of Health Communication*, 2nd ed. New York: Routledge; 2011: 414–28.
11. Emanuel E, Emanuel L. Four models of the physician-patient relationship. *JAMA* 1992;**267**(16): 2221–7.
12. Van den Berg M, Timmermans D, ten Kate L, et al. Informed decision making in the context of prenatal screening. *Patient Education and Counseling* 2006;**63**: 110–17.
13. van den Huevel A, Chitty L, Dormandy E, et al. Will the introduction of non-invasive prenatal diagnostic testing erode informed choices? An experimental study of health care professionals. *Patient Education and Counseling* 2010;**78**:24–8.
14. Press N, Browner C. Why women say yes to prenatal diagnosis. *Social Science and Medicine* 1997;**45**(7): 979–89.
15. Macer DR. Ethics and prenatal diagnosis. Milunsky A (ed.). *Genetic Disorders and the Fetus: Diagnosis, Prevention and Treatment*. Baltimore, MD: Johns Hopkins University Press; 1998: 999–1024.
16. Harrison D, Cooke C. An elucidation of factors influencing physicians' willingness to perform elective female sterilization. *Obstetrics and Gynecology* 1988;**72** (4):565–70.
17. Young age a factor in sterilization regret. *Contraceptive Technology Update* 1999 Oct;**20**(10):116–17.
18. Moseman C, Robinson R, Wright Bates Jr G, Propst A. Identifying women who will request sterilization reversal in a military population. *Contraception* 2006;**73**(5):512–15.

Index